Management of
Patients with
Neuromuscular
Disease

Management of Patients with
Neuromuscular Disease

John R. Bach, MD
Professor and Vice Chairman
Department of Physical Medicine and Rehabilitation
Professor of Neurosciences
University of Medicine and Dentistry of New Jersey
New Jersey Medical School

Director of Research and Associate Medical Director
Department of Physical Medicine and Rehabilitation
Medical Director, Center for Ventilator Management
    Alternatives and Pulmonary Rehabilitation
Co-director, UMDNJ-New Jersey Medical School's
    Jerry Lewis Muscular Dystrophy Association Clinic
University Hospital
Newark, New Jersey

HANLEY & BELFUS
An Affiliate of Elsevier

HANLEY & BELFUS
An Affiliate of Elsevier

The Curtis Center
Independence Square West
Philadelphia, Pennsylvania 19106

Note to the reader: Although the techniques, ideas, and information in this book have been carefully reviewed for correctness, neither the authors nor the publisher can accept any legal responsibility for any errors or omissions that may be made. Neither the publisher nor the authors make any guarantee, expressed or implied, with respect to the material contained herein.

Library of Congress Control Number: 2003105543

MANAGEMENT OF PATIENTS
WITH NEUROMUSCULAR DISEASE   ISBN: 1-56053-604-7

All quotations by Gustav Mahler are from Henry de La Grange: *Gustav Mahler*. Paris, Fayard, 1979. English translations by the author.

Printed in the United States

Last digit number is the print number: 9 8 7 6 5 4 3 2 1

This book is dedicated to the health care organizations that not only raise money for research to seek cures for neuromuscular diseases but also train and encourage health care professionals to provide the high-quality care necessary to prevent mortality while cures are being sought. The following deserve recognition in this regard: Famiglia Atrofia Muscolare Spinale in Rome, Domenico Marchetti, Director; The Duchenne Parent's Project in Rome, Filippo Buccella, Director; Unione Italiana Lotta alla Distrofia Muscolare; Families of SMA in Libertyville, Illinois, Audrey Lewis, Director; The Jennifer Fund, Anita Macauley, Director; Tori's Buddies, Toronto, Tracy Lacy, Director; and Project ALS in New York, Valerie Estess, Director.

The book is also dedicated to the health care professionals and patients of the University of Medicine and Dentistry of New Jersey–New Jersey Medical School (UMDNJ–NJMS) Center for Ventilator Management Alternatives and Pulmonary Rehabilitation. The center was founded at University Hospital, Newark, New Jersey, in 1992. It consists of health care professionals dedicated to the holistic and comprehensive care of people with neuromuscular weakness. The center's physicians have developed orthopedic approaches that prevent musculotendinous contractures and prolong brace-free ambulation. They have developed surgical and anesthetic techniques that permit vital interventions, such as gastrostomy, while avoiding general anesthesia for both infants and adults. In conjunction with the center's respiratory therapists, they have developed inspiratory and expiratory muscle aids that, regardless of the extent of ventilatory impairment, can prevent respiratory complications, permit surgical correction of scoliosis without resort to tracheotomy, and permit the removal of tracheostomy tubes. In fact, the center has removed over 100 tracheostomy tubes from ventilator users with little or no ability to breathe and has taught alternative methods of breathing without ventilators. The physicians have developed cardioprotective interventions that preserve heart function for patients with cardiomyopathy. Indeed, thanks to the center's physicians and therapists, patients do not have "terminal illnesses" when they are offered the management options that prevent cardiopulmonary complications.

The center's therapists and nurses have been instrumental in teaching, training, and equipping patients, families, and care providers in its life-sustaining methods. These health care professionals include Louis Saporito, R.R.T., Brian Weaver, R.R.T., and Pat Dillman, R.N. Their unparalleled knowledge, skill, and dedication and their willingness to instruct these methods all over the world have spared suffering and given new life to people left with no hope by their physicians.

The center's patients and care providers have developed many of the practical interventions that we use. They have taught us common sense rather than reliance on invasive and high-technology solutions for their physical problems. The Piazza, Schepis, and Swanson families taught us that children with SMA type 1 can survive (Fig. 1) and thrive without tracheostomy tubes. People like Mr. Jeffrey Gray, webmaster for non-invasiveventusers.net, and the late Mr. James Starita taught us that people with Duchenne muscular dystrophy

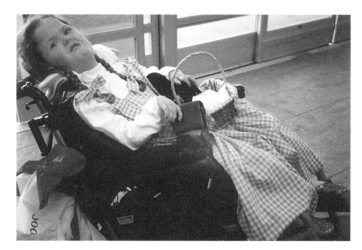

Figure 1. Lisa Hoover, 8-year-old girl with SMA type 1 who cannot eat candy but can still "trick or treat" as Dorothy of Oz.

should never need tracheostomy tubes. Makoto Katahashi and Kazuhiro Kawakami of the rock group DMD (Dream Music Directory) (Fig. 2) taught us that people can become professional musicians and singers despite ventilator dependence. DMD was made up of five musicians with muscular dystrophy, four with Duchenne muscular dystrophy, three of whom required continuous noninvasive mechanical ventilation. The late Makoto Takahashi of DMD died on Christmas morning, 2001, of a gastric hemorrhage associated with stress after unnecessary tracheotomy at the age of 27. Before his death the group had released its second compact disk.

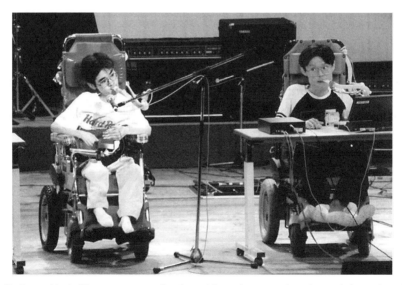

Figure 2. Dream Music Directory, a group of rock musicians who cannot breathe on their own but who still sing, write, and perform, thanks to noninvasive inspiratory aids.

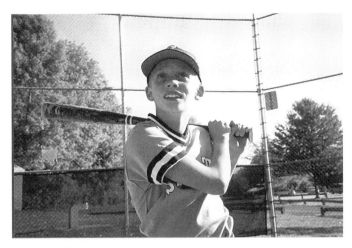

Figure 3. Gaveric Alexandre Bach hitting a home run.

I also dedicate this book to my greatest sources of inspiration, my wife Anne-Marie Bach, my son Gaveric (Fig. 3), and Colía and Leila-Danaë, my new daughters. All too often we strike out when we can only guess. This book will take the guess work out of caring for patients with neuromuscular disease.

Men will have to work
a long time at cracking
the nuts that I'm shaking
down from the tree for them.

Gustav Mahler, *Briefe*[1]

Contents

Contributors

Karen J. Dikeman, M.A., C.C.C.-S.L.P.
AVP, Rehabilitation Services
Silvercrest Center for Rehabilitation and
  Nursing
Briarwood, New York
New York Hospital Queens
Flushing, New York

Jill A. Gaydos, R.D.
Clinical Dietitian–Pediatrics
Newark, New Jersey

Anne E. Gulyas, M.A., C.C.C.-S.L.P
Adjunct Instructor
Department of Speech-Language
  Pathology
Kean University
Union, New Jersey
Manager, University Hospital
Newark, New Jersey

Irving I. Haber, D.O.
Clinical Assistant Professor
Department of Physical Medicine and
  Rehabilitation
Indiana University School of Medicine
Indianapolis, Indiana

Ira E. Holland, M.A.
Former President
Concepts of Independence, Inc.
Department of Rehabilitative Medicine
New York University Medical Center
Department of Occupational Therapy
New York University School of Education
New York, New York

Yuka Ishikawa, M.D.
Department of Pediatrics
National Yakumo Hospital
Hokkaido, Japan

**Marta S. Kazandjian, M.A., C.C.C.-
  S.L.P**
Director
Department of Speech Pathology
Silvercrest Center for Rehabilitation and
  Nursing
Briarwood, New York
New York Hospital Queens
Flushing, New York

**Angela King, B.S., R.R.T., R.P.F.P.,
  C.P.H.Q.**
Clinical Director
Pulmonetic Systems Inc.
New York, New York

Barbara Rogers
President, Respiratory Resources, Inc.
Director, Breethezy
New York, New York

Kenneth G. Swan, M.D.
Professor, Department of Surgery
New Jersey Medical School
Attending Surgeon, University Hospital
Newark, New Jersey

Cees van der Schans, P.T., Ph.D.
Department of Rehabilitation
University Hospital Groningen
Groningen, The Netherlands

After completing studies in science and engineering at Stevens Institute for Technology in Hoboken, New Jersey, Dr. John R. Bach received his medical degree from the UMDNJ–New Jersey Medical School in 1976. He completed postgraduate studies in pediatrics and in physical medicine and rehabilitation at the New York University–Howard Rusk Institute in 1980. In 1979, as a house physician on the Howard Rusk Ventilator Unit at Goldwater Memorial Hospital, he reported the long-term use of non-invasive positive pressure ventilation by patients with Duchenne muscular dystrophy. He managed the ventilator unit from 1980 to 1981. He then became the technical advisor to Professor Yves Rideau, working to develop a service for noninvasive ventilation for the Faculté de Médecine et de Pharmacie de Poitiers, France, from 1981 to 1983. During the winter of 1981–1982 he, along with Drs. Rideau and Delaubier, first used nasal ventilation. He joined the faculty of the UMDNJ–New Jersey Medical School in June 1983.

Dr. Bach is a fellow of the American Academy of Physical Medicine and Rehabilitation, the American College of Chest Physicians, the Association of Academic Physiatrists, the American Paraplegia Society, the New Jersey Association of Electromyography and Electrodiagnosis, l'Association Francaise d'Actions et de Recherches sur les Dystrophies Musculaires, Sigma Xi, Alpha Omega Alpha National Honor Society, the American Spinal Injury Association, and the Institut Duchenne pour la Recherche dans les Maladies Neuromusculaires. He is a Professor of Physical Medicine and Rehabilitation, Department of Physical Medicine and Rehabilitation, Professor of Neurosciences, Department of Neurosciences, Vice Chairman of the Department of Physical Medicine and Rehabilitation, UMDNJ-New Jersey Medical School; Director of Research and Associate Medical Director of the Department of Physical Medicine and Rehabilitation at University Hospital, Newark, New Jersey; Codirector of the UMDNJ–New Jersey Medical School's Jerry Lewis Muscular Dystrophy Association Clinic; and Medical Director of the Center for Ventilator Management Alternatives and Pulmonary Rehabilitation, University Hospital, Newark, N.J. He has written over 160 peer-reviewed scientific articles, 80 book chapters, and 9 books about neuromuscular and pulmonary medicine and has lectured on these topics in 37 countries around the globe.

Dr. Bach has received the following awards:

American Journal of Physical Medicine and Rehabilitation:
    Award for Excellence in Research Writing in 1990
    Award for Excellence in Research Writing in 1994

William H. McLean UPTAM Alumni Honor Award, Stevens Institute of Technology in 1994

American Academy of Physical Medicine and Rehabilitation:
    Award for the Best Research Paper Published by a Physiatrist, 1994

University of Medicine and Dentistry of New Jersey:
  University Excellence Award for Patient Care, 1994
  New Jersey Medical School, Special Faculty Achievement Award presented by
    the Faculty Organization, October 1996
American Academy of Physical Medicine and Rehabilitation:
  Education and Research Fund Best Scientific Research Paper for 1997
Newark Beth Israel Health Care Foundation Humanism in Medicine Award, May 17,
  1998
The American Paraplegia Society A. Estin Colmarr Memorial Award for Clinical Service,
  September 9, 1999
New Jersey Society for Respiratory Care/American Association of Respiratory Care:
  A. Gerald Shapiro, M.D. Award for Outstanding Leadership in the Field of Respiratory
  Care, October 2000

Dr. Bach is an internationally recognized pioneer in the rehabilitation of patients with neuromuscular conditions and in the use of physical medicine interventions as noninvasive alternatives to intubation and tracheostomy for these patients. He brought the Rideau protocol for prolongation of brace-free ambulation by early lower extremity musculotendinous release surgery to the United States. He was part of the group that defined indications for spinal instrumentation to treat scoliosis. He was the first to describe the use of robot arms to facilitate activities of daily living for people with neuromuscular disease. He first tried nasal ventilation in 1981, was first to use it for patients with no autonomous breathing ability in 1984, and was first to report it in 1987. He was also first to report the nocturnal use of IPPV via a mouthpiece for a large population of ventilator users with no autonomous breathing ability. He defined criteria for extubation and tracheostomy tube decanulation and described normalization of ventilatory drive and blood carbon dioxide levels by conversion of patients from tracheostomy to noninvasive ventilatory support methods. He is responsible for the re-introduction of mechanical insufflation-exsufflation and mechanically assisted coughing (MAC). He described the mechanisms whereby open, noninvasive systems of ventilatory support can be successful for patients with no autonomous breathing ability. Along with Dr. Ishikawa, he first reported the effective medical management of cardiomyopathy in patients with neuromuscular cardiomyopathy. He developed the respiratory muscle aid protocol that spares people with respiratory muscle weakness from respiratory complications, hospitalizations, intubations, and tracheostomies. He developed the intensive care extubation protocol that permits the successful extubation without tracheotomy of infants who are unable to breathe. He has treated celebrities and statesmen, including a former Prime Minister of Greece. He also published key studies of quality of life and cost-effectiveness issues concerning mechanical ventilation and rehabilitation for lung disease and neuromuscular disease patients.

His work continues to be recognized in Who's Who, Strathmore's Directories, Ltd.; The National Registry of Who's Who; America's Top Doctors, Castle Connelly Guide; Top Doctors in the New York Metro Area, Castle Connelly; and the New York Magazine's Best Docs in the New York, Metropolitan Area.

Neuromuscular diseases (NMDs) can affect anyone at any time. They cause muscle weakness that can affect the heart, breathing, coughing, swallowing, speech, and limb muscles, all of which can cause disability and compromise quality of life. Untreated, heart muscle weakness can be prematurely fatal. Swallowing difficulties can cause under-nutrition, respiratory complications, and loss of the pleasure of eating a meal. Weakness of breathing and coughing muscles, however, continues to be the major cause of re-peated hospitalizations and loss of life. For the great majority of people with these disor-ders, the need for repeated hospitalizations, resort to invasive ventilatory support (tracheostomy), and death due to breathing complications are avoidable.

People with NMD can benefit from cardiopulmonary, orthopedic, gastrointestinal, nutritional, and other interventions. No physician can be familiar with all therapeutic possibilities. Most physicians are too specialized to be able to provide holistic multidisci-plinary management options at every stage of NMD. It is impossible for neurologists to be abreast of the respiratory and rehabilitation as well as the neurologic literature. Likewise, pulmonologists rarely read neurology and orthopedic literature. Therefore, the specialist may not be aware of all possible management options. As a result, the patient and family are usually presented only with the single approach taken by the consulting specialist for any particular problem.

Physical medicine and surgical interventions can prolong walking and normal mobil-ity for up to 5 years, prevent back deformity, optimize independent functioning, and greatly prolong meaningful life without resort to tracheotomy. With the methods taught in this book, the crisis decision of whether or not to undergo tracheotomy can be avoided. Management of NMD deserves to be a medical specialty in its own right be-cause once the diagnosis is established, the practitioner then needs knowledge of physia-try (physical medicine and rehabilitation); orthopedics; respiratory medicine; otolaryngology; cardiology; physical, occupational, and respiratory therapy; augmenta-tive communication; nutrition; sexual counseling; and psychology.

This book is not meant to be a compendium of diagnostic information for every NMD. Although there are few effective medical treatments for specific NMDs, there are many beneficial, and even life-saving, physical medicine interventions that can be used for virtually all of these conditions. This book is published so that patients no longer will need to die from preventable complications before effective medical treatments become available. It offers the interventions that the researchers and clinicians of the UMDNJ–NJMS Center for Ventilator Management Alternatives and Pulmonary Rehabilitation have found most effective as well as the interventions offered by other investigators so that the clinician can choose among all available options. It is a comprehensive guide for the day-to-day management of these conditions.

Commonly Used Abbreviations

A/C:	assist control
ACE:	angiotensin-converting enzyme
ADL:	activities of daily living
AHI:	apnea/hypopnea index
ALS/MND:	amyotrophic lateral sclerosis/motor neuron disease
ANP:	atrial natriuretic peptide
BMD:	Becker muscular dystrophy
BNP:	brain natriuretic peptide
BUN:	blood urea nitrogen
CMT:	Charcot-Marie-Tooth disease
CHF:	congestive heart failure
CNEP:	continuous negative expiratory pressure
CNS:	central nervous system
COPD:	chronic obstructive pulmonary disease
CPAP:	continuous positive airway pressure
CPF:	cough peak flow
DAG:	dystrophin-associated glycoprotein
DCM:	dilated cardiomyopathy
DMD:	Duchenne muscular dystrophy
$dSpO_2$:	oxyhemoglobin desaturation
EDMD:	Emery-Dreifuss muscular dystrophy
EMG:	electromyography
EPAP:	expiratory positive airway pressure
EPP:	equal pressure point
EPR:	electrophrenic respiration
$EtCO_2$:	end-tidal carbon dioxide
FEV_1:	forced expiratory volume in 1 second
FRC:	functional residual capacity
FSH:	facioscapulohumeral muscular dystrophy
GPB:	glossopharyngeal breathing
HME:	heat and moisture exchanger
IAPV:	intermittent abdominal pressure ventilator

ICU:	intensive care unit
I/E:	inspiratory/expiratory (ratio)
IPAP:	inspiratory positive airway pressure
IPPB:	intermittent positive pressure breathing
IPPV:	intermittent positive pressure ventilation
IQ:	intelligence quotient
LGMD:	limb-girdle muscular dystrophy
LVDd:	left ventricle end-diastolic dimensions
LVEF:	left ventricular ejection fraction
MAC:	mechanically assisted coughing, a combination of mechanical insufflation-exsufflation and manually assisted coughing with an exsufflation-timed abdominal thrust
MDA:	Jerry Lewis Muscular Dystrophy Association
MIC:	maximum insufflation capacity
MI-E:	mechanical insufflation-exsufflation
MND:	motor neuron disease
MUGA:	multigated radionucleotide angiography
NMD:	neuromuscular disease
NPBV:	negative pressure body ventilator
OSAS:	obstructive sleep apnea syndrome
PAP:	positive airway pressure
PAS:	personal assistance services
PEEP:	positive end-expiratory pressure
PEF:	peak expiratory flow
PNE:	norepinephrine
REE:	resting energy expenditure
REM:	rapid eye movement
ROM:	range of motion
SaO$_2$:	oxyhemoglobin saturation measured by arterial blood sampling
SpO$_2$:	oxyhemoglobin saturation by pulse oximeter
SCI:	spinal cord injury
SIMV:	synchronized intermittent mandatory ventilation
SMA:	spinal muscular atrophy
SONI:	strapless oral nasal interface
SPECT:	thallium-201 single-photon emission computed tomography
VC:	vital capacity

GENERAL EVALUATION AND MANAGEMENT CONCERNS

People who want to make a living from the treatment of nervous patients must clearly be able to do something to help them.[2]

—S. Freud, M.D. (1909)

Chapter 1

Disease Assessment and Evolution

The test of a first-rate intelligence is the ability to hold two opposed ideas in the mind at the same time, and still retain the ability to function.

⋅◉⋅ F. Scott Fitzgerald. *The Crack-Up*. New York, James Laughlin, 1956, p 69.

Neuromuscular diseases (NMDs), which include both hereditary and acquired diseases of the peripheral neuromuscular system, affect over 400,000 people in the United States.[3] They are diseases of the peripheral nerves (neuropathies and anterior horn cell diseases), the myoneural junctions (myasthenia gravis), or the muscles (myopathies) themselves (Table 1). The pathologic processes affecting the nerves and muscles can be anatomic, metabolic, electrical, inflammatory, or immunologic as well as idiopathic. These conditions cause muscle weakness but do not usually affect sensory functions.

Natural Histories

La primera reacción no está en manos de los hombres.

⋅◉⋅ Don Quixote de la Mancha

Prenatal and General Diagnostic Considerations

Prenatal diagnosis of Duchenne and Becker muscular dystrophies, spinal muscular atrophy (SMA), and some other NMDs can now be done by DNA analysis of cells taken from amniotic fluid. Muscle biopsies cannot be used to distinguish between muscular dystrophies for which specific gene defects have not yet been discovered or for which it is not yet possible to stain for the presence of specific disease-associated proteins such as emerin or dystrophin. In such cases, the diagnoses are usually determined by the pattern of muscle weakness and by nonmuscular findings in the examination of the patient; no prenatal diagnosis is possible.

The Floppy Newborn

Most children who are floppy at birth develop normally. When floppiness persists and the infant does not attain the ability to raise the head or sit by 7 months of age, 70% have central nervous systems disorders (cerebral palsy), 15% have inherited NMD (Table 2), and 15% ultimately develop essentially normally, although at least some of these children may have mild myopathies that we are as yet unable to diagnose. Congenital bilateral adductor vocal cord paralysis presenting with symptoms of upper airway obstruction may be the first recognized sign of NMDs such as SMA type 1, congenital myasthenia gravis, and facioscapulohumeral myopathy.[4]

Table 1.	Neuromuscular Conditions with Functional Bulbar Musculature That Result in Physical and Ventilatory Impairments[110]

Myopathies
1. Muscular dystrophies
   - Dystrophinopathies (Duchenne and Becker dystrophies)
   - Other muscular dystrophies (limb-girdle, Emery-Dreifuss, facioscapulo-humeral, congenital, childhood autosomal recessive, oculopharyngeal, and myotonic dystrophy
2. Myopathies exclusive of muscular dystrophy
   - Congenital and metabolic myopathies (e.g., acid maltase deficiency, acid alpha glucosidase deficiency, carnitine deficiency, myotubular myopathy mucopolysaccharidoses, mitochondrial myopathies, arthrogryposis) Inflammatory myopathies such as polymyositis
   - Diseases of the myoneural junction (e.g., myasthenia gravis, congenital myasthenic syndromes, mixed connective tissue disease)
   - Myopathies of systemic disease (e.g., carcinomatous myopathy, cachexia/anorexia nervosa, medication-associated myopathy)

Neurologic disorders
1. Spinal muscular atrophies
2. Motor neuron diseases
3. Poliomyelitis
4. Neuropathies: hereditary sensory motor neuropathies, including familial hypertrophic interstitial polyneuropathy, Guillain-Barré syndrome
5. Multiple sclerosis, Parkinson's disease, Down's syndrome, familial dysautonomia
6. Disorders of supraspinal tone, such as Friedreich's ataxia
7. Myelopathies of rheumatoid, infectious, spondylitic, vascular, traumatic, or idiopathic origin
8. Tetraplegia associated with pancuronium bromide, botulism
9. Static encephalopathies associated with Arnold-Chiari malformation and syringomyelia, myelomeningocele, encephalitis
10. Phrenic neuropathies: associated with cardiac hypothermia, surgical or other trauma, radiation, phrenic electrostimulation, familial, paraneoplastic or infectious etiology, and lupus erythematosus

Myopathies

Duchenne and Becker Muscular Dystrophy

Muscular dystrophies are myopathies that tend to be progressive with ongoing degeneration and regeneration and fatty infiltration of muscle fibers. Duchenne muscular dystrophy (DMD), the most common NMD (Fig. 1), occurs in 1 of every 3500 male births.[5] A case of DMD was first reported in Italy in 1836, and in 1852 it was recognized and beautifully described as an inherited disorder of boys by the English physician Meryon.[6] The condition was inappropriately named after Duchenne, a neurologist practicing in Paris, who, disparaging Meryon's work, first wrote about the condition in 1868 and confused it with cerebral palsy, poliomyelitis, and other conditions.[7] Becker muscular

Table 2.   Neuromuscular Diseases of Floppy Infants in Order of Incidence
Spinal muscular atrophy Congenital myopathies Congenital muscular dystrophies Congenital myotonic dystrophy Congenital myasthenic syndrome Acid maltase deficiency (Pompe's disease) Debranching enzyme deficiency (type 3 glycogen storage disease) Branching enzyme deficiency (type 4 glycogen storage disease) Carnitine deficiency Mitochondrial myopathies Congenital peripheral neuropathies

dystrophy (BMD) is caused by essentially the same genetic defect as DMD, but it is about 5 times less common and generally milder.

In both DMD and BMD, the single gene defect is on the small (petit) arm of the X chromosome (Xp21 site). This gene is normally responsible for the manufacture of the cell wall protein dystrophin. In DMD no dystrophin is found in muscle or other body tissue cell walls. In BMD, severity depends on how abnormal the dystrophin is and how little is present. At times patients have undetectable levels of dystrophin but are still able to walk even in adulthood; thus, other factors are involved.[8] Although about two-thirds of patients with DMD and BMD receive the abnormal Xp21 gene from their mothers,

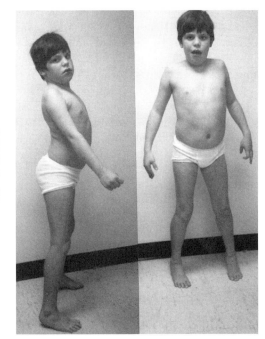

Figure 1. Seven-year-old child with Duchenne muscular dystrophy demonstrates the typical contractures seen in this disorder as well as in many patients with Becker muscular dystrophy, limb-girdle muscular dystrophy, polymyositis, and spinal muscular atrophy types 3 and 4 (see text).

in about one-third of cases the mother does not carry the abnormal gene in all of her cells; a spontaneous mutation occurs in the germ cell that affects only the child.

Blood samples for DNA linkage studies are required from family members, or, at times, a muscle biopsy is necessary to determine the carrier or disease status of the siblings of affected children for whom the defect is too small to be identified by direct analysis. These studies can indicate that the patient's and carrier's Xp21 DNA are identical, thereby establishing the carrier status of the family member. When DNA of the patient and other family members' DNA is not available and a deletion cannot be seen in the possible carrier, the presence of elevated levels of muscle enzymes and electromyographic (EMG) evidence of myopathy can signal carrier status for over one-half of actual carriers. About 70% of DMD carriers have serum muscle enzyme elevations of 2–5 times normal, especially after exercise, and about 8% of carriers also have some skeletal muscle weakness and occasionally heart muscle weakness (cardiomyopathy). When the mother is not a carrier, there is extremely little risk that siblings or others in the family will be affected.

Both utrophin and dystrophin are proteins found at the cytoplasmic face of muscle cell membranes. They also occur in the cell walls of most other body tissues, including nerve cells. The utrophin content of cell walls naturally decreases after birth and is gradually replaced by dystrophin. When this replacement does not occur, the cell wall becomes fragile and porous to the passage of calcium, other electrolytes, and cell body enzymes such as creatine kinase, especially during muscle contractions. This process progressively damages the cells. They attempt to hypertrophy like normally exercising muscle cells, but the leakage of vital substances and degeneration overwhelm the cells' efforts to regenerate and they become progressively weaker.

Although muscle strength can be slightly decreased from birth, typically infants with DMD are thought to have no physical problems. On the average, affected children begin to walk at 18 months of age, but 35% can walk independently before 15 months of age, and some begin to walk only when they are 3 years old. There is no correlation between late walking and rapid progression or severity. For patients with BMD, onset of muscle weakness can be early as for patients with DMD, or it may first be noted well into adulthood. It is not unusual for BMD to be recognized first because of complications during general anesthesia or as shortness of breath due to cardiomyopathy.

In DMD, muscle weakness is usually first recognized between ages 3 and 5 years. It progresses symmetrically and linearly until age 14, when progression slows and occurs in a predictable pattern, with extensor muscles being weaker than flexor muscles.[9] Children tend to walk on their toes from outset and may never be able to walk with the feet flat. They also tend to waddle and have to climb up their legs, thighs, and hips (Gower's sign) when getting up from the floor or from a chair. The ability to run, which is normally achieved by 2 years of age, is not attained. Although walking velocity normally reaches 3.44 m/sec in males, for DMD it begins to decrease linearly between ages 4 and 6 at a rate of 0.0308 m/sec/month and is about 29% of normal by age 10.[10] Patients with BMD have the same pattern of muscle weakness and calf muscle thickness.

Left untreated, these patients develop an imbalance in muscle strength at every joint. Hip flexors remain stronger than hip extensors (Fig. 2); knee flexors (hamstrings) remain stronger than knee extensors (quadriceps) (Fig. 3); and ankle plantarflexors remain stronger than ankle dorsiflexors (Fig. 4). Imbalance in strength at any joint leads to

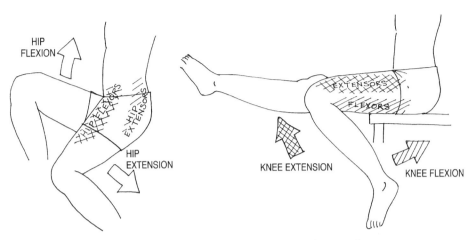

Figure 2. Hip flexors and extensors.

Figure 3. Knee flexors and extensors.

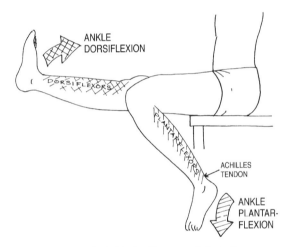

Figure 4. Ankle dorsiflexors and plantarflexors.

musculotendinous contractures and loss of joint range of motion (ROM) (Fig. 5). The stronger muscles on one side of the joint stretch their weaker antagonists. This action not only causes contractures but also makes the weaker muscles get weaker even faster because they are no longer at their ideal length for contracting. Although very severe muscle weakness can prevent ambulation, these patients and many others with NMDs lose the ability to walk prematurely because of joint contractures.

To understand the rationale behind therapeutic interventions, one must understand pathokinesiology.[11] Iliotibial band tightness plays an important role. The iliotibial band is the thickened lateral extension of the fascia lata; it descends the outer aspect of the thigh to insert at the knees (Fig. 6). The fascia lata forms a "stocking" of connective tissue around the thigh. It splits to cover the superficial and deep surfaces of the gluteus maximus and tensor fascia lata, enveloping and, at least in DMD and other myopathies, compressing the muscles of the thigh. When tight or contracted, it is responsible for the

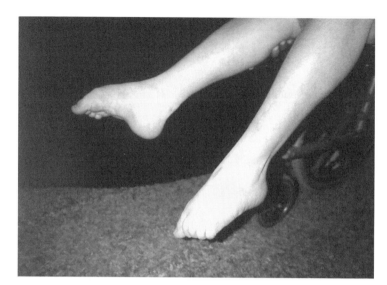

Figure 5. Ankle muscle and soft tissue contractures (equinus deformity) due to greater strength of the plantarflexors compared with the dorsiflexors.

typical wide base of walking and the inward rotation of the lower legs and feet seen in many people with NMD.

Hip extensor weakness leads to muscle contractures at the hip and increased lumbar lordosis (see Fig. 2). The child has to bend his trunk backward to keep the center of gravity behind the hips and to prevent jack-knifing at the waist. Connective tissue, the fascia lata and iliotibial bands, tighten (Fig. 7), leading to a wide-based gait, inward rotation of the knees, further flexion contractures of the hips, and, eventually, flexion contractures of the knees (see Fig. 1). With increasing knee extensor (quadriceps) weakness the child

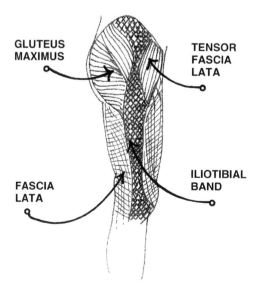

GLUTEUS MAXIMUS

TENSOR FASCIA LATA

FASCIA LATA

ILIOTIBIAL BAND

Figure 6. The iliotibial band is the lateral thickening of the fascia lata (see text) from the tubercle of the iliac crest to the lateral condyle of the tibia.

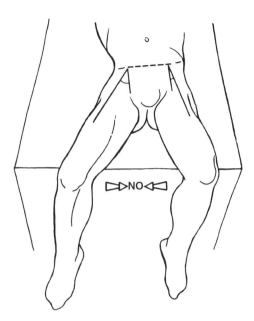

Figure 7. Examination for iliotibial band tightness. (From Rideau Y, Duport G, Delaubier A, et al: Early treatment to preserve quality of locomotion for children with Duchenne muscular dystrophy. Semin Neurol 15:9–17, 1995, with permission.)

must stabilize the knee by keeping the center of gravity in front of the knee. It becomes increasingly difficult to keep the center of gravity both behind the hips and in front of the knees. The stronger calf muscles (ankle plantarflexors) encourage toe walking and lead to worsening of ankle contractures (equinus deformity) (see Fig. 5). Eventually knee flexion contractures prevent the child from keeping the center of gravity both behind the hip and in front of the knee, and ankle instability leads to falls on uneven, and eventually on all, walking surfaces. Untreated, such children lose the ability to walk between 8 and 12 years of age, most between 8.5 and 9.5 years of age.[12]

By age 13, boys with DMD find it increasingly difficulty to feed themselves. The weight of the arms can eventually make it difficult to move the shoulder and the elbow. Substitute movements, such as bending the trunk forward to meet the hand and using objects as levers for the forearm, become increasingly difficult. Some patients use their fingers to crawl up the opposite arm, dragging up the affected arm. Some take advantage of the fact that a vertical forearm balanced on the tip of the elbow requires less effort to move. Despite the eventual development of severe shoulder and elbow weakness, however, virtually all people with DMD retain sufficient finger and other muscle use to be able to operate computers, environmental control systems, robotics, and motorized wheelchairs.

There are also nonmuscular findings in DMD. Head circumference tends to be increased; stature tends to be small; and intelligence can be affected. The average verbal and performance intelligence quotients (IQ) for children with DMD are between 85 and 90 (within normal range). There is a high incidence of hyperactivity, attention deficit disorder, and dyslexia, including impairment in reading non-words.[13] Deficits in verbal comprehension and expressive language are present in almost one-half of children. Short-term memory can also be impaired. Despite these problems, IQs over 130 occur—and IQs remain constant over time. Some evidence indicates that patients with

DMD and higher IQs have a better prognosis. People with DMD have worked as physicians, lawyers, accountants, teachers, musicians (see Dedication), and in other professions (Chapter 13). Some of our patients have married, in some cases more than once, and their children are not affected.

Because the smooth muscle of the intestines (Chapter 4) and the heart (Chapter 5) can be affected, constipation and cardiomyopathy are common. About 85–90% of children with DMD develop scoliosis that warrants surgical intervention (Chapter 7). In 15% of cases the scoliosis begins while the child is still walking.[9] It progresses rapidly once the child is confined to a wheelchair. When not prevented surgically, it progresses throughout life.

In 1852 Meryon described a 16-year-old boy with "DMD" who died from respiratory failure during a febrile episode with "profuse secretion of mucus from the trachea and larynx."[6] One hundred fifty years later, most people with progressive NMDs still die prematurely from bronchial mucus plugging during otherwise innocuous colds. All conventionally managed people with childhood-onset NMD eventually develop respiratory failure. In 90% of cases, the respiratory failure occurs during otherwise benign upper respiratory tract infections (chest colds) because of an ineffective cough.[14] About 10% of the time, ventilatory failure (coma) develops when the symptoms of alveolar hypoventilation (see Table 1 in Chapter 11) are ignored or inappropriately managed with supplemental oxygen. Fortunately, respiratory failure is virtually always preventable for patients with DMD and normal cognition; but without proper management people with NMD continue to die prematurely or are subjected to respiratory failure and tracheostomy tubes. Eighty to 90% of conventionally managed people with DMD without tracheostomy tubes needlessly die from respiratory failure between 16 and 19 years of age and rarely after age 25.[5,15] One study of "conventionally" managed patients with DMD reported that once the vital capacity (VC) has decreased below 1 liter, the 5-year survival rate is 8%.[16] Comparable morbidity and mortality figures are not available for patients with BMD, but clearly, as with DMD, many die needlessly from respiratory complications of unmanaged respiratory muscle weakness.

Other Muscular Dystrophies

Emery-Dreifuss muscular dystrophy (EDMD) is an X-linked recessive condition linked to the mutant color blindness gene located on the distal long arm of the X chromosome at Xq27-28.[17] Autosomal dominant EDMD has also been defined by a defect in the gene 1q21 (Fig. 8).[18] Xq27-28 muscular dystrophy causes emerin deficiency, whereas the 1q21 defect results in the absence of lamin A and lamin C, both nuclear membrane proteins whose exact roles are unknown. Many publications in the neurology literature note that flexion contractures develop at the elbows and heel cords before muscle weakness becomes prominent. The cervical spine tends to be hyperextended and the entire spine rigid. Most patients are able to walk until the third decade. Cardiac arrhythmias are common and often life-threatening when not adequately treated (Chapter 5). They are probably related to the fact that emerin is normally expressed in the heart's adhesive junctions.[19]

The predominantly autosomal recessive muscular dystrophies include limb-girdle muscular dystrophy (LGMD) and the congenital muscular dystrophies. Defects have thus far been found at at least 13 locations on various chromosomes for LGMD. At least

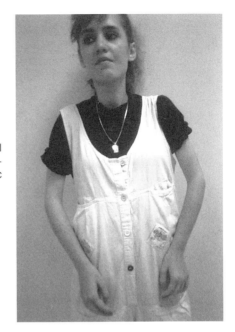

Figure 8. Twenty-two-year-old woman with autosomal dominant Emery-Dreifuss muscular dystrophy demonstrates a stiff, hyperextended spine and characteristic elbow contractures.

three of the chromosomal defects associated with LGMD result in autosomal dominant inheritance. When no genetic abnormalities are found, the diagnoses of these conditions must be made by examining muscle biopsy material and the patient's pattern of muscle weakness. These conditions are equally expressed in either sex. Deficiency in sarcoglycans, muscle cell glycoproteins in a dystrophin-glycoprotein complex, occur in several of the LGMDs.

Onset of LGMD is between 1 and 30 years of age. Initial involvement is of the shoulder and pelvic girdle muscles; however, the pattern of muscle weakness can be clinically indistinguishable from that of DMD. Rate of progression is highly variable. Calf thickness can occur. Some patients walk only on their toes from infancy. Severe disability, muscular contractures, skeletal deformities, cardiomyopathy,[20] and chronic alveolar hypoventilation are common (Fig. 9). Such patients appear to have no intellectual or cognitive impairment, but the incidence of cardiomyopathy is similar to that in other muscular dystrophies.[21]

Childhood-onset autosomal recessive muscular dystrophy, including LGMD, can be confused with DMD or BMD.[22] However, muscle dystrophin is normal, and there is no Xp21 defect. In the childhood-onset autosomal recessive dystrophy associated with a chromosome 13q12 defect, gamma-sarcoglycan is completely absent and alpha- and beta-sarcoglycans are greatly reduced in the dystrophin-glycoprotein complex.[23] History of parental consanguinity may help in establishing the diagnosis. Wheelchair dependence begins from age 10 to middle age. If untreated, scoliosis can become severe and ventilatory impairment can begin as early as age 20, although it more commonly appears after age 25.

Congenital muscular dystrophy without central nervous system (CNS) involvement usually presents as hypotonia at birth or soon thereafter (Fig. 10).[24] Static to rapidly progressive forms have been described.[25–27] Patients usually develop predominantly proximal

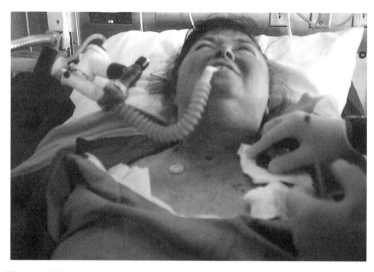

Figure 9. Woman with limb-girdle muscular dystrophy. Onset of disease was at age 5. The patient was diagnosed at age 10, became wheelchair-dependent at 22, and was tracheostomized for continuous ventilatory support at age 37. After 6 years of 24-hour tracheostomy IPPV, she was converted to daytime mouthpiece IPPV (see Case Study 5 of Chapter 11 for details).

muscle weakness, joint contractures, and occasionally facial muscle weakness. Bulbar musculature is generally spared. About 50% of patients never achieve the ability to walk. Scoliosis and chronic alveolar hypoventilation can become early and severe problems.

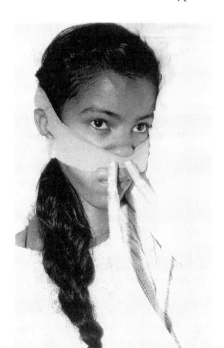

Figure 10. Twenty-eight-year-old woman with congenital muscular dystrophy required continuous nasal ventilation in 1983 before CPAP masks became commercially available.

Predominantly autosomal dominant forms of muscular dystrophy include, most commonly, facioscapulohumeral muscular dystrophy (FSH) and myotonic dystrophy. Autosomal recessive forms have also been described for FSH.[22] FSH can present in adult, juvenile, or infantile forms.[28] In 95% of cases it is associated with a small deletion on chromosome 4 that can be detected by using a DNA test. It is unclear what genetic defect may be associated in the other 5% of cases. Although 90% of patients can be accurately diagnosed by the DNA test, in some families asymptomatic individuals also appear to have the deletion. Future children of unaffected parents of a sporadically affected child have a 20% chance of expressing FSH due to mosaicism for the FSH deletion in one parent. Prenatal testing is possible. The cause of FSH is unknown. It can vary greatly in severity, and each form can lead to the development of life-threatening hypoventilation. The pattern of weakness is distinct. Facial muscles are usually markedly weakened, and scapular winging becomes prominent. Limb weakness usually begins in the upper arms but typically spares the biceps. Weakness in the legs may be more prominent in distal musculature. Patients can lose the ability to close their eyes; speech can become indistinct and smiling and whistling impossible. Occasionally myalgic pain can be severe and associated with sleep disturbance.[29] About 35% develop spinal deformity. Seventy-seven percent of patients have abnormal electrocardiograms, mostly bradycardias (56%), abnormal Q waves (40%), and increased R/S ratio in lead V1 (28%); the incidence of abnormalities increases over time. Intellectual and memory functions are normal.[30]

Myotonic dystrophy is common, with an incidence of 13 per 100,000 (Fig. 11).[31] The defective gene, a triplet repeat sequence of DNA abnormally expanded many times, is located on chromosome 19.[32] A second group of patients has a gene defect on chromosome 3q. Clinical severity increases as the number of nucleotide triplet repeats exceeds 40; the number of repeats can reach into the thousands. An increase in the size of the expansion occurs in succeeding generations, particularly when the affected parent is the

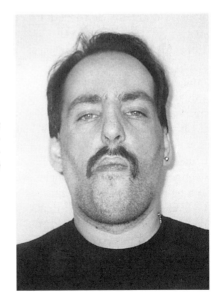

Figure 11. Forty-year-old man with myotonic dystrophy demonstrates typical dolicocephalic facies, temporal atrophy, and frontal balding. He also has cataracts, cardiomyopathy, and chronic alveolar hypoventilation, for which he uses nocturnal nasal IPPV.

mother. With few exceptions, the most severe form, congenital myotonic dystrophy, is inherited from the mother.[33]

Myotonic dystrophy can present from birth until 50 years of age with some combination of mandibulomaxillary disproportion, myotonic facies, myotonia, hand weakness, gait difficulties, facial muscle atrophy, baldness (in males), complaints of poor vision, ptosis, weight loss, impotence, occasionally fecal incontinence,[34] increased hair growth, and cognitive impairment. Occasionally it presents as velopharyngeal incompetence.[35] Cataracts, testicular and ovarian atrophy and other endocrine anomalies, cardiomyopathy, bony changes, chronic alveolar hypoventilation, and daytime drowsiness are common. Hyperkalemia secondary to hypoaldosteronism associated with elevated renin activity has been described in 3 patients.[36] Cognitive impairment, including mental retardation, can be especially pronounced in congenital myotonic dystrophy. Seventy-five percent of patients have cognitive impairment that is usually severe, whereas only mild impairment is present in 35% of noncongenital patients.[37] Mean verbal and performance IQs of people with myotonic dystrophy are in the low 90s, but there is no change in IQ over time. Fecal incontinence has been reported to be successfully treated by mexiletine, a local anesthetic and antiarrhythmic, structurally similar to lidocaine.[38]

Myotonia may be due to a reduction in membrane permeability to chloride. Diphenylhydantoin (200 and 300 mg/day), quinine, procaine amide,[39] carbamazepine (600 and 800 mg/day), n-propyl-ajmalin, troglitazone,[40] disopyramide,[41] and amitriptyline[42] have been used to decrease myotonia.[43]

As for people with other myopathies, episodes of respiratory failure and mortality result from ineffective coughing out of airway secretions during respiratory tract infections,[14] and conventional management outcomes (without respiratory muscle aids) are quite poor.[44] In addition, because they are usually able to walk and tend to have difficulty tolerating noninvasive ventilation, both during daytime hours and overnight, patients with myotonic dystrophy tend to present with cor pulmonale. It should be noted that patients with myotonic and other muscular dystrophies often have elevated liver enzymes without any evidence of liver disease.[45]

Other Myopathies

The term *congenital myopathy* relates to conditions defined by specific abnormalities observed in muscle biopsy specimens. Such patients are often floppy at birth. The best-characterized congenital myopathies include central core disease, centronuclear myopathies, and nemaline myopathies. Central core disease usually presents as hypotonia at birth, is usually autosomal dominant, and is generally a mild, nonprogressive condition.[24,46] Centronuclear and nemaline myopathies can have mildly to rapidly progressive courses leading to severe disability and chronic alveolar hypoventilation. Nemaline myopathy also has a rapidly progressive adult-onset form.[47] Spheroid body myopathy can also be rapidly progressive and lead to ventilatory failure.[48] Cardiomyopathies can also be severe. Most other congenital myopathies are less well characterized and have mild or nonprogressive courses (Fig. 12). It is possible that some severe myopathies thought to be congenital are actually of viral etiology.[49]

Metabolic myopathies are usually autosomal recessive disorders for which defects have been identified (or are suspected) in muscle metabolism. The defects may be in lipid, glycogen, or purine metabolism. Most patients with metabolic myopathies present with

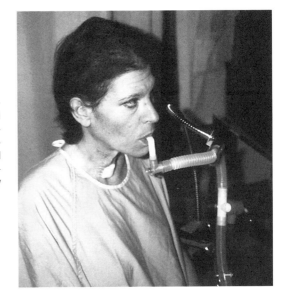

Figure 12. Woman with a congenital myopathy. She was able to walk until age 16 and was well until age 49, at which point respiratory failure led to tracheostomy for ventilatory support. After 5 months of unsuccessful ventilator weaning attempts, she was converted to noninvasive IPPV (see Case Study 8, Chapter 11 for details).

fatigue, muscle cramps, and exercise intolerance; ultimately they have only mild muscle weakness. However, progressive generalized muscular weakness resembling LGMD is characteristic of acid maltase deficiency; both branching and debranching enzyme deficiencies, which are disorders of glycolysis; and carnitine deficiency.[50] Key findings in these disorders may include generalized, predominantly proximal, often painless muscle weakness and possibly severe cardiomyopathy. Acid maltase deficiency, which leads to accumulation of glycogen in lysosomes, not uncommonly presents with hypercapnia and cor pulmonale due to respiratory muscle involvement, particularly in the adult-onset form (Fig. 13).[51]

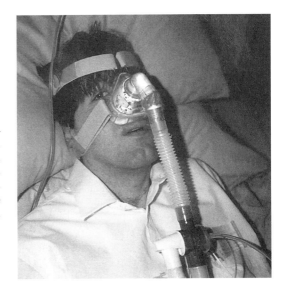

Figure 13. Man with acid maltase deficiency. He was a successful high school athlete. Onset of weakness was noted at age 24; diagnosis was made at age 28; and severe dyspnea and chronic alveolar hypoventilation led to rocking bed ventilator use for nocturnal ventilatory assistance from 30 to 35 years of age. At this point the rocking bed was minimally effective, and he required periods of daytime ventilatory assistance. He was switched to daytime mouthpiece IPPV and nocturnal nasal IPPV, which he has used for 9 years.

Mitochondrial myopathies are metabolic disorders in which abnormalities are suspected in mitochondria. Most commonly, patients have progressive weakness of eye and eye lid muscles that result in ptosis.[52] This condition can be treated by medial tarsal suspension, a surgical intervention that elevates the medial lower eyelid;[53] frontalis suspension; or the use of silicone slings for patients with less than 8 mm of levator function.[54] Patients can also have cataracts, visual disturbances, cardiac arrhythmias, cardiomyopathy, intestinal pseudo-obstruction, short stature, diabetes, goiter, deafness, ataxia, neuropathy, seizures, and strokes. Kearns-Sayre syndrome is a common mitochondrial myopathy (Fig. 14).[52]

Polymyositis is an inflammatory myopathy that does not affect more than one member of a family. It uncommonly presents before age 20; however, childhood and infantile cases do occur (Fig. 15).[55] Progression may be quite rapid or insidious, with symmetric muscle weakness, predominantly of the hip, shoulder, and neck. Dysphagia is also common. Inflammation is not always seen in the muscle biopsies. Such patients are susceptible to both acute and late-onset ventilatory failure.

The prevalence of myasthenia gravis is about 1 in 10,000, with females predominating (Fig. 16).[56] The disease usually occurs around 20 years of age, but the incidence is highest in young women and middle-aged men. The onset is usually insidious but can be sudden. Diagnosis is made on the basis of the characteristic clinical picture, which often includes asymmetric ptosis and ophthalmoplegia, characteristic electrodiagnostic findings, and therapeutic response to anticholinesterases. Myasthenia gravis is characterized by intermittent exacerbations of muscle weakness following repetitive muscle activation and fatigue. There is at least partial recovery after a period of inactivity, especially with treatment. Bulbar and respiratory muscles can be markedly affected, particularly during acute exacerbations, and patients often have moderate irreversible involvement of both. Nonetheless, bulbar muscle function is usually adequate for effective physical medicine interventions.

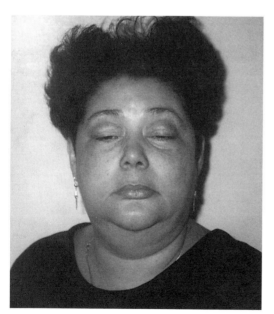

Figure 14. External ophthalmoplegia (PEO) and ptosis due to Kearns-Sayre syndrome. The patient had both depressed ventilatory drive and respiratory muscle weakness, which led to severe chronic alveolar hypoventilation and four episodes of respiratory failure before institution of respiratory muscle aids.

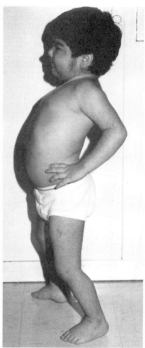

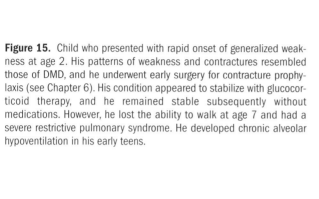

Figure 15. Child who presented with rapid onset of generalized weakness at age 2. His patterns of weakness and contractures resembled those of DMD, and he underwent early surgery for contracture prophylaxis (see Chapter 6). His condition appeared to stabilize with glucocorticoid therapy, and he remained stable subsequently without medications. However, he lost the ability to walk at age 7 and had a severe restrictive pulmonary syndrome. He developed chronic alveolar hypoventilation in his early teens.

Many systemic diseases cause generalized muscle weakness that is associated with neuropathies, anterior horn cell damage, or myopathic changes in muscle. Successfully treating the primary medical disorder can reverse the neuromuscular pathology that,

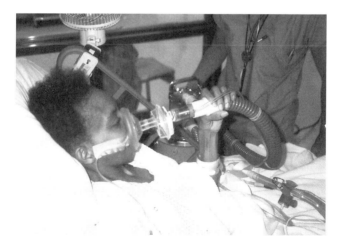

Figure 16. Patient with myasthenia gravis who has relied heavily on auto-administration of mechanical insufflation-exsufflation, nocturnal nasal IPPV, and continuous noninvasive IPPV during acute exacerbations for 9 years, during which she has been free of hospitalization despite intermittent exacerbations. Before this time she was hospitalized and underwent endotracheal intubation on numerous occasions during exacerbation-associated episodes of respiratory failure.

when severe, can necessitate the use of respiratory muscle aids. The physical and ventilatory impairments due to the neuromuscular pathology associated with cancer, HIV infection, collagen disease, or endocrine disease can also be exacerbated by advanced age, obesity, cardiopulmonary disease, malnutrition, ongoing glucocorticoid therapy, or the use of certain chemotherapeutic agents or agents, such as penicillamine and cimetidine, that can produce an inflammatory myopathy.[44]

Motor Neuron Diseases

SMA, amyotrophic lateral sclerosis (ALS), and poliomyelitis are motor neuron diseases (MNDs). The biopsies of patients with motor neuron disorders demonstrate well-defined areas of muscle atrophy. The causes of the deaths of these cells have never been fully determined, but cell death may result from destructive intracellular events and deregulated apoptosis. Apoptosis is an essential physiologic cell death for selective elimination of cells. Deregulation of apoptosis can result in cancer and autoimmune diseases as well as degenerative neurologic diseases. Bcl-2 proteins that regulate apoptosis may be implicated in SMA.[57] SMN1 mutants seen in SMA have been shown to lack antiapoptotic activity.[58] Glutamate is a neurotransmitter that permits communication between motor neurons but under certain circumstances can be toxic to nerve cells. Factors under consideration to explain MNDs include increased activation of glutamate receptors, excessive glutamate, reduced glutamate uptake, or normal glutamate levels with excessively vulnerable cells as well as increased free radical production or reduced inactivation, increased intracellular free calcium, and reduced neurotrophic (nerve growth factor) support.

Spinal Muscular Atrophy

Spinal muscular atrophy is the most common inherited NMD of the floppy newborn (see Table 2). Gene deletions are detectable in 98% of patients with SMA. The other 2% of children with SMA, like children with many other NMDs, may need to undergo EMG and a muscle biopsy to establish the diagnosis. When gene deletions are not detectable, conditions such as polyneuropathies, myopathies, myasthenia gravis, syringomyelia, and ALS need to be ruled out. Direct DNA observation and linkage studies are now very helpful for determining the carrier status of SMA. The incidence is about 1/5,000.[59] SMA is caused by a defect on chromosome 5 at 5q13 at exons 7 and 8 of the survival motor neuron (SMN) 1 gene and occasionally are due to a defect on chromosome 11q13-q21.[60] Although both SMN 1 and 2 genes encode the same protein, their transcription patterns (splicing) are different. Genes are composed of exons that are spliced together to make messenger RNA that is ultimately transcribed into the gene product's full-length protein. The SMN 2 gene produces some full-length messenger RNA, but most of the product lacks the exon 7 segment. The more complete the SMN 2 gene product messenger RNA, the milder the disease severity. Medications are being sought to increase SMN 2 gene expression of exon 7 complete messenger RNA. Loss of neuronal apoptosis inhibitory protein gene and two other genes adjacent to SMN (four in all) appear to play a role in the severity of SMA.[61] Defects in mitochondrial metabolism similar to those seen in mitochondrial myopathies have been identified (Chapter 3). Interestingly, mitochondrial myopathies can closely resemble infantile SMA.[62]

SMA ranges from severe generalized weakness and need for ventilatory support from birth to relatively mild, static conditions presenting in the young adult. Proximal weakness is typically greater than distal weakness, and the legs are weaker than the arms. The SMAs have been arbitrarily separated into five types based largely on severity. Despite attempts to categorize this disorder, there is a great deal of overlap among types. With any type, weakness tends to affect all major muscle groups, including, to a lesser extent, the bulbar muscles. In general, muscle function tends to be best maintained in the face, hands, wrists, ankles, and feet.

In infantile SMA type 1 (Werdnig-Hoffmann disease) the infant never attains the ability to sit (Fig. 17). In this book, SMA type 1 is also defined by failure to attain the ability to roll, loss of the ability to take nourishment by mouth before 2 years of age, paradoxical chest wall movement from the time of diagnosis, and the development of acute respiratory failure (usually during chest infections) before 2 years of age. Affected children also have fine muscle tremors and twitching. They have periods of perspiration and flushing, especially during sleep, that can be relieved by proper management (Chapters 3 and 12). Often after a period of sleeping well overnight, they have ongoing frequent arousals that necessitate nocturnal nasal ventilation for relief. Some patients exhibit episodic bradycardias (Chapter 5). Patients with SMA type 1 rarely lose the ability to move the fingers or to use certain facial muscles, although occasional patients lose eye muscle movements and develop ptosis during adolescence. Eighty to 85% who do not

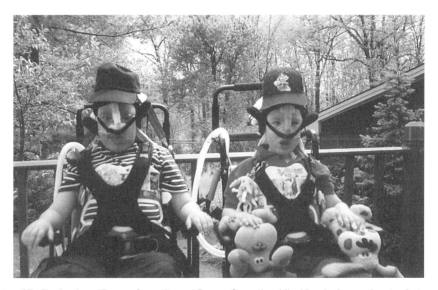

Figure 17. Two brothers (7 years 4 months and 5 years 6 months old) with spinal muscular atrophy type 1. The older brother developed respiratory failure at 5 months of age and required continuous nasal ventilation before weaning to nocturnal-only high span bilevel PAP. A second episode of respiratory failure occurred at 11 months of age, from which time he has required nasal ventilation continuously. He has a VC of 90 ml and has received all nutrition via nasogastric tube since 5 months of age. His brother has been continuously dependent on high-span bilevel PAP and nutrition via nasogastric tube since 4 months of age but has never been hospitalized. He has a VC of 70 ml. Both are averbal but communicate via computer voice synthesizer. They are happy children with their own personalities and do extremely well with school work. Neither has any sign of pectus excavatum or significant irreversible back curvature.

undergo tracheotomy develop the ability to speak and maintain the ability to breathe unassisted at least throughout childhood (Chapter 12).

Patients with conventionally managed SMA type 1 die from respiratory failure before 2 years of age (median: around 7 months), and about 80% die by 12 months of age.[63] Only two such children with SMA type 1 have been described to survive beyond 2 years of age—both with the use of continuous tracheostomy IPPV.[64,65]

Some infants with infantile SMA can never sit but may roll, take food orally well into adulthood, and have clearly milder courses. Such children are considered to have SMA type 1+ rather than SMA type 1. Some of them can feed themselves and breathe independently and are stronger when they at 20 years of age than some children with type 2 SMA and later onset of disease.[64] A least one 27-year-old woman with SMA type 1+ has had a successful pregnancy despite severe kyphoscoliosis and a VC of 270–400 ml.[66]

Children with SMA type 2 at least temporarily attain the ability to sit independently or are more mildly affected than those defined as type 1 (Fig. 18). Seventy-three percent of children sit within the normal age range of up to 9 months; the remainder sit between 10 and 30 months. Rarely can type 2 patients come to sitting on their own or hold their hands above their heads.[67] In a study of 10 children with SMA type 2, overall strength was determined to be 35–40% of normal. Six children were capable of at least one-half pound of force in pinch or gross grasp, and four children had zero force in one of these measures. Repeated measures revealed no changes over time in proximal or distal strength. Ability to produce a measurable force in pinch or gross grasp was found to be associated with independence in mobility, hand function, and activities of daily living (ADLs).[68] Likewise, from ages 10 to 19, when measured dynametrically, muscle strength

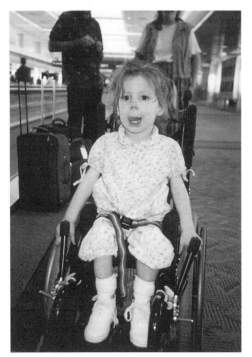

Figure 18. Whereas children with SMA type 3 generally have normal physiognomy (other than possible generalized muscle atrophy and scoliosis), children with type 2 SMA can have facies and high arched palates similar to type 1 children or, in milder cases, minimal abnormality (seen here).

can remain constant and SMA can be considered a nonprogressive disease.[69] Thus, such patients have weak but stable muscle force. Without any ongoing access to respiratory muscle aids, the survival rate among 240 children with type 2 SMA was 98.5% at 5 years and 68.5% at 25 years.[70]

Children with SMA type 3 (Kugelberg-Welander disease) attain the ability to walk independently. For 10% this ability is delayed past the upper limit of normal (18 months).[71] Children with SMA type 3 who sit late also tend to walk late. The ability to walk is subsequently lost. The probability of being able to walk 10 years after onset of SMA type 3 before 3 years of age is 70%; it is 22% at 40 years. For type 3 with onset after 3 years of age the probability of walking 10 years after onset is 97%; it is 59% at 40 years.[14] The median age for becoming chair-bound does not differ between SMA 3 patients who walk with delay and those who walk at less than 18 months (10.2 vs. 10.5 years).[71] In another study, 50% of children who could walk without assistance and whose onset was prior to age 2 lost the ability to walk independently by age 12. Fifty percent who walked and whose onset was between 2 and 6 years of age lost walking ability by age 44. Patients who can walk only with assistance lose any ability to walk by age 14. Eighty-five percent of patients who could walk independently could not negotiate stairs without holding onto a rail. As patients lost the ability to walk, they also lost the ability to raise the hands over the head.[67]

Although most people with SMA type 3 retain functional use of the arms and the ability to feed themselves independently into adulthood, 80% with an onset of symptoms at age 17.4 ± 14.2 months, lose the ability to walk before adulthood.[72] Unlike people with Xp21 muscular dystrophies, patients with SMA type 3 have weak iliopsoas and strong gluteus maximus muscles. However, type 3 SMA can be extremely variable. Some patients have earlier and more severe weakness than children with DMD, whereas others do not require wheelchair use until late middle age. Musculotendinous contractures and scoliosis are inevitable in patients with childhood SMA (Chapters 6 and 7).

Life expectancy is about normal for patients with SMA type 3. For type 2 and type 3 patients, bulbar musculature usually remains adequate for speaking and for taking at least some nutrition by mouth throughout life; however, about 50% of type 2 children eventually require gastrostomy tubes for supplemental nutrition. Many type 2 children also exhibit muscle tremors and episodic arousals and perspiration, particularly when paradoxical breathing is present. Muscle strength and function (motor milestones) can improve during childhood, and strength should remain constant during adolescence.[59] Hand and facial muscle function and usually some upper limb function are retained throughout life.

In a study of 25 patients with SMA between 5 and 32 years old, excessive vertical development, particularly of the lower face, was noted. There was relatively larger anterior than posterior facial height due to a smaller cranial base angulation and a more anteriorly positioned mandibular ramus. Patients also had a protrusive maxilla, retrusive mandible, and other abnormal craniofacial growth patterns.[73]

Strength and function can plateau and then begin to decrease for children with SMA. This decrease may be due to some combination of limb growth that outstrips muscle strength or to suboptimal nutrition (Chapter 3) not directly related to the primary anterior horn cell pathology. Actual strength does not decrease over 5-year periods during adolescence once the limbs are nearly fully grown.[59] Undernutrition and other metabolic factors may also be responsible for strength and bulbar musculature weakening during intercurrent illnesses, after surgical anesthesia, and during other periods of physiologic stress (Chapter 3).[74,75] After 19 years of age, our natural physiological peak, anterior horn cells and muscle strength gradually diminish. Although the primary pathologic processes have not been demonstrated to affect the heart directly, neural input to the heart can be affected (Chapter 5).

SMA type 4 presents after adolescence. It may be caused by deletion of the (telomeric) SMN 2 gene.[76] Patients usually become wheelchair users in middle age and may not require nocturnal ventilator use until old age. Kennedy's disease is now considered SMA type 5. This sex-linked, recessive MND predominantly affects males. It presents after adolescence and is slowly progressive. Affected men have muscle weakness, arm tremors, muscle twitching and cramps, abnormal breast enlargement, small testicles, and diminished fertility.

Amyotrophic Lateral Sclerosis/Motor Neuron Disease

Throughout the ALS process, I have learned many things. I have learned that having ALS does not necessarily mean a death sentence, that I am not living with a life-threatening disease, but rather with a life-enhancing condition.

•✿• Sam Filer

The Honorable Justice Sam Filer, who uses a computer-activated communication system, has been employed as a municipal court judge despite having only eyelid movements and requiring ventilatory support via tracheostomy for 15 years.[77] ALS is a disease of unknown etiology that occurs in about 1 in 1800 people. It is at times associated with a small autosome 14 defect, a chromosome 2 defect that carries instructions for a protein called alsin, or a mutation in a gene on chromosome 21 that encodes the protein superoxide dismutase. About 5–10% of cases are inherited as an autosomal dominant disorder. It usually presents between ages 25 and 75 years with a mean age at onset of about 57 years. Disease limited to one limb and juvenile forms exist. ALS is associated with derangements in cytoskeletal protein and glutamate metabolism, mitochondrial function, and glial interactions. Some patients also have a defect in the IgG subclass expression of T-cells, and some patients with this defect have low IgG levels overall.[78] Potentially reversible (with antiretroviral therapy) anterior motor neuron degeneration also occurs in association with AIDS,[79] renal cell carcinoma,[80] and, rarely, certain systemic cancers. In one group of 14 patients with MND and cancer, 3 developed a rapidly progressive MND, less prominent symptoms of involvement of other areas of the nervous system, and anti-Hu antibodies; 5 women with breast cancer developed upper MND without antineuronal antibodies with symptoms occurring within 3 months of cancer diagnosis or tumor recurrence; and 6 patients developed ALS, probably coincidentally, within 4 years before or after the diagnosis of cancer. Lymphoproliferative disorders including macroglobulinemia, multiple myeloma, chronic lymphocytic leukemia, follicular cell lymphoma, and Hodgkin's disease, have also been associated with MND. Occasional cases are associated with the presence of anti-GM1 ganglioside antibodies. Interestingly, there also appears to be a relationship with the etiology of SMA. Homozygous deletion of SMN 2 gene was reported to be a prognostic factor in sporadic ALS. In patients with

SMA, the SMN 1 gene product is eliminated and disease severity is an inverse function of the quantity of full-length messenger RNA produced by the SMN 2 gene. In ALS, although no SMN 1 deletions were noted in 110 patients, 16% had deletions of SMN 2 (as opposed to 4% of controls), and presence of an SMN 2 deletion was independently associated with diminished survival time. Therefore, the SMN 2 gene appears to be a phenotypic modifier in sporadic ALS.[81]

Thus, various processes, including immunologic processes, are involved in the deterioration of motor neurons.[82] Immunologic involvement is evidenced by the association of ALS with cancer, lymphoma, and monoclonal gammopathies and with the presence of serum antibodies to neural antigens. Furthermore, occasional patients, especially those with purely lower motor neuron findings (multifocal motorneuropathy), respond to immune or cytostatic therapies.[83] Female patients with primary lateral sclerosis should undergo mammography.

ALS affects both the anterior horn cells (as does SMA and poliomyelitis) and the lateral tracks of the spinal cord; occasionally it affects the brain itself. Twenty percent of inherited cases are associated with mutations in the gene for superoxide dismutase type 1 (SOD-1).[84]

Because there are no specific tests for making the diagnosis, ALS is a diagnosis of exclusion. "El Escorial Revisited" is a revised set of criteria developed at a 1998 World Federation of Neurology ALS meeting in Warrenton, Virginia; these criteria are available on the Internet at www.wfn-als. The following conditions must be ruled out: multiple sclerosis, polyneuropathy (especially multifocal motor neuropathy), SMA, myelopathies, Alzheimer's disease, AIDS and other immune system diseases, cancer, syphilis, Lyme disease, thyroid disorders, and parathyroid disease. Patients with multifocal motor neuropathy—that is, those with lower MND and electrodiagnostic evidence of conduction block—can be treated (Chapter 2).[85,86]

The first complaints are usually muscle cramps, twitching, and weakness; however, fatigue, shortness of breath, slurred speech, difficulty in swallowing, vocal cord paralysis, muscle spasticity, pain, numbness, and tingling can be among the presenting symptoms. Disease that begins in one limb, several limbs, or the respiratory muscles is nonbulbar-onset ALS/MND. Disease that begins in the muscles above the neck and affects speech and swallowing at onset is bulbar-onset ALS. Sometimes people have pure skeletal ALS or pure bulbar ALS for many years before those with nonbulbar ALS develop bulbar muscle weakness or those with bulbar ALS develop respiratory and skeletal muscle weakness (Fig. 19). Most patients, however, have some combination of both skeletal and bulbar ALS almost from the outset. ALS can at times present as ventilatory failure and/or dementia.[87] In one study, 11 of 23 patients with bulbar-onset ALS/MND were cognitively impaired with frontotemporal involvement, memory impairment, alteration of judgment and reasoning, reduced speech, and behavioral dyscontrol. Cognitive impairment was five times more likely in male as opposed to female patients.[88] Impairment can often be ameliorated by nocturnal ventilatory assistance.[89]

The rate of disease progression is usually linear initially. The rate of decline in pulmonary function most closely correlates with death for patients not managed with respiratory aids. For such patients, mean survival is 4 years. In one study, untreated patients with onset between 25 and 44 years survived 71.5 months and those with later onset survived 32.5 months.[90]

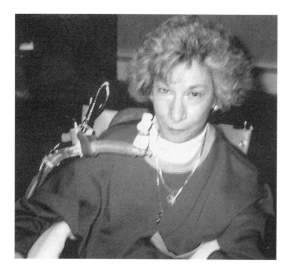

Figure 19. A woman with onset of amyotrophic lateral sclerosis at age 59, diagnosed 6 months later, developed hypophonia from diminished tidal volumes and alveolar hypoventilation 13 months from onset and quickly became dependent on daytime mouthpiece and nocturnal nasal IPPV with no breathing tolerance. She lost bulbar function 6 months later and died after refusing tracheotomy.

After establishment of the diagnosis of ALS, the VC typically remains normal for several years. However, ventilatory failure and death occasionally occur in as little as 2 months from onset of symptoms and can occur at the time of initial presentation to a physician.[91] The mean survival from onset of symptoms without the use of ventilatory support has been reported as 2.4,[92] 3.1,[93] and 2.5–5.9 years, depending on age at onset.[94] Mean survival from the point of diagnosis was reported as 15–20 months in studies of 708[94] and 194[95] patients, respectively. Jablecki et al., on the other hand, reported that about 20% of 194 patients survived 10 years without ventilatory support.[93]

Typically, people become weaker until some point at which they plateau. Usually, but not always, the plateau occurs when the person is already dependent on wheelchair use and has little remaining limb function. Often, plateaus occur once the VC is between 200 and 400 ml. On some occasions, patients show spontaneous improvement in major muscle groups, and the original diagnosis is usually put into question. We and others have had patients with typical ALS/MND who have had stabilization or persistent improvement in VC and in strength of large muscle groups beginning 6–7 years after onset. On rare occasions, overall spontaneous improvement has been reported. In one report, 4 patients with a clinical syndrome and electrodiagnostic studies consistent with ALS recovered completely and without treatment 5–12 months after onset.[96]

About 4–20% of people with ALS have a relatively benign course and do not require the use of any inspiratory or expiratory muscle aids for over 5 years.[94,97] Such patients can then often use noninvasive ventilation for many years before requiring tracheotomy. Even for patients with typical ALS, however, who have used invasive IPPV for 10 years or more, 70–90% retain the ability to blink the eyes or control other volitional muscle activity. Most patients, therefore, retain the capacity to operate voice synthesizers and other computer-activated communication and environmental control systems.

Loss of emotional control can require treatment (Chapter 2). For patients with bulbar ALS, drooling may occur, and dysphagia can result in continuous aspiration of saliva. This syndrome can cause airway spasm and coughing. With increasing severity it results in microscopic atelectasis, oxyhemoglobin desaturation, macroscopic atelectasis, and finally pneumonia and respiratory failure. Medical management of airway secretions is noted in Chapter 8. The indication for tracheotomy in patients with bulbar ALS is a decrease in SpO_2 baseline below 95% because of severe aspiration of airway secretions (Chapter 10).

An interesting study of 1600 hospitalizations for patients with ALS found that the most common concurrent diagnoses were dehydration and malnutrition (574 patients; 36%), pneumonia (506 patients; 32%), and respiratory failure (398 patients; 25%). Only 38% of patients were discharged home without health care, and average hospital stays were 8.4 days as opposed to 5.4 days for non-ALS admissions.[98] Thus, 57% of admissions were for respiratory morbidity.

As for all other neurologic NMDs, such as SMA, since the primary pathology does not directly affect the heart; thus, life is usually threatened only by respiratory complications, which can be avoidable for many years. When asked in advance and when noninvasive options are not presented, 95% of patients with ALS think that they will decide against using a ventilator (tracheotomy) and may sign an advanced directive to this effect. However, for at-home users of noninvasive ventilation whose bulbar muscle function severely deteriorates or for people intubated in the intensive care setting because acute respiratory failure was not avoided in the first place, the great majority agree to tracheotomy for continued ventilatory support and survival.[99] In retrospect, the great majority of patients and families who choose ventilatory assistance say that it was worthwhile and that they would make the same decision if they had to do it over again (Chapter 13).[100]

With nonbulbar ALS, ventilatory failure is usually caused by ill-advised treatment of advancing respiratory muscle weakness with oxygen therapy or sedatives (which exacerbate hypercapnia) or by ineffectively low-span bilevel positive airway pressure (BiPAP)—that is, low-span positive inspiratory pressure plus positive end-expiratory pressure limited to nocturnal-only use. Sometimes respiratory failure is triggered by the inability to cough out airway secretions during a chest cold. As for other patients with conventionally managed NMD, the inevitable respiratory failure is then either treated by emergency translaryngeal intubation and, ultimately tracheotomy or by oxygen and narcotics to hasten death. Once a tracheostomy tube has been placed, patients with ALS also quickly lose any ability to breathe on their own. As described later, when the assisted cough peak flows (CPF) of patients with ALS can exceed 160 liters per minute, tracheotomy should rarely need to be considered. Unfortunately, bulbar muscle function is not usually quantitated, nor are nonbulbar and bulbar types treated differently. Outcomes of conventional care using nocturnal-only low-span BiPAP are poor, extend tracheostomy-free survival by only a few months, and are summarized elsewhere.[101] We have found that patients survive a mean of over 5 years and occasionally over 15 years when they receive ventilatory support via tracheostomy.[97] Ultimately, death is usually caused by complications resulting from the tracheostomy itself (Chapter 8). Proper evaluation and management of ALS/MND are described in Chapter 11.

Poliomyelitis

Poliomyelitis is an acquired anterior horn cell disease caused by infectious agents, most commonly one of three strains of the poliomyelitis virus. Many poliomyelitis survivors have required continuous noninvasive ventilatory support since contracting acute poliomyelitis over 45 years ago (Fig. 20). There are even more poliomyelitis survivors who, weaned from ventilator use after acute polio, once again require ongoing ventilatory assistance. In general,

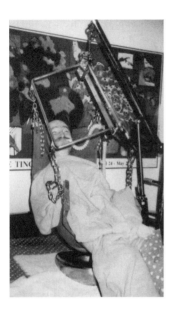

Figure 20. Patient with poliomyelitis who uses 24-hour-per-day mouthpiece (daytime)and Lipseal IPPV (during sleep). He has had no measurable VC and no volitional extremity movement since 1952 but has not been intubated and has been hospitalized only once for respiratory management of acute bronchitis since 1952. He uses a Hoyer lift to facilitate bowel movements. This approach has reduced the time needed to complete bowel movements from 3 hours to 15-20 minutes.

as opposed to the normal rate of loss of VC with aging (about 30 ml per year), post-polio survivors lose VC at a rate of 70% greater.[102] As for patients with inherited NMD, respiratory morbidity and mortality are extremely high and almost always avoidable because bulbar muscle function and assisted CPF almost invariably remain much more than adequate. Because both nonrespiratory and respiratory management have been comprehensively described elsewhere, the reader is referred to other sources.[103,104]

Other Neurologic Conditions

Neuropathies

The most common hereditary motor and sensory neuropathy is Charcot-Marie-Tooth disease, a slowly progressive, autosomal dominant disorder with variable penetrance. It is associated with symmetric distal greater than proximal weakness and atrophy and sensory involvement. Electromyography (EMG) typically demonstrates severe nerve conduction slowing; in the axonal form, however, conduction can be within normal limits while amplitudes are diminished. Ankle deformities, distal extremity weakness, and sensory loss are usually the predominant impairments; occasionally (five patients in the author's experience) weakness progresses to severe generalized paralysis and the need for permanent ventilatory support. In one study, 12 of 86 patients had histories of respiratory complications. Expiratory muscles tended to be weaker than inspiratory muscles. Thirty percent of patients had abnormal electrocardiograms, and 7% had a history of cardiovascular complications. Kyphoscoliosis was the major spine deformity. Intellectual and neuropsychologic profiles were normal.[105]

Familial hypertrophic interstitial polyneuropathy (Dejerine-Sottas disease) is a rare disease of generalized weakness. It is diagnosed by peripheral nerve biopsy. Bulbar muscle involvement often precludes the optimal use of noninvasive inspiratory muscle aids because the lips are often too weak to grasp a mouth piece, and scoliosis can prevent the effective use of an intermittent abdominal pressure ventilator (IAPV) (Chapter 10). Expiratory muscle aids, however, can be very helpful to assist cough.

A multitude of conditions can cause phrenic nerve trauma and neuropathies (see Table 1). Phrenic neuropathy is often the initial sign of ALS/MND or multiple sclerosis. Such patients, who may otherwise have normal musculature, insidiously develop shortness of breath when reclining. Patients can use accessory breathing muscles when sitting but not when supine, and the diaphragm becomes unable to adequately ventilate the lungs. A common, new cause of phrenic nerve pathology is iatrogenic damage during coronary artery bypass surgery. Ventilatory failure occurs during the first few days after surgery. Although with bulbar and expiratory muscle sparing, such patients require only the use of inspiratory muscle aids, typically these aids are not offered. Patients are conventionally managed by invasive means, often with dire consequences (see Case 20 of Chapter 15 of reference 103).

Acute postinfectious polyneuropathy (Guillain-Barré syndrome) is an acquired inflammatory segmental demyelinating neuropathy. Two-thirds of cases present with a history of preceding viral infection, immunization, surgery, or immunologic disorder. Sensory loss is usually slight and is absent in one-third of patients. Ascending weakness and paresthesias begin in the hands and feet and usually progress for 1–2 weeks. Partial to almost complete recovery usually takes 3–6 months. The diagnosis is made on the basis of the history, clinical features, and laboratory picture, including the elevation of cerebrospinal fluid protein and the observation of characteristically severe nerve conduction slowing. With recovery, residual weakness ranges from mild ankle dorsiflexion impairment to severe paralysis (uncommon) that necessitates permanent ventilatory support. Ventilatory support often can be provided noninvasively.

Skeletal Pathology and Other Conditions or Nonneuromuscular Diseases with Physical and Ventilatory Impairments

The kyphoscoliosis that develops in children with NMD is due to paraspinal muscle weakness and the inability of weak paraspinal muscles to hold up the spine (Chapter 7). The development of scoliosis is almost ubiquitous in pediatric patients with NMDs. It is also seen frequently in neurofibromatosis, osteogenesis imperfecta, tuberculosis of the spine, rigid spine syndrome, and familial dysautonomia. People without generalized muscle weakness can also develop kyphoscoliosis as a result of severe osteoporosis, systemic diseases (such as ankylosing spondylosis), or unknown causes (idiopathic).[103]

Table 1 lists other conditions for which the management principles described in this book can be pertinent. For patients with inherited NMD, this text is the only comprehensive management guide available, whereas there are comprehensive texts for the evaluation and management of certain other conditions, such as for post-poliomyelitis,[104,106] myelopathies and spinal cord injury,[107] multiple sclerosis,[108] and chronic obstructive pulmonary disease.[109] In many such texts, however, the use of respiratory muscle aids is not fully described but can be found in a recent publication by the present author.[103]

No ande buscando tres pies al gato!
(Don't go looking for a cat with 3 legs!)

◦✿◦ Don Quijote de La Mancha

Chapter 2

Medical Therapies and Research

No tengas pena, amigo, porque yo haré ahora el balsamo precioso, con el que sanaremos en un abrir y cerrar de ojos.

Don't worry, my friend, because I now have a precious balm that will make you healthy in the blink of an eye.

・◉・ Don Quijote de La Mancha

General Therapeutic Strategies

Thus far, numerous medical therapies have been attempted in treating spinal muscular atrophy (SMA), amyotrophic lateral sclerosis (ALS), Duchenne muscular dystrophy (DMD), and other neuromuscular diseases (NMDs) with little or, at times, controversial success. Medications used for specific conditions are discussed below.

Some medications are thought to benefit more than one or perhaps all NMDs. For example, creatine is a molecule derived from two amino acids. Normally about one gram is synthesized in the liver and kidneys, and another gram is taken in with food each day. Creatine enters the blood and is taken up by the muscles. Exercise, thyroid hormone, and substances such as insulin can greatly increase muscle creatine uptake. When the diet is supplemented with creatine, its concentration and the concentration of its phosphorylated form, phosphocreatine, become elevated. This increased concentration serves to prevent depletion of adenosine triphosphate, a substance needed to maintain physiologic processes such as muscle contraction; to protect tissue from hypoxia-induced damage; to stimulate protein synthesis or reduce protein degradation; and to stabilize biologic membranes. Normal young exercising males who receive 20 gm/day for 4–28 days increase total body mass significantly more (by 1–2 kg) than males not receiving supplementation.[111] For small children, creatine supplementation has been recommended at a dose of 0.1 gm/kg.

Total creatine is greatly reduced in the skeletal muscle of patients with muscular dystrophy and congenital, inflammatory, and mitochondrial myopathies. The beneficial effect of creatine on cell wall membrane stabilization, leakage prevention, myotube formation, and survival has been demonstrated in cell cultures from mammals with correlates of muscular dystrophy, ALS, and mitochondrial disease.[112] Creatine has also been reported to prolong survival in mice with MND.[113]

In studies of humans with muscular dystrophy, supplementation of 10 gm/day for adults and 5 gm/day for children for 8 weeks resulted in a 3% increase in strength and a 10% improvement in symptom score. Significant improvement in muscle strength and ADL also has been reported with the same doses in humans with neuropathic disorders and mitochondrial, inflammatory, and congenital myopathies.[112,114] The patients also had small but significant increases in body weight.[115] Twenty of 28 patients with ALS who took 20 gm/day of creatine had significant temporary increases in the strength of major muscle groups. After the first week the patients received 3 gm/day for up to 6 months.

Creatine, an end-product of muscle contraction, stimulates muscle protein synthesis. Supplementing the diet with creatine enhances this effect. Side effects of creatine supplementation include weight gain, gastrointestinal distress, renal dysfunction that is reversible with cessation of supplementation, and possibly muscle cramps; there has been a report of hepatic dysfunction in one person. Liver enzymes and glomerular filtration are not normally elevated with supplementation. Creatine may be cytotoxic because it can ultimately be converted to formaldehyde and hydrogen peroxide. Formaldehyde can cross-link proteins and DNA. Creatine supplementation does increase urinary formaldehyde excretion. In addition, byproducts in the manufacture of creatine, including arsenic and dicyandamide, can contaminate commercial preparations. As a dietary supplement, manufacture is not regulated by the Food and Drug Administration (FDA).

Coenzyme Q10 is synthesized in the body and active in antioxidation reactions, bioenergetics, and growth control. Coenzyme Q10 is an essential cofactor of the electron transport chain as well as a potent free radical scavenger in lipid and mitochondrial membranes. It has been shown to increase cardiac (Chapter 5) and cerebral cortex mitochondrial concentrations, attenuate striatal lesions produced by systemic administration of 3-nitropropionic acid, and significantly increase the life span of transgenic mice with ALS, suggesting that it may have a protective effect in the treatment of neurodegenerative diseases.[116]

Gene therapy or use of carriers (vectors) to introduce dystrophin, emerin, or other missing substance into muscle or other body tissues in which it is deficient appears promising. Adenoviruses, adeno-associated viruses, herpes viruses, retroviruses, and lentiviruses are candidates. Other types of delivery systems, such as the use of liposomes and myoblasts, are being tried. When adenoviruses are used to deliver the dystrophin gene into affected muscle, only about 2% of the muscle fibers use the dystrophin gene. This low efficiency may be a result of the method of delivering the gene as well as the immune system's recognition of foreign material in the cells containing the adenovirus. Viral vectors have been used successfully to slow the course of cystic fibrosis. In treating cystic fibrosis, however, one has the advantage that the target organ, the bronchial membranes, can be reached by simply breathing.

Embryonic stem cells multiply and differentiate into all of the specialized cells of the body, including muscle and nerve cells. Stem and early precursor cells from umbilical cord blood, muscle, or bone marrow are able to disperse to sites of nerve or muscle damage via the vascular system and to participate in repair. Thus, like gene therapy, stem cells may have the potential to treat or cure all NMDs. The problem is to get them to divide into the required cells and not into tumors and to avoid elimination by the immunologic system. Stem cells—in particular, mononuclear cells from embryonic cord blood—have been reported in two studies to slow the progression of ALS in mice.[117,118] They also regenerate damaged muscle in dystrophic mice.[119] We are currently organizing studies in humans.

Myopathies

Medical and surgical strategies for treating DMD date back to 1845.[6] For DMD alone, medical trials have been conducted with selenium, laevodosin, antioxidants (e.g., desferrioxamine, penicillamine, vitamin E), isaxonine (a nerve growth stimulator), the xanthine oxidase inhibitor allopurinol, adenylate or adenine, mazindol and cyprohepta-dine (for growth hormone release), isoniazid and adenosine triphosphate, the amino acid leucine, tolmetin, imipramine, theophylline, phenytoin, antiserotonin agents (methyl-sergide and pizotifene), antioxidant superoxide dismutase, L-carnitine, vasodilators, calcium channel blockers (e.g., verapamil, flunarizine, nifedipine, diltiazem), plasma infusions, dantrolene sodium, gentamicin, the metabolite adenylosuccinate, cromolyn, bemitil, and myoblast transfers.[109] None of these attempts have yielded positive results in humans.

The story of myoblast transfers deserves to be told. Immature mouse muscle cells (myoblasts) from normal mice, when implanted into mice with muscular dystrophy, multiplied and combined with the abnormal immature mouse muscle cells to produce more normal muscle fibers. When normal myoblasts were injected into the little toe of a 9-year-old boy with DMD, some implanted myoblasts survived, developed, and pro-duced dystrophin; dystrophin-positive muscle fibers developed in clusters. There were no complications over the 3 months after the myoblast injection, and the strength of the toe may have increased temporarily to a slight degree. Subsequently, 32 boys with DMD, aged 6–14 years, were injected with no change in force 3, 6, or 9 months later.[120] Myoblasts can be produced by the billions, but the problems are how to deliver them to a wide range of affected muscles and how to deal with the body's immune response to foreign tissues. Jerry Lewis MDA investigators reported that increases in the amount of force generated by the injected muscle cells and the amount of dystrophin have not been significant in humans as opposed to mice. This finding has not discouraged charlatans from charging desperate families $150,000 for useless myoblast transfer treatments de-spite the absence of clinical effectiveness.

Diethylstilbestrol and corticosteroids such as prednisone, which have been taken by many people with DMD since 1974,[121] temporarily increase muscle strength and de-crease the subsequent rate of loss of muscle strength for many patients. Prednisone has been shown to protect muscle against exercise-induced damage, probably by stabilizing muscle cell wall membranes. It has not been shown to reduce creatine kinase levels,[121–123] but, when taken at 0.75 mg/kg/day for 6–8 weeks, it has been shown to increase strength by 15%, to increase 24-hour creatinine excretion (an index of muscle mass), to decrease 3-methylhistidine excretion (like urinary acid soluble proteins,[124] an index of muscle breakdown), and thereby to increase muscle mass.[125] Prednisolone at 0.35 mg/kg/day[122] and 0.75 mg/kg/day for 6 months has yielded similar results for DMD and BMD.[126]

Corticosteroids can prolong the ability to walk for 2 years in children with DMD.[127] A recent report suggests that some patients with BMD can have a dramatic and sus-tained improvement in strength with therapeutic use of prednisone.[128] It has even been suggested to benefit patients with SMA and hereditary sensory and motor neuropa-thy,[129] although a study using 1.5 mg/kg/day of prednisone for 12 weeks for patients with FSH did not result in increased strength or any measurable benefits.[130] Optimal dosage schedule for prednisone is unclear, but 0.75 mg/kg/day for at least 6 months be-tween ages 4 and 8 years appears to be highly beneficial. When tolerated, treatment can be begun by age 3 years and extended indefinitely. Intermittent or "pulsed" prednisone therapy for several weeks 6 or more times per year from age 3 to 17 years has also been reported to be beneficial. Alternate-day dosing and 10 days on, 10 days off dosing seem beneficial while minimizing side effects.

Unfortunately, all users experience side effects, and often steroid use cannot be tolerated very long. Users experience weight gain and reshaping of the fat layer under the skin. In addition, steroids affect the immune system, bone development, metabolism, protein synthesis, and mood. They can cause intestinal disturbances, excessive hair growth, and cataracts. Patients must be followed closely for high blood pressure, adequate growth, and urinary and blood glucose levels. Supplemental calcium and vitamin D are taken to allay the effects on bone metabolism. Evaluation must also be done for typical side effects, including vertebral compression fractures,[131] cushingoid appearance, acne, behavioral changes (e.g., hyperactivity, irritability, insomnia, euphoria, depression), easy bruising, increased appetite, nausea, stomach discomfort, excessive hair growth, and intercurrent infections. Low sodium and sugar diets are prudent, and supplemental calcium carbonate is recommended with each meal.[123] Glucocorticoids may increase surgical and anesthetic risks.

A synthetic steroid called deflazacort is now used outside the United States. It has been reported to provide the same benefits as prednisone but with fewer side effects, particularly on weight gain and bone development, an important concern in growing children.[132,133] With 0.9 mg/kg/day of deflazacort vs. 0.75 mg/kg/day of prednisone, muscle strength increased equally, but weight gain was 18% in the prednisone group vs. 5% in the deflazacort group. In one study, 24 untreated boys stopped walking at 9.8 ± 1.8 years of age, whereas 7 of the 30 treated boys stopped walking at 12.3 ± 2.7 years of age and of the 23 who were still walking, 21 were over 10 years of age. At age 15, VC was 88% of normal in treated but only 39% of normal in untreated boys (Fig. 1).[133] Untreated boys lost weight faster than treated boys after 13 years of age. Unfortunately, deflazacort has not been approved by the Food and Drug Administration.[134] Glucocorticoids such as prednisone can also be effective in treating polymyositis, multiple sclerosis, and

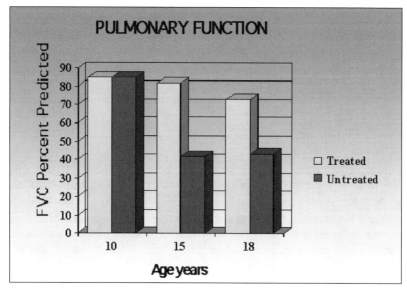

Figure 1. Comparison of the vital capacities of patients with Duchenne muscular dystrophy receiving and not receiving deflazacort.

myasthenia gravis. Certain other medical treatments directed at the immune system have also been shown to be at times helpful in treating these conditions.[135]

Mice with DMD-like conditions have been effectively treated by enhancing muscle cell wall utrophin levels[136] and receiving muscle creatine kinase promoter as well as by gene therapy. The advances demonstrated in mice have not yet been reproduced in humans, but MDA-sponsored human protocols are under way.

Dystrophic mice have also had decreased net muscle catabolism with improved muscle morphology, strength, and function when receiving high protein diets.[137] Furthermore, in a randomized, 6-month, double-blind, placebo-controlled study of oxandrolone, an anabolic steroid, in boys with DMD, the mean change in grades on manual muscle testing was 0.035, whereas for controls it was –0.140.[138] It was suggested that, because oxandrolone is safe, accelerates linear growth, and may have some beneficial effect in slowing the progression of weakness, it may be useful before corticosteroid therapy is initiated. Likewise, one study suggested that oral glutamine had a protein anabolic effect by sparing nitrogen precursors for six 8- to 13-year-old boys with DMD.[139] Other studies suggested that Chinese herbal medications[140] and green tea[141] can benefit mdx mice and possibly humans with DMD.

Recently a trial of albuterol, 8 or 16 mg twice daily for 1 year, in patients with FSH resulted in a significant improvement in grip and a significant increase in lean mass compared with placebo but not in a significant increase in general muscle strength.[142] Certain myopathies, such as those due to carnitine palmityl transferase deficiency, can respond to treatment with oral L-carnitine. There is no medical treatment for acid maltase deficiency. The use of small frequent meals is recommended for patients with debranching enzyme deficiency, and liver transplantation has been highly effective in treating branching enzyme deficiency.[51] Some patients with carnitine deficiency respond well to restrictions in dietary fat and treatment with oral L-carnitine.[50] In one pilot study, dehydroepiandrosterone sulfate, 200 mg/day for 8 weeks, was reported to improve activities of daily living (ADL) and muscle strength and to reduce myotonia in 11 patients with myotonic dystrophy.[43] Conduction block and premature beats also improved in the 4 patients with cardiac involvement in this study.

Patients with myasthenia gravis can respond well to corticosteroid therapy, anticholinesterase administration, plasmapheresis, and thymectomy. In one study, 91 patients (69%) had a good response to thymectomy, whereas 41 (31%) had a poor response. Fifty patients went into remission, 41 improved, 34 had no change, and 7 became worse. Patients who had the disease for more than 3 years had a tendency toward a bad prognosis. Other variables associated with poor prognosis were high doses of pyridostigmine, use of steroids before surgery, total duration of the disease, duration of the disease between diagnosis and surgical procedure, and discovery of thymic atrophy and thymoma in histopathologic studies.[143]

Anterior Horn Cell Diseases and Neuropathies

Amyotrophic Lateral Sclerosis

Many medications have been tried to treat ALS. In patients for whom anti-GM1 ganglioside antibodies have been found, cyclophosphamide, an immunologic system suppressant, has been temporarily effective.[144] In ALS associated with immunodeficiency, intravenous immunoglobulin has been shown to ameliorate symptoms and increase general physical well-being.[145] For others without anti-GM1 ganglioside antibodies or immune deficiency, however, other treatments aimed at the immunologic system (e.g., plasmapheresis, azothioprine and other AIDS medications, prednisolone, cyclosporine, total lymphoid irradiation) have not helped. Medications used to treat AIDS continue to be used for medical trials, however, because AIDS-associated anterior horn cell loss has resolved with effective medical treatment of AIDS.

Riluzole has been reported statistically to prolong life or delay tracheotomy by 1 week in mice and by several months in people with ALS.[146] It has been reported to be safe for up to 7 years.[147] It has been suggested that patients receiving vitamin E along with riluzole may remain more mildly affected for longer periods than those taking riluzole alone.[148] However, riluzole is quite expensive and has no observable effect on muscle strength. Likewise, medications designed to reduce neurotoxins such as branch chain amino acids, dextromethorphan, quinidine, and the immune system stimulant interferon, have not helped. Gabapentin is an anticonvulsant that may act like riluzole to prevent secondary damage to nerve cells from the leaking of glutamates, but it has not yet been shown to be beneficial.

Although lamotrigine has not been effective,[149] other medications that more effectively block release of or eliminate glutamate are being investigated. Celecoxib (Celebrex), a nonsteroidal anti-inflammatory medication, prostaglandin inhibitor, and possibly a protector of motor neurons from toxic effects of glutamate, is under study. Glutathione peroxidase and aromatic amines such as iminostilbene are superior neuroprotective antioxidants and have promise.[150] Diaminopyridine (an enhancer of acetylcholine release), phthalazinol, verapamil[151] and nimodipine[152] (calcium channel blockers), L-threonine (used to increase glycine levels),[153] selegiline (an antioxidant used to treat Parkinson disease symptoms), and other antioxidants (e.g., vitamin E,[154] thyrotrophin-releasing hormone, growth hormone) have also proved ineffective. Pimozide, a calcium blocker, was reported to statistically slow the course of ALS in one study.[155] Nerve growth factors, such as ciliary neurotrophic factor, insulin-like growth factor 1, brain-derived neurotrophic factor, and glial cell line-derived neurotrophic factor (GDNF), are natural nervous system chemicals with neuroprotective effects. Studies so far, however, have demonstrated questionable benefit.[156] Tamoxifen, an estrogen inhibitor; minocycline, an antibiotic and inhibitor of caspase (a substance that normally helps eliminate motor neurons in the developing brain); and other substances with better or worse theoretical rationales are also under study.[157] Patients with lower motor neuron disease and electrodiagnostic evidence of conduction block can be treated with immunoglobin therapy or glucocorticoids.[85] Age at onset, number of affected limb regions, and creatine kinase level greater than 180 U/L were significantly lower in those who responded to therapy. Elevated anti-GM1 antibodies and definite conduction block were also found significantly more often in responders.[86]

Emotional lability has been treated by administration of lithium carbonate, 300 mg 1–3 times daily, or levodopa. Medications used for decreasing cramps include baclofen, diazepam, and quinine; however, highly sedating medications such as diazepam can cause ventilatory depression and should be avoided. It has been suggested that marijuana has many properties that may be beneficial in managing ALS, including analgesia, muscle relaxation, bronchodilation, saliva reduction, appetite stimulation, and sleep induction.

In addition, it is strongly antioxidative and neuroprotective. Where legal, further investigation is warranted.[158]

In one report, 20 of 41 patients with ALS had subclinical sympathetic hyperactivity with elevated norepinephrine levels unrelated to respiratory status. This finding may result in autonomic spells that lead to the circulatory collapse and sudden death described in patients with advanced disease. Tamsulosin hydrochloride, a selective alpha1 blocker, markedly decreased norepinephrine levels in such patients. It may be useful, therefore, for suppressing the central sympathetic hyperactivity that can occur as a primary pathomechanism.[159]

Expensive unorthodox treatments have been used. Dr. Rajka Medenica, who has given interferon along with sandostatin and growth hormone, reports that some patients have improved but has neither published his work nor done any scientific analysis. The American Association of Ayurvedic Medicine has reported improvement in 7 patients with ALS after use of an "internal purification system," including massage during body immersion in sesame oil, transcendental meditation, and herbs to address "imbalances." The Edgar Cayce Foundation in Virginia recommends a five-part treatment, including (1) changing mental attitudes by reading specific verses of scripture; (2) attaching battery plates to the body; (3) massage for 30 minutes using olive oil, peanut oil and lanolin; (4) drinking a potion of gold chloride and bromide of soda; and (5) an alkaline-forming diet low in carbohydrates without alcohol. Others have tried coffee enemas and bee venom. No positive results have been reported. Vegetarian diets, calves' liver extract, multivitamins, pancreatic extract, amino acids, vaccinations, snake venom, acupuncture, and avoidance of aluminum as much as possible have also been tried.

Spinal Muscular Atrophy

Fewer attempts have been made at medical treatment of SMA compared with DMD and ALS. A recent placebo-controlled trial of gabapentin did not yield positive outcomes.[160] Guanidine hydrochloride was tried earlier,[161] and anabolic steroids and hexahydrocoenzyme Q4 have been of questionable benefit.[162] In a recent blinded and controlled study, 9 patients were reported to have had increases in muscle strength after receiving thyrotrophin-releasing hormone intravenously over the course of 1 month.[163] Improvements in strength appeared to have lasted up to 6 months. This medication is now available for oral delivery, and its effects are under study. Folic acid, vitamin B12, and creatine have been beneficial in animal models of NMD and may be useful for SMA.

Aclarubicin and sodium butyrate (500 mg/kg of body weight) promote the expression of the SMN 2 gene exon 7 in mice lymphoid cells. They decreased the birth rate of severe types of SMA-like mice and ameliorated the course for all mice in the study.[164] Aclarubicin induced incorporation of exon 7 into SMN2 transcripts from the endogenous gene in type 1 SMA fibroblasts as well as into transcripts from a SMN2 minigene in motor neuron cells.[165] It may soon be on the market for treating SMA. About 50 compounds that have the potential to modify the gene expression of SMN 2 are now under study. Interferon has recently been reported to have promise for treating SMA by promoting the transcription of both SMN1 and SMN2 genes.[166] Even when compounds show promise, however, efficacy must first be demonstrated in animals, and both short- and long-term safety concerns must be addressed. A recent pilot study suggested that albuterol therapy may result in increased strength in children with SMA type

2 or 3.[167] In addition, nutritional modifications are promising (Chapter 3). In the future, gene therapy may be useful to correct for the absence of SMN1 and to restore superoxide dismutase type 1 for people with SMA and this defect.

A pulmonologist who considers the airways but who ignores the respiratory muscles is like a cardiologist who considers the blood vessels but who ignores the heart.

Peter Maclem, M.D.

Nutrition

With Contributions from Irving Haber, M.D., and Jill Gaydos, B.S.

It is the character of the true philosopher to hope all things not impossible, and believe all things not unreasonable, so is it the character of the physician to hope and believe that the term vis medicatrix naturae (the healing force of nature) does not represent a nonentity; and that there is in the animal body, when in a state of disease, a tendency to return to its healthy state, and that he has means and appliances to assist this curative process.

> Edward Meryon (1809–1880), the physician who first described, accurately and comprehensively, what came to be known as Duchenne muscular dystrophy[6]

People with neuromuscular diseases (NMDs) have little lean body mass with small protein and mineral reserves and are, therefore, highly susceptible to periods of undernutrition. Malnutrition can exacerbate muscle weakness and decrease lung and immunologic function. Malnutrition and weight loss are independent and significant determinants of morbidity and mortality from respiratory causes.

Nutritional Requirements

Recommended daily allowances (RDAs) are used to estimate nutrient needs.[168,169] They are designed to provide a margin of safety. Even in the general population, however, RDAs may not be adequate. The elderly often have inadequate gastrointestinal absorption of specific nutrients. Younger patients can also develop malabsorption abnormalities, especially with the presence of gastrointestinal or certain other complicating conditions. In addition, many people eating overly processed foods and few vegetables and fruit may simply not receive enough of many nutrients. It has also been estimated that up to 70% of all children do not receive adequate calcium from their daily diets.

Nutrient requirements of the normal infant and child are determined by taking into consideration rate of growth and physical activity as well as basal energy expenditure. The RDAs for children were estimated using intakes of normally growing infants and the nutrient content of human milk (Table 1). Nitrogen balance studies were used to establish amino acid requirements. The needs for children with NMD or generalized medical conditions can be quite different. The best way to measure adequacy of nutrient intake is to monitor growth.

Fluid needs are determined by the amount of water lost through the skin, lungs, urine, and feces and also the amount needed for growth. The renal-concentrating capacity of

Table 1. Normal Calorie and Protein Needs: Requirements per Day per Kilogram of Body Weight		
Age	Calories (kcal)	Protein (gm/kg Body Weight)
0-5 months	108	2.2
6-12 months	98	1.6
1-3 years	102	1.2
4-6 years	90	1.1
7-10 years	70	1.0
11-14 years (males)	55	1.0
15-18 years (males)	45	0.9
11-14 years (females)	47	1.0
15-18 years (females)	40	0.8
Adults	25-35	0.8
Adults over 60		1.0-1.1

the infant is less than that of an older child, making infants at greater risk for water imbalance. Small children require 100 ml of fluid/kg per day, whereas older children and adults require about 1000 ml of fluid plus 50 ml/kg when they weigh more than 10 kg. Calorie and protein needs per unit of body weight are also greater than those of an adult (see Table 1 and www.nal.usda.gov/fnic/dga/rda.pdf) but decline as the rate of growth slows.

Breast milk is usually ideal, but when it is contraindicated, infant formulas provide the appropriate distribution of essential nutrients under normal conditions. As for human milk, it is recommended that infants receive at least 30–50% of total calories from fat. The calories from fat help to spare protein for tissue synthesis. Infant formulas are grouped into standard, soy, protein hydrolysate, and elemental formulas. When non-infant elemental formulas are used for infants, they must be supplemented to ensure that the RDA is achieved for all essential nutrients.

The RDAs and, in particular, requirements for calories and micronutrients differ for adults of different ages and activity levels and in different circumstances. For example, a 25-year-old woman requires 800 micrograms of vitamin A, whereas a man of the same age requires 1000 micrograms. Other RDAs of micronutrients for typical healthy adults include:

- Vitamin D, 5–10 µg
- Vitamin E, 8–10 mg
- Vitamin K, 60–70 µg
- Vitamin C, 60 mg
- Thiamine, 1–1.5 mg
- Riboflavin, 1.2–1.7 mg
- Niacin, 13–19 mg
- Pyridoxine, 2 µg
- Calcium, 800–1200 mg
- Phosphorous, 800–1200 mg
- Magnesium, 280–350 mg
- Iron, 10–15 mg
- Zinc, 12–15 mg
- Iodine, 150 µg
- Selenium, 45–70 µg

Pathophysiologic Effects of Weight Loss or Gain

As little as 10% weight loss from ideal levels can be associated with high morbidity.[170] Short-term starvation depletes muscle protein and decreases lung connective tissue, protein synthesis, and lung surfactant.[171–173] It also diminishes the body's response to illness or injury.[174] This effect is particularly detrimental for patients with respiratory or ventilatory impairment, who have a high risk of lung injury when intercurrent respiratory infections result in pulmonary infiltrates and scarring because of impaired pulmonary defense mechanisms.

Prolonged food or nutritional deprivation impairs muscle function by reducing available energy substrates. With prolonged fasting, branched-chain amino acids, a component of muscle tissues, become an important energy substrate for diaphragm activity. The rate of the degradation of branched-chain amino acids by the diaphragms of semistarved rats is 10–20 times greater than normal (Fig. 1).[175] In certain NMDs associated with impaired fatty acid oxidation, even a few hours of fasting can result in degradation of muscle protein.

Malnutrition impairs immunity and white cell function.[176–179] Bacterial adherence to the lower airways increases in undernourished patients with indwelling tracheostomy tubes.[180] In addition, deficiencies in specific nutrients can have repercussions for respiratory function. Hypophosphatemia, which can be due to malnutrition or rapid glucose loading, can trigger acute respiratory insufficiency or difficulty in weaning from assisted ventilation.[181] Similarly, carbohydrate intake can increase carbon dioxide production and carbon dioxide levels in already hypercapnic patients.

Besides leading to weakening and wasting of skeletal and respiratory muscles, semistarvation also blunts both the hypoxic[182,183] and hypercapnic[184] drive to breathe. Ventilatory failure and hypercapnic coma can result from starvation alone.

Tilton, Miller, and Khoshoo reported that 54% of 7- to 13-year-old patients with NMD are obese.[185] The most obvious explanation for the obesity is that more calories

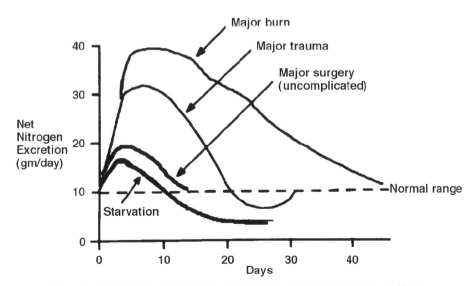

Figure 1. Nitrogen loss associated with undernutrition, major surgery, trauma, and burns.

are taken in than expended; however, this explanation is still debated. As NMD progresses, a loss of lean muscle tissue reduces the resting energy expenditure. Hankard et al. reported reductions of muscle mass by up to 71% in DMD despite obesity.[186] Resting energy expenditure is reduced by 13%, and postabsorptive fat utilization is also reduced in DMD.[186] Furthermore, obesity does not indicate adequate protein stores or adequate vitamin and mineral status. In fact, obesity can mask deficiency states, making the food intake record and biochemical evaluation a vital component of assessment for obese as well as undernourished patients. Obesity can compromise both ventilatory dynamics and central regulation of both spontaneous and assisted ventilation; it also impairs mobility and leads to skin pressure problems.

Thus, a combination of the direct biochemical effects of undernutrition and the indirect effects of under- or overnutrition can predispose patients to respiratory tract infections, atelectasis, chronic alveolar hypoventilation, and impaired pulmonary defense mechanisms and lung repair.

Causes of Malnutrition and Wasting

The underlying mechanisms for muscle wasting include the primary pathologic processes of NMD combined with decreased oral intake, malabsorption, and altered metabolism of nutrients. In addition, many patients are treated with glucocorticoids. Glucocorticoids can further potentiate loss of muscle mass. Rat studies show a significant decrease in diaphragmatic muscle strength even with minimal dosing of methylprednisone over a relatively short period.[187]

Decreased nutrient intake can also be related to eating difficulties resulting from upper limb muscle weakness and contractures,[188,189] cognitive impairments, infections, psychiatric abnormalities (e.g., depression), dysphagia, or loss of appetite, which can be associated with medications, bloating, and shortness of breath. Decreased nutrient intake can also result from vomiting or diarrhea. Indwelling tracheostomy tubes also impair swallowing (Chapter 4).

Although patients with NMD require fewer calories than normal because of sedentary lifestyles and decreased muscle mass, they may require more protein to help prevent muscle catabolism. In addition to having many reasons for malnutrition, patients with NMD, especially children, may have little tolerance for fasting. They have low muscle buffering capacity with little muscle carbohydrate, protein, and mineral stores. Normally, liver glycogen is metabolized to glucose to sustain blood glucose levels for 6–8 hours after a meal. With continued fasting, muscle degrades its protein to amino acids that enter the blood and are converted to glucose by the liver. Within 3 hours of a normal meal, blood glucose and amino acid levels of infants with SMA decrease to levels that would not be reached until after at least 8 hours of fasting in unaffected children.[190] Such patients, therefore, tend to have low blood glucose levels. When blood glucose and amino acid levels are low, muscle protein is catabolized; when they are high, muscle protein is synthesized. Furthermore, infants with SMA type 1 do not efficiently metabolize fatty acids, another major source of energy during fasting. As seen below, such children can have high levels of fatty acid byproducts in their urine and blood after overnight fasting. For the average unaffected child or adult, the amount of muscle protein that is degraded in one day of fasting may be only 1% of total muscle mass, whereas for a child with NMD who may have less than 10% of normal mass, a much greater proportion is sacrificed. Thus, even the small net loss of protein that occurs during normal overnight fasting may be significant for a child with SMA.

Although vitamin supplements can be critical for children on modified elemental amino acid diets, the fat-soluble vitamins A, D, and K should be administered with caution. Excessive levels of these vitamins stored in the liver and adipose tissues can reach toxic levels.[191]

Because of inadequate bone buffering, serum potassium and phosphate levels quickly decrease to hazardous and potentially lethal levels during respiratory tract infections or episodes of fever and diarrhea or vomiting (Chapter 2).[192] Thus, electrolytes and metabolites are particularly important to monitor and replace during intercurrent illnesses.

Bone Integrity

Greater than the RDA intake of vitamins, minerals, and protein may also be necessary.[193] Vitamin D functions in the absorption of calcium and phosphorous. Deficiencies of vitamin D, calcium, and magnesium lead to reduced bone mineral content. Even though intake of vitamin D and calcium may be adequate, decreased intestinal absorption of calcium and vitamin D, along with drug interactions and lack of physical activity and weight-bearing, can decrease bone calcium adsorption and greatly increase the risk of fracture with minor trauma. Decreased exposure to sunlight also impairs the conversion of skin 7-dehydrocholesterol into 1,25-dehydroxycholecalceferal (vitamin D).

The use of exercise, range-of-motion mobilization, and active assistive exercises can help prevent musculoskeletal contractures (Chapter 6) and may also have a beneficial effect on preserving bone integrity. Osteoporosis has been recognized in nonambulatory boys with DMD, even in weak but still ambulatory boys, and is proximally in the femurs and lumbar spine.[194] Upper limbs can also decalcify when losing function, thus increasing the risk of fracture with minor trauma.[195] Medications used for increasing bone density in postmenopausal women may play a role in preventing this problem.[195] Such medications include alendronate sodium (Fosamax, Merck, Inc., West Point, PA), risedronate sodium (Actonel, Procter & Gambel, Inc., Cincinnati, OH), and zoledronic acid (Zometa, GlaxoSmithKline, Inc., Research Triangle Park, NC). These biphosphonates bind to the hydroxyapatite of bone and act as a specific inhibitor of osteoclast-mediated bone resorption. Their use may be particularly important to counter the osteoporosis-inducing effects of glucocorticoid therapy. Bone densitometry can be useful for monitoring bone decalcification and recalcification with treatment.[185]

These medications are now under study and appear to be beneficial for children. Since no evidence indicates that they are metabolized by the body, they are also unlikely to be harmful for children. Products that contain calcium are likely to interfere with the absorption of alendronate. Contraindications include hypocalcemia and inability to stand or sit upright for at least 30 minutes, at least for patients who cannot receive the medications via gastrostomy tubes. This contraindication is due to the fact that biphosphonates may cause esophageal and gastrointestinal mucosal irritation; they should be discontinued if symptoms of heartburn occur. For postmenopausal women, alendronate, 70 mg once weekly or 10 mg daily, is taken with 8 ounces of water 30 minutes before breakfast. A daily dose of 5 mg is used for prophylaxis of osteoporosis. Recommended dosages are the same for risedronate sodium. Zoledronic acid can be used by injection on a less frequent treatment schedule.

Abnormalities in Fatty Acid Oxidation and SMA

There is a curious overlap in the clinical and biochemical features of SMA and mitochondrial myopathies.[62,196] In addition to decreased muscle nutrient stores, metabolic aspects of immobility, systemic illness, and muscle denervation and atrophy, children with SMA also have abnormalities in muscle mitochondrial fatty acid oxidation and carnitine metabolism and impaired insulin regulation, all of which can lend to muscle atrophy and progressive weakening.[190] Any process that increases cytoplasmic free fatty acid levels, such as fasting or defects in fatty acid transport or beta-oxidation, can increase the liver and kidney's production and excretion of possibly toxic dicarboxylic acids. Fasting ketosis reflects normal ketogenesis by the liver's utilization of free fatty acids. However, children with SMA can be catabolic without developing ketosis because of enhanced gluconeogenesis at the expense of muscle mass and a downregulated insulin response.

Dicarboxylic acid levels are elevated in the urine of infants with SMA and in their blood and urine after fasting overnight. The extent of dicarboxylic aciduria is a function of SMA severity. Patients with SMA type 1 tolerate the briefest fasting without ketosis and dicarboxylic aciduria, whereas patients with SMA type 3 express these abnormalities only during prolonged fasting, illness, and periods of physiologic stress. The quantity of fatty acid metabolites generated in SMA type 3 may be considerably lower than in SMA types 1 and 2, reflecting a lower percentage of atrophic muscle fibers. Furthermore, these metabolites may be taken up by liver and metabolized, whereas in the more severe types of SMA the absolute levels of the metabolites are higher or the capacity of the liver is saturated so that the excess is detected in serum and urine.[197] Metabolic analyses, including the appearance of relatively early ketosis, selective renal loss of carnitine,[197] and fatty vacuolization of the liver, suggest that the abnormalities are caused by changes in cellular physiology related to the molecular defects of the SMA-pathogenic survival motor neuron gene or neighboring genes. Abnormal fatty acid metabolism also appears to resolve with age independently of disease severity.[198]

Motor function can improve and developmental milestones be achieved for infants with SMA.[199] However, often before 10 years of age or during periods of physiologic stress, such as intercurrent respiratory tract infections, patients with SMA suddenly lose muscle strength at a high rate.[69] During these episodes loss of strength tends to become progressive and is most severe in infants. Infants with SMA also weaken rapidly when nutrition is compromised by swallowing impairment. It is quite possible that the sudden exacerbations of muscle weakness are due to relative fasting and that the weakening can be abated or averted with proper nutrition.

Evaluation and Monitoring

History and Physical Examination

Appetite and nutrient intake are monitored for deficits. A baseline weight is obtained. Weight should be in the 10th to 25th percentile. Braces, casts, catheter bags and tubing, clothing, wheelchair weight, seat cushions, pillows, blankets, and time since the patient has eaten or been fed must be considered during the weighing process. Weight can also be affected by hydration and edema.

The patient's height is important for understanding the effects of nutrition on growth and for comparison with predicted normal values. When height is difficult to assess because of kyphoscoliosis or other musculoskeletal abnormalities, knee height measurements from under the foot to the top of the femoral condyle have been proposed to estimate height using published formulas of questionable validity.[200,201] Alternate techniques for assessing body size have been suggested, such as arm span and single arm length.[202]

The appearance of the hair, eyes, skin, and teeth is noted. Changes in skin or hair color and texture and tongue or gingival lesions can signal specific nutritional deficiencies. Swallowing ability, taste, and smell are evaluated. Bowel routines are reviewed. Mouth dryness can indicate dehydration or suboptimal vitamin C or zinc levels.[203] Dehydration due to compromised fluid intake can be exacerbated by excessive fluid losses such as from vomiting and drooling. In one study, salivary losses of an 8-year-old girl were 320 ml per day, or 25% of the girl's maintenance fluid requirement.[185] Urine specific gravity is assessed to determine hydration status. A 24- to 72-hour food and fluid intake diary can be helpful.

Caloric requirements vary significantly for normal and NMD children alike. However, calorie and nutrient ingestion is quantitated and almost invariably compared with average quantities for age, sex, and height when matched with the general population. Caloric and nutrient assessments are expressed as a percentage of the RDA over a 3-day period.[204]

A number of indices have been developed to assess nutritional status and quantitate body fat and lean mass[205]:

- Determination of skin-fold thickness
- Midarm circumference
- Bioelectric resistive impedance
- Creatine-height index
- Body mass index (BMI), which is weight divided by height squared
- Total body conductivity
- Biophotonic absortiometry
- Underwater weighing
- Isotopic dilution
- Gamma camera
- X-ray computed tomography
- Echography
- Neutron activation
- Weight for zero muscle mass (ZMM), which is described below
- Estimation of body composition by magnetic resonance imaging

The parameters analyzed, patient acceptance, cost, precision, technical difficulties, and various studies using 12 of these methods have been previously summarized.[206]

Tape and caliper anthropometry is the most commonly available and cost-effective method; the results are accurate to ±3%. Suprailiac and subscapular skin folds are often easier to obtain and can be more reliable than the triceps fold measurement because of the often present contractures of the upper arm. If obtainable, midarm muscle circumference (midarm circumference minus 3.14 × triceps skinfold) can be used as a muscle mass indicator. Standards for anthropometric measurements are available.[201] The 50th percentile for fat stores is considered ideal for children with NMD.[185] Weight, height, and anthropometric measurements are complementary.

Clinical anthropometry is complicated for patients with NMD by the fact that the largest body compartment, the muscle mass, is affected by the primary pathologic processes. Therefore, generally accepted anthropometric equations for determining body fat mass[207,208] are not reliable for patients with NMD.[209,210]

A recent study demonstrated that ZMM more effectively takes into account muscle fat composition and more successfully indicates overweight status (excessive body fat composition) than BMI for patients with DMD and ALS.[211] To calculate ZMM, one must provide a creatine-free diet for 6 days and then measure total urinary creatinine excretion for the next 3 days. This measurement permits the estimation of total lean muscle mass. It can be subtracted from the patient's body weight, and the weight at zero muscle mass is divided by the theoretical body weight for zero muscle mass to determine presence of any excessive body fat. Of a total of 7 patients with ALS and 34 patients with DMD, BMI was normal (20–25 kg/m^2) for all 7 patients with ALS and for 29 patients with DMD, whereas 5 patients with ALS and 30 patients with DMD were classified as overweight by ZMM.

In summary, assessment for pediatric patients with NMD is complicated by altered growth dynamics and metabolism as well as by atrophied muscle mass, diminished nutrient buffer, and limb contractures and weakness. Children require more frequent assessment by physical examination, assessment of caloric and nutrient intake, anthropometric measurements, and biochemical analyses because of deficiency in the muscle mass "buffers." Concomitant abnormalities of fatty acid metabolism and insulin regulation can also complicate the clinical picture for patients with SMA and certain other pediatric conditions.

Laboratory Evaluation

Undernutrition reduces liver protein synthesis. Serum levels of albumin and iron transport protein (transferrin) reflect protein availability to the liver for protein synthesis. Both protein and transferrin have half-lives just under 2 weeks. Therefore, their serum levels reflect long-term but not short-term changes in protein status. Prealbumin and retinol-binding protein are more useful for assessing short-term nutritional interventions because of their shorter half-lives of 2 days and 12 hours, respectively.[212] Measures of the urinary nitrogen level, a measurement of nitrogen metabolism, are usually accomplished by a 24-hour urine collection.[213] Other tests that assess nutritional status include total iron-binding capacity, cholesterol, and serum vitamin levels, especially of vitamins A, C, and E. Vitamin levels are especially important because patients with NMD have a high incidence of vitamin deficiencies. In addition, because of the minimal muscle protein reserves, it may be beneficial to monitor blood amino acid levels. Glucose, potassium, and phosphorus levels need to be monitored closely during acute illnesses.

Nutritional Interventions

The goals of nutritional management of patients with NMD are to limit wasting, lean body mass depletion, and loss of muscle strength; to enhance well-being; and to preserve energy reserves to help resist respiratory complications. Possible additional benefits are also discussed.

Spinal Muscular Atrophy and Other Neonatal Neuromuscular Diseases

Caloric needs for infants with NMD are 80–100 cal/kg; older children with NMD also require less than normal caloric intake. In addition, sufficient fluid intake is required to prevent dehydration, urinary system calculi, and constipation. It is especially important to prevent constipation, which can cause fever, urinary retention, and difficulty in breathing for infants and older children with NMD. Fluid intake is often insufficient because of decreased thirst, difficulty to obtain or swallow fluids, or communication impairment.

Three general dietary goals have been identified: (1) increase in dietary complex carbohydrates, (2) about 2 grams of protein per kg per day, and (3) a feeding schedule that limits overnight fasting to 4 hours for a young infant and 8 hours for older children. A minimum of 5% of calories need to come from essential fatty acids. Infants are awakened for feeding at 4-hour intervals or placed on continuous drip or 4-hour interval boluses via gastrostomy tubes. Some children grow nicely with as little as 50–60 calories/kg and 1.2 gm of protein per day.

In addition to avoiding hypoglycemia and muscle protein catabolism by avoiding prolonged fasting, infants with SMA have also been anecdotally reported to benefit from taking elemental or semielemental formulas such as Tolerex and Pediatric Vivonex (Novartis, Inc., Minneapolis, MN), which provide high quantities of amino acids and small-chained polypeptides.[197] These formulas are easier to digest and may allow better utilization of nutrients and spare muscle protein while avoiding hypoglycemia. A late evening supplement of complex carbohydrates such as uncooked corn starch (1 gm/kg) can sustain blood glucose levels and reduce the effects of overnight fasting.[190] In addition, considering that denervation itself can cause a decrease in muscle carnitine concentrations and the abnormalities in fatty acid metabolism associated with infantile SMA, supplemental riboflavin, coenzyme Q10,[116] and L-carnitine have been suggested along with 200–300 mg/kg of glutamine and 250 mg/kg of arginine.[197] The elemental formulas, glutamine, and arginine provide extra essential amino acids to shift the ketoacid/amino acid equilibrium in favor of muscle protein retention and synthesis. The glutamine may simultaneously remove ketoacids from degradative pathways. Glutamine supplementation is well established for patients with inborn errors of amino acid and organic acid metabolism, for burn patients, and for postsurgical care.

Both Tolerex and Pediatric Vivonex have essential fatty acids, but the former has only 1 gm of fat per 300 calorie packet as opposed to 5 gm per 200 calorie packet for the latter. Tolerex also has twice as many complex carbohydrates per pack as Pediatric Vivonex. For children, both Tolerex and Pediatric Vivonex are low in calcium, iron, iodine, potassium, vitamin C, B complex, fat-soluble vitamins, and folic acid. Supplements are necessary.

Recent evidence gleaned from animal models indicates that such children may also benefit from receiving more than the RDA of folic acid and vitamin B12. Folic acid should be provided daily, 65 micrograms for children from 0 to 6 months of age, 80 micrograms from 7 to 12 months of age, 150 micrograms from 1 to 3 years of age, 200 micrograms from 4 to 8 years of age, 300 micrograms from 9 to 13 years of age, and 400 micrograms for older people. At the same ages vitamin B12 is provided at 0.5, 1.5, 2, and 2.5 micrograms, respectively; 3 micrograms should be provided from 9 to 13 years of age and subsequently.

In addition to corn starch and mineral and vitamin supplements, the low fatty content of these elemental formulas is often compensated by adding several grams of primrose or safflower oil with water or white grape juice. It is necessary to make these formulas palatable for patients without gastrostomy tubes. Jars of baby fruit and vegetables can round out the diet, along with sufficient fluids for good hydration to prevent thickening of airway secretions.

Diets high in carbohydrate, amino acids, and polypeptides and low in fat provide muscle with utilizable energy substrates, thereby decreasing dependence on fatty acid oxidation and decreasing dicarboxylic acids.[197] This diet maintains more normal blood glucose levels during fasting, delays fasting-associated ketoacidosis, and has been noted to normalize liver function enzyme levels. Provision of amino acids and short-chained peptides instead of complex dairy proteins facilitates glucogenesis. Most tube-fed children using this dietary strategy do not receive any whole protein foods such as eggs, meats, soy, or grains because these products are often said to exacerbate thickness and possibly quantity of airway secretions as well as to increase sweating and constipation. Harpey et al. believed that there was a significant improvement in strength and function for 13 patients treated in this manner, and in a survey that we took of the parents of 53 children with SMA type 1, virtually all concurred with this assessment.[214]

Caution has been recommended in making empirical changes to a diet that may lead to unintended consequences.[198] Because of limited muscle stores and rapid changes in blood levels, there is a narrow window of optimal blood protein levels. Excessive levels leading to high blood nitrogen content may be hazardous. Furthermore, the use of protein-hydrolysate formulas containing modified cornstarch results in high levels of oxtenylsuccinic aciduria,[215] the pharmacokinetics, drug interactions, and long-term effects of which are unknown. It may be that the avoidance of fasting rather than nutrient manipulation itself plays the largest role in preventing ongoing muscle weakening. Although caution is always in order, it should be considered that up to 80% of conventionally managed infants with SMA type 1 are dead by 12 months of age, and virtually all without tracheostomy tubes have died by age 2 years.[63] Yet, of 53 infants with SMA type 1 who received these dietary modifications and for whom death and tracheostomy are avoided with the use of respiratory muscle aids (Chapter 12), 24 are already over age 3 and 10 over age 6; only three have died. No children are known to have died or suffered from receiving these formulas. Parents report increasing motor function or stabilization of previously deteriorating motor function and benefits for secretion management, flushing, diaphoresis, bowel motility, and weight. Clearly, these children either have fewer life-threatening respiratory tract infections or handle them better. Thus, it is hard to imagine what can be lost by at least briefly attempting an elemental diet. Table 2 outlines a typical "modified" diet given to children with SMA via gastrostomy tube drip. Children with SMA type 2 without tubes drink the formula in fruit juices, slowly throughout the day; however, cooperation can be a problem.

Based on recent studies (Chapter 2), it may be prudent to provide supplemental creatine monohydrate at 0.1 gm/kg daily, divided into 2 doses. Creatine, a 2-amino acid peptide, is similar in nature to the elemental amino acid preparations that seem to be beneficial for children with SMA. Sodium butyrate also appears to be beneficial (Chapter 2).

Because patients with SMA are often hypoglycemic and blood glucose levels can fall 3.4 to 2.7 mmol/L during a 12-hour fast,[216] it may be tempting to treat them with glucose administration. However, hyperglycemia can be severe because of inadequate insulin release. This finding indicates need for insulin therapy (0.05 units/kg/hr) to increase glucose utilization, block protein catabolism, and enhance protein synthesis.

Table 2. **Typical Modified Diet**	
Pediatric Vivonex, 2 packs	L-glutamine, 300 mg/kg
Sodium butyrate acid, 9 gm	Acetyl L-carnitine, 500 mg
Water, 1400 ml warm water divided into	Creatine, 1 gm
700 ml each	Calcium, magnesium, iron, zinc, manganese
Vitamin C, 1 gm	Choline and inositol, 500 mg each
Vitamin E, 400 units	Flax/borage oil combination, 7 ml
Vitamin B complex	Amino Fuel, 25 ml, or Amino 75 with 75 mg
Methyl B12, 500 µg	of each essential amino acid
Folic acid, 400 µg	Mannatech* Phytaloe, 2 capsules
Coenzyme Q, 100 mg	Mannatech Sport, 2 capsules
Mineral supplements, Miracle 2000, 20 ml	Mannatech Ambrotose, $\frac{1}{4}$ teaspoon
Lactobacillus, 25 ml	Fruit juices, 100%, to make 2 liters

* Mannatech (www.mannatech.com) is a dehydrated, plant-based supplement similar to Shaklee and Amway products.

For a 5 year old girl with SMA type 2, 44 inches, 39 lbs, for 24 hours via continuous drip via gastrostomy. Sodium butyrate is available only by prescription and only from specific pharmacists (http://www.iacprx.org/). Some children take fatty acid supplements from primrose (about 1000 mg) and safflower oil (1/2 tsp) before bedtime.

Cyclic vomiting may respond quickly to glucose plus insulin administration, whereas it may not respond to intravenous glucose alone. Rather than assume a respiratory etiology, hypoglycemia must be suspected and treated when patients with severe muscle wasting due to chronic neuromuscular disorders are admitted in a comatose state.[216]

Because the avoidance of fasting is crucial to maintain muscle strength, fasting and undernutrition must be avoided when children with SMA are acutely ill. Virtually all children with SMA type 1 and many with SMA type 2 require gastrostomy tubes before 2 years of age. It may be an important strategy to provide them prophylactically before acute illness or dysphagia-associated weight loss causes muscle deterioration. It should be remembered that nasogastric tubes can interfere with the use of nasal ventilation (Chapter 12). Patients who require surgery and have periods without oral nutrition should receive nutrition parenterally.

Many tube-fed infants with SMA type 1 receive enough packets of elemental formula for 80–90 cal/kg over 24 hours, initially at 60–90 ml per hour. Eventually small boluses are provided during the day along with a slow drip overnight. Two- to 3-year old children receive 60–70 cal/kg/day and larger boluses. Supplements are prepared in a blender every morning and individualized for each child, taking into account patient tolerance along with effects on strength and function, secretions, and respiratory status.

Duchenne Muscular Dystrophy

Although some studies suggest that DMD is a hypercatabolic disease and that patients with DMD have a higher than normal basal metabolic rate, higher maintenance protein requirements, and a higher daily excretion of urinary 3-methylhistidine per unit muscle mass,[217] other studies report that basal metabolic rate is either similar to or slightly lower than controls.[218] Functional defects of skeletal muscle mitochondria have been cited as a possible cause of hypercatabolism.[219] However, 24-hour energy expenditure is about 25% lower than controls because of the reduction in physical activity. Therefore, it is important to take this fact into account when supplementing diets and calculating caloric needs. Of interest, consistent with suggestions for nutritional intervention for SMA, branched-chain amino acid treatments have been reported to result in prolonged righting ability and increased pectoral muscle mass and protein content with a reduction in degenerating fibers for avian muscular dystrophy. Such benefits, however, have not been duplicated in humans.[220]

The caloric needs of relatively inactive patients with NMDs have been estimated from an equation developed to guide the recommended caloric intake of children with DMD:

$$\text{Daily energy intake in kcal} = 2000 - \text{age (years)} \times 50$$

An ideal weight percentile chart for boys with DMD has been reported (Fig. 2). For advanced patients who require ventilatory support, caloric needs may not exceed normal resting energy expenditure, which is estimated to be 110% of basal metabolic rate. This finding is due to the fact that the oxygen cost of breathing and the energy substrates needed for respiratory function are greatly reduced in people for whom ventilators substitute for inspiratory muscle function.

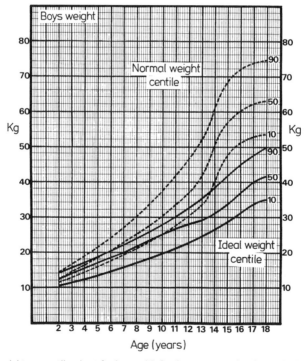

Figure 2. Ideal weight percentile chart for boys with Duchenne muscular dystrophy based on data from Edwards et al.,[221] Edmonds et al.,[226] and Tanner et al.[209] It assumes a 4% per year decline in muscle bulk. (From Griffiths RD, Edwards RHT: A new chart for weight control in Duchenne muscular dystrophy. Arch Dis Child 63:1256–1258, with permission.)

Caloric needs must be modified for obese or undernourished patients as well as during respiratory tract infections and after surgical interventions. In obese patients, many physicians hesitate to recommend an overly restrictive diet for fear of aggravating muscle atrophy by relative fasting. However, surveillance of the body composition of two patients with severe caloric restrictions demonstrated no deleterious effects on either body composition or muscular function.[221] Accordingly, it seems reasonable to advise a 20% reduction in caloric intake and a monthly weight reduction of 2 kg for obese patients with DMD and perhaps for other obese patients with NMD. Moderate rather than severe dietary restriction is more likely to favor lean muscle sparing over fat sparing.

Cookbooks are available that contain recipes for appetizing and attractive texture-adapted meals that facilitate swallowing and minimize aspiration.[222,223] Patients ultimately can subsist on a pureed food diet or commercially prepared thick liquids that provide complete balanced nutrition. Currently, anecdotal reports suggest that, as for children with SMA, dietary supplementation with bioarginine and glutamine (about 2 gm/day) and creatine (100 mg/kg) can result in clinical improvements. Investigative studies are under way.

Psychosocial Issues

Most children and adolescents with NMD attend school. Adolescents want to eat the same foods and in the same manner as their peers. Failure to do so and weight extremes can decrease self-esteem and cause depression. Depression can also decrease appetite or lead to overeating. Adolescents and children may also use eating as a control tactic. Unfortunately, schools are often not equipped or staffed to deal with the special needs of feeding children with NMD, and this factor can contribute to malnutrition. Time constraints and schedules can also adversely affect feeding and eating in the school setting. Such issues need to be explored with a child psychologist.

Amyotrophic Lateral Sclerosis/Motor Neuron Disease

As in pediatric NMD, patients with ALS/MND lose lean body mass from the primary disease process as well as from decreased oral intake secondary to loss of appetite and dysphagia signaled by jaw weakness and fatigue, drooling, choking on fluid and food, and slow eating. Even before laboratory evidence of malnutrition occurs, it may be most prudent to recommend gastrostomy as an alternative or supplemental route for oral nutrition. A gastrostomy is indicated when patients with ALS have severe dysphagia with accelerated weight loss due to insufficient caloric intake, dehydration, and choking despite a pureed or thick liquid diet.[224] All patients whose bulbar dysfunction necessitates tracheotomy also require gastrostomies. When reflux is a problem, the tubes are passed into the jejunum. The immediate benefits of gastrostomy are adequate nutritional intake, weight stabilization, and an alternate route for medication. People with gastrostomies can often continue to swallow some liquids and solids. The only study of energy metabolism and caloric intake for a group of patients with ALS using tracheostomy IPPV and gastrostomy tubes for nutrition highlighted the problems of adjusting caloric intake because three-quarters of the patients had excessive weight gain.[225]

Es menester que andemos por el mundo, como en aprobación, buscando aventuras.

•◉• Don Quijote de La Mancha

Chapter 4

Swallowing and Gastrointestinal Concerns

With contributions by Ken Swan, M.D., Marta Kazanjian, M.A., S.L.P., and Ann Gulyas, M.A., S.L.P.

The SpO$_2$
on my pulse-ox meter
Tells me I've inhaled
what was fed by my feeder

               Richard L. Clingman, Sr.,
               Webmaster of DoctorBach.com

Neuromuscular disorders can affect swallowing, speech, and gastrointestinal motility. Gastroesophageal reflux and aspiration may be increased, both of which can affect respiratory function.

Swallowing and Breathing

The great majority of ventilator users with neuromuscular disease (NMD) have some degree of dysphagia. Dysphagia can hamper nutrition and result in aspiration and respiratory impairment. The symptoms of dysphagia include drooling, difficulty with initiating swallowing, nasal regurgitation, difficulty with managing secretions, choking and coughing, and the sensation of food sticking in the throat. Despite its high occurrence in NMD, diagnosis of dysphagia is often delayed and considered to be of secondary importance.

The tongue, epiglottis, pharynx, larynx, and intrinsic and extrinsic laryngeal musculature are innervated by bulbar nerves and participate in both breathing and swallowing. Until 1 year of age deglutition is characterized by suction, propulsion, deposition in the posterior pharynx, and initiation of the swallowing, pharyngeal, and esophageal reflexes that complete the swallowing process. Even when the swallowing process is severely dysfunctional, aspiration of food and saliva does not occur because the neonatal larynx is higher than the base of the tongue and the central position of the epiglottis deviates liquids laterally into a large funnel-shaped continuation of the pharynx over the esophageal sphincter.[227] Thus, at birth there is no pharyngeal intersection of food and air, and newborns can breathe and swallow simultaneously. During the first months of life the larynx descends. At about 8 months of age the airways cross the digestive track, and aspiration becomes possible. By this time, the funnel-shaped area below the larynx and over the esophageal sphincter has been reduced to the size of a thimble. Between the base of the tongue and the epiglottis a ridge forms that channels flow toward the valleculae to help protect the airway. In the small child, tracheal aspiration tends to occur only when the pharyngeal reflex is not promptly triggered after the oral phase or when the security reservoirs are full or abnormally shortened.

After 1 year of age, deglutition occurs 600 times per day. Mouth opening must be sufficient for entry of nutrients. The tongue functions in the preparation, control, and transport of the bolus to a point at which the pharyngeal swallow, an involuntary reflex, is triggered. As the tail of the bolus moves toward the base of the tongue, the base of the tongue and the pharyngeal walls make contact with each other and apply pressure to the bolus to drive it through the pharynx and into the esophagus. The epiglottis moves downward to meet the arytenoids as the larynx elevates and moves anteriorly to move the larynx out of the path of the descending bolus and to contribute to the closure of the airway.[228] The false and true vocal folds close to provide another level of airway protection. When airflow stops, subglottic airway pressures increase sharply. The rise in airway pressure is important for normal glottic closure and movement of the bolus through the pharynx.

The upper esophageal sphincter is pulled open by the combined mechanical traction of the tongue and larynx, allowing the bolus to move through it and into the esophagus. Esophageal peristalsis then moves the bolus past the lower esophageal sphincter into the stomach. The esophagus is 23–25 cm long. It has striated muscle in the upper third, which often is most involved in myopathic conditions. Esophageal action is also involuntary.

The precisely timed movements of a normal swallow ensure airway protection. The passage way through which the bolus travels, the pharynx, is shared with air for respiration. Shaker et al. reported that in most normal subjects, the swallow interrupts expiration rather than inspiration.[229] The pharyngeal swallow triggers, and the bolus moves through the pharynx; when the larynx opens again, expiration continues. The post-swallow expiration is a pulmonary defense mechanism to reduce the risk of aspiration. However, patients with concomitant chronic obstructive pulmonary disease (COPD) swallow more during inspiration than normal age-matched controls.[229,230] A higher incidence of post-swallow inspiration is associated with large volume, liquid swallows, and rapid breathing.[231] Thus, patients with compromised respiratory systems have altered coordination of breathing and swallowing that may predispose them to aspiration and further respiratory compromise. Such patients also often have difficulty in the generation and timing of an effective cough.

Dysphagia in Pediatric Neuromuscular Disease

Infants with NMD such as spinal muscular atrophy (SMA) type 1 experience swallowing difficulties that involve both the oral and pharyngeal phases of swallowing. The breakdown includes weak sucking, weak or slow movements of the tongue, and pooling of the food in the pharynx with no movement of the epiglottis.[232] The utilization of artificial alimentation methods may be necessary during infancy, and all patients with SMA type 1 require gastrostomy tubes before 2 years of age. Swallowing difficulties are much milder in SMA types 1+ and 2 and other SMAs, with fewer such patients requiring gastrostomy tubes. In a sampling of 15 such patients compared with age-matched controls, maximal bite forces, opening, and protrusion were one-half normal values. Fatigue times of patients were reduced by 30% (from 17.9 seconds to 11.1 seconds).[233]

Children with Duchenne muscular dystrophy (DMD), SMA, and other pediatric NMDs have difficulty in the oral stages of swallowing due to both muscle weakness and abnormal facial bony structures. The structural impairments often include shortening of the mandible[234] and impairment of the temporomandibular joint. These impairments can result in insufficient mouth opening for food entry, a not uncommon problem in DMD and SMA type 2. Spinal instrumentation and fusion to reverse spinal deformity, common in this patient population, can also hamper swallowing by altering the position and decreasing the flexibility of the neck.

Because of the high prevalence of dysphagia and malnutrition in DMD, this disorder is a good model for understanding other pediatric NMDs. By 12 years of age all patients with DMD have dysphagia.[235] Masticatory and deglutition impairment stages are summarized in Tables 1 and 2. Besides abnormalities of temporomandibular joint motion, dental malocclusion is common. Moderate swallowing dysfunction appears between ages 9 and 18 years because of muscle deficits, especially of the lip and cheek muscles and tongue elevators. The muscles of the soft palate and chewing are relatively preserved. Chewing muscle strength is highly functional, with a mean force of 5.4 kg at age 18. This force is well maintained subsequently. By age 15 years, however, head instability due to neck flexor weakness tends to cause the patient to eat with a hyperextended neck, a position that can predispose to aspiration. Protrusion of the mandible seems to be associated with an enlarged tongue and weakness. Jaw opening is often reduced to 3 cm or less.

Advanced weakness and structural impairment occur after age 18.[236] Dysphagia symptoms, weight loss, and aspiration become common at this point. The incidence of respiratory complications and weight loss correlate with deglutition impairment stage[206] and inversely with maximum assisted cough peak flows (the best measure of bulbar function). Untreated tachypnea in patients with DMD decreases oral phase time and breathing-related fatigue. This effect further hampers swallowing efforts. Many patients eventually reach the point of subsisting on thick hypercaloric fluids and requiring long periods to complete each liquid meal because of increased oral phase times. If adequate nutrition cannot be maintained in this manner, a gastrostomy is warranted. Ten to 15% of patients with DMD eventually require gastrostomies. To avoid the complications of general anesthesia, the tubes can be placed under local anesthesia (see below).

Table 1.	**Functional Classification of Deglutition Impairment**
Stage 0:	no difficulty
Stage 1:	little difficulty (hard or large pieces of solids must be excluded)
Stage 2:	moderate difficulty (thin liquids and hard solids must be excluded; aspiration rare)
Stage 3:	considerable difficulty (alimentation limited to blended and pureed foods and moist bread; occasional aspiration)
Stage 4:	great difficulty (alimentation limited to thick liquids; aspiration usually frequent)

Table 2.	Functional Classification of Masticatory Impairment

Stage 0: no difficulty (intact ability to bite, crunch, and tear)
Stage 1: little difficulty (moderate difficulty in biting; relatively intact crunching, munching, and tearing)
Stage 2: moderate difficulty (loss of functional biting and crunching; ability to tear bread)
Stage 3: severe difficulty (inability to bite, crunch, and tear; ability to malaxate and mix in the mouth)

Dysphagia in Adult Neuromuscular Disease

Alimentation problems occur in 41% of patients with myotonic dystropy.[237] Chewing difficulties can be caused by myotonia of chewing muscles, weakness, and jaw deformity. Aspiration is common and often underestimated by patients and their care providers. Mechanical abnormalities include long bolus transit times, significantly delayed onset of some swallow gestures, and prolonged upper esophageal sphincter opening.[238] Pharyngeal pooling and irregular clearing of the pharyngeal recesses also occur.[239] Silent aspiration can cause respiratory infections and death.[240]

Dysphagia is the first sign of myasthenia gravis in 6–15% of adult patients.[241] The infant-onset forms are characterized by problems in sucking, swallowing motility, and weak or absent crying. Symptoms vary greatly from one patient to another and often from one hour to the next. Dysphagia is frequently encountered with the first signs of acute respiratory distress and is often a harbinger for myasthenic crises.[241]

Abnormalities were found in swallowing for 31 of 32 post-poliomyelitis patients reporting recent decreases in limb strength.[242] Examples include tongue-pumping to initiate swallow; delayed initiation of the swallowing response; uncontrolled bolus flow into the pharynx; diminished laryngeal elevation and epiglottic tilt; delayed, diminished, or absent pharyngeal contraction; unilateral transport of boluses through the pharynx; vallecula and pyriform sinus residuals; "silent" laryngeal penetration; and laxity of pharyngeal walls.[242–244]

Virtually all patients with amyotrophic lateral sclerosis (ALS) and MND develop swallowing dysfunction. About 73% of patients with ALS experience swallowing difficulties before using ventilatory assistance.[245] Despite differences in presentation, a general scheme of progression has been suggested, beginning with dysfunction of the lips and tongue, followed by dysfunction of the palate, chewing weakness, and weakness of the constrictors of the pharynx and the cheek muscles.[246] Initial complaints may be postnasal congestion or choking on saliva while reclining. Such problems can progress to difficulties with liquid intake and eventually with solids.

Clinical Presentation of Dysphagia

Initial difficulties are usually limited to chewing and temporomandibular joint motion and, for pediatric patients, dental malocclusion and a forward jaw thrust. Even in the presence of severe chewing impairment, however, the risk of aspiration of food or saliva into the lungs is very low when swallowing motility is intact (see Table 1). Weakness of lip and cheek muscles and tongue elevators can become more pronounced subsequently. The often-present excessive cervical lordosis stretches the muscles that close the jaw and retract the mandible, retract the upper lip, and reduce neck flexion and rotation. Likewise, lumbar hyperlordosis, sitting imbalance, and scoliosis cause or exacerbate dysphagia.

Initially, patients experience difficulty with managing liquids secondary to a delay in triggering of the pharyngeal swallow reflex. Eventually, laryngeal penetration and/or aspiration of liquids occurs. Compensatory head positions are often used to protect the airway; however, reduction in flexion and rotation of the cervical spine eventually hampers this strategy.

Appetite reduction by medications, diminished appreciation of taste, impaired emptying of the stomach and intestines, salivary insufficiency, aspiration of food and saliva, weight loss, and pulmonary complications may occur. Loss of sense of smell may be linked to repeated nasal infections or, rarely, may be part of the clinical picture of certain conditions. Because air does not pass through the upper airway, ventilator use via an indwelling tracheostomy tube prevents patients from smelling and, therefore, appreciating the taste of food. The chronic pathogenic bacterial colonization associated with indwelling tubes and impairment of physiologic mechanisms for airway secretion clearance alter taste. Additionally, the presence of a tracheostomy tube interferes with swallowing (see Tracheostomy Tube Considerations below). This, too, can affect the desire to eat.

Although not part of the swallowing mechanism, intestinal hypomotility can contribute to poor appetite and reduced nutritional intake by causing nausea, retching, bloating, and vomiting (see below).

Clinical and Instrumental Assessment

Because chewing and swallowing difficulties often are underestimated by the patient, family members are also interviewed about such problems. Factors that trigger eating difficulties, such as food textures and bolus sizes, are determined. In patients with abdominal distention, satiety can occur after little food intake because the food displaces the raised diaphragm and causes a sensation of fullness. Inability to finish meals because of difficulties with breathing, endurance, or airway secretions is explored. Any history of respiratory complications and pneumonia not resulting from colds may be due to aspiration of food or saliva as a result of dysphagia. Pneumonias affecting the right lung suggest aspiration because aspirated material is more likely to enter the right airways.

Any previous intubation may explain the presence of dysphagia. Swallowing motility impairments associated with surgical procedures and intubation can result from decreased base of tongue strength and elevation.[247] Impairments may result from the continuous pressure of the endotracheal tube resting on the base of the tongue, which reduces the tongue's function as a driving force for the bolus. Vocal changes after surgery should alert one to potential airway protection problems. As a result of aspiration, some patients expel food from or around the tracheostomy tubes while eating. A tracheostomized patient's increased frequency of suctioning and a more inspissated character of secretions can signal repeated aspiration or infection.

Good oral hygiene is important for minimizing bacteria in the oral cavity that eventually may be aspirated. The mouth, therefore, is examined for caries, gingivitis, ulcers, or other lesions. In addition, tongue movement can be assessed for ability to manipulate a food bolus. Repeated neck flexion and extension may be observed as the patient attempts to compensate for difficulty in manipulating the bolus. Oral retention may be observed. The patient's ability to chew and to break a solid bolus into pieces is also observed. Nasal regurgitation can indicate an incomplete velopharyngeal seal. The chewing muscles, soft palate, lips, tongue, and cheek muscles are evaluated for strength, function, and ability to create intraoral pressure. Tongue weakness is also significantly related to articulatory imprecision and can be quantitated.[248]

Saliva and secretion management provides information about general oral motor status, swallowing, and expectoration ability. Drooling is a result of inadequate lip and tongue control. The presence of a tracheostomy tube increases the secretions produced in the airway and impairs swallowing and expectoration. In addition, an inflated tube cuff eliminates the airflow needed to clear secretions effectively from the pharynx and larynx.

Further evaluation includes assessment for contractures, jaw structure, lateral jaw movement and opening, and strength of lip occlusion. Neck stability and mobility, especially flexion and extension, posture, positioning, and sitting balance and stability, need to be evaluated and optimized.

The senses of smell and taste are evaluated. Gag and cough are assessed along with coordination of breathing patterns during swallowing. Accessory muscle use indicates increased absolute or relative work of breathing, and the resulting fatigue can hamper swallowing efforts.

Although only the oral phase of swallowing can be assessed clinically, some observations can be made about the pharyngeal component. Coughing or a wet vocal quality during the presentation of oral materials may indicate aspiration. A patient's subjective complaint of food sticking in the throat and the habit of taking frequent sips of fluid after a swallow of solid food suggest pharyngeal retention. During a clinical assessment, the larynx is felt for timing and elevation. The pharyngeal stage of swallowing is most accurately assessed by a modified barium swallow.

The presence of airway congestion can be highly suggestive of aspiration. Other suggestive signs include throat clearing, choking, nasal speech, and sudden episodes of spitting, dyspnea, and oxyhemoglobin desaturation ($dSpO_2$).[249] When aspiration is not recognized by the patient's physicians in a timely manner (before a sustained decrease in baseline SpO_2 less than 95%), it will cause respiratory distress due to extensive airway encumberment, pneumonia, and acute respiratory failure. It is usually not recognized early because the patient optimizes food preparation, takes great care during the oral phase of swallowing, and may still have a sufficiently effective cough to avoid a sustained decrease in baseline SpO_2.

Cervical auscultation can be performed to listen to the sounds of the swallow. This procedure assesses the ability to achieve and maintain airway closure[250] during the passage of the bolus through the pharynx.[251] Lack of coordination between breathing and swallowing can also be identified. Laryngeal palpation determines the onset of the swallow. The extent and duration of airway closure can be identified by the cessation of breathing. Additionally, pharyngeal secretion management can be evaluated prior to trial swallow attempts. Cued by vocal changes or audible airflow through a secretion-filled pharynx, cervical auscultation may first be used to assess saliva swallows, secretion management, and candidacy to advance to trial bolus swallows. If secretions that cannot be cleared by the patient, in-exsufflation or suctioning are heard in the airway, trial swallows are deferred. Cervical auscultation has particular relevance for the user of tracheostomy intermittent positive-pressure ventilation (IPPV) because it assists in identifying upper airway flow during tracheostomy IPPV, especially when the tube is cuffed and flows are insufficient for audible speech.

Trial Swallows

Initial trial swallows can consist of ice chips that provide lubrication and permit assessment of the swallow response. Then food is presented, and any subsequent coughing, wet vocal quality, increased mucus production, or $dSpO_2$ can indicate aspiration. Although coughing can be an indication of aspiration, it is also a protective mechanism to clear aspirate from the airway. A less sensitive larynx may not respond to penetrated or aspirated material.

For the tracheostomized patient, the cuff, if present, must be deflated and the tube occluded to determine vocal fold status and ability to generate airflow past the tube for vocalizing, coughing, clearing the throat, and expectorating. Assessment with an inflated cuff is limited to oral phase management and the ability to trigger a pharyngeal swallow.

Aspiration without an accompanying cough is called "silent aspiration." Aspiration can result from pooling of foods in the valleculae, the space between the base of tongue and the epiglottis, and pyriform sinuses when the initiation of pharyngeal swallow is delayed. It can occur with all food consistencies and may be accompanied by a reflex laryngeal cough. The tendency to aspirate can increase during a meal when the pooled material builds up as the patient fatigues.

Blue Dye Test

When a tracheostomy tube is present, a methylene blue or vegetable dye test can be performed to assess for aspiration and expulsion of material through the tracheostomy. Because aspirated food material is difficult to differentiate from secretions, food is dyed blue. Several drops of the colored substance are placed into a glass of water. After the patient drinks the water, mechanical insufflation-exsufflation (MI-E) or suctioning is immediately performed through the tracheostomy tube with the cuff inflated and then at 15-minute intervals for 1 hour. If no colored material (suctionate) is extruded, it is appropriate to proceed with trial swallows of foods and liquid mixed with blue dye. If, with suctioning or MI-E, the suctionate is correspondingly colored (positive blue dye test), further assessment of aspiration is undertaken with a videofluoroscopic modified barium swallow study.

If an inflated tracheostomy tube cuff is used for IPPV, the blue dye test is first performed with the cuff inflated. Then, if the test is negative, the cuff is deflated as the patient is simultaneously suctioned or insufflated-exsufflated. Colored fluid is then again swallowed, the cuff is re-inflated, and MI-E is repeated to observe the suctionate. Care must be taken to increase the ventilator-delivered volumes to compensate for excessive insufflation leakage out of the mouth and nose when a tracheostomy tube cuff is deflated. Shortness of breath must be avoided, or swallowing cannot be accurately assessed. It should be understood that any patient who has a patent upper airway and can swallow without aspiration to an extent that decreases baseline SpO_2 does not need a tracheostomy tube for ventilatory support and should be formally evaluated for decannulation.

During the administration of trial bolus swallows with dye, only one food consistency is used at a time, and the patient is suctioned or insufflated-exsufflated several times at intervals. When the thickness of the bolus is increased, the potential for pharyngeal retention can be increased. The presence of blue dye in the suctionate hours after ingestion may signal such retention and eventual aspiration, although the etiology of the aspiration remains unclear and its extent is not very significant unless the baseline SpO_2 is less than 95%. A standard test format is used to assess the types of food that are swallowed or aspirated.[252]

Cuff deflation is important during the blue dye test. If the test is performed with the tracheostomy tube cuff inflated and the patient aspirates, most of the aspirated material will collect in the trachea above the cuff. This area must be suctioned, and the cuff must then be deflated and the airway suctioned to clear this material before reinstituting the test. The presence of the cuff itself, even when deflated, hampers swallowing. As for patients without tubes, whether the cuff is inflated or not, coughing, throat clearing, and vocal changes are possible signs of aspiration.

Because aspirated food is difficult to differentiate from secretions, the results of a blue dye test are not definitive. However, a recent study comparing the use of the methylene blue test in water and custard with a barium swallow in water and paste confirmed good correlation between the two methods for 15 of 20 patients. The liquid methylene blue test and the liquid barium swallow produced equivalent results in 18 of the patients. The results using the custard methylene blue test, however, were not as reliable. Four patients had positive results for the paste barium but were negative for the custard with methylene blue.[253]

Patients who are only tube-fed but who are suspected of aspiration due to reflux may also benefit from a version of the blue dye test. The blue dye can be added to enteral feedings. MI-E is then used through the tracheostomy tube immediately upon cuff deflation to observe the suctionate. Airway suctioning is used only if a Cough-Assist (J. H. Emerson Company, Cambridge, MA) is not available.[254]

A helpful addition to the blue dye test is placing glucose oxidase strips into secretions obtained from the tracheostomy tube or from around the stoma. The glucose level can signal the presence of aspirated food or formula. Standard directions provide the user with guidelines for interpretation. Glucose oxidase strips have been reported to be more sensitive than blue dye visualization in detecting food or formula in pulmonary secretions.[255]

Fiberoptic Endoscopic Evaluation

A fiberoptic endoscopic evaluation of swallowing provides objective information about swallowing and airway protection capabilities. Airway patency, glottic competence, vocal cord mobility, the presence of any infectious or traumatic lesions, and any pooling of food or secretions are observed. Pooling of secretions in the pharyngeal area or entry of secretions into the larynx can be noted before food is administered. Pooling and aspiration of food boluses that are not immediately detected with a blue dye procedure can be documented.

Direct visualization of the pharynx and larynx is done during swallowing.[256] The ability to close the airway at the appropriate time during the swallow, to maintain airway closure, and to manage secretions is documented.[257] Fluid or food with dye is usually taken while the scope is in position; if aspiration is present, the dyed material is detected in the airway before or after the swallow takes place. Fiberoptic endoscopic evaluation not only provides a method of assessing management of various bolus consistencies but also allows visualization of the impact of respiratory patterns on swallowing, including tachypnea and structural and positional impairments. By using a specialized scope that releases a burst of air, the sensitivity of the laryngeal closure mechanism can also be tested.[258] Sensitivity is vital for normal laryngopharyngeal protective reflexes.[259]

Videofluorography

The most frequently used diagnostic evaluation tool for assessing swallowing is videofluorography,[228] also known as a modified barium swallow study. It permits the identification of swallowing motility throughout the oral cavity, velopharynx, and pharynx. It can be used to quantitate pharyngeal transit times.[260] It identifies the presence of anatomic and physiologic abnormalities and detects aspiration, along with the anatomic and physiologic causes. Although esophageal motility can be viewed during this study, it is best studied with a standard barium swallow.

The modified barium swallow is typically carried out with a variety of barium consistencies and bolus sizes. Oral preparation, bolus propulsion, initiation of the swallowing reflex, the presence and timing of aspiration, and pharyngeal passage of the bolus can be documented. Therapeutic maneuvers and postural changes are evaluated to optimize the patient's ability to swallow safely and to minimize the potential for aspiration. For example, if aspiration occurs before the initiation of the swallow reflex because of weakness of the base of the tongue or poor bolus control, the patient may be instructed to flex the neck in an effort to protect the airway. This maneuver widens the valleculae so that more material can collect there until the pharyngeal swallow is triggered and the bolus is cleared.

Other Tests

A decrease in baseline SpO_2 levels observed by oximetry during trial swallows or especially during meals alerts the clinician to fatigue, increased work of breathing, or, most often, severe aspiration.[258,261-263] Finger Bobs (Braun JLB, Ltd., Cornwall, England) can be used to retain the oximetry pick-ups or electrodes conveniently and comfortably, minimizing the need for tape. As material enters the airway, SpO_2 and lung ventilation are reduced because of bronchospasm and airway obstruction that reduces functioning respiratory exchange membrane. Thus, SpO_2 should be monitored during meals when severe aspiration is suspected.[264] Chronic aspiration of saliva or food that causes a sustained decrease in the baseline SpO_2 from normal levels is associated with a greater than 90% risk of aspiration pneumonia in less than 2 months for patients with ALS (ongoing data analysis from 98 patients) and perhaps an equally high risk of pneumonia and acute respiratory failure for other patients with NMD (Chapter 8). Pulse rate, as conveniently monitored by oximetry, increases even before SpO_2 begins to decrease for patients having difficulty with oral intake. Thus, dysphagia can result in decreases in SpO_2 and increases in blood carbon dioxide tensions, respiratory rate, accessory muscle use, and heart rate. Other useful tests include assessment of CPF with a peak flow meter (Chapter 11),[265] assessment of maximum inspiratory and expiratory pressures, and ultrasound of the oral cavity to observe tongue function.

Treatment for Dysphagia

A management program for dysphagia involves education and dietary counseling. Oral muscle and temporomandibular joint mobilization exercises may be helpful. In one study of 21 patients with various conditions and jaw opening limited to 21 mm, manual stretch with finger pressure, tongue depressor stretching, and use of the Therabite System (Therabite Corp., West Chester, PA, www.therabite.com) resulted in increases in jaw opening of 4.4 ± 2.1, 6 ± 1.8, and 13.5 ± 1.6 mm (SE), respectively.[266] The Therabite System is a manual traction system; as a result of grip pressure on the lever, mouthpiece cushions apply stretch to the dentition to open the mouth in the arch of normal mouth opening. Although this system has been used for a variety of patients, studies have not yet been performed in patients with primarily muscle weakness. The untoward effect of malocclusion on mastication can also be offset by dental prosthetics.[267]

Food is prepared with consideration of swallowing limitations. The variety of food flavors and odors may be widened for greater pleasure in eating. Soft, easy-to-chew foods reduce fatigue. Caution is taken to avoid large boluses. Thickened liquids may be helpful. Soft (semisolid) foods such as custards tend to bind together and can be swallowed as a single bolus. Sticky foods, such as white bread, and substances that combine with saliva to create thick mucus, such as milk products and chocolate, may need to be avoided. Books of adapted recipes are available.[222] Care providers are given a list of foods to be avoided. Pills can be placed in Jello cubes or custard to be swallowed as a single bolus[269] or crushed and delivered with fluid. Since a patient may fatigue during a large meal, smaller more frequent meals may need to be recommended.[235]

Abdominal distention associated with delayed gastric emptying and dyspnea can also occur and may be an indication for use of intestinal prokinetic medications such as metoclopramide (Reglan). Metoclopramide stimulates motility of the upper gastrointestinal tract without stimulating gastric, biliary, or pancreatic secretions. It seems to sensitize tissues to the action of acetylcholine, and its effect can be abolished by anticholinergic drugs.

To optimize swallowing, the patient should be seated upright at 90°, the head and trunk should be supported to prevent fatigue, and the neck should be flexed slightly forward. Many patients can use upper extremity assistive devices, including robotics,[189] for self-feeding. Seat belts can assist with body stabilization. If present, airway and nasal congestion, sinusitis, dyspnea, and fatigue are treated. Pharyngeal pooling can be cleared manually (Fig. 1), provided that the patient can swallow quickly enough to avert excessive aspiration.

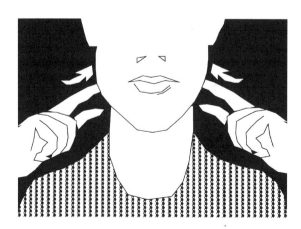

Figure 1. Clearing of the pharynx.

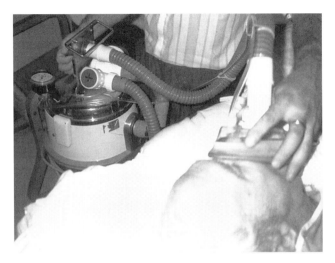

Figure 2. Seventy-two-year-old man with C2 complete tetraplegia and no ventilator-free breathing tolerance. He had hypomobility of the left vocal cord and severe dysphagia, which resulted in extensive aspiration of food. For humanitarian reasons, limited oral intake was permitted with instructions to use mechanical insufflation-exsufflation after every few swallows to eliminate the aspirated food and reverse aspiration-induced oxyhemoglobin desaturations. When aspiration of food and airway secretions was excessive and mucus production increased, oral feeding was suspended for a few days until airway secretions (and, at times, mean pulse oxyhemoglobin saturation levels) returned to normal.

As dysphagia progresses, it is especially important to monitor the nutritional value and caloric adequacy of meals, to alert caregivers to observe for the signs and symptoms of aspiration, and to monitor oximetry for feedback using mechanically assisted coughing (MAC) as needed.[270] SpO_2 is normalized as airway debris is cleared by MAC. MAC can be crucial to permit some degree of oral intake in patients with severe dysphagia (Fig. 2).

When tachypnea and dyspnea hamper swallowing efforts, the use of high-tidal volume mouthpiece IPPV facilitates swallowing by decreasing the respiratory rate, giving the patient more time to chew and swallow without dyspnea. It increases oral phase times, decreases fatigue, and relieves hypercapnia-associated decreases in appetite. It can also normalize SpO_2 and end-tidal carbon dioxide ($EtCO_2$) levels as patients coordinate deep assisted breathing with swallowing. Weight loss correlates with swallowing impairment, but weight typically increases once noninvasive IPPV and MAC are provided. As weight improves with better nutrition, ventilator use is required for shorter periods of time during daytime hours, and many patients can sit in wheelchairs longer (better endurance), manage their airway secretions more effectively, and feel better clinically. Occasional myopathic patients with dysphagia, regurgitation, or aspiration due to a tight upper esophageal sphincter have been reported to benefit from surgical release of the sphincter.[271]

Supplemental nutrition becomes necessary when adequate calories and fluid cannot be taken by mouth despite swallowing interventions. An orogastric tube can be passed for each meal for supplemental feeding. Patients have passed these tubes for 6 months or more, up to 5 times a day, without apparent ill effects.[269,272]

Nonoral Feeding

Nonoral nutrition can be provided via nasogastric, cervical esophagostomy, pharyngostomy, gastrostomy, or jejunostomy tubes. Nasogastric tubes cause discomfort and irritation and interfere with normal esophageal motility, gastroesophageal sphincter function, and use of nasal ventilation. They also increase the incidence of gastroesophageal reflux and esophagitis.[273] The size of the tube does not seem to matter.[274] To minimize the risk of esophageal injury, patients should maintain a semirecumbent position. Strategies that improve gastric emptying and prevent gastroesophageal and duodenogastric reflux, such as the use of metoclopramide,[275] should be considered. Although we have seen children with SMA type 1 who require nasal ventilation continuously (see Fig. 17 of Chapter 2) retain nasogastric tubes for over 9 years, when the need for nonoral feeding is indefinite, gastrostomy is recommended.

Anesthesia Concerns

Patients with NMD pose anesthetic challenges. Local or epidural anesthesia should be preferred over general anesthesia whenever possible.[276] Most paralytic, analgesic, and inhalation agents have a depressive effect on muscle function. Hazards have been reported with the use of thiopentone, suxamethonium, neostigmine, and halothane.[277] However, general anesthesia can be provided without using muscle relaxants.[278,279] Postoperative atelectasis and an increase in airway secretions are common. Most postoperative complications in patients with muscular dystrophy (16 of 18 in one study[277]) are respiratory. Respiratory complications can be largely avoided by preanesthesia training in and postoperative use of MAC and noninvasive IPPV as needed (Chapter 11).

The use of volatile anesthetics or succinylcholine can result in malignant hyperthermia. In one study, about 70% of 29 patients with NMD, including 2 of 3 patients with DMD, were found to be susceptible to malignant hyperthermia by the in vitro contracture test.[280] Impaired inspiratory and expiratory musculature, cardiac compromise due to cardiomyopathy, and increased susceptibility to anesthetic induced malignant hyperthermia and rhabdomyolysis[281] should encourage every effort to avoid general anesthesia. Intravenous sedation is also often poorly tolerated because of chronic ventilatory impairment. In addition, esophageal intubation with the gastroscope may sufficiently compromise ventilation to prohibit percutaneous endoscopic gastrostomy (PEG).

Modified Stamm Gastrostomy

For the above reasons, the Stamm gastrostomy[282] was modified so that it can be performed easily under local anesthesia. Noninvasive IPPV can also be provided during these procedures for patients with little ventilatory reserve.[283] The modification passes the gastrostomy tube through the omentum en route to the abdominal wall. The omentum ensures a seal to the site and eliminates the need for tacking sutures between the stomach and peritoneum. Because this simplification enables the use of a smaller midline incision, less intra-abdominal manipulation, and no peritoneal sutures, it can be performed comfortably under local anesthesia. In our center over the past 10 years, the technique of open gastrostomy under local anesthesia has been used in more than 40 patients with NMD, almost one-half of whom were infants with SMA type 1, with no documented leaks or respiratory morbidity.[284]

In preparation for the procedure, patients who have marginal inspiratory and expiratory function but who do not use noninvasive aids on an ongoing basis are trained in their use (Chapters 10 and 11). Infants as young as 3 months of age can become accustomed to using bilevel PAP. In this way, in the event that intubation is required, they can be extubated whether or not they are capable of autonomous breathing (Chapter 11).

The patient is placed in supine position with the table in reverse Trendelenberg position to allow the stomach to fall below the costal margin. Patients requiring ventilatory support, either via tracheostomy or via mouthpiece or nasal interface,[285] continue this support throughout the procedure.

The skin is prepared and draped in the routine and sterile manner for an upper abdominal midline procedure. A 5- to 7.5-cm vertical midline incision is placed midway between the umbilicus and xyphoid process after infiltration with local anesthetic (1% lidocaine) (Fig. 3). The incision is carried through the linea alba and into the peritoneal cavity. Babcock forceps are used to grasp the mid-anterior gastric wall and bring it into the surgical field (Fig. 4). One 3-0 silk pursestring suture is placed in this region of the stomach (Fig. 5). A gastrotomy is created within the pursestring suture, and a 22F Malecot catheter is inserted into the stomach. The pursestring suture is then tied (Fig. 6). Next, the proximal end of the catheter is trimmed to allow easy passage through the abdominal wall (Fig. 7). It is then passed through an avascular site in the omentum, and the omentum is draped over the stomach (Fig. 8).

A point on the left anterior abdominal wall lateral to the midline incision is selected that corresponds to the exit site of the gastrostomy tube from the stomach. This area is infiltrated with local anesthetic, and a 4-mm stab wound is made through the abdominal wall. A tonsil clamp is passed through the stab wound into the peritoneal cavity. The

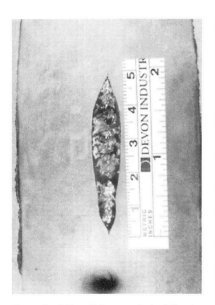

Figure 3. A 5- to 7.5-cm vertical midline incision is placed midway between the umbilicus and xyphoid process.

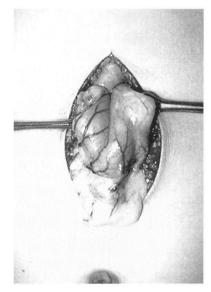

Figure 4. Babcock forceps grasp the mid-anterior gastric wall and bring it into the surgical field.

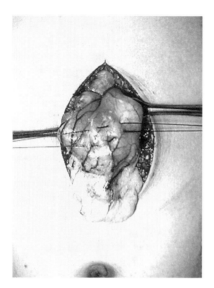

Figure 5. One 3-0 silk pursestring suture is placed in this region of the stomach.

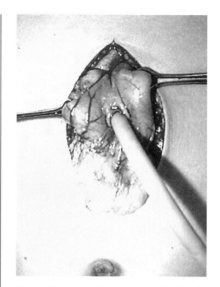

Figure 6. A gastrotomy is created within the pursestring suture, and a 22F Malecot catheter is inserted into the stomach.

gastrostomy tube is pulled through the stab wound, and the stomach is drawn toward the abdominal wall (Fig. 9). The omentum will lie between the stomach and the peritoneum (Fig. 10). Placement of the tube through the omentum ensures a watertight seal to the exit site and eliminates the need for tacking the stomach to the abdominal wall. This

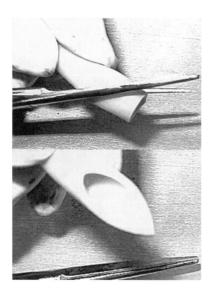

Figure 7. The proximal end of the catheter is trimmed.

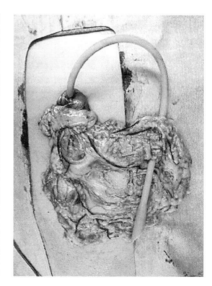

Figure 8. The catheter is passed through an avascular site in the omentum, and the omentum is draped over the stomach.

Figure 9. A point on the left anterior abdominal wall lateral to the midline incision that corresponds to the exit site of the gastrostomy tube from the stomach is selected, and a 4-mm stab wound is made through the abdominal wall. A tonsil clamp is passed through the stab wound into the peritoneal cavity. The gastrostomy tube is pulled through the stab wound, and the stomach is drawn toward the abdominal wall.

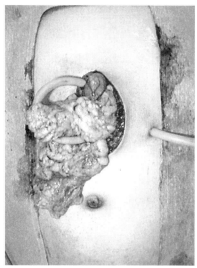

technique allows less intra-abdominal manipulation and, in turn, a smaller midline incision. These factors greatly reduce the discomfort of the procedure. Suturing the Malecot catheter to the skin is not necessary because the exit site is small enough to encircle the tube tightly. The midline incision is then closed in the standard fashion (Fig. 11).

The gastrostomy tube is taped securely to the abdominal wall and placed for gravity drainage overnight. Its location within the stomach is verified on the first postoperative day using water-soluble contrast and bedside radiography. The gastrostomy tube can be

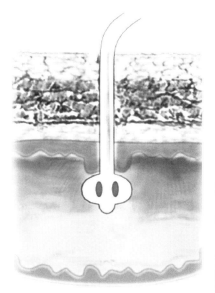

Figure 10. The omentum lies between the stomach and the peritoneum.

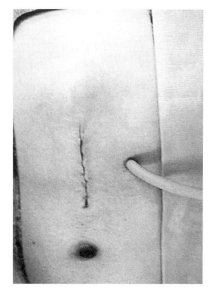

Figure 11. The midline incision is then closed in the standard fashion.

used on the same day. Thus, the modified Stamm technique makes it possible to perform an open gastrostomy comfortably under local anesthesia. The enteral tube should be regularly evaluated for signs of obstruction, rigidity, or deterioration, and it is changed regularly. Other difficulties with gastrostomy tubes include infection and accidental dislodgment.

For patients with gastrostomy tubes, feedings are administered with the patient upright, or at least somewhat vertical, for continuous overnight infusion to minimize the risk of gastroesophageal reflux. Continuous infusions are used initially and are generally well tolerated. However, intermittent bolus infusions are more practical during daytime hours and better preserve stomach volume. Volumetric infusion pumps or gravity drip methods are available and are especially important for infants with SMA who tolerate overnight fasting poorly. The volumes and concentrations of solutions to be infused are increased gradually, and electrolytes should be checked regularly.

The sodium content of the formula is reduced for patients who develop edema. Hyperglycemia can necessitate insulin administration. Clogged tubes are flushed or replaced by tubes with larger tip holes. Complications from tube feedings include diarrhea and cramping. They usually are best managed by decreasing the infusion rate, diluting or changing the feeding formula, verifying sanitation and storage procedures, and possibly adding antibiotics. Antibiotic therapy can result in *Candida albicans* infection. The risk of this infection may be decreased by providing probiotics such as lactobacilli and bifido bacteria. For the patient with congestive heart failure, the infusion rate is decreased, the sodium content is reduced, and medical treatments may be required (Chapter 5).

The use of tube feeding does not preclude oral feedings; however, oximetry is used to ensure rapid detection of excessive aspiration. MAC can be used after every few swallows and for every aspiration-triggered $dSpO_2$ until the aspirated material has been eliminated and the SpO_2 returns to normal (see Fig. 1 in Chapter 4).

Tracheostomy Tube Considerations

The presence of a tracheostomy tube hampers swallowing and predisposes to aspiration by fixing the trachea and larynx to the skin, thereby decreasing laryngeal elevation and neck excursion. The tube also decreases neck muscle movement,[286,287] hampering glottic closure and increasing laryngeal penetration. It interferes with relaxation of the cricopharyngeal sphincter, compresses the esophagus, changes intratracheal pressure,[286,287] and reduces hypopharyngeal and laryngeal sensitivity.[288] Videofluoroscopic swallowing studies revealed abnormal findings in 80% of patients receiving tracheostomy IPPV, even without concomitant NMDs.[289,290]

The degree of laryngeal fixation can be affected by the location and size of the tracheotomy incision. To allow the tracheostomy tube to move easily with the larynx, vertical tracheotomy incisions are preferred over horizontal incisions.[291] However, individual surgical technique and patient anatomy can affect the choice of incision. Additionally, scarring around the stoma site can occur, more frequently with long-term tracheostomy. Decreased laryngeal excursion is also possible after oral intubation from pressure of the tube on the base of the tongue.[292]

The tube cuff also contributes to dysphagia.[286,293] Cuff inflation drags along the tracheal wall, anchoring the larynx and impairing pharyngeal swallow.[286,292] Shortening of the pharynx and contraction of the arytenoids with the base of the epiglottis are diminished, and the larynx does not move out of the path of the descending bolus. In addition, the mechanical leverage that normally assists in pulling open the cricopharynx is decreased. Tracheomalacia or destruction of the trachea itself is also a potential hazard because of the friction of the cuff on the tracheal wall. Cuff impingement on the esophagus can create a physical barrier to the passage of a bolus. A finding related to esophageal compression by a tracheostomy tube cuff is expulsion of saliva, secretions, or food particles from the stoma after the material has been aspirated into the trachea.

Although cuff deflation can facilitate safer swallowing, crucial timing aspects of the swallow remain disrupted by tracheostomy IPPV. Loss of the normal apneic interval occurs in patients who have difficulty in timing airway closure with a swallow and the mandatory mechanical breath supplied by the ventilator.[294] Videofluoroscopic studies and scintigraphy confirm that the loss of positive subglottic pressure can be a major contributor to aspiration. Cuff deflation and placement of a one-way speaking valve, such as a Passy-Muir valve or an expiratory valve cap, can help coordinate swallowing with expiration after the ventilator-delivered breath. With speaking valves, subglottic pressure peaks average 10 cmH$_2$0. The restoration of positive subglottic air pressure may reduce aspiration.[295] Therefore, unless aspiration with the tracheostomy tube cuff deflated is severe (as indicated by decreases in SpO$_2$), the patient should eat only with the cuff deflated and use of a one-way value or expiratory valve cap. Again it is important to note that unless the upper airway is obstructed, all patients with NMD who can eat should be strongly considered for decannulation.

Upper airway flows that generate pharyngeal pressures help propel the bolus into the esophagus.[294] The reduction or cessation of airflow through the upper airway in patients using tracheostomy IPPV thus impairs swallowing and can result in the accumulation of pharyngeal residue and possibly aspiration.[296] Even patients with open, unoccluded tracheostomy tubes experience expiratory air leakage from the tube that decreases subglottic pressure during the pharyngeal swallow.[228]

The great majority of tracheostomy IPPV users with sufficient bulbar muscle function to speak have speech and swallowing difficulties and airway damage because of the tracheostomy tube. Infants with SMA and probably other NMDs who undergo tracheotomy do not develop the ability to speak, whereas infants with the same disease severity who are managed noninvasively do develop the ability to speak (Chapter 12).

Loss of airflow through the upper airway by using tracheostomy IPPV with an inflated cuff also decreases the sensitivity of the larynx to penetrating and aspirated material and impairs the cough reflex[292,293]—especially for people who have inflated tracheostomy tube cuffs for long periods. If upper airway flow is restored by cuff deflation or decannulation, the reflexive cough is often initially absent in response to airway penetration.[297,298]

Oral Secretion Management and Prevention of Aspiration

Oral secretions include saliva and serous and mucoid fluids from the nose and airways. Stimulation of cholinergic receptors produces thin serous secretions, whereas beta-adrenergic receptors produce thick protein and mucus-rich secretions. The control of these secretions can be difficult for patients with bulbar dysfunction.

Sialorrhea is excessive saliva production or loss of control of saliva. Inability to manage saliva and other oral secretions can result in aspiration or drooling. Drooling occurs because of decreased oropharyngeal muscle function. It usually becomes a problem only for some patients with bulbar ALS or SMA type 1.

Although drooling causes social stress, it is not usually harmful in itself. Many people who drool maintain clear airways and normal SpO_2. Others who drool less appear to have essentially continuous aspiration of saliva, a decrease in baseline SpO_2 below 95%, and recurrent pneumonias. Although patients with bulbar muscle dysfunction appear to produce a larger than normal quantity of secretions, saliva production is actually decreased in patients with ALS.[299] It is also important to recognize that mucus that stagnates in the oropharynx can become inspissated.

The goals of management strategies are to decrease secretion production, improve handling of secretions, and divert and remove saliva and other secretions. Glycopyrrolate has been reported to be useful to decrease oral secretions for children with central nervous system disorders.[300–302] Decreased drooling in patients with cerebral palsy has also been reported with benzotropine,[303] trihexyphenidyl hydrochloride,[304] and transdermal hyoscine.[305–307] The latter has also been useful for patients with oropharyngeal carcinoma.[302] Atropine reduced sialorrhea in a crossover study of patients with closed-head injury but exacerbated constipation, especially in patients already prone to this problem.[308]

There have been few medical trials, controlled or uncontrolled, for managing secretions for patients with NMDs. In one pilot study, 12 of 16 patients with bulbar ALS experienced relief from thick secretions with the use of beta agonists.[309] Antihistamines and anticholinergics, including atropine, benzotropine, scopolamine, propantheline, amitriptyline (10 mg every 8 hours), imipramine, methantheline, glycopyrrolate, trihexyphenidyl, and methylphenidate, may also be helpful in decreasing secretions. Scopolamine can be given as a tablet or delivered via a patch on the user's skin. Although these medications are usually only a little effective and can cause dry mouth and exacerbate constipation,[224] some of our patients with NMD have responded well to the use of scopolamine patches; others have responded well to glycopyrrolate (Robinul).

External beam irradiation of the parotid, submandibular, and sublingual glands can reduce sialorrhea by 50% or more for 6 months[269] and decrease symptoms in about 50% of patients with ALS.[310] One study suggested that the lowest effective dose was 8 Gy.[311]

Surgical interventions, such as transtympanic sectioning of the corda tympani and tympanic plexus and parotid duct ligation[269] or rerouting,[272] can be done under local anesthesia. These procedures have been tried for patients with ALS without consistent evidence of efficacy.[299,312] Botulinum toxin injections, generally 25–50 units per parotid, are now used for patients with ALS.[313] Botulinum toxin A blocks the release of acetylcholine in motor and autonomic nerve terminals. It has been noted to decrease saliva production by up to 90% in young patients for 6 months or more. Results in older patients are less impressive, and the saliva becomes thicker. Recurrent jaw dislocation following botulinum toxin injection was described as a complication for one patient with ALS.[314] An intraoral "lip plumper" prosthesis has been developed that approximates incompetent lips and creates an oral seal to dam saliva for convenient suctioning to decrease drooling.[315]

For sialorrhea with thick mucus, hydration, oral hygiene, and beta blockers such as propranolol or metoprolol can be useful.[224] When ongoing aspiration of saliva causes choking and persistent $dSpO_2$ and vocal cord dysfunction precludes verbal communication, whether or not ventilatory assistance is needed, tracheotomy and laryngeal diversion are indicated. This approach may permit cuff deflation. In one study it returned 4 of 5 patients to oral food intake.[316,317] It also eliminates any residual verbal ability. In this procedure, the trachea is transected to about the third ring, and its distal portion is sutured to the skin. Then, either the esophagus is dissected and sutured to the proximal portion of the trachea, or the proximal portion of the trachea is folded upon and sutured to itself.[316,318]

Cricopharyngeal myotomy can be used to decrease aspiration from pyriform sinus and vallecula pooling[269,319] caused by failure of the upper esophageal sphincter to open. It is useful only in patients with dysfunction of the cricopharyngeal muscle and conservation of sufficient pharyngeal propulsion to carry the food to the back of the pharynx. In general, dysphagia is due to upper esophageal sphincter spasm in only a minority of patients with ALS.[320] A cricopharyngeal myotomy will not assist safe swallowing when failure to open the sphincter is caused by reduced laryngeal elevation or decreased traction forces on the upper esophageal sphincter. In one study, 64% of 100 patients with ALS were said to have benefited from the procedure.[321] Another 13 of 92 patients with ALS and pseudobulbar symptoms and signs underwent cricopharyngeal myotomy with a satisfaction rate of 89%.[322] Two patients with limb-girdle muscular dystrophy (LGMD) were reported to benefit from cricopharyngeal myotomy.[260] In a study of 205 general patients undergoing cricopharyngeal myotomy, there was a 5.3% infection rate (11 patients) with fistula in 2 patients. Three patients died from the surgical intervention itself.[323]

Another procedure that can diminish aspiration and improve cough flows is apposition of vocal cords paralyzed in abduction. Several groups have also proposed orthodontic treatment or maxillofacial surgery for mandibular deformations and problems with dental articulation in patients with DMD or myotonic dystrophy.[324]

Gastroesophageal Reflux

Many patients with NMD, including most infants with SMA, have gastroesophageal reflux that may result in episodes of aspiration pneumonia. These patients almost invariably have weak diaphragms. Lower esophageal sphincter pressures decrease with diminished diaphragmatic contraction, especially the diminished diaphragmatic contraction associated with mechanical ventilation.[325] In addition, most infants with SMA and many others with NMD require gastrostomy tubes for nutritional support. The tube results in the lowering of the fundus of the stomach, changing the angle of His, and compromising the integrity of the gastroesophageal sphincter. These effects, and perhaps other factors, can increase reflux. For example, a high-protein diet tends to facilitate sphincter function, whereas high-fat regimens tend to decrease it. By traversing the lower esophageal spincter, nasogastric tubes are also likely to increase reflux. Reflux can result in aspiration of stomach contents. Glottic dysfunction can also cause aspiration of upper airway secretions.

The symptoms and signs of reflux typically include heartburn, productive cough, chest pain, bronchospasm, nausea, regurgitation, vomiting, and weight loss or failure to thrive. Reflux can be diagnosed by monitoring the pH of the esophagus. It is more sensitively diagnosed by ingestion of radioactive colloid, after which scintigrams of the thorax are obtained to determine whether gastric contents can be detected in the esophagus or lungs.[326] Scintigraphic images of the chest are recommended 5 minutes, 4 hours, and the day after colloid ingestion.[327] Scintigraphy performed on 50 newborns admitted to intensive care with cyanosis, apnea, bradycardia, laryngeal stridor, or wheezing not thought to be of cardiopulmonary origin demonstrated gastroesophageal reflux in 40 cases. Thirty-nine of 40 cases had respiratory symptoms, but no radiation was observed in the pulmonary fields.[328] This finding implies that the symptoms frequently associated with gastroesophageal reflux may depend on involuntary vagal stimulation rather than on pulmonary aspiration. For patients who reflux, barium, too, can be radiographically demonstrated in the esophagus or in the lungs in the event of aspiration after oral ingestion as part of an upper gastrointestinal series.

Nissen fundoplications have been performed since 1991 to reinforce the gastroesophageal sphincter and decrease reflux. Laproscopic Nissen fundoplication involves lengthening the abdominal esophagus (if necessary), retroesophageal dissection at the gastroesophageal junction, closure of the esophageal hiatus, retroesophageal wrap, suturing, and fixation of the wrap to the crura.[329] It has been reported to relieve reflux,[330,331] and, more recently, has been used extensively for infants and children with NMD.[332]

Eight of 10 children with SMA type 1 whom we studied were experiencing reflux. Seven of the 8 underwent Nissen fundoplications, but only 1 of the 10 children had a history of pneumonia that did not appear to be associated with an upper respiratory tract infection. Furthermore, other patients who were not studied for reflux and did not undergo fundoplication have not had pneumonia due to aspiration—in some cases, for at least the first 7 years of their lives. Thus, it is unclear whether fundoplications are usually necessary. In addition, one child who used only nocturnal high-span bilevel PAP before fundoplication required continuous bilevel PAP after the procedure. This finding may have been due to lack of adequate nutrition in the 4 pre- and postoperative days. It may be important to provide hyperalimentation and to avoid fasting even for this relatively brief period. No studies have been performed, and as yet no clinical evidence indicates that patients who undergo Nissen procedures fare better than those who do not. Occasionally, after having no symptoms and even testing negative for reflux, infants with SMA develop vomiting and regurgitation and clearly require and benefit from fundoplications. Now that patients with NMD are living longer because of respiratory muscle aids and children with SMA type 1, with and without fundoplications, are living for many years, it may be possible to compare the outcomes of those who undergo the procedure and those who do not.

Gastrointestinal Hypomotility

Complaints of malaise, anxiety, epigastric discomfort, and vomiting by patients with myopathies may be due to gastrointestinal hypomotility. When abdominal distention, pain, constipation, and vomiting are severe and mechanical obstruction is excluded by abdominal radiography, contrast studies, and colonoscopy, intestinal pseudoobstruction is diagnosed. Manometric and cineradiographic findings of abnormal intestinal motility confirm the diagnosis. This condition can be treated conservatively by using laxatives and motility-enhancing agents such as metoclopramide (Reglan). In one study, 15 of 16 patients with myotonic dystrophy had delayed gastric emptying of a solid meal, and 10 had delayed emptying of a liquid meal. Esophageal emptying was also markedly delayed in 15 of 16 patients. No relationship was found between gastrointestinal symptoms and severity of skeletal muscle weakness.[275]

Occasionally gastroparesis and dilatation necessitate acute decompression by passing a nasogastric tube.[333] A gastrostomy tube, when present, can be burped. Occasionally, when the distention is in the large intestine and megacolon is severe, persistent and un-relieved by mobilization or passing a rectal tube, colostomy becomes necessary. Although one patient described in the literature did not fare well postoperatively and a perioperative complication rate of 8.2–42.9% was noted for patients with myotonic dystrophy,[334] we have had patients who survived for years after colectomy with ileorectal stapled anastomosis. This finding applies particularly to patients requiring mechanical ventilation (Chapter 10). One patient with myotonic dystrophy and gastric distention developed gastric volvulus with pyloroantral obstruction that was successfully treated by emergency gastrectomy.[335]

Symptoms of gastrointestinal hypomotility are often associated with congestive heart failure and left ventricular ejection fractions (LVEFs) below 15%. Acute episodes of gastric and intestinal distention and tenderness, vomiting, diarrhea, and tachycardia can result in dehydration, impaired diaphragm excursion, and hypoventilation, and, if not caused by it, can lead to cardiopulmonary failure.[336] Hypokalemia and hypoglycemia, which commonly occur during respiratory tract infections, can result in or exacerbate abdominal distention. It has been noted that such episodes can follow anesthesia, complicate chest colds, and be associated with emotional factors and fatigue. Intestinal obstruction, pseudoobstruction, malabsorption, and volvulus can also occur in patients with NMD and can cause or contribute to ventilatory insufficiency.[293] Nausea, retching, vomiting, and tachycardia also may be associated with uncomplicated ventilatory insufficiency.

Mechanical ventilation, especially with positive end-expiratory pressure (PEEP), increases intrathoracic pressure and decreases venous return by reducing the systemic-venous pressure difference. This effect decreases cardiac preload and right atrial pressure and results in decreased cardiac output,[337] particularly for patients with cardiomyopathies who receive beta-blocker and angiotensin-converting enzyme inhibitor medications. Splanchnic blood flow decreases in parallel with PEEP-induced reductions in cardiac output. This decrease can lead to gastrointestinal mucosal damage and altered gastrointestinal motility.[338]

Constipation

Constipation is common in NMD and can cause abdominal distention, which, in turn, cause ventilatory failure. One must be aware, however, that nausea, vomiting, and abdominal pain and distention can be a sign of anatomic abdominal obstruction or cardiac failure and, thus, should be evaluated before assuming that symptoms are due to simple constipation.

For treating constipation, high fluid and fruit intake is encouraged, but laxatives are often required. Bulk-forming laxatives are derived from agar, psyllium seed, kelp, plant gums, and cellulose. They facilitate passage of intestinal contents and reflexively stimulate bowel wall activity. They exert a laxative effect in 12–24 hours. The components of

Metamucil (G. D. Searle & Co., Chicago, IL), a bulk-forming vegetable laxative, are psyllium and dextrose. Metamucil is usually provided in dosages of 30 mg (two tablespoons) per day. Its use can result in highly fibrous and bulky stools that may be increasingly difficult to evacuate as bowel weakness progresses. It also necessitates additional fluid intake, which can be difficult for people with dysphagia.

Salt laxatives include Fleet Phospho-Soda (Fleet, Inc., Lynchburg, VA), magnesium citrate, and Milk of Magnesia (Roxane Laboratories, Inc., Columbus, OH). These laxatives cause water to be retained in the intestines. Up to 20% of ingested magnesium can enter the blood stream and may cause confusion and coma in people with poor kidney function. Likewise, excessive sodium intake can be hazardous for people with edema, high blood pressure, or heart disease. Dehydration can also be a problem with the use of saline laxatives.

Osmotic agents, such as saline laxatives, also cause water to be retained with the stool. Polyethylene glycol (MiraLax, Braintree Laboratories, Braintree, MA) is a synthetic glycol with a high molecular weight. It increases the water retention of stools and thereby softens them and increases the frequency of bowel movements. It has no effect on the absorption or secretion of glucose or electrolytes, and no tachyphylaxis is associated with its use. However, prolonged use requires monitoring of serum electrolytes, and some patients are allergic to polyethylene glycol. It can be used either daily at doses of about 17 gm (1 tablespoon of powder in 8 ounces of water) to effect daily bowel movements or every second to fourth day in larger doses (about 65 gm) for patients wanting to avoid constipation but not wanting daily bowel movements. Some of our patients with muscular dystrophy and severe constipation have done quite well with prolonged use of this medication.

Surface active agents increase the wetting efficiency of intestinal water and tend to soften stools. The most commonly used medication in this class is bioctyl sodium sulfosuccinate gels (Colase, Bristol-Myers Squibb Co., Princeton, NJ). Two gels (200 mg), taken once a day, can make stool more slippery and facilitate bowel evacuation. Colase can help prevent constipation but does not appear to have any effect on existing constipation. There are no side effects.

Mineral oils soften and lubricate stools. Examples include liquid petroleum and plant oils such as olive oil. Large doses should not be taken with food because they can retard stomach emptying. Since large doses can cause oil to leak out of the anus, doses should be divided or taken only before bedtime. Long-term mineral oil use can also lead to oil deposits in the lungs (and, thereby, lipid pneumonia) or lymph nodes, liver, and spleen, where they can cause chronic inflammation.

Stimulant laxatives can stimulate both small and large intestines. They increase the activity of the intestinal wall muscles by irritating the mucus lining or by stimulating local nerve reflexes to increase wall muscle activity. This effect may cause griping, increased mucus secretion, evacuation of fluid produced in the bowel, and loss of potassium. Anthraquinone laxatives include rhubarb root powder and aloe vera, substances that act to irritate the bowel wall, as well as cascara and senna. These substances act only on the large intestine (colon). The way in which they increase bowel activity is not entirely clear. Senokot (Purdue Frederick Co., Norwalk, CT) is one of the most common preparations of senna. It can be provided as granules, in tablet form, as a syrup, or as a suppository. Rhubarb and senna cause excretion of chrysophanic acid in the urine. Depending on the acid content of the urine, this substance colors the urine either yellowish-brown or reddish-violet.

Herbal laxatives include Herb-lax (Shaklee Corporation, San Francisco, CA), a senna leaf powder preparation with numerous other organic laxative substances, including rhubarb root powder. Another example is Aloe Vera Herbal Stimulant Laxative (Nature's Way Products, Inc., Springville, UT). One Herb-lax tablet includes 175 mg of senna powder. Four or more tablets can be used at bedtime. Aloe Vera capsules include 200 mg of aloe vera resin, 50 mg of aloe barbadensis (aloe vera leaf), and other ingredients, including fennel and beet root. One or two tablets of these products usually produce a bowel movement in 6–12 hours.

Phenolphthalein was once the main ingredient of many preparations. It is a colorless, odorless substance that primarily stimulates the large intestine, but the small intestine also may be stimulated to some degree. Its mechanism of action is not known. Because it can cause serious systemic effects, products containing phenolphthalein have been withdrawn from the market. Bisacodyl (Dulcolax tablets or suppositories, Ciba-Geigy Corporation, Summit, NJ) is related to phenophthalein but continues to be widely used. Although its action on the small intestine is negligible, a soft, formed stool is usually produced 6–8 hours after oral ingestion or often after 15 to 30 minutes when taken as a suppository. Griping, diarrhea, and, from the use of suppositories, rectal burning can occur.

In addition to bisacodyl, glycerin, and senna concentrates, carbon dioxide-releasing compounds can also be used as laxative suppositories. These substances are primarily effective in evacuating the lower bowel. They are easier to administer and aesthetically and psychologically more acceptable than enemas and, therefore, should be used before resort to enemas.

Tap water, salt water, soap suds, vegetable oils, and milk enemas add bulk to the descending colon and rectum, thereby stimulating the intestines and initiating the defecation reflex. Soap suds and hydrogen peroxide also produce a bowel movement by irritating the bowel. Enemas, however, should not be overused. Excessive use of enemas can result in fluid and electrolyte imbalances, worsening constipation, and colonic perforation. The recipient should be horizontal. If an enema is applied to someone who is sitting, only the rectum will be cleared. The container holding the fluid should also be above the hips to allow free but not forced entry of the fluid. Properly introduced, a pint of fluid will cause evacuation if it is retained until lower abdominal cramping is felt.

Besides surface active laxatives, gastrointestinal prokinetic agents such as Reglan can be helpful (see above).[339] There is one report of a patient with SMA whose constipation improved with administration of erythromycin.[340]

Not having daily bowel movements can be especially desirable because, once begun, completion of the movement may take hours. The patient may have to remain in bed for hours to await completion. This problem can be alleviated by the use of a Hoyer or Easy Pivot Lift (Rand-Scot, Inc., Fort Collins, CO) (Fig. 12). Such a lift facilitates bowel evacuation by hoisting the user over a commode. The feet on the floor force the thighs into the abdomen as a substitute for abdominal muscle contraction, and with the buttocks in the most dependent position over a commode, gravity helps complete the bowel movement up to 10 times faster (according to some of our patients) than when they are lying in bed.

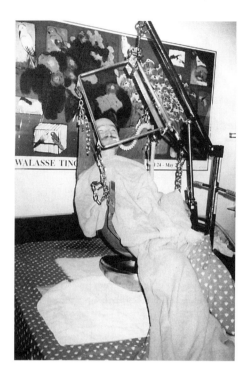

Figure 12. 24-hour noninvasive IPPV user in position to have bowel movement with Hoyer lift.

I can not see
I can not pee
I can not chew
I can not screw
Oh My God,
What can I do?
My memory shrinks
My hearing stinks
No sense of smell
I look like hell
My mood is bad—can you tell?
My body's drooping
Have trouble pooping
The Golden Years have come at last
The Golden Years can kiss my ass.

~~~ Dr. Seuss

Chapter 5

Cardiac Management

Yuka Ishikawa, M.D., with contributions by John R. Bach, M.D.

C'est vrai que je me tape la tête contre les murs, mais ce sont toujours les murs qui cèdent.
It is true that I am beating my head against walls, but it is always the walls that give way.

•❥• Gustav Mahler

In addition to deconditioning due to lack of exercise and the common occurrence of right ventricular hypertension because of failure to maintain normal lung ventilation, neurologic disorders can also affect the heart's electrical system, and myopathies affect the heart muscle directly. Cardiomyopathy commonly results in global hypokinesis along with valve abnormalities, heart wall muscle thinning or thickening, and, when hypokinesis is severe, increased risk of life-threatening arrhythmias.

Cardiac complications have been second only to respiratory dysfunction as the leading cause of death for people with neuromuscular disease (NMD). However, since the use of noninvasive respiratory muscle aids can all but eliminate respiratory mortality except for patients with severe bulbar amyotrophic lateral sclerosis (ALS), patients with myopathy are increasingly experiencing cardiac morbidity, and congestive heart failure (CHF) is an increasingly prevalent cause of death. Nonetheless, because of inactivity, mild-to-moderate heart failure is usually not recognized; in addition, with often severe spine and chest wall deformities, it is also difficult to diagnose by physical and radiographic examinations. Fortunately, there are new methods both to detect early cardiomyopathy and to alleviate it. As a result, cardiac status should be reassessed yearly or more frequently, depending on the extent of cardiac involvement and its rate of progression in a particular patient. Only when evaluated and treated in a timely manner can many patients obtain the full benefits of the use of respiratory muscle aids in terms of survival and quality of life.

Cardiopulmonary Pathophysiology

Because the heart and lungs are integrated both mechanically and functionally,[341] abnormalities of one quickly affect the physiology of the other.[341] Acute CHF results in an increase in extravascular lung water, a reduction in lung volume and respiratory system compliance, and an increase in airway resistance.[342] The consequent lung compression, pulmonary venous hypertension, and low cardiac output result in reduced lung volume, airway obstruction, diffusion abnormality, ventilation/perfusion mismatching, low mixed venous pO_2, and respiratory muscle fatigue. Tests of pulmonary function can indicate obstructive and restrictive pathology along with bronchial hyperresponsiveness, reduced carbon monoxide diffusion, hypoxemia, and decreased respiratory muscle strength.[343]

Just as lung function can be impaired by left heart failure, ventricular function can deteriorate because of blood gas alterations and the stress of intercurrent respiratory tract infections. Respiratory muscles are also weakened during respiratory infections[75] as well as during exacerbations of cardiac dysfunction. During an episode of pneumonia, one of our patients demonstrated an acute drop in left ventricular ejection fraction (LVEF), which returned to baseline after recovery. In such patients with vulnerable cardiac status, frequent exacerbations of respiratory muscle dysfunction and the often inadequate daytime or nighttime use of ventilatory assistance can lead to cardiac compromise. Likewise, the stress of surgery can decrease left ventricular function.

Left ventricular dilation allows maintenance of stroke volume when the ventricle has diminished contractility, but only at the expense of increasing wall stress and myocardial oxygen requirement.[343] Such dilation can lead to increased myocardial dysfunction or arrhythmogenicity.[344] Because massive left ventricular dilation is associated with poor outcome for patients with low LVEFs, it is important to prevent it.

Cardiomyopathy and Myopathic Disease

Conte and Gioia first described cardiac involvement in a patient with Duchenne muscular dystrophy (DMD) in 1836.[345] DMD cardiac histopathology was described in 1883.[346] Cardiomyopathy has subsequently been found to be a common finding in most generalized myopathies, and CHF is occasionally the initial reason for medical referral.[347] Seay described two patients whose muscular dystrophy was initially signaled by cardiac arrest during anesthesia.[348]

Most patients with myopathies who die before developing chronic ventilatory insufficiency or who die suddenly despite effective use of noninvasive respiratory muscle aids die from complications of cardiomyopathy.[349] Cardiomyopathies can range from subclinical in patients with otherwise advanced disease to severe in female carriers of DMD[350–352] as well as in patients with Becker,[353,354] Emery-Dreifuss,[355] myotonic,[356] and limb-girdle muscular dystrophies (LGMDs).[357] Dilated cardiomyopathy (DCM) can be found in one-fifth of carriers of DMD and Becker muscular dystrophy (BMD). If left-ventricular dilatation is taken into account, the proportion of carriers with symptoms is as high as 40%.[358] X-linked cardiomyopathies associated with abnormalities of cardiac dystrophin without skeletal muscle involvement have also been described.[359–361] In fact, DCM leading to CHF is inherited in over 30% of cases.[362] Thus, the etiology of some idiopathic cases of DCM appears to be the same as that of DMD cardiomyopathy.[363] Genetic defects in specific nuclear envelope proteins, lamin A and lamin C, which play an important role in cardiac conduction and contractility,[364] also selectively cause DCM with conduction system disease in autosomal dominant Emery-Dreifuss muscular dystrophy (EDMD).

DCM is defined as left ventricular dysfunction as indicated by LVEF less than 40% or fractional shortening less than 0.20, high left ventricular end-diastolic dimensions, and normal coronary arteries.[359,367–369] DCM can often be present without clear increases in cardiothoracic ratio (CTR), but serum neuroendocrine levels usually increase. Cor pulmonale and right ventricular failure also commonly result from untreated ventilatory insufficiency.[371] In addition, patients with DMD develop a decrease in parasympathetic activity, an increase in sympathetic activity, or both as the disease progresses.[372]

In addition to CHF, valvular dysfunction and coagulation abnormalities are common. Left ventricular thrombi can occur in association with valvular dysfunction as well as with severe ventricular hypokinesis and can result in systemic emboli.[373,374] One report associated hypercoagulability with a separately inherited protein C factor V deficiency in a 46-year-old patient with myotonic dystrophy who had experienced episodes of deep venous thrombosis at ages 19 and 20.[375] Even without a concomitant condition, however, a hypercoagulable state would be anticipated for patients with so little mobility, left ventricular dysfunction, and the elevated serum levels of tumor necrosis factor that are associated with elevated levels of creatine kinase (CK).[376] It is most likely that the very low incidence of deep venous thromboses and pulmonary emboli in patients with DMD is due to a deficiency of platelet adhesion and ristocetin-induced aggregation as well as a 50% reduction in expression of glycoprotein IV.[377] The excessive blood loss that occurs in patients with DMD during surgery may also result from poor vascular smooth muscle vasoconstrictive response due to a lack of dystrophin.[378] Thus, with platelet defects and vascular smooth muscle dysfunction, patients with muscular dystrophy are prone to excessive blood loss, as during surgery, and highly resistant to thromboses under normal circumstances. When they are left in bed with severe scoliosis, poor nutrition, and inadequate medical therapy for cardiac dysfunction and encumbered with airway secretions, hypercapnia, frustration, and stress, they may then be more susceptible to venous thrombosis and pulmonary emboli. Although pulmonary emboli are commonly considered, almost invariably airway secretions—not emboli—are the cause of oxyhemoglobin desaturation (dSpO$_2$) and respiratory distress.

X-Linked Muscular Dystrophies

DMD cardiomyopathy is the best studied cardiomyopathy associated with myopathic disease. A specific deficiency of the 50-kDa dystrophin-associated glycoprotein (DAG) was found in cardiac and skeletal muscles of cardiomyopathic dystrophic hamsters.[366] In these hamsters other dystrophin-associated proteins were also decreased in heart but not in skeletal muscle, explaining, perhaps, why the cardiomyopathy is more severe than the general myopathy.[366] Human Xp21 gene deletions may also cause loss of DAG and other cardiac proteins,[353,359,366] along with diminished or absent cardiac dystrophin.[379,380]

Angiotensin-converting enzyme (ACE) genotype DD has been described as a risk factor for severe cardiomyopathy.[369] ACE genetic variants may contribute to the onset of heart muscle disease or may act to cause disease progression after an initial precipitating event.[369] However, neither the extent of Xp21 gene deletion nor ACE genotype can as yet be used to predict severity of DMD cardiac involvement. Thus, factors influencing the severity of DMD-associated DCM appear to be epigenetic in origin.[367] This observation helps to explain the fact that, although cardiac degeneration is progressive,[381,382] there is little correlation between its severity and age, skeletal muscle involvement, physical condition, vital capacity (VC), or respiratory status (Fig. 1).[383,384] The anatomic and histopathologic findings in DMD cardiomyopathy have been described.[385]

Nigro et al.[382] monitored 328 DMD patients over a 3- to 11-year period. Preclinical cardiac involvement was found in 25% of patients under 6 years of age and in 59% of those between 6 and 10 years of age. After the age of 10, clinically apparent cardiomyopathy

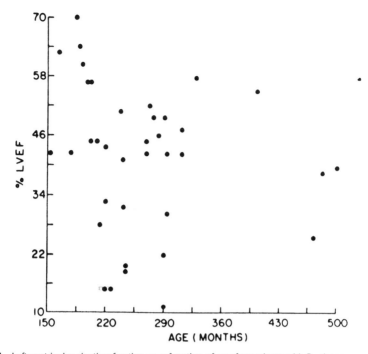

Figure 1. Left ventricular ejection fraction as a function of age for patients with Duchenne muscular dystrophy demonstrating no correlation between cardiac and musculoskeletal or respiratory muscle function. (From Stewart CA, Gilgoff I, Baydur A, et al: Gated radionuclide ventriculograhy in the evaluation of cardiac function in Duchenne's muscular dystrophy. Chest 1998;94:1245-1248, with permission.)

continued to increase in incidence. Fewer than 15% of patients with detectable cardiac involvement had symptoms before 14 years of age, and after age 18 only 57% were symptomatic.[382] The incidence of CHF was reported to be 9.4% (5 of 53 cases) in DMD,[386] despite the fact that at some time at least 96% of patients with DMD have myocardial involvement.[387]

As myocardium is gradually replaced by fibrous tissue, the left ventricular walls become thin and show decreased systolic contraction and diastolic relaxation.[388] Because the fibrosis involves the posterior papillary muscle, the mitral valve can prolapse into the left atrium with or without mitral regurgitation. Mitral valve prolapse can also occur in the presence of severe thoracic deformities. Its reported incidence ranges from 25%[389] to 55%[390] in DMD. Atrial enlargement can result from mitral regurgitation or poor left ventricular contractility.

As the conduction system is increasingly affected by fibrous replacement, conduction defects (Fig. 2) and arrhythmias (Fig. 3) develop. Virtually all patients with DMD have electrocardiographic (EKG) abnormalities.[356] The sum of the R-S amplitude in lead V1 and the R/S ratio in leads V1 and V2 have been shown to be significantly greater than in age-matched controls, even for female carriers of DMD.[391] Serial changes in EKG have been noted over time and have been associated with disease progression.[392,393] The incidence of heart block, bundle-branch block, and other arrhythmias remains low (6–13%) until DCM is severe. It has been reported that left ventricular dysfunction is associated

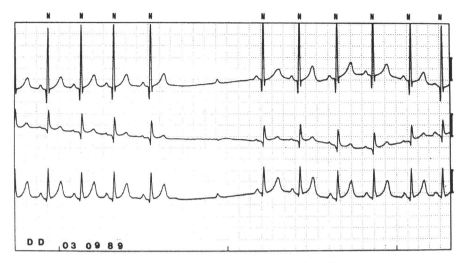

Figure 2. Holter monitoring showing an unconducted P-wave.

with the presence of late potentials on the signal-averaged EKG that correlate with ventricular arrhythmias.[394]

Hilton et al.[395] observed that only about 10% of patients with DMD develop symptomatic cardiomyopathy before overt respiratory failure. Others have estimated that 9–50% of patients with DMD die from cardiac failure.[15,382] On our service, since respiratory mortality has been reduced, we have seen three deaths due to cardiomyopathy and no other deaths over the past 9 years in 62 ventilator users with DMD.

For patients with EDMD, cardiac involvement is a dominant and often presenting feature. Initially cardiac arrhythmias usually include premature atrial contractions and

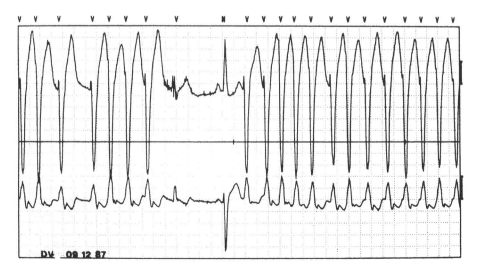

Figure 3. Holter monitoring demonstrating premature ventricular contractions between episodes of ventricular tachycardia.

sinus bradycardia. Later, permanent atrial standstill, atrial fibrillation, or atrial flutter develops. Atrioventricular heart block is common and may be progressive.[355,396] Some patients present with syncopal episodes and atrial arrest.[397] Sudden death can occur in as many as 50% of patients.[398] Because most patients have no cardiac symptoms prior to sudden death, cardiac monitoring and follow-up are indicated. Implantation of a pacemaker has been recommended if the heart rate falls below 50 beats/minute. Cardiac pacemaker placement and at times radiofrequency ablation conduction system interventions can be life-saving. One patient with EDMD also underwent transvenous implantation of a single-unit biventricular cardioverter defibrillator for progressive heart failure with ventricular arrhythmia and permanent atrial fibrillation. The unit was effective for pacing and control of ventricular tachyarrhythmia.[399]

Myotonic Dystrophy

Patients with myotonic dystrophy develop myocardial fibrosis and fatty infiltration, especially of the conducting tissue, and also patchy involvement of other regions of the myocardium.[400] Whereas as many as 80% of 236 patients with myotonic dystrophy have EKG abnormalities, including prolonged PR and QRS intervals, only about 16% have cardiac symptoms.[356] Conduction impairment and tachyarrhythmias commonly occur.[401,402] Ventricular arrhythmias may be linked to the high incidence of sudden death in such patients. When bundle-branch re-entry is the mechanism of tachycardia, radiofrequency catheter ablation of the bundle branch can eliminate ventricular tachycardias. Myotonic dystrophy should always be considered in patients with sustained ventricular tachycardia, and a high clinical suspicion of bundle-branch re-entrant tachycardia is justified in patients who exhibit wide QRS complex tachycardia—especially if no apparent heart disease is found.[403]

The main clinical concern is the development of complete heart block and the role that it plays in sudden death. As many as 30% of patients die suddenly, with Stoke-Adams syncope, conduction block, or ventricular arrhythmias.[404] Left and right bundle-branch blocks are seen in 5–25% of patients. The His-to-ventricle interval is increased in 56% of cases,[405] and the PR interval is increased in 21–40%.[406,407] Sinus bradycardia has been noted in 5–25% of patients,[407] often in conjunction with other abnormalities such as abnormal sinus node function and various degrees of heart block; thus, it is important to monitor the evolution of conduction system abnormalities.

Atrial flutter and fibrillation are the most common tachyarrhythmias and are found in up to 25% of patients.[407] Because such patients have a tendency to fall and their cognitive and physical disabilities can make it difficult for them to attend to anticoagulant therapy, one must be very cautious about prescribing warfarin.

Echocardiography reveals mitral valve prolapse in 25–40% of patients.[402] Although investigation of the role of possible myocardial myotonia has been limited, delayed myocardial relaxation has been reported.[408] Occasional cases of subacute DCM and focal myocarditis have been reported, but most of the abnormalities are subclinical.[409] Many patients have abnormalities of ventricular wall motion during exercise, as assessed by radionuclide angiography.[410]

Thirty-seven patients were followed for progression of disease over 6 years. At entry, 9 had first-degree atrioventricular (AV) block, 2 had left anterior hemiblock, and 1 had complete left bundle-branch block. Six years later 6 additional patients had bundle-branch block, four had new left anterior hemiblock, and 10 more had first-degree AV block.

Atrial flutter or fibrillation developed in 2 patients. The PR interval increased in 90%, and the QRS interval increased in 74%. In addition, one patient manifested complete heart block and needed a permanent pacemaker, and another who had worsening of first-degree block and an increasing QRS interval died suddenly.[405] Subsequently there have been similar reports of Adam-Stokes syndrome, sick sinus syndrome with sinus arrest, atrial flutter, right bundle-branch block, and marked sinus bradycardia in 3 patients requiring cardiac pacemakers.[411]

All patients with myotonic dystrophy should be examined for symptoms such as palpitations, syncope, and feelings of faintness. They require a yearly EKG and, if symptomatic, should have Holter monitoring. Patients with progressive AV block or widening QRS intervals are also questioned about syncope or presyncope to determine the need for a cardiac pacemaker. Intracardiac electrophysiologic studies may be warranted. A high clinical suspicion of bundle-branch re-entrant tachycardia is justified in patients with myotonic dystrophy who exhibit wide QRS complex tachycardia or tachycardia-related symptoms. Ablation via cardiac catheterization can effectively abolish the problem. Extra care is taken before, during, and after use of general anesthetics that carry a high frequency of cardiorespiratory complications.

There have been few studies of heart disease in congenital myotonic dystrophy. A study of the natural history of congenital myotonic dystrophy showed that 3 of 44 deaths were due to cardiac disease and that 6 were due to sudden death.[412]

Other Non-Xp21 Myopathies and Sleep Breathing Disorders

Cardiomyopathy can also be severe in the other muscular dystrophies and the congenital, metabolic, and mitochondrial myopathies. The cardiomyopathies in these conditions have not been as well characterized. Nevertheless, affected patients can also manifest cardiac arrhythmias and DCM.[52] Kearns-Sayre syndrome (Chapter 1) can present with DCM and heart block. The cardiac conduction disturbances in this syndrome are slowly progressive and potentially fatal and may necessitate pacing. Many patients with these myopathies can walk and work despite cardiopulmonary insufficiency. As a result, cor pulmonale can be especially difficult to reverse because such patients tend not to use respiratory muscle aids enough to normalize alveolar ventilation.

People with NMDs have an increased risk of sleep-disordered breathing (Chapter 9). Complications of sleep-disordered breathing and congenital central alveolar hypoventilation include cor pulmonale,[413] systemic hypertension,[414] and death from cardiac arrhythmias.[415,416] Although cardiac involvement is not a primary feature of diseases of the myoneural junction, anterior horn cell diseases, or other generalized neuropathic conditions, untreated ventilatory insufficiency often leads to cor pulmonale.

Spinal Muscular Atrophy

Although sinus tachycardia is commonly recognized, sinus bradycardia can also be severe in SMA types 1 and 2. Sinus bradycardia may occur after $dSpO_2$ secondary to respiratory difficulties, in which case it resolves with effective high-span bilevel PAP and airway secretion management. However, for some children, the SpO_2 decreases as a result of bradycardias that may be due to autonomic dysfunction similar to that seen in many premature infants. Children's heart rates can normally decrease to 60–80 beats per minute, but some children with SMA lose consciousness and are thought to have seizure disorders when their heart rates descend into the 30s. Bradycardias and desaturations can also cause flushing, diaphoresis, and skin blanching. Although bradycardias can be triggered by airway suctioning or tracheal stimulation, they can also occur without apparent warning, often during sleep. Bradycardias or other arrhythmias may also be responsible for sudden deaths. Most bradycardias that precede decreases in SpO_2 resolve spontaneously or with stimulation of the child. Bradycardias associated with loss of consciousness and refractory to stimulation of the child may respond to atropine or cardiac resuscitation efforts. Cardiac pacemakers may be warranted for patients with persistent, symptomatic episodes of bradycardia.

About 80% of children with SMA have tremors of the isoelectric line in electrocardiogram tracings.[417] More recently, atrial hyperexcitability with varying degrees of AV block were described in one of 8 patients with SMA type 3. This patient required cardiac pacing. Another of the 8 patients died from dilated cardiomyopathy.[418] There is another report of 2 children with SMA and congenital heart disease.[419] Thus, the cardiac status of patients with SMA requires increased attention.

Detection and Monitoring of Cardiac Involvement

There is marked variation in the clinical presentation of cardiac involvement in NMD.[420,421] Symptoms can include palpitations, dyspnea, cough, syncopal episodes, chest discomfort atypical of angina, stridor, sputum, general malaise, epigastric or abdominal pain, diarrhea, sweating, pallor, cyanosis, arthralgias, chills, loss of appetite, constipation, weight gain, generalized edema, decreased urine output, irritability, difficulties with concentration, sleep disturbance, nausea, and retching. Shortness of breath can occur on exertion or at rest or may be positional (in the sitting, supine, or side-lying position). Orthopnea may be due to cardiac or diaphragm dysfunction. When dyspnea is due to ventilatory insufficiency, it can be relieved by assisted ventilation. Dyspnea that persists despite adequate alveolar ventilation suggests cardiac etiology. Clinicians should be attentive to the possibility of myopathic disease in patients presenting with symptoms or signs of cardiomyopathy.

Physical Examination

Although there may be abnormal heart sounds and murmurs, most often there are no abnormal auscultatory findings in moderately affected patients with cardiomyopathy. Perloff[422] described the presence of a soft, mid-systolic murmur in the second left intercostal space as well as a loud pulmonic component of the second heart sound associated with pulmonary hypertension. A murmur of mitral regurgitation is usually due to mitral valve prolapse. Mitral valve prolapse may also be signaled by the presence of systolic clicks.[423] When CHF is present, a third heart sound, jugular venous distention, and pulmonary rales may be detected. In nonambulatory patients, extremity edema can suggest cardiac insufficiency, dependent edema, or immobility. Blood pressure is usually normal or slightly low. The heart rate can vary with the presence of arrhythmias. Persistent tachycardia, which is most often an early manifestation of cardiomyopathy and sleep-disordered breathing or chronic ventilatory insufficiency that stresses the myocardium, is common in patients with neuromuscular cardiomyopathy.[392,422,424,425] Arrhythmias, cardiomegaly, pulmonary edema, and thromboembolism occur with advanced cardiomyopathy.

Laboratory Tests and Neurohormones

Monitoring of cardiac and liver enzymes and neuroendocrines can be useful. The neuroendocrines include atrial natriuretic peptide (ANP),[426] brain natriuretic peptide (BNP),[427] and plasma norepinephrine (PNE).[428,429] Neuroendocrines are peptides that are thought to be secreted by the heart in response to increasing atrial and ventricular pressures. Because peripheral venous plasma concentrations are increased in most cases of CHF, cardiac neuroendocrine activation is a highly sensitive indicator of DCM or incipient or manifest CHF.[428,430–440] PNE concentrations have been shown to be an independent predictor of prognosis for patients with CHF.[428,429] ANP levels, normally about 10 pg/ml in young adults, increase as a function of CTR and with the ratio of the pre-ejection period to left ventricular ejection time. Plasma concentrations of BNP and ANP are sensitive indicators of moderate-to-severe left ventricular dysfunction. Both peptides are superior to PNE for identifying patients with LVEF less than 35%.[440] There are strong negative correlations between LVEF and the logarithms of BNP and ANP levels.[441] BNP now appears to have a higher positive predictive value for DCM and CHF than the other peptides. In one study, 70% of patients in the general population with high plasma BNP concentrations had CHF.[431] In our studies, in which plasma ANP[439] and BNP[432] concentrations were monitored for patients with DMD, plasma BNP concentrations were high in patients who subsequently developed overt CHF.[442] In another recent study, plasma BNP levels were more sensitive and specific than either LVEF or plasma ANP in identifying heart failure.[442]

These simple neuroendocrine radioimmunoassays can be used to screen patients with suspected ventricular dysfunction to reduce the need for more expensive echocardiography and radioscintigraphy studies.[443] Because it is difficult to evaluate clinically for cardiac overload, the measurement of BNP and ANP can assist greatly in the recognition of CHF.[441] The ANP/BNP ratio is also increased in patients with primary lung disease compared with patients in heart failure with or without lung disease.[441] Thus, BNP measurements can be used as a screening test to decide which patients need further studies and as a monitor for treatment outcomes.

Electrodiagnostic Testing

The EKG is the simplest tool for detecting cardiomyopathy.[391,444–449] The typical EKG demonstrates tall R waves and an R/S ratio greater than 1 in the right precordial leads.[424] An rSr′ pattern can be seen in lead V1 in some patients.[445] Q waves greater than 4 mm deep in lead 1, aVL, and/or V5 and V6, which mimic anterolateral myocardial infarction, and a prolonged QT segment (QT/PQ ratio = cardiomyopathic index)[450] can be present. These Q waves are considered to reflect the amount of fibrous replacement of the myocardium. Axis deviation is less often seen.

Conduction defects can occur anywhere between the sinus node and the His-Purkinje system. Intra-atrial conduction defects, Mobitz type 1 blocks, nonconducted atrial premature beats, and right ventricular conduction delays are most common.[425] A short P-R interval without delta waves can be frequently seen. We are managing a patient who presented with only a short P-R interval at initial evaluation but who later manifested the pre-excitation pattern of Wolff-Parkinson-White syndrome. The prognostic value of EKG, however, is not good because it has no consistent correlation with clinical course or cardiac enzyme elevation.[391]

Labile or persistent sinus tachycardia is the most common arrhythmia found on Holter monitoring.[392,425] Sinus pauses, premature atrial contractions, AV nodal block, and atrial flutter are also common. These abnormalities are usually not deleterious. Premature ventricular beats and ventricular tachycardia are less common unless DCM is severe.

Chest Radiography

If thoracic deformity is not severe, heart size (CTR) and pulmonary vasculature can be assessed in both posteroanterior and lateral projections of a chest radiograph. The presence of a straight back, pectus excavatum, or kyphoscoliosis helps to explain mitral valve prolapse. In a severely deformed patient, the chest radiograph is of limited value and often of no use for diagnosing cardiomegaly and CHF.

Echocardiography

Echocardiography is simple and easy to use at bedside, but quantitative measurements can be accurate only in the absence of severe chest and spinal deformities.[386,393,449,451–455] When a good-quality recording is obtained, M-mode echocardiography can evaluate for mitral valve prolapse, posterior wall systolic and diastolic velocities, and left ventricular wall thickness, mass, fractional shortening, and ejection fraction. Two-dimensional echocardiography (2DE) with Doppler and color flow mapping gives a realistic viewing of the cardiac chambers, valvular anatomy and function, regional and global left ventricular contraction patterns (wall motion),[456] and any intracardiac masses or thrombi. Serial measurements of left ventricle end-diastolic dimensions (LVDd), fractional shortening, and LVEF are useful to monitor progression of cardiomyopathy and response to therapy.[457–459] CHF with LVEFs lower than 25% and elevated ANP levels are observed only in patients with high LVDd.

Color kinesis is a new technique based on acoustic quantification that improves the qualitative and quantitative evaluation of spatial and temporal aspects of global and regional ventricular wall motion. It has been incorporated into a commercial ultrasound system (Sonos 2500, Hewlett-Packard, Cupertino, CA).[460,461] It may prove to be more useful than the monitoring of BNP levels in the detection of early NMD-associated cardiomyopathy and, therefore, may be useful in indicating treatment.

Radionuclide Studies

Nuclear medicine procedures can be used to evaluate myocardial perfusion, ventricular function, and the extent of cellular necrosis or other damage. Technetium-99m pyrophosphate scintigraphy, which is routinely used to study myocardial infarction, can be used to assess patients with cardiomyopathy. Myocardial perfusion imaging using thallium-201 single-photon emission computed tomography (SPECT) is useful for early diagnosis of myocardial damage, but it does not correlate well with LVEF, LVDd, or cardiac function in general. We have found that SPECT with transesophageal pacing of the left atrium can be quite useful for evaluating cardiac reserve. Patients with poor cardiac reserve developed larger perfusion defects with pacing and showed reversibility with rest. Myocardial perfusion imaging during pharmacologic stress demonstrated an improvement in perfusion with dipyridamole infusion,[462] suggesting a role for vasodilator therapy.

Multigated radionucleotide angiography (MUGA), sometimes called resting gated radionuclide ventriculography, is a reliable method for determining LVEF, LVDd, and wall motion.[383] It is more accurate than M-mode echocardiography for the measurement of LVEF. Because MUGA determinations are based on changes in count rates within defined areas rather than changes in geometric shapes, they are less affected by the unusual ventricular positioning in patients with thoracic abnormalities. MUGA has been shown to be useful both in determining myocardial function and in predicting morbidity in DMD-associated cardiomyopathy.[383] It can also be used to follow progression of cardiomyopathy and response to therapy.[463]

A newer nuclear medicine technique, positron emission tomography (PET), demonstrates regional alterations in myocardial metabolism and wall motion abnormalities.[464] Although PET imaging is expensive, not readily available, and difficult to perform in severely deformed or ventilator-assisted individuals, it may be useful for following the progression of cardiomyopathy.

Pulmonary Function

Vital capacity, maximum insufflation capacity (MIC), SpO_2, and end-tidal carbon dioxide ($EtCO_2$) should be monitored for all patients with cardiomyopathy associated with NMD. It has been known since 1919 that the VC of patients with incipient CHF diminishes before any complaints of dyspnea, signs of pulmonary edema, auscultatory evidence of lung congestion, or other signs of impending failure.[465] It should also be noted that, although elevated $EtCO_2$ indicates alveolar hypoventilation, sudden, unexpectedly low levels of $EtCO_2$ may signal the effects of severe cardiomyopathy on cardiac output and pulmonary perfusion rather than inexplicable hyperventilation. When the issue is in doubt, an arterial blood gas sampling can be useful.

Treatment

There is as yet no treatment to prevent metabolic and structural cardiac abnormalities. The asymptomatic patient with only typical EKG abnormalities, mild sinus tachycardia of about 100 beats per minute at rest, good left ventricular function, and normal alveolar ventilation may not require treatment. However, if tachycardia is more severe, LVEF is less than 40%, or neuroendocrines are elevated, treatment may avert the development of DCM.

Dilated Cardiomyopathy

ACE inhibitors, beta blockers, digitalis, and spironolactone are important in the treatment of patients with primary or secondary DCM and mild-to-moderate heart failure.[385,456,467–470] ACE inhibitors inhibit the conversion of angiotensin I to angiotensin II. They are used as antihypertensives but can provide sustained hemodynamic and clinical improvement in CHF.[471,472] Long-term ACE inhibitor therapy slows or reverses left ventricular dilation in patients with asymptomatic DCM.[473] The use of ACE inhibitors also appears to improve respiratory muscle strength, as indicated by increases in maximum inspiratory and expiratory pressures measured at the mouth.[474] In dogs with reduced LVEF, early long-term therapy with enalapril and beta blockers prevents or retards deterioration of left ventricular systolic function and the progression of left ventricular chamber enlargement.[475] BNP levels decreased significantly toward normal (Fig. 4) in association with an increase in LVEF (Fig. 5) and decreases in LVDd (Fig. 6) with ACE inhibitor therapy in patients with CHF.[435]

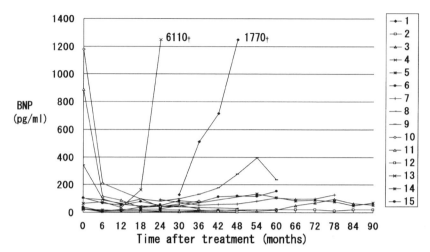

Figure 4. Changes in plasma brain natriuretic peptide (BNP) as a function of ACE inhibitor and beta-blocker administration. (From Sanyal SK, Leung RKF, Tierney RC, et al: Mitral valve prolapse syndrome in children with Duchenne's progressive muscular dystrophy. Pediatrics 1979;63:116–122, with permission.)

Beta blockers reduce heart rate.[476] In a meta-analysis of randomized clinical trials, beta blockade reduced all-cause mortality in patients with CHF.[477] With initiation of beta-blocker therapy, plasma ANP, BNP, and PNE levels further decreased (Figs. 4, 7, and 8), lymphocyte beta-adrenoreceptor density increased in as little as 2 weeks, LVDds and LVEFs improved, and CHF resolved in patients with idiopathic or ischemic DCM.[478]

Others have confirmed similar benefits of long-term beta blockade on mortality for patients with idiopathic DCM.[479–481] In addition, a reduction in total beta-adrenoceptor density and, in particular, a selective reduction in beta1 adrenoceptors have been demonstrated in BMD.[482] Long-term beta-blocker therapy has been shown to increase

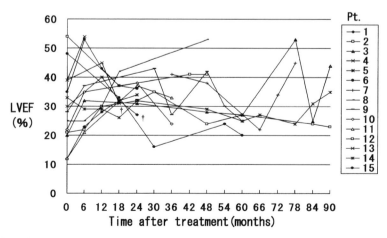

Figure 5. Left ventricular ejection fraction during treatment with ACE inhibitors and beta blockers in 15 patients with DCM and DMD. (From Sanyal SK, Leung RKF, Tierney RC, et al: Mitral valve prolapse syndrome in children with Duchenne's progressive muscular dystrophy. Pediatrics 1979;63:116–122, with permission.)

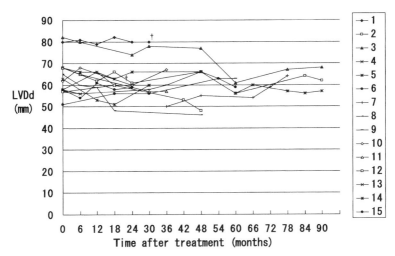

Figure 6. Left ventricular end-diastolic diameter (LVDd) during treatment with ACE inhibitors and beta block-ers for 15 patients with DCM and DMD. (From Sanyal SK, Leung RKF, Tierney RC, et al: Mitral valve prolapse syndrome in children with Duchenne's progressive muscular dystrophy. Pediatrics 1979;63:116–122, with permission.)

myocardial beta-receptor density in such patients.[482,483] Beta-blocker therapy may cor-rect the imbalance in sympathetic-parasympathetic activity—that is, the sympathetic predominance and increased susceptibility to ventricular arrhythmias[484] that develops in late-stage muscular dystrophy.[372]

Xi et al. reported that beta-adrenergic stimulation induces dystrophin breakdown fol-lowed by apoptosis. They suggested that beta-blocker therapy can be beneficial by low-ering norepinephrine for patients with dystrophin-related cardiomyopathy.[485] It can also

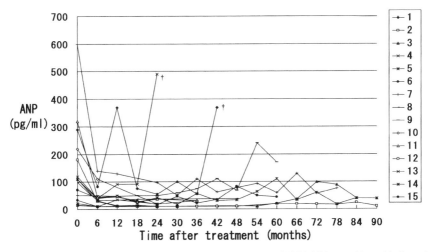

Figure 7. Changes in atrial natriuretic peptide (ANP) as a function of ACE inhibitor and beta-blocker admin-istration. (From Sanyal SK, Leung RKF, Tierney RC, et al: Mitral valve prolapse syndrome in children with Duchenne's progressive muscular dystrophy. Pediatrics 1979;63:116–122, with permission.)

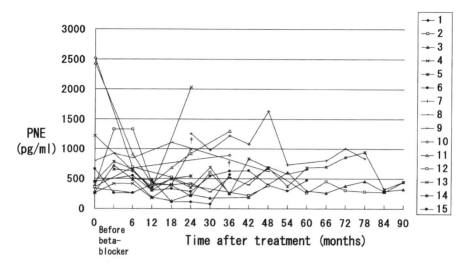

Figure 8. Changes in plasma norepinephrine levels (PNE) as a function of ACE inhibitor and beta-blocker administration. (From Sanyal SK, Leung RKF, Tierney RC, et al: Mitral valve prolapse syndrome in children with Duchenne's progressive muscular dystrophy. Pediatrics 1979;63:116–122, with permission.)

significantly improve left ventricular systolic performance and passive diastolic relaxation properties, resulting in more complete myocardial relaxation and increased contractility.[486] Beta-blocker therapy significantly decreases left ventricular chamber stiffness.[486] Thus, whereas maximal insufflation therapy reduces lung stiffness and extremity mobilization reduces articular stiffness,[487] beta-blocker therapy increases end-diastolic volumes and decreases heart muscle stiffness.[486] Despite its negative inotropic effects, the initiation of beta-blocker therapy can be well tolerated by patients with CHF, including those with idiopathic[488] or NMD-associated cardiomyopathies. Beta blockers also increase total cardiac creatine, another potentially beneficial effect.[111]

Fatty acids contribute 60–90% of the energy used by the normal heart. The remainder comes from glucose and lactate oxidation.[489] Regional myocardial fatty acid intake decreases in DCM. SPECT with I231-BMIPP demonstrated abnormal lipid metabolism for all of our DMD patients with DCM. It has been hypothesized that switching the heart's substrates from fatty acids more toward glucose and lactate may ameliorate many of the hemodynamic and biochemical alterations associated with heart failure.[490] Recent studies have indicated that the administration of metoprolol decreases fatty acid oxidation and increases carbohydrate oxidation.[491] Inhibition of fatty acid oxidation by etomoxir, an inhibitor of carnitine palmityl transferase, has been shown to decrease contractile dysfunction, myosin isozyme shift, and deterioration in the ability of the sarcoplasmic reticulum to manage calcium transport in rat models.[492,493] Metoprolol administered to dogs in heart failure leads to a decrease in carnitine palmityl transferase activity and an associated increase in triglyceride content.[488] The potential decrease in fatty acid oxidation may optimize cardiac energetics and assist in decreasing the decompensatory effects of heart failure. Thus, the improved cardiac function observed with beta blockers may be due, in part, to a decrease in fatty acid oxidation by the heart.[494] It remains to be demonstrated whether directly inhibiting fatty acid oxidation improves contractile function in CHF.[491]

A recommended dosage schedule for the administration of ACE inhibitors and beta blockers is indicated in Figure 9. Therapy is instituted in the outpatient setting except for markedly symptomatic, wheelchair-bound patients with an LVEF below 25% or ANP levels over 150 pg/ml. For patients symptomatic for CHF, ACE inhibitors, digoxin, and diuretics can be used to alleviate CHF on hospital admission. Intravenous infusion of diuretics is also effective for CHF, provided that one is careful to avoid excessive potassium loss.

For more severe CHF it has been suggested that milrinone, a III phosphodiesterase inhibitor with inotropic and vasodilatory actions, causes less tachycardia and has fewer side effects than catecholamines (including dopamine or dobutamine).[495] Once severe symptoms are relieved, beta-blocker therapy is re-instituted before the patient is discharged from the hospital. With alleviation of symptoms and neuroendocrine levels essentially stabilized, further increases in beta-blocker medication can usually be done safely at home.

We initiate treatment with enalapril in daily doses of 1.25 mg. The dose is gradually increased to 10 mg twice daily. Provided that the patient is asymptomatic or minimally symptomatic for CHF and systolic blood pressure and urinary output are adequate, the beta$_1$-adrenoreceptor blocker metoprolol or bisoprolol is added to ACE inhibitor therapy.[496] The ACE inhibitor and beta-blocker dosages are increased as tolerated. Metoprolol is initially administered at 5 mg per day in 2–3 divided dosages for 1 week. The dose is increased by 5 mg per day every 1–2 weeks until reaching a total of 25–50 mg per day in 3 divided dosages. Patients are then switched from metoprolol to bisoprolol for the more convenient dosing schedule of 1 or 2 tablets per day.

Patients can be initially treated with bisoprolol instead of metoprolol beginning at 0.5 mg per day. This dosage is increased by 0.5 mg per day per week in divided doses until it reaches 2.5–5 mg per day. Almost all patients can reach the maximum dosing levels of both ACE inhibitors and beta blockers but it can take 5–8 weeks to reach the maximum for the latter because of temporary side effects, including hypotension.[494]

Side effects of ACE inhibitors may include hypotension (systolic pressure less than 85 mmHg),[497] renal dysfunction,[498] hyperkalemia, hyponatremia, reduction in hemoglobin

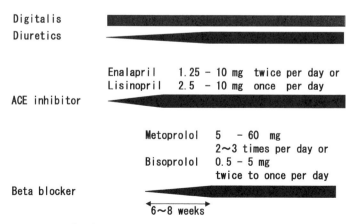

Figure 9. Dosage schedule for ACE inhibitors and beta blockers in addition to digitalis and diuretics. (From Sanyal SK, Leung RKF, Tierney RC, et al: Mitral valve prolapse syndrome in children with Duchenne's progressive muscular dystrophy. Pediatrics 1979;63:116–122, with permission.)

concentration,[497] and dry cough. These side effects can be particularly troublesome for patients with heart failure.[498,499] Sometimes reduction of diuretic dosage prior to introduction of ACE inhibitors can protect against initial dose hypotension.[500] An occasional patient may also experience severe hypotension during acute infections and dehydration, during which ACE inhibitor therapy may need to be temporarily suspended.

Monitoring of creatinine clearance is not adequate to assess renal function for myopathic patients because creatinine titers do not increase significantly in the presence of inadequate muscle mass. Blood urea nitrogen (BUN), cystatine C, and beta-microglobulin are better monitors. Swedberg et al. suggested that an increase in BUN less than 30% from pretreatment levels is not harmful.[499] If severe hypotension, renal dysfunction, hyperkalemia, or hyponatremia occurs, adequate salt administration and possibly reduction in diuretics are warranted before reducing the dosages of ACE inhibitors.[499]

Side effects of beta-blocker therapy can include sinus bradycardia (less than 40 beats/min when awake), hypotension, and possible exacerbation of heart failure. However, these side effects can be avoided during the first few months of therapy and cardiac function well preserved when dosages are increased gradually and the patient is carefully monitored for heart rate, blood pressure, sleep dysfunction, urinary output, and symptoms and other signs of cardiac decompensation. Complete blood cell counts, electrolytes (sodium, potassium, chloride), BUN, and liver function enzymes are drawn twice weekly for the first two weeks, then weekly while increasing dosages, and finally at 3-month intervals. Beta$_2$-microglobulin levels are drawn initially and when BUN is found to be elevated. Evaluation of CTR is done every 3 months and whenever signs of cardiac decompensation are suspected. LVEF and LVDd are determined by echocardiography every 6 months during the first year of treatment and then annually. ANP, BNP and PNE are drawn monthly during the period of increasing dosage and then at 6-month intervals.[479,480,494]

Improved 5-year survival has been reported for patients with DCM treated with beta blockers in conjunction with diuretics, digitalis, and ACE inhibitors by comparison with patients treated with diuretics, digitalis, and ACE inhibitors alone.[501] This combination has been shown to relieve symptoms and signs of CHF and significantly reduce ANP, BNP and PNE levels for patients with DMD[442] and others[501] with cardiomyopathy for over 5 years (see Figs. 4, 7, and 8). In the DMD study, LVEF increased and remained stable or decreased very gradually;[442] in most patients, LVDd decreased initially and remained stable or increased only slightly with time; and survival was improved.[442] This approach has also been reported to be successful for a 42-year-old patient with BMD and a LVEF of 11%.[502] Thus, although the life expectancy of untreated patients with DMD is less than 20 years, concomitant beta-blocker, ACE inhibitor, and digoxin therapy effectively prolongs survival for DMD (Fig. 10) and is effective over the long term for BMD cardiomyopathy as well (Table 1).[442,503]

Although salt restriction, diuretics, and cardiac glycosides are useful in the treatment of NMD cardiomyopathy, they have not been reported to prolong survival.[424,476,504] Digitalis should be instituted after ACE inhibitor therapy is begun. For patients with NMD, low-dose digitalis therapy is recommended even if serum levels are low because digitalis can still be effective and higher dosages tend to increase the risk of severe side effects such as lethal arrhythmias. The therapeutic role of digoxin in patients with CHF and normal sinus rhythm is now well documented.[505] Patients with NMD and moderate-to-severe

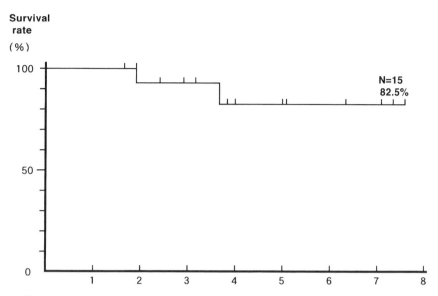

Figure 10. Kaplan-Meier survival curve for 15 patients with DMD and DCM treated with ACE inhibitors and beta blockers from age 17.3 ± 4.4 years (range: 10 years 3 months to 24 years 4 months) showing a cumulative survival of 92.9% at 3 years and 82.5% at 7 years. The longest duration of treatment was 91 months. These patients had improvements in neuorendocrine levels from pretreatment values of 302 ± 433 (BNP), 145 ± 160 (ANP), and 822 ± 789 pg/ml (PNE) to 26 ± 21 (BNP), 20 ± 14 (ANP), and 291 ± 197 pg/ml (PNE). The LVEFs improved from 33.3 ± 12.0% (range: 14–54%) to 42.9 ± 7.5% (range: 33–54%), and LVDd improved from 62.5 ± 6.5 mm (range: 53–75 mm) to 56.4 ± 6.7 mm (range: 48–74 mm) with treatment. Two patients had sudden severe re-elevations of ANP and BNP levels before death due to worsening congestive heart failure after 44 and 23 months of therapy. Six patients had symptoms of chronic alveolar hypoventilation that were relieved by nocturnal noninvasive IPPV. The thirteen surviving patients are currently 22.8 ± 3.8 years old (range: 14–27 years) and have BNP of 70.8 ± 77.1, ANP of 42.2 ± 43.4, PNE of 742.2 ± 487.5 pg/ml, LVEF of 35.0 ± 10.4% (range: 23–54%), and LVDd of 60.1 ± 8.4 mm (range: 46–80 mm).

cardiomyopathy despite absence of gross symptoms were more likely to decompensate soon after digoxin discontinuation than were patients with less severe disease.[506] Therefore, digitalis therapy is continued throughout treatment. The risk of digitalis toxicity is increased in the presence of hypoxia, poor renal function, or low serum potassium, a common finding in patients with NMD and low muscle potassium reserves, especially during respiratory tract infections.[192] The use of bilevel PAP has also been reported to improve the left ventricular function of patients with chronic congestive heart failure.[507]

Aldosterone plays an important role in the pathophysiology of heart failure.[508] It promotes the retention of sodium, the loss of magnesium and potassium, sympathetic activation, and parasympathetic inhibition; prevents the uptake of norepinephrine by the myocardium;[508,509] causes myocardial and vascular fibrosis,[510] baroreceptor dysfunction,[511] and vascular damage; and impairs arterial compliance.[508,511,512] It had been assumed that inhibition of the renin-angiotensin-aldosterone system by an ACE inhibitor would suppress aldosterone production. However, evidence now suggests that ACE inhibitors suppress only transiently the production of aldosterone.[513,514] Treatment with the aldosterone-receptor blocker spironolactone, in conjunction with an ACE inhibitor and loop diuretic, is well tolerated and decreases ANP concentrations without leading to

Table 1.   Change of Cardiac Function after Treatment with Ace Inhibitor and Beta Blocker in 15 Patients with DCM and Duchenne Muscular Dystrophy

Pt	Age		Time After		ANP		BNP		PNE		LVEF		LVDd	
	At Onset	At Last	ACEI	Beta-Blocker	Pre	After	Pre	After	Pre	After	Pre	After	Pre	After
(No.)	(years.months)		(months)		(pg/ml)		(pg/ml)		(pg/ml)		(%)		(mm)	
1	17y4m	21y9m†	44†	36†	290	56		127		80	24	36	75	74
2	15y4m	22y8m	88	87	180	10		11.4	370	155	21	35	68	56
3	19y7m	27y3m	91	89	110	10		6.7	278	112	35	44	68	61
4	12y7m	14y6m†	23†	21†	32	41	45.7	34.1	260	179	42	45	58	60
5	12y10m	19y11m	85	89	110	10		25.4	626	42	33	39	68	54
6	15y10m	20y5m‡	61	62	72	18	105	50.4	453	283	38	33	54	56
7	16y2m	22y7m‡	76	75	600	23		52.5		737		45		50
8	22y10m	26y10m	48	48	99	32	340	28.3	798	624	25	53	65	46
9	13y10m	18y10m‡	60	36	51	19	101	62.6	256	189	37	43	63	56
10	19y3m	22y4m	35	34	220	19	1180	40	2522	676	22	38	62	60
11	21y6m	24y8m‡	38	37	320	27	887	26.4	2437	420	14	37	68	57
12	21y2m	26y5m	46	46	14	10	23.6	2.5	361	219	54	41	57	48
13	22y0m	24y5m‡	29	29	16	10	26.2	8.8	1218	333	33	54	53	56
14	24y4m	26y4m	23	9	22	10	21.4	9.5	446	296	30	40	63	51
15	10y3m	14y1m	20	16	33	10	37.3	7.5	662	252	35	53	55	54
mean	17.3	22.8	51.1	47.6	144.6	20.3	302.4	26.2	822.1	290.8	33.3	42.9	62.6	56.4
SD	4.4	3.8	24.6	26.8	160.0	13.7	432.5	21.2	782.4	187.0	12.0	7.5	6.5	6.7
P value					(0.008)		(NS)		(0.013)		(0.033)		(0.005)	

† Deceased
‡ Nocturnal noninvasive ventilation successfully cleared symptoms of chronic alveolar hypoventilation for 6 patients.

serious hyperkalemia.[515] In a recent double-blind study, treatment with spironolactone reduced the risk of death from all causes, death from cardiac causes, hospitalization for cardiac causes, and the combined end-point of death from cardiac causes or hospitalization for cardiac causes among patients who had severe heart failure as a result of left ventricular systolic dysfunction and who were receiving standard therapy, including an ACE inhibitor.[516] Spironolactone also relieved the symptoms of heart failure, as noted by changes in the New York Heart Association (NYHA) functional class.

Spironolactone was originally thought to have primarily hemodynamic effects due to urinary sodium excretion and also to prevent excessive potassium loss when used in combination with loop diuretics. However, in a recent study, these effects were found to be minor with the use of typical daily dosages of 25 mg or less.[515] More importantly, spironolactone appears to be cardioprotective by reducing myocardial and vascular fibrosis. The reduction in the risk of mortality associated with spironolactone may be due primarily to prevention of progressive heart failure, myocardial fibrosis, and sudden death by increasing the myocardial uptake of norepinephrine as well as by averting arrhythmias associated with excessive potassium loss. Spironolactone may prevent myocardial fibrosis by blocking the effects of aldosterone on the formation of collagen.[517] Myocardial fibrosis may predispose patients to variations in ventricular conduction times and, hence, to re-entry ventricular arrhythmias and sudden death.[517]

Gynecomastia or breast pain was reported by 10% of men taking spironolactone. Serious hyperkalemia was seen in 2%.[516] Eight percent of patients discontinued treatment because of adverse effects.[516] We had to discontinue spironolactone because of liver transaminase increases in two patients. Furthermore, one must take extreme caution when using aldosterone-receptor blockers in conjunction with ACE inhibitors because of the potential for hyperkalemia.[518]

Arrhythmias

Routine antiarrhythmic therapy does not appear to be indicated. Most arrhythmias are associated with DCM and appear to abate with its successful treatment. Beta-blocker therapy for DCM also decreases the tendency for sinus tachycardia and ventricular ectopy. Furthermore, it is uncertain whether suppression of ventricular arrhythmias would improve the prognosis for patients with DMD because antiarrhythmic therapy with encainide or flecainide appears to have lowered the survival rate of patients who had ventricular arrhythmias after myocardial infarction.[519] The incidence of AV nodal block is low in patients with DMD.[476] If a high-degree AV block is observed in a patient receiving digitalis, digitalis blood levels should be monitored carefully.

Lidocaine or procainamide can terminate runs of ventricular tachycardia, premature ventricular beats, and other arrhythmias. Procainamide has been given intravenously to control paroxysmal supraventricular tachycardia. Oral maintenance doses of procainamide must be carefully adjusted to avoid exacerbating both muscle weakness and drug-induced elevations of antinuclear antibodies. Use of quinidine sulfate is also reasonably safe with close monitoring for muscle weakness, EKG changes such as prolongation of the QRS complex and Q-T interval, and possible worsening of the arrhythmia.

Bradycardias, short periods of sinus arrest, and AV conduction blocks may respond to intravenous atropine, especially if they are precipitated by suctioning or other airway manipulation. The need for a pacemaker is infrequent in these patients. Presence of the catheter in the right ventricle can produce serious ventricular arrhythmias, and patients with pacemakers should be carefully followed by Holter monitoring. Supraventricular tachyarrhythmias often also respond to intravenous digitalis. When hemodynamic status is deteriorating, emergency cardioversion can be used.

Acute Exacerbations of Cardiac Failure

In acute exacerbations of DCM, the patient is placed in Fowler's position or in any position that relieves symptoms. In severe cases of CHF, diuretic therapy can be increased by oral and/or intravenous administration. Sometimes increasing the dosage of beta blockers is effective. EKG, blood pressure, SpO_2, plasma levels of sodium, potassium, and chloride, total protein, hemoglobin, liver function enzymes, BUN, ANP, BNP, PNE, and intake/output are monitored. When myogenic serum transaminases are elevated, isocitrate dehydrogenase is useful to monitor liver function.

The chest X-ray often shows cardiomegaly and pulmonary edema with congestion, especially in the right middle and lower lobes. In this case, diuretics are begun or increased and ACE inhibitors (e.g., enalapril, 1.25–2.5 mg) are added. Liver dysfunction is often due to liver congestion and combination drug therapy. Because the effect of enalapril is decreased with liver dysfunction, 2.5–5 mg of lisinopril can be initiated along with digitalis, 0.125–0.25 mg/day, when the patient is not at high risk for digitalis toxicity. The beta blocker metoprolol (5 mg) or bisoprolol (0.5 mg) may be added. Nitrites can be used concomitantly to treat chest pain. Hypokalemia (potassium level less than 4 mEq/L) increases the risk of lethal ventricular arrhythmias for patients receiving digitalis.[520] However, rapid potassium replacement can also result in cardiac arrest.

Once ventricular tachycardia occurs, 50 mg of lidocaine hydrochloride is injected intravenously. If ventricular tachycardia occurs more than once over a few hours, lidocaine hydrochloride drip infusion of 720–1440 mg/24 hours is administered until the potassium level exceeds 4.0 mEq/L. If blood pressure is low or urinary output is poor even with high-dose intravenous diuretics, dopamine and sometimes dobutamine may be administered at 3 µg/kg/min. If systolic blood pressure remains below 80 mmHg, heart rate is less than 160/min, and ventricular premature contractions are infrequent, dopamine and dobutamine can be increased up to 5 µg/kg/min with care to avoid ventricular tachycardia.[484]

Once CHF is relieved, patients are weaned from catecholamine therapy. With long-term use, these medications are cardiotoxic. Patients who cannot wean from catecholamine therapy have particularly poor prognoses. If beta blockers are discontinued because of acute deterioration, they are readministered from initial doses once the patient becomes stable in the post-acute period. Thus, early detection of CHF and medical prevention of severe CHF are important to avoid acute deterioration and the need for catecholamines.

Hypoproteinemia can be treated by an infusion of 25% albumin (50 ml) over a 2-hour period, taking care not to volume-load the heart. High caloric preparations containing glucose, lipid, protein, vitamins, and essential minerals are provided in low-intake volumes (about 800 ml/day). H_2 blockers can be provided to prevent gastric and intestinal ulcers.

Two patients with advanced DCM receiving ACE inhibitors presented with severe hyponatremia, hyperkalemia, and metabolic acidosis. They had abdominal pain, hematuria, diarrhea, and disorientation. Combination treatment with hydrocortisone, glucose-insulin therapy, and bicarbonate rescued one patient, but the second patient fell into shock with a sodium level of 108 mEq/L and BUN level of 60 mg/dl and died.[521] Thus, life-threatening metabolic alkalosis can occur in patients receiving ACE inhibitors, particularly in the presence of renal dysfunction or CHF. Hyponatremia, hypovolemia, nonsteroidal anti-inflammatory drug therapy, and potassium-sparing diuretics appear to be risk factors. In treating this condition, glucocorticoids are administered and water and sodium intake are restricted.

Since at least 1952 it has been known that the use of IPPV for patients with pulmonary edema of any etiology decreases edema and airway resistance and improves ventilation-perfusion relationships. IPPV increases pulmonary compliance, the alveolar-arterial (A-a) oxygen difference, and alveolar ventilation while decreasing work of breathing.[465] Much more recently, a number of studies have demonstrated the value of providing high-span bilevel PAP, as opposed to CPAP or no ventilation, for patients with severe acute cardiogenic pulmonary edema (ACPE), a common cause of respiratory failure. ACPE is defined by a past history of cardiovascular disease, predisposing factors, cardiomegaly, bilateral alveolar and interstitial opacities, and presence of crepitations on auscultation. Such patients often require intubation on the basis of having a respiratory rate greater than 30 per minute, SpO_2 less than 90% despite 6–10 L/m of supplemental oxygen via nasal cannula, and severe dyspnea with the use of accessory respiratory muscles or paradoxical abdominal motion.

One prospective clinical study of 26 consecutive patients with ACPE reported a 79% success rate (21 of 26 patients) in avoiding intubation with the use of IPAP, 20.5 ± 4.7 cmH_2O, and EPAP, 3.5 ± 2.3 cmH_2O, via a face mask with an initial fractional inspired oxygen of 93.0 ± 16%. For the successful group SpO_2 increased from 84% to 96%, the respiratory rate decreased from 36 to 22 breaths/min, and PaO_2, $PaCO_2$, and pH normalized (p < 0.001 for all measures) in 15–60 minutes. The only differences between the successful and unsuccessful groups were in initial $PaCO_2$ (54.2 ± 15 vs. 32 ± 2.1) and creatine kinase (176 ± 149 vs. 1282 ± 2080 IU/L). Thus, 4 of the 5 patients in the unsuccessful group had had myocardial infarctions as opposed to 2 of 21 patients in the successful group, and hypercapnic patients with ACPE were more likely to benefit.[522] Patients experiencing a decrease in dyspnea by using bilevel PAP also tended to avoid intubation.[523]

In a controlled, prospective study of patients with ACPE, intubation was required in 1 of 19 patients using bilevel PAP, but in 6 of 18 patients not using it. The bilevel PAP user requiring intubation was not hypercapnic at the initiation of therapy. Bilevel PAP also improved respiratory rate, SpO_2, CO_2, work of breathing, pH, and other physiologic parameters, but there were no differences in hospital length of stay or mortality rates.[524] Of 29 other patients with ACPE treated with bilevel PAP via oral-nasal interfaces at IPAPs of 13–24 cmH_2O and EPAPs of 2–8 cmH_2O, only one required intubation. These patients had similar normalization of physiologic parameters.[525] A number of other studies of patients with ACPE treated with bilevel PAP have yielded similar outcomes.[523,526–529] Unfortunately, simple mouthpiece or lipseal IPPV was not attempted in any of these studies.

Heart Transplantation

Criteria for heart transplantation for patients with idiopathic DCM include LVEF less than 25%.[369] Symptoms can be portentous and prognosis equally bleak for wheelchair-bound patients with DMD once LVEFs are observed to be below 25%. However, of a total of 582 heart transplant recipients in one study, only 6 had muscular dystrophy associated with end-stage cardiomyopathy. Three had DMD, one had BMD, one had EDMD, and one disorder was not precisely characterized. A more recent study reported the use of heart transplantation in patients with myotonic dystrophy.[530] Mean age was 25 years (range: 9–45 years). Mean follow-up was 40 months (range: 10 months to 7 years). One patient died suddenly at 27 months postoperatively. Recatheterization studies showed normal LVEF, and no signs of coronary artery disease were found.[531] In the U.S., although heart transplantation has been performed for several ambulatory patients with BMD, it has not been attempted for patients with DMD-associated cardiomyopathy.[395] Thus, since respiratory morbidity and mortality can be prevented, heart transplantation should no longer be ruled out as an effective means to prolong survival.

Other Treatments

Mural thrombi and embolic complications of DCM may be prevented by warfarin or aspirin when these drugs are not contraindicated.[373,532] However, Forst et al. reported that therapeutic warfarin levels are difficult to maintain in such patients. Since there are no reports of pulmonary emboli in uncomplicated patients with NMD and only one of our over 250 patients with DMD has had thrombotic complications even without anticoagulation therapy,[377] resort to warfarin therapy should be restricted to patients with cardiac arrhythmias or other complicating medical conditions that predispose to embolic phenomena.

Coenzyme Q10 (ubiquinone) has been reported to improve myocardial mitochondrial function, prevent cellular damage during myocardial ischemia and reperfusion, and ameliorate idiopathic DCM. It is taken by many patients with NMD, cardiovascular disease, and hypertension as well as by millions of unaffected Japanese.[533] In doses of 33 mg 3 times per day, it was reported to improve the cardiac function of patients with DMD.[534] Improvement was measured by impedance cardiography. Two double-blind trials of 100 mg per day in 27 patients, mostly with muscular dystrophy, resulted in "definitely improved physical performance," and higher dosages were recommended clinically.[535] Coenzyme Q has also been reported to improve myocardial mitochondrial function, prevent cellular damage during myocardial ischemia and reperfusion, and ameliorate idiopathic dilated cardiomyopathy. Nigro et al. have reported its use along with an ACE inhibitor, ramipril, to treat DCM.[467] Further research is necessary before routinely recommending this over-the-counter agent to patients with NMD

Creatine supplementation, which results in increases in phosphocreatine levels, has been reported to have a protective effect on cardiac tissues during ischemia, and it may have antiarrhythmic effects. Creatine also helps to protect diseased cardiac tissue from metabolic stress. Indeed, the hearts of patients with DCM have about 50% less creatine than normal.[111] For patients in heart failure taking creatine, ejection fractions are not increased, but exercise performance is improved. Creatine also lowers blood plasma cholesterol and triglycerides.

The indications for cardiac pacing are generally based on EKG abnormalities such as sick sinus syndrome or AV block with or without associated symptoms. However, a few recent articles investigated the use of pacemaker therapy as an alternative treatment for idiopathic DCM refractory to medical therapy.

Hochleitner et al. examined 16 patients with idiopathic DCM who presented with CHF and dyspnea at rest, severe hypotension, and pulmonary edema. All of them had a history of multiple hospital admissions during the previous year with at least one ICU admission. Coronary artery disease was excluded, and medical therapy with diuretics, digitalis, and vasodilators was unsuccessful. Seven patients were accepted as candidates for heart transplantation. All were evaluated by EKG, chest radiograph, MUGA, 24-hour Holter monitoring or telemetry, and M-mode and two-dimensional echocardiography within 1 week before and 2–14 days after pacemaker implantation. Permanent dual-chamber pacemakers with AV interval set at 100 ms in the DDD mode were implanted.[536]

After pacemaker implantation, clinical symptoms improved (a decrease from NYHA class IV to class III; $p < 0.0001$). LVEF increased from $16 \pm 8.4\%$ to $25.6 \pm 8.6\%$ ($p < 0.001$). Left atrial and right ventricular echocardiographic dimensions decreased from 48 ± 5 mm to 45 ± 5 mm and from 21 ± 4 mm to 25 ± 4 mm ($p < 0.01$), respectively. Systolic and diastolic blood pressures increased from 108 ± 29 mmHg to 126 ± 21 mmHg ($p < 0.01$) and from 67 ± 15 mmHg to 80 ± 11 mmHg ($p < 0.01$), respectively. No major complications from pacemaker implantation or DDD pacing were reported. All patients were discharged from the hospital within 3 weeks after implantation and returned to a relatively normal life.[536]

At 1-year follow-up, 12 patients maintained their clinical amelioration. Four of the heart transplant candidates were able to locate donor hearts. Strikingly, the remaining three candidates did not require the transplantation as the result of clinical amelioration. The other four patients died suddenly or from cerebrovascular disease.[536] In November of 1992, Hochleitner et al. published a similar 5-year longitudinal study of 17 patients refractory to medical therapy who were implanted with DDD mode pacemakers and noted similarly beneficial effects.[537]

The mechanism for the beneficial effects of DDD pacing is unknown. Postulated theories include decreases in preload, which may improve left ventricular function; decreases in ventriculoatrial flow with a resultant decrease in mitral valve regurgitation; and a reduction of the time delay between atrial systole and ventricular contraction to 100 ms. This time delay shift may correct the missed timing of atrial contraction that is believed to result in a loss of atrial contribution to ventricular outflow, thereby optimizing cardiac output.[536]

Case Reports

Case 1

A 21-year-old patient with DMD complained of loss of appetite, palpitations, frequent need for postural adjustments, and dyspnea when recumbent. He had been wheelchair-bound since 10 years of age. He was admitted to the hospital with complaints of cough, rapid breathing, general malaise, easy fatigability, palpitations, tachycardia (120 beats/min), sweating, pale lips and face, nausea, loss of appetite, abdominal discomfort, constipation, lower leg and facial edema, decreased urinary output, irritability, difficulties with concentration, and sleep disturbance. He exhibited a loud holosystolic murmur and a gallop rhythm. His CTR was 65.0%, and his chest radiograph demonstrated pulmonary congestion. No arrhythmias were seen on the EKG or with Holter monitoring. His LVEF was 17%; FS was 0.06; and LVDd was 68 mm on echocardiography, compatible with a diagnosis of DCM. ANP levels were 320 pg/ml; BNP levels were 887 pg/ml; and PNE levels were 2437 pg/ml. His VC was 660 ml (16% of predicted normal). His SpO_2 was 96%, and $EtCO_2$ was 32 mmHg when he sat. During sleep his SpO_2 mode was 96% with a low of 80%; the ratio of major $dSpO_2$ time to total sleep time was 1.3%; the mode of $EtCO_2$ was 38 mmHg with a high of 47 mmHg; and the mode of pulse was 120/min with a high of 162/min.

DCM and CHF were diagnosed. Lisinopril and digitalis were begun. Furosemide was added to balance intake and output. Serum levels of sodium and chloride and total protein were low and, therefore, supplemented intravenously. In 3 weeks, most cardiac symptoms were relieved, and neurohormone levels had decreased to 58 pg/ml for ANP, 210 pg/ml for BNP, and 911 pg/ml for PNE. Then metoprolol was administered and the dosage increased gradually. When the metoprolol dose was 20 mg per day, he once again complained of nausea, sleep disturbance, and palpitations. Metoprolol was decreased to 15 mg per day. After 2 weeks, 20 mg of metoprolol was tolerated. Ultimately, one 2.5 mg tablet of bisoprolol, 5 mg of lisinopril, 0.125 mg of digitalis, and 60 mg of furosemide twice daily resulted in relief of all cardiac symptoms and stabilized ANP at 58 pg/ml, BNP at 210 pg/ml, and PNE at 911 pg/ml.

During follow-up sleep monitoring, a SpO_2 mode of 93% and a low of 82% were noted. The ratio of major $dSpO_2$ time to total sleep time became 6.3%. The $EtCO_2$ mode became 47 mmHg with a high of 53 mmHg. The mode of the pulse was 92/min with a high of 128/min. Noninvasive IPPV was begun at night using a custom nasal interface and a PLV-100 portable volume ventilator (Respironics, Inc). In 3 weeks he could sleep through the night using nasal IPPV, and his nocturnal SpO_2 mode became 97% with a low of 86%. The ratio of major $dSpO_2$ time to total sleep time became 2.2%. The $EtCO_2$ mode during sleep became 43 mmHg with a high of 52 mmHg. His pulse mode during sleep decreased to 61/min with a high of 96/min. ANP levels became 68 pg/ml; BNP, 149 pg/ml; and PNE, 908 pg/ml. After 1 year 8 months, he has no cardiac symptoms and continues to have almost normal neurohormones (ANP = 36 pg/ml, BNP = 27 pg/ml, and PNE = 684 pg/ml). His CTR decreased to 51%. He could continue his daytime craft work and work with his computer. His mother was freed from having to change his position frequently.

Case 2

A 22-year-old patient with DMD had been wheelchair-bound since 10 years of age. His IQ was 119 (WISC-R). He attended a university. When he was 21 years old, his VC was 390 ml (9% of predicted normal), but he had no remarkable symptoms. Sleep monitoring demonstrated a SpO_2 mode of 93% with a low of 77%, a ratio of major $dSpO_2$ time to total sleep time of 16.8%, an $EtCO_2$ mode of 60 mmHg with a high of 68 mmHg, and a pulse mode of 90/min with a high of 137/min. Nocturnal noninvasive IPPV was begun using a custom nasal interface and a PLV-100 volume ventilator. Ventilator settings were adjusted for the first 3 nights to optimize SpO_2 and $EtCO_2$ levels, at which point his SpO_2 mode became 98% with a low of 91%; the ratio of major $dSpO_2$ time to total sleep time became 0%; $EtCO_2$ mode became 30 mmHg with a high of 42 mmHg; and pulse mode became 54/min with a high of 114/min.

No remarkable arrhythmias were observed on EKG or with Holter monitoring. His LVEF was 39%, and LVDd was 53 mm on echocardiography. ANP level was 15 pg/ml;

BNP, 20.9 pg/ml; and PNE, 1776 pg/ml. These levels decreased with nocturnal nasal IPPV to 11 pg/ml for ANP, 18.9 pg/ml for BNP, and 1218 pg/ml for PNE. This picture was compatible with latent cardiomyopathy with mild cardiac dysfunction.

After 10 months of nocturnal use of nasal IPPV, he was admitted to the hospital with complaints of increased bronchial secretions in the morning and difficulty in clearing them. His heart rate was 100/min; blood pressure, 121/77 mmHg; and CTR, 51% without obvious pulmonary congestion. Severe scoliosis, however, was noted on x-ray. His VC was 470 ml (11% of predicted normal); his SpO_2 was 97%; and his daytime $EtCO_2$ was 43 mmHg. During sleep using nasal IPPV, his SpO_2 mode was 98% with a low of 82%; the ratio of major $dSpO_2$ time to total sleep time was 3.7%; $EtCO_2$ mode was 22 mmHg with a high of 41 mmHg; and the pulse mode was 60/min with a high of 120/min. Therefore, his $EtCO_2$ was noted to be considerably lower than previously. Echocardiography demonstrated DCM with a LVEF of 37% and LVDd of 58 mm. Neurohormones were only slightly greater than normal with an ANP of 16 pg/ml, BNP of 26.2 pg/ml, and PNE of 367 pg/ml.

Mild CHF was diagnosed, and enalapril and digitalis were begun along with furosemide. In 3 weeks, sputum and cough were relieved. Then metoprolol was added. Four weeks later he was receiving one 2.5-mg tablet of bisoprolol, 5 mg of lisinopril, 0.125 mg of digitalis, and 60 mg of furosemide twice daily. This regimen stabilized neurohormone levels to an ANP less than 10 pg/ml, BNP of 8.8 pg/ml, and PNE of 333 pg/ml. Beta$_2$-microglobulin was 1.4 pg/ml (normal). Echocardiography performed after only 7 weeks of treatment by the same cardiologist demonstrated an improvement in LVEF to 54% and LVDd to 56 mm.

At 7 weeks, while continuing to use nocturnal nasal IPPV, his SpO_2 mode was 97% with a low of 90%, the ratio of major $dSpO_2$ time to total sleep time was 0%, $EtCO_2$ mode was 38 mmHg with a high of 46 mmHg, and pulse mode was 65/min with a high of 116/min. Therefore, the low $EtCO_2$ caused by his CHF was corrected by therapy for cardiac dysfunction.

In addition, it should be noted that this patient became an excellent glossopharyngeal breather. He learned the technique on his own to speak more loudly and to sing songs. Although his VC was only 470 ml, his $GP_{max}SBC$ and MICs were 2000 ml compared with 1400 while he had CHF. Likewise, his maximum unassisted CPF had increased from unmeasurable levels to 150 L/m, and assisted CPF had increased from 170 L/m during CHF to 260 L/m. Because of his earlier cough inadequacy, he had been unable to clear effectively the bronchial secretions that had increased in quantity because of CHF.

Case 3

A 19-year-old boy with DMD associated with Xp21 exon 43-45 deficiency developed a cough and increased sputum production. The condition was treated as a common cold, but the cough and sputum persisted for 1 month and his appetite diminished. On referral to us, in addition to cough, sputum, and loss of appetite he requested frequent change in body position and was pale, tachycardic (129/min), tired, and irritable. The patient's cardiac status was NYHA class IV. His blood pressure was 115/65 mmHg. His EKG demonstrated sinus tachycardia, and Holter monitoring showed frequent premature ventricular complexes (PVCs), 928 of 154,148 total beats, with 7 couplets and 1 run of PVCs. His CTR was 63.5%. He had no scoliosis. The LVEF was 22%, LVDd was 62 mm, and left atrial dimension/aorta diameter was 34/22 by echocardiography (greater than 1 indicates dilated atrium). BNP was 1180 pg/ml; ANP, 220 pg/ml; and PNE, 2522 pg/ml.

His respiratory function was unremarkable with a VC of 2900 ml (68.9% of predicted normal), PCF of 220 L/min, and sleep SpO_2 mode of 97% with a low of 88%. His ratio of major $dSpO_2$ time to total sleep time was 4.2%, but the $dSpO_2$s were frequent with each lasting less than a few minutes. Mode of $EtCO_2$ was 42 mmHg with a high of 47 mmHg. The mode of the pulse was 85/min with a high of 150/min.

Thus, his symptoms were attributed to CHF due to DMD-associated cardiomyopathy, and therapy was introduced with lisinopril, digitalis, furosemide, and potassium supplements. In 2 weeks, most cardiac symptoms were relieved, and neuroendocrine levels had decreased to BNP of 260 pg/ml, ANP of 140 pg/ml, and PNE of 439 pg/ml. Then metoprolol was administered, and the dosage was increased gradually. He ultimately received one 2.5-mg tablet of bisoprolol, 5 mg of lisinopril, 0.125 mg of digitalis, 40 mg of furosemide, and 60 mg of azosemide as a long-acting loop diuretic, potassium supplements, and 81 mg of aspirin daily with complete symptomatic relief. His pulse settled between 70 and 90 beats per minute (sometimes 40 during sleep), and blood pressure became 80–120/40–60 mmHg. He had no potentially hazardous arrhythmias. His CTR decreased to 58.9%. The LVEF increased to 35%, LVDd to 68 mm, and LA/AO was 39/23. Neuroendocrines stabilized at 211 pg/ml (BNP), 110 pg/ml (ANP), and 676 pg/ml (PNE).

His CPF improved to 465 L/min, and his MIC was found to be 3060 ml. Sleep desaturation, hypercapnia and tachycardia disappeared, and the mode of his pulse decreased to 70/min. He was not hospitalized and remained asymptomatic, and cardiac status remained stable over at least the next 5 years with BNP of 40 pg/ml, ANP of 10 pg/ml, PNE of 894 pg/ml, LVEF of 38%, and LVDd of 60 mm 5 years later.

Case 4

A 12-year-old boy with DMD had normal neuroendocrine levels and a CTR of 53.5%. One year later he complained of mild fatigue and dyspnea. His CTR was 60.0%, BNP had increased to 167 pg/ml, ANP to 100 pg/ml, and PNE to 616 pg/ml. He had no scoliosis, and his respiratory examination was unremarkable, including sleep oximetry and $EtCO_2$ monitoring. He had no renal dysfunction with normal serum beta$_2$-microglobulin.

One month later, an echocardiogram revealed a LVEF of 16%, LVDd/Ds of 65/60 mm, and LA/AO of 38/15 mm. He also developed tachypnea (32–42 breaths/min) along with dyspnea, especially when sitting up straight; facial pallor, especially during bowel movements; diaphoresis; loss of appetite; frequent need for changing body position; tachycardia (125–135 beats/min at rest); and decreasing urine volume. His cardiac status was NYHA class IV, blood pressure was 106/57 mmHg, and SpO_2 ranged from 94% to 97%. EKG demonstrated only sinus tachycardia. The CTR was 64% with pulmonary congestion. Neuroendocrines were elevated to BNP of 1130 pg/ml, ANP of 800 pg/ml, and PNE of 653 pg/ml.

He was diagnosed with severe CHF secondary to DMD-associated cardiomyopathy, and treatment was begun with lisinopril, 5 mg; digitalis, 0.125 mg; furosemide, 80 mg; spironolactone, 25 mg; and potassium supplements. In 1 week, most cardiac symptoms were relieved, and metoprolol was added. At 3 weeks his CTR had become 54%, congestion was cleared, BNP decreased to 49.9 pg/ml, ANP to 60 pg/ml, LVDd to 58 mm, LA to 20, and LVEF to 21%. After 2 months of therapy, LVDd was 60 mm and LVEF was 25%. He returned to junior high school.

Case 5

A twenty-three-year-old man with DMD was asymptomatic with normal neuroendocrines. One year later his BNP increased to 21.4 pg/ml, ANP to 22 pg/ml, and PNE to 446 pg/ml. His respiratory status remained unremarkable, but echocardiography demonstrated a LVEF of 30% and a LVDd of 63 mm. At that time, he did not note any cardiac symptoms, although he thought that he was fatiguing easily because of progressive muscle weakness. Treatment was initiated for cardiomyopathy with enalapril, 2.5 mg; digitalis, 0.125 mg; and bisoprolol, 2.5 mg. He reported that his fatigue was relieved. Eight months later his BNP was 9.5 pg/ml and ANP was less than 10 pg/ml. At 15 months LVDd was 51 mm, and LVEF was 40%.

Case 6

During a routine evaluation a 12-year-old boy with DMD had BNP of 101 pg/ml, ANP of 51 pg/ml, and PNE of 256 pg/ml. His echocardiogram demonstrated LVEF of 37% and LVDd of 63 mm. He complained of no cardiac symptoms, but DMD-associated cardiomyopathy was diagnosed and treatment begun. He received enalapril, 5 mg; lisinopril, 2.5 mg; digitalis, 0.125 mg; furosemide, 160 mg; and bisoprolol, 2.5 mg. BNP decreased to 62.6 pg/ml, ANP to 19 pg/ml, PNE to 189 pg/ml, and LVDd to 56 mm; LVEF increased to 43%. Neuroendocrines increased gradually over the next few years without symptoms. When he was 18 years old, BNP increased to 494 pg/ml, ANP to 480 pg/ml, and PNE to 407 pg/ml. LVEF was 32%, and LVDd was 64 mm. VC was now only 940 ml. He had many episodes of dSpO$_2$ and hypercapnia during sleep and began using nocturnal nasal high-span bilevel PAP. BNP decreased to 219 pg/ml, ANP to 120 pg/ml, and LVDd to 61 mm; LVEF remained at 32%. He is currently 21 years old and asymptomatic with stable neuroendocrine levels.

Cardioprotection

Cardioprotection is defined as preserving cardiac integrity by reducing or preventing myocardial damage.[538] Long-term pharmacotherapeutic cardioprotective interventions in patients with CHF and DCM cannot be explained exclusively by the hemodynamic effects of the pharmacologic agents. Cardioprotection is also facilitated by inhibition of the sympathoadrenergic and renin-angiotensin-systems by prevention of ventilatory insufficiency.

In ventilator users with ALS, circulatory collapse and sudden death have been related to sympathetic hyperactivity associated with high PNE levels.[539] Despite potential sympathoinhibitory mechanisms, it has been difficult to demonstrate any effect of ACE inhibitors (enalapril) on mean PNE concentration.[429,430] We have observed that patients with left ventricular dysfunction secondary to coronary artery disease have an increase in neurohormonal activity after several years of ACE inhibitor therapy. This finding is consistent with previous work suggesting that patients may become refractory to the effects of ACE inhibitors with time.[430,540] In a trial of vasodilator therapy for CHF, PNE levels increased from baseline after 5 years of ACE inhibitor therapy, and once they exceeded 900 pg/ml, the risk of mortality increased significantly.[429]

The sustained decrease in PNE levels in our patients with DMD after addition of beta blockers to a therapeutic regimen including ACE inhibitors is consistent with previous studies that demonstrated decreased arterial levels of PNE in response to concomitant use of these medications in patients with heart failure.[541] Beta blockers reduce sympathetic activity and restore more nearly normal levels of beta receptors in patients with CHF.[542] In addition to shielding the heart against the potentially toxic effects of increases in neurally released or circulating catecholamines, beta blockers may dampen central sympathetic outflow and improve the temporal coordination of excitation and contraction between innervated and denervated segments by restoring the uniformity of neural stimulation of the heart.[430] The lower levels of PNE may be secondary to improved myocardial function.[542] The reduction in total beta-adrenoceptor density in patients with CHF due to BMD[482] suggests both a causative mechanism linking sympathetic activation with adverse outcome and a therapeutic opportunity to improve prognosis by inhibiting sympathetic outflow and restoring normal beta-receptor levels.

Early detection and treatment of hypercapnia and DCM (Table 2) can have a cardioprotective effect and prolong the survival of patients with NMD and cardiomyopathy.[543] Hypercapnia is treated by noninvasive ventilation. Ventilatory insufficiency begins and is worst during sleep. Aggressive efforts are made to maintain normal alveolar ventilation around the clock to prevent cor pulmonale, to ensure effective clearance of airway secretions, and to avoid unnecessary oxygen administration.[544–546] Besides VC, SpO_2 and $EtCO_2$ are evaluated diurnally and overnight on a regular basis. Nocturnal nasal IPPV is instituted when patients are symptomatic for hypercapnia. With sufficient use of noninvasive IPPV, SpO_2 can be maintained within normal limits around the clock.[544,547]

Table 2.   Parameters for Cardiopulmonary Evaluation and Management

Pulmonary function
  Vital capacity
  Maximum insufflation capacity
  Cough peak flows, unassisted and assisted (Chapter 10)
  Capnography awake and asleep for peak values and respiratory rates
  Oximetry awake and asleep for mean, mode, and lowest values and heart rate

Cardiac function
  Radiographs for cardiothoracic ratio (CTR), chest diameter, deformity, Cobb angle
  Neuroendocrines: brain natriuretic peptide (BNP), atrial natriuretic peptide (ANP), plasma
    norepinephrine (PNE)
  Echocardiography for left ventricular ejection fraction (LVEF) or fractional shortening (FS),
    left ventricular diastolic diameter (LVDd), and left atrial diameter/aortic diameter
    (LA/AO)
  Electrocardiogram
  Holter EKG for heart rate (mean, maximum, minimum) and arrhythmias

Renal function
  $Beta_2$-microglobulin or cystatin-C

DCM, even when asymptomatic, is treated with ACE inhibitors and beta blockers in addition to diuretics and digitalis. Measurement of left ventricular size can help guide management decisions, including timing of the initiation of ACE inhibitors, diuretics, and beta-blocker therapy. Further study is required to establish that early medical intervention for subclinical cardiomyopathy can prevent DCM. In general, use of ACE inhibitors and beta blockers in patients with LVEFs below 35% appears to be helpful for stabilizing cardiac status.

In conclusion, we recommend ongoing monitoring of neuroendocrine levels and Holter monitoring at least annually in patients with generalized myopathic disease who are at risk for cardiomyopathy or conduction abnormalities. This recommendation is tempered by considerations for specific diagnoses. Although it is more difficult to suggest monitoring guidelines for patients with most forms of myopathic disease, reasonable recommendations can be made for the more common and severe cases of DMD. CHF can develop in patients with DMD as early as age 10 years and DCM as early as age 8 years. Thus, it may be reasonable to suggest cardiac screening of such patients from age 9 years. Because valvular dysfunction and other anatomic abnormalities may be present and echocardiograms tend to be more accurate in assessing early disease before spinal deformities become severe, echocardiograms may be appropriate every 3 years until signs of decreased cardiac contractility are present. At this point, yearly neuroendocrine monitoring is more cost-effective for monitoring cardiac deterioration and response to treatment. A similar strategy can be devised for other conditions.

Como quiera que sea eso, esa gente va por fuerza y no de su voluntad. De esa manera, aqui encaja la ejecución de mi oficio, que es deshacer las fuerzas y socorrer a los miserables.

Wherever it be that people go by force and against their wishes [as when coerced to undergo tracheostomy], it is my duty to undo the ignorance and save the unfortunate.

·❦· Don Quijote de La Mancha

THE PHYSICAL INTERVENTION STAGES

There is no doubt that all these [physicians] in their hunt for popularity by means of some novelty, did not hesitate to buy it with our lives. Hence, these wretched, quarrelsome consultations at the bedside of the patient, no consultant agreeing with another but he should appear to acknowledge a superior. Hence, too, that gloomy inscription on monuments: "It was the crowd of physicians that killed me."

—Pliny the Elder, AD 50

General management concerns often cut across clinical stages. For example, nutritional well-being, cardiac monitoring and management, and the use of medications often need to be considered throughout the clinical course. However, the deterioration in muscle strength that occurs in everyone with normal aging can occur at an accelerated pace in patients with neuromuscular diseases (NMDs). As a result, most patients with NMD go through three physical management stages in which orthopedic, habilitation, and respiratory concerns can be organized and addressed. Throughout these stages, the intelligent, self-directed patient needs to be prepared to assume responsibility for his or her own management decisions.

Chapter 6

Stage 1: The Ambulatory Stage

Stage 1 is the stage up to and including the period during which a patient walks. The goals are as follows:

1. Early diagnosis to facilitate family planning (Chapter 1)
2. Optimal nutrition (Chapter 3)
3. Early and informed counseling and psychological support to prevent counter-productive family psychodynamics, to encourage goal-oriented activities, and to prepare the patient for self-direction and decisions concerning therapeutic options
4. Prevention or reduction of soft tissue contractures of the chest and extremities
5. Prolongation of brace-free ambulation
6. Monitoring and prevention of cardiac complications (Chapter 5)

Early and Informed Counseling and Psychological Support

Because neuromuscular diseases (NMDs) are usually inherited, parents may feel inappropriately guilty. The affected child may be overly sheltered or infantilized, "spoiled" or favored over other children in the family. Such treatment can impede the child's emotional and intellectual maturation and cause resentment and adjustment difficulties in the other children. To make matters worse, parents of children with Duchenne muscular dystrophy (DMD) or infantile spinal muscular atrophy (SMA) often read or are told that their children will die young. As a result, goal-oriented activities are avoided, and achievement in school may not be encouraged. The stress of caring for a disabled child can also put enormous strains on financial resources, family dynamics, and the parents' marriage.

First of all, it is important to realize that many children with typical DMD or infantile SMA can live well into middle age if the intervention options are presented and used wisely. Thus, it should be assumed that the child will outlive his or her parents and, therefore, should learn how to make decisions and take responsibility for his or her own care. Goal-oriented activities should be encouraged; the child should be treated like siblings and encouraged to work hard in school. Guilt feelings should be resolved, with the help of psychotherapy if necessary, so that they do not interfere with the child's maturational process. Thus, early and informed counseling and, at times, psychological support are important to prevent counterproductive family psychodynamics, to encourage goal-oriented activities, and to prepare the patient and family for current and future physical medicine interventions. An overly protective environment should be discouraged.

Exercise

Skeletal Muscle

The muscle strength of children with DMD and other NMDs can be significantly increased by the use of strengthening exercises, provided that the strength of the muscle groups being exercised is greater than antigravity when the exercises are begun.[548] For example, straightening the legs with weights placed on the ankles substantially increases the strength of the quadriceps for patients with DMD.[549] Likewise, the muscles of people with any but the most rapidly progressive conditions (e.g., rapidly progressive amyotrophic lateral sclerosis [ALS]) can also be strengthened with resistance-type exercises, provided that the exercises are performed at least every other day or so while strength is good.[550–552] In a study of dynamic weight training 3 times per week for 9 weeks, arm strength increased by 19–34%, from −14% to 25% in the control arm and from 11% to 50% in the exercised leg for 5 patients with SMA, limb-girdle muscular dystrophy, or fascioscapulohumeral (FSH) muscular dystrophy. Endurance was also increased. Most of the gains in strength were believed to be due to neural adaptation rather than muscle hypertrophy.[553]

A study of strength training for 29 patients with hereditary motor and sensory neuropathy was consistent with the above results, whereas one study reported no beneficial or untoward effects of exercise for 33 patients with myotonic dystrophy.[554] In another study, however, 9 patients with myotonic dystrophy had a 35% increase in quadriceps strength with a supervised, progressive high-resistance training program using free weights (3 times per week for 12 weeks).[555] In yet another study of 12 patients with myotonic dystrophy, the combination of 50 mg of amitriptyline nightly with weight training resulted in significant improvements in strength for major limb muscles with greater than antigravity strength and decreases in myotonia, as quantified by measuring relaxation times.[42]

At 3 months, 14 patients with ALS who performed a program of moderate daily exercise showed less deterioration on a functional rating scale and Ashworth spasticity scale than 11 patients with ALS who did not exercise. At 6 months there was no significant difference between the groups, although a trend toward less deterioration was seen in the treated group. At 9 and 12 months there were too few patients in the groups for any meaningful comparison. Thus, a regular moderate physical exercise program apparently has a short-lived positive effect on disability in patients with ALS.[556]

Despite the ability to strengthen muscles that are still relatively strong, it has not been shown that, with the loss of strength due to age or advancing pathology, the strengthened muscles retain their strength for functional activities longer than muscles that are not exercised. Thus, it is possible that the subsequent rate of loss of strength in exercised muscles is correspondingly greater than the rate of loss in unexercised muscles so that both groups lose function at about the same time (Fig. 1). It is even possible that exercised muscles lose function somewhat sooner. Certainly, it is clear that muscles with less than antigravity strength cannot benefit and may actually be weakened by exercise. Furthermore, any discontinuation of exercise for even short periods results in rapid loss of the improved strength. In addition, for people with myopathies, serum muscle enzymes are increased after exercise. This increase may indicate muscle damage. Of interest, the muscles on the more frequently used dominant or preferred side are usually weaker than the muscles on the nondominant side.[548] Such findings do not point to long-term benefits from exercise.

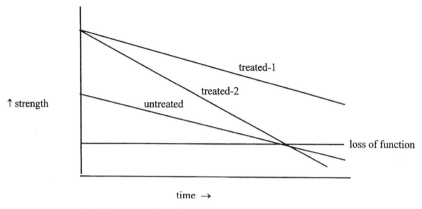

Figure 1. Possible rates of loss of strength of unexercised and exercised muscles.

In general, therefore, neither long-term benefit nor harm has been demonstrated for the muscles of people with any NMDs provided that muscles are not overstrained. If someone wishes to undertake a muscle-strengthening program, the program should be started early in the course of the disease and restricted to patients with slowly progressive disorders; furthermore, only submaximal resistance or aerobic exercise should be used. Vignos advised that patients undertake 2–3 hours per day of standing, walking, or swimming as long as they feel rested after a night's sleep.[557] Of course, it is hardly necessary to ask a child to keep active in this manner. All patients, however, should be encouraged to keep as active as possible with activities that they enjoy while avoiding muscle strain. It has been argued that endurance-type exercise may be more reasonable to recommend than resistance exercise training. However, in addition to muscle weakness, there are other physiologic limitations to exercise for patients with NMD. For example, for children with DMD vs. unaffected children of the same age, maximum work capacity is 400 vs. 600 kg/min; maximum oxygen consumption, 0.37 vs. 1.35 L/min; maximum heart rate, 136 vs. 189 beats per minute; cardiac stroke volume, 41 vs. 60 ml; perfusion, 5.2 vs. 11 L/min; and maximum ventilation, 8.2 vs. 36.9 L/min, respectively.[558] Once respiratory muscle dysfunction is also severe, however, poliomyelitis survivors and patients with ALS have been shown to have increased exercise tolerance and slower motor decline by exercising while using nocturnal noninvasive bilevel PAP or IPPV.[559] On the other hand, a recent study suggested that the use of mouthpiece IPPV was not beneficial during exercise for patients with severe scoliosis.[560]

Respiratory Muscle

Inspiratory resistive exercises include voluntary isocapnic hyperpnea, inspiratory resistive loading, and inspiratory threshold loading. These exercises are provided by breathing through inexpensive training devices, typically for 15–20 minutes daily for 8–10 weeks. With inspiratory resistive loading, subjects breathe through narrow orifices with adjustable diameters. While doing so, however, subjects consciously or unconsciously reduce their inspiratory flow rates and lengthen inspiratory time to reduce the severity of the imposed loads, thereby decreasing the effort. Isocapnic hyperpnea is hyperventilation with rebreathing of exhaled air to avoid hypocapnia. It is less convenient and often impossible for people with primarily ventilatory impairment. Consequently, of the three methods, "targeted" or threshold inspiratory muscle training has been recommended. This method ensures adequate intensity of inspiratory muscle activity throughout training by making the patient unable to generate flow through the device until a predetermined pressure is achieved. The patient is also provided feedback about the inspiratory flow rates through the resistor or the inspiratory pressure generated by flow through the resistor. The settings of the device are adjusted to increase difficulty as patients improve.

The many studies employing these devices for people with lung disease concluded that, although lung function could not be improved in general, breathing endurance improved because trained patients could breathe at 30% to 90% of their maximum voluntary ventilation or against greater pressures for longer periods. Three studies also reported a significant increase in maximal sniff or global inspiratory muscle strength.[561–563] Results of studies of patients with NMD were positive, provided that the patient's vital capacity (VC) was greater than 30% of predicted normal and carbon dioxide levels were normal when the exercises were begun.[557] Likewise, a recent study of post-polio nocturnal ventilator users, in which nine of 10 patients had VC greater than 30% of normal, demonstrated improved inspiratory endurance and claimed generally improved functioning despite lack of better total body endurance.[564] In another study of 21 children with DMD who were about 12 years old and used respiratory muscle training with both resistive inspiratory and expiratory loads daily for 6 months, maximum inspiratory and expiratory pressures and respiratory load perception (Borg scale) were monitored for 1 year. Training resulted in improvements in both maximum inspiratory pressures (mean improvement of 20 cmH$_2$O) and maximum expiratory pressures (mean improvement of 27 cmH$_2$O), whereas controls showed no improvement. Although benefits in maximum pressures were lost 3 months after termination of the exercise, respiratory load perception decreases were maintained for at least 1 year.[565]

Another study suggested possible benefits in expiratory muscle strength from resistance exercise training.[566] Ten patients with multiple sclerosis, a condition with clinical severity that can vary from day to day, completed a 10-week course of daily use of a threshold training device and showed an increase in maximum mouth expiratory pressures from 19.4 cmH$_2$O to 72 cmH$_2$O. Unfortunately, it is unclear how this increase translates into improved CPF either when the patient is well or, more importantly, in the presence of chest infections.

Evidence indicates that inspiratory muscle training is ineffective in rapidly progressive conditions. In one study, only patients whose VC decreased by less than 10% per year benefited from training.[562] Thus, physiologic ameliorations would not be expected for patients with rapidly progressive motor neuron diseases (MNDs). Likewise, no evidence suggests that any benefits can be achieved by patients with VC below 30%, nor has inspiratory or expiratory resistive exercise been shown to improve VC, delay the need for ventilator use, or decrease the risk of respiratory failure during intercurrent chest infections. Indeed, patients often begin to require inspiratory muscle aids (ventilatory assistance) once VC declines below 30%.[567] Episodes of respiratory failure in such patients are due primarily to expiratory (cough) muscle weakness rather than inspiratory muscle dysfunction.[14] There have been few attempts at increasing expiratory muscle function for patients with NMD.

Early Intervention to Prevent Muscle, Joint, and Chest Wall Contractures

The goals of therapy are to optimize function, maintain functional mobility, and maximize quality of life. For people with NMD, loss of function is caused by both muscle weakness and musculotendinous contractures. Many patients with much less than anti-gravity strength at all lower-limb pivots can remain on their feet and walk, provided that they have little contracture. On the other hand, people with good strength may not be able to walk if hip, knee, and ankle contractures are severe. These contractures hamper ambulation and other lower-limb activities, and immobility can result in bony under-development, articular deformities, and joint dislocations. Upper-limb contractures, too, can hamper activities and result in discomfort.[568] Joint contractures were one of the most common causes of pain in patients with slowly progressive NMDs and have been found to be associated with fatigue, decreased social and physical functioning, sleep disturbance, and difficulties in coping.[569]

The physical and orthopedic treatment goals are to prevent or assuage pain, to prevent contractures, to maintain the balance of strength at each joint, to prolong the ability to walk safely with minimal or no bracing, and to increase or substitute for arm function. Patients who cannot walk can benefit from improved cosmesis and greater function and comfort through relief of contractures, whereas in ambulatory patients appropriate management can prolong the period of brace-free ambulation.[12,570] These approaches are particularly important for children with DMD as well as people with milder muscular dystrophies, certain children with type 3 SMA, and poliomyelitis survivors.

Even more important than limb range of motion (ROM) is ROM of the chest wall and lungs. Patients do not die from having tight ankles, whereas a tight chest wall that does not permit sufficient insufflation volumes to optimize lung recoil for effective coughing can result in pneumonia and acute respiratory failure.

Lower-limb Contractures in Ambulatory Patients

There are at least four physical approaches to minimize lower-limb contractures and preserve the ability to walk: the use of supportive physical and occupational therapy mobilization techniques; therapy plus splinting; late surgical correction of contractures with bracing and physical therapy; and contracture prevention by early surgery.

Supportive Physical and Occupational Therapy

Because the use of strengthening exercises has not been shown to be beneficial over the long term and because children with NMD usually do not have the physiologic capabilities to perform aerobic conditioning exercises,[558] the most important goal of physical therapy is to instruct patients and care providers in how to perform active-assistive exercises and ROM. Any normal limb joint has a certain arc of movement (ROM) through which it can normally move or be moved. However, there is usually an imbalance of strength at joints, and joints may be kept in attitudes that utilize only a small fraction of their ROM (e.g., patients who sit in a wheelchair most of the day). Results may include skin, muscle, tendon, and ligament shortening, which over time result in joint "contractures" (e.g., knee and hip flexion contractures in wheelchair users). Many of the exercises and joint mobilization techniques taught by physical and occupational therapists are designed to limit the development of joint contractures.

ROM exercises involve putting (weak) limb joints actively or passively through full normal movement (ROM). When the muscle strength of the limb is less than the strength needed to move the joint through its full ROM, personal assistance is required (active-assisted exercises). Diligent performance of full ROM exercises to stretch tightening tissues decreases the rate at which joint contractures develop. Although ROM may be performed on weak limb joints for at least a few minutes several times a day, no amount of ROM can entirely prevent contractures from developing when muscle strength imbalance is severe or the patient becomes confined to a chair. When done less than several times per day, ROM exercises have not been reported to make a significant difference.

The stronger, tighter muscles that cause joint contractures need to be stretched. It is equally important to stretch the plantarflexors (Fig. 2), hamstrings (Fig. 3), and hip flexors (Fig. 4). Some indirect evidence suggests that the regular use of stretching has prolonged the ability to walk for children with DMD. In 1954, before the use of ROM became more systematic, one-third of 90 children with DMD ceased to walk before 6 years of age.[571] Now, however, virtually all children undergo regular stretching, and even without other treatment (prednisone therapy or surgery), loss of the ability to walk generally occurs between 8.5 and 9.5 years of age and rarely before age 6 years.

Physical Therapy and Leg Splinting

A second approach is to combine ongoing lower-limb stretching with splinting of lower limb joints at rest to discourage the progression of contractures and loss of ROM. The joints of weak limbs are splinted in maximum extension or, for the ankle, conventionally in neutral position. Resting splints are most often used for the entire lower limbs during sleep and for the ankles when the patient is in a wheelchair and can no longer

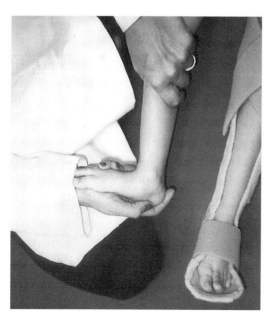

Figure 2. Passive stretching of the right ankle joint to its maximum dorsiflexed position—in this case, neutral. This position is about 35° less than normal maximum dorsiflexion. A long leg resting splint is also used on the left leg to stretch the hamstrings and ankle dorsiflexors.

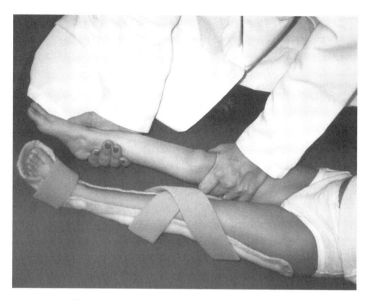

Figure 3. Passive stretching of the right hamstrings.

walk. One study reported 23% less contracture development in patients with DMD treated by passive stretching combined with the use of night splints vs. passive stretching alone.[572] In another study of 246 patients with DMD, the ability to walk was reportedly prolonged to a mean of 10.3 years of age by the combined use of daily stretching and resting splints.[573] Nevertheless, many patients, especially children, are resistant to the use of resting splints. Splints can be expensive, and contractures may progress despite stretching and splinting. Because of growth, long-term casting of full-length lower limb

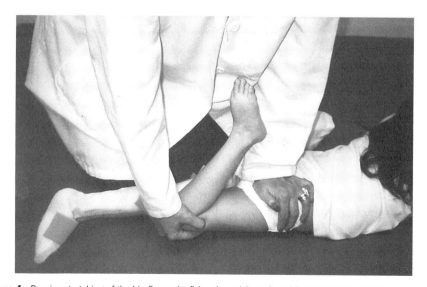

Figure 4. Passive stretching of the hip flexors by fixing the pelvis and applying pressure to extend the hip joint.

splints needs to be repeated about every 6 months. Short-term progressive serial casting can provide sustained stretching of the joint at the maximal angle tolerated. Casts can be reapplied every few days to change the angle and progressively stretch the joint. This process can temporarily increase ROM for joints without fixed contracture.

Late Surgery, Bracing, and Physical Therapy

The only way to restore full normal ROM to a contracted joint is through surgery that stretches or "releases" the joint and its tightened soft tissues. The most commonly used surgical protocol to reverse lower-limb contractures in muscular dystrophy was essentially described in 1845 for an 11-year-old patient with DMD;[6] the protocol was redescribed in 1959.[574] It includes surgical release of tight flexor muscles at the hips, knees, and ankles (Achilles tendon) and release of the iliotibial bands at the knees and hips once the child begins to fall frequently and to require a wheelchair (Fig. 5). Surgical iliotibial band releases followed by physical therapy and long leg bracing (Fig. 6) have been shown to prolong the ability to stand and walk for some children with DMD (Fig. 7). After "late" surgical intervention in this manner, long leg bracing is always required for continued ability to stand and walk. With this approach, Vignos et al. reported a prolongation of standing and independent ambulation to age 11.5 ± 1.2 years and of walking with assistance to age 12.7 ± 1.4 years for children with DMD treated at the mean age of 9.9 years.[575] More recently, a review was published of 30 publications reporting the outcomes of 35 studies of the use of knee-ankle-foot orthoses, mostly following lower limb tendon release surgery. Seven of the studies reported continued ability to stand for at least 1 year in 75.1% of patients, for 2 years in 47.9%, and for 3 years

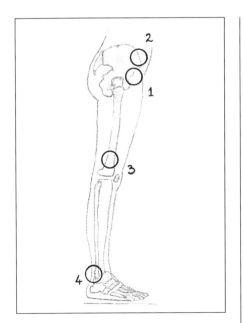

Figure 5. Typical sites for subcutaneous releases of the tensor fascial lata (1), iliotibial band (2 and 3), hamstrings (3), and heel cord (4).

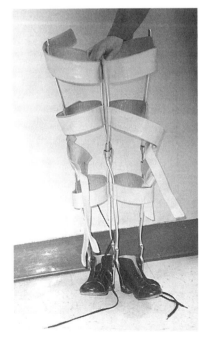

Figure 6. Long leg braces.

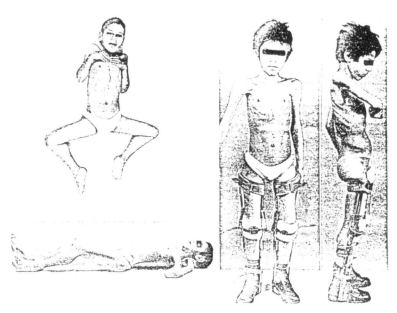

Figure 7. Although some patients can walk using long leg braces after late subcutaneous lower-limb musculotendinous releases, many patients can stand but not attain functional ambulation.

in 24.3%. Of these patients, the median for independent walking was 24 months; for assisted walking, 36.2 months; and for standing, 50.5 months.[576] It was unclear how long the patients would have remained on their feet without the interventions and whether the interventions prolonged functional walking. The boys who benefited most had a relatively slow rate of deterioration and were highly motivated. Unfortunately, it is not possible to predict when any particular patient will benefit from late surgery and tolerate long leg bracing.

In addition to release of lower-limb contractures, some surgeons also transfer the tibialis posterior, normally a plantarflexor and inverter of the foot (Fig. 8), to insert into the second or third cuneiform on the dorsum of the foot. This procedure makes a dorsiflexor out of a plantarflexor and normalizes the active ROM of the previously contracted ankle.[12] Since 1970 up to 40% of Muscular Dystrophy Association clinics[577] have reported patients who underwent tibialis posterior transfers in combination with Achilles tendon and iliotibial band releases when it was believed that the "children were about to lose their independent walking." One study reported satisfactory results in 26 of 28 transfers for patients with DMD.[578] In another study of 57 patients with DMD, the 34 patients undergoing tibialis posterior transfers stopped walking at 11.2 years of age compared with 10.3 years of age for patients who did not have the surgery. Ninety-four percent of the operated feet continued to have clinically satisfactory results at a mean of 8.5 years after surgery. The investigators believed that, regardless of the desire to continue ambulation, all patients with DMD should undergo tibialis posterior transfers.[579]

Physical therapy can be of paramount importance after late lower-limb orthopedic surgery. Joint-stretching, general strengthening, and conditioning exercises are important for recovery as well as for resumed ambulation and training in the use of long leg bracing.

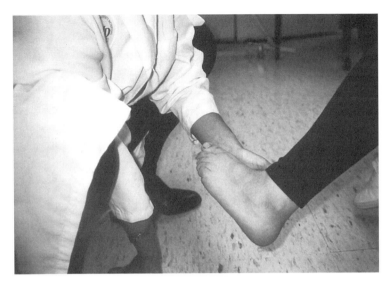

Figure 8. Examining the strength of the tibialis posterior with the foot plantarflexed and inverted.

Progressive creeping, crawling, rolling, and walking can make the difference between the success or failure of this procedure. When the tibialis posterior is transferred, the physical therapist re-educates the patient in the new use (dorsiflexion) of the muscle.

The disadvantages of this approach include the need for surgery, the expense of bracing, the time needed to don and remove the braces, the weight of the braces on already weak legs, the possibility that despite the expense and effort the patient will not tolerate the braces or will fail to benefit from them, the several months of daily physical therapy required to train the patient in their use, and the fact that the braces can be outgrown. In one study, modular long leg braces were 23% lighter, resulted in 10% energy savings during ambulation, and increased walking speed by 8% while reducing cost and requiring only 1 hour to fabricate.[580] Despite the disadvantages of long leg bracing, 115 of 166 MDA clinics (69%) reported at least the occasional use of long leg bracing with or without precedent orthopedic surgery.[577] The use of swivel walkers can be an alternative to surgery and long leg bracing for continued verticalization and walking for patients no longer able to walk safely otherwise.[581]

Short leg bracing—that is, bracing the ankle at about 90%—can prevent foot drop and tripping on the toes; it can also increase ankle stability and thereby decrease falls. Thus, ankle-foot braces can be quite useful for patients with mild NMDs, especially Charcot-Marie-Tooth disease, that predominantly cause weakness of the ankles and feet. Their use, however, is less effective and often ineffective in helping to maintain ambulation in children with DMD, SMA, or other NMDs. The reason is simple: there is no effective bracing for hip and trunk weakness, which are the predominant problems for most people with NMD. In the presence of severe weakness at the hips, fixing the angle of the ankle with a brace can make it more difficult to rise from a chair because this activity normally requires bending the knees and ankles. The procedure also slows walking, and the additional weight at the ankle can be a hindrance. For people with good strength in plantarflexion but not dorsiflexion, braces with ankle joints should be used if at all possible. They can be spring-loaded to assist the dorsiflexors yet permit plantarflexion by allowing continuing activity of the plantarflexor muscles. After late surgical release of contractures, the use of ankle-foot braces along with Lofstran crutches can be an alternative to long leg bracing for prolongation of standing and walking in some patients (Fig. 9).

Prophylactic Surgery

It was first recognized in 1971 that lower-limb surgery "need not be delayed until bracing becomes inevitable."[557] Various musculotendinous releases and tibialis posterior transfers were followed by physical therapy in 16 children with DMD aged 8–14 years (average age: 9 years). Four children were able to continue brace-free ambulation. The French physiatrist Yves Rideau and his group subsequently described the use of lower-limb surgical interventions much earlier, usually for children between 4 and 6 years of age.

The early surgical approach is indicated at the onset of lower-limb contracture development—typically at the point when ankle dorsiflexion cannot exceed 15°, lumbar lordosis is greater than normal with passive hip extension less than 20°, and iliotibial band contracture causes hip abduction to greater than 25° from the sagittal plane with the knee flexed 90° (Fig. 10). The release procedure includes wide resection of the fascia lata and iliotibial bands, tensor fascia lata, hamstrings, and heel cords (Fig. 11). The tibialis posterior need not always be transferred initially, but the removal of the iliotibial bands and fascia lata requires a more extensive outer thigh incision than simple iliotibial band resection at the knees.[582] When simple subcutaneous resections are performed and the iliotibial bands and fascia lata are not thoroughly removed, connective tissue overgrows the resections and the contractures redevelop in a matter of weeks to months. Although the hamstrings may not be very tight and knee ROM may be essentially intact at the time of surgery, if the hamstrings are not lengthened along with the releases at the hips, thighs, and ankles, knee flexion contractures eventually become the limiting factor in prolonging ambulation.

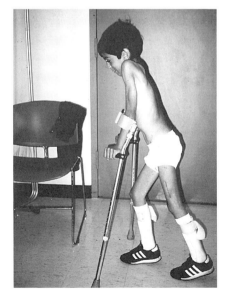

Figure 9. Patient with Duchenne muscular dystrophy undergoing late intervention that included wide resection of the iliotibial bands and tibialis posterior transfers. However, because the procedure was delayed, he could ambulate only by using Lofstran crutches and molded ankle-foot orthoses.

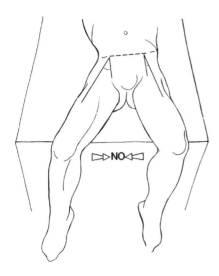

Figure 10. Iliotibial band tightness is estimated by the angle between the thigh and the sagittal plane with the knee flexed 90°. (Courtesy of Dr. Yves Rideau.)

In addition to being indicated at onset of contractures, the surgery is also indicated while quadriceps retain greater than antigravity strength and before Gowers time begins to increase.[582] Gowers time is the time required for a patient to rise to a standing position from a sitting position on the floor. Patients tend to "climb up themselves." As weakness develops after 4 years of age, it eventually takes longer to climb up. As Gowers time increases, the benefits of early lower extremity surgery diminish.

Earlier intervention can essentially prevent development of contractures, eliminate the need for ongoing physical therapy or splinting, help preserve the strength of the weaker muscles (muscles that otherwise would have been stretched out of their optimal length for contraction by the stronger contralateral muscles), normalize standing balance, eliminate any tendency to fall, preserve quality of movement, and prolong the ability to walk without bracing.[582] Early surgical intervention was also found to be safer and better tolerated

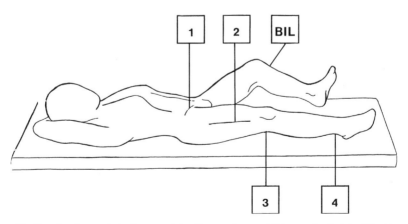

Figure 11. The sites for prophylactic musculotendinous releases: (1) tensor fascia lata, (2) wide resection of the iliotibial band and fascia lata, (3) hamstrings release, and (4) heel cord release with all procedures done bilaterally. (Courtesy of Dr. Rideau.)

than late approaches. The postsurgical rehabilitation process is much shorter, and the vicious cycle of weakness, contracture, further weakness, and further contracture with difficulty in walking is broken.

Whereas the late surgical approach requires long leg bracing and several months of intensive daily physical therapy to permit continued ability to walk, the protocol after early surgical intervention is simpler. No particular activity is undertaken for about 2–3 days, and the ankle is maintained in dorsiflexion by a simple elastic wrap or a light provisional splint for about 2 weeks. Free walking is permitted by postoperative day 3. General conditioning exercises and progressive resumption of ambulation are undertaken for 2 weeks. No lower-limb bracing is used; regular outpatient or home physiotherapy is continued for 2 months. Normal daily activities are encouraged. Fatigue is avoided. Joint stretching, strengthening, and reconditioning exercises are important for quick recovery. Tibialis posterior transfers necessitate ankle casting for 1 week before bivalving the cast or using a splint.

In a study of over 200 patients undergoing early lower-limb releases, Forst et al. reported prolongation of brace-free ambulation by a mean of 1.25 years for patients with DMD and longer for patients with less rapidly progressive conditions.[570] In another study of 32 children with DMD who underwent surgery at a mean of 6.1 years of age, all children had complete and durable correction of contractures and were still ambulating 3.4 years later.[583] In a prospective evaluation of duration of ambulation in patients with DMD, seven patients were treated with early lower-extremity musculotendinous surgery, followed by a definitive course of rehabilitation for contractures. They ambulated with little difficulty. Six others were treated just before or after becoming wheelchair-dependent. Predicted posttreatment duration of ambulation was calculated from established clinical criteria. Actual prolongation of brace-free ambulation after treatment was a mean of 0.8 years greater than predicted for the group as a whole but 1.16 ± 0.63 years for the group treated early compared with 0.65 ± 0.55 years for the group treated later. The number of falls significantly decreased from 84 ± 87 to 1 ± 1 per month postoperatively ($p < 0.05$), but the speed of ambulation over a distance of 10 yards decreased from 10.2 ± 4 to 12.1 ± 7.3 seconds/10 yards. Three patients who had tibialis posterior transfers retained greater than antigravity dorsiflexor strength and continued to wear normal footwear 2.5, 3.7, and 4.0 years after loss of ambulation. Thus, ambulation becomes more stable and brace-free ambulation is prolonged by a comprehensive program of early orthopedic surgery and rehabilitation (Figs. 12 and 13).

Patients with DMD, BMD, LGMD, polymyositis, and SMA type 3 have presented with similar pathokinesiology and a similar pattern of musculotendinous contractures. Patients with all of these conditions have benefited from the "prophylactic" (early) surgical approach at our institution. Patients with greater hip and knee strength and minimal hip or knee contractures may require only Achilles tendon lengthening and possibly tibialis posterior transfers without tendon releases at the hips and knees. Surgical releases should never be limited to the ankles for patients with DMD.

Despite the clear advantages and patient and parent satisfaction,[12] few clinicians offer the early intervention approach for children with DMD. In a recent survey of NMD clinic neurologists, no early form of lower-limb surgery was offered to children with DMD in 94% of clinics, whereas late surgery with long leg bracing was performed in 62 clinics (37%).[577] Unfortunately, many physicians are apprehensive about performing surgery on children who as yet have little difficulty in walking.

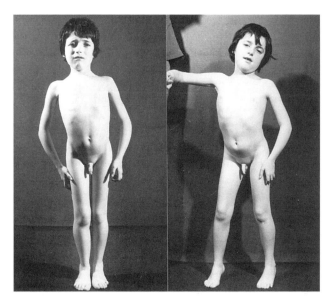

Figure 12. Patient with Duchenne muscular dystrophy before (*right*) and after (*left*) early surgery, including wide resection of iliotibial bands and fascia lata. The child regained standing balance and fall-free ambulation with this intervention.

Lower-limb Contractures in Nonambulatory Patients

Once a patient is wheelchair-dependent, soft tissue surgery will not result in functional restoration of ambulation. Residual foot and ankle deformities secondary to persistent muscular imbalance around the ankle and foot can still be remedied surgically. Releases to relieve equinus deformity should be considered in patients with severe ankle or foot pain, skin breakdown and/or ulceration, and inability of the foot and ankle to

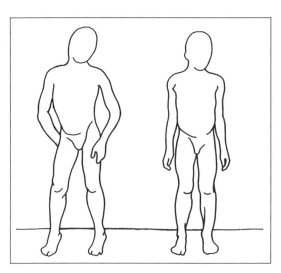

Figure 13. Attitude of typical 9-year-old child with Duchenne muscular dystrophy untreated (*left*) and after prophylactic musculotendinous releases (*right*).

accept reasonable costing and available shoe wear. Resting ankle-foot splints need to be worn after surgery to prevent recurrence of contractures.[584] Keeping the feet flat on foot rests, even off-set foot rests, can be helpful.

After loss of the ability to walk, iliotibial band contractures tend to accelerate. Use of a custom-made dry flotation (ROHO) wheelchair cushion with a sunken middle portion and separately inflated lateral portions to provide adduction to the thighs has been reported to reduce iliotibial band contractures by 13° or 34% after 9 weeks.[585]

Standers, both prone and vertical, can give support to the trunk, hips, knees, and ankles of nonambulating patients, both to stretch lower extremity contractures and to provide weight-bearing to impede osteoporosis (Grandstand II, Prime Engineering, Fresno, CA; Giraffe and Buffalo Tilt Systems, Snug Seat Inc., Mathews, NC; Kaye Products Inc., Hillsborough, NC). Standers can be especially useful for children who are unable to procure or operate standing motorized wheelchairs.

Hip Dislocation

Hip dislocation is common in infants with NMDs. The incidence is especially high in those who are never able to walk and who do not receive standing therapy by being provided with standers and standing wheelchairs (Chapter 7). In one study, 31% of the hips of 35 patients with SMA type 2 were normal, 38% had unilateral or bilateral subluxation, and 11% had dislocation. There was a linear correlation between migration percentage and age and between migration percentage and scoliosis. Of 14 patients with SMA type 3, 50% had normal hips, 28% had unilateral or bilateral subluxation, and 22% had dislocation.[586] In a study of long-term follow up of 4 patients with SMA after hip relocation surgery, all hips dislocated again.[587] Considering this finding and the fact that we have found no adult patients with SMA type 2 who were symptomatic from hip dislocation, surgical intervention for hip dislocation is of questionable utility. In patients with SMA type 3 who were still able to walk and in patients with SMA type 2 who were provided with orthotics for standing or walking, no hip dislocations were reported.[576] The best current treatment approach is to maximize standing time and, for small patients constrained to using wheelchairs, to foster hip abduction with the use of pommels or, at least, by putting pillows between the legs.

Hip dislocation once was thought to be uncommon in DMD. In one study of 54 patients, however, hip radiographs revealed unilateral subluxation in 15 patients, bilateral subluxation in 1 patient, and unilateral dislocation in 3 patients. The possible relationship between subluxation and pelvic tilt calls for better control of sitting posture to prevent tilt. Maintenance of sitting balance and comfort, in addition to early spinal stabilization for scoliosis and pelvic tilt, may delay or prevent progressive subluxation of the hip.[588] Although spinal surgery can decrease pelvic tilt, hip surgery does not.[589]

Scapular Winging

Scapular winging can be prominent in patients with FSH muscular dystrophy and occasionally in patients with SMA or nerve injury. As the deltoid contracts, the arm attempts to move in a normal fashion. However, because the scapula is no longer stable, it wings and rotates under the forces of the long lever arm of the upper limb and scapula complex. Mechanical fixation of the scapula to the thoracic wall provides a stable fulcrum on which the deltoid can exert its action on the humerus and abduct the arm without rotation of the scapula.[590] Scapular stabilization has been performed by scapulocostal fusion. This procedure often permits the deltoids to raise the arms over the head. Two studies reported an average gain in shoulder flexion and abduction of 30° and excellent improvements in function.[590,591] Another study reported an improvement in abduction of 60° and gains in strength for carrying and lifting.[592] Complications included a temporary brachial plexus palsy and a frozen shoulder, but all but one patient was pleased with the results. A modified method of operative fixation of the scapula to the chest or interscapulo-scapulocostal scapulopexy, using polyester laces, preserves greater mobility between the scapula and the chest wall and conserves VC by comparison with scapulothoracic arthrodesis.[593] Another approach is to stabilize the scapula by using an inflatable orthosis placed between the scapula and an external restraint, such as a spinal jacket. In one patient using this device, arm elevation increased by 35° or 37%, and functional improvement was achieved in the use of the hand around the head and face.[594]

Charcot-Marie-Tooth Disease

Patients with Charcot-Marie-Tooth disease (CMT) have stocking-glove weakness and sensory deficit that often result in severe ankle and foot deformities. Both pes cavus and equinocavovarus deformities occur. Such patients tend to trip on their feet. Because proximal muscle strength is usually good, they walk better using molded ankle-foot orthotics (MAFOs). The MAFOs also more evenly distribute weight and relieve excessive pressure, most often on the metatarsal heads.

In addition to orthotics, patients with CMT usually benefit from soft-tissue releases to correct foot deformities. Release of tight intrinsic foot muscles can delay or obviate the need for triple arthrodesis or ankle fusion.[595] One study advised against tibialis posterior transfers as part of staged treatment that includes a possible future hindfoot stabilization.[578]

Triple arthrodesis prevents mobility of the tarsal joint and consequently increases stress on the ankle joint. Among patients who eventually undergo triple arthrodesis, 20-year follow-up assessments have been rated as good to excellent for 24%, fair for 30%, and poor for 47%. Patients with poor results had severe impairment in function and required orthotics to walk. Progressive muscle imbalance resulted in recurrent cavovarus deformity after a period of satisfactory alignment. Degenerative joint changes of the ankle and intrinsic foot joints were noted in two-thirds of the feet. Results in patients with CMT have been much inferior to those in post-polio patients who have intact sensation. Thus, good position sense is important before recommending triple arthrodesis or any other surgical procedure.[596] It has been suggested that triple arthrodesis should be reserved as a salvage procedure limited to patients with severe, rigid deformity.[597,598]

Upper-limb Contractures

Arm, hand, and finger weakness, tightness, and resulting deformities are commonly neglected problems. Some infants with SMA present with severe contractures at all major joints at birth, a condition known as arthrogryposis. More commonly, infants with

SMA have no contractures at birth but develop them subsequently. In patients with DMD, limitations of wrist movement begin by 8 years of age, and wrist, elbow, and shoulder contractures begin between 8 and 14 years of age. People with adult-onset conditions such as ALS may not develop significant contractures until the stage of prolonged survival. Deformities accelerate loss of strength and function.

A recent survey of the parents of children with infantile SMA or birth-onset muscle diseases, as well as a survey of children and adolescents with these conditions, revealed that the risk for long-term arm discomfort correlated with extent of joint contractures. Elbow flexion contractures greater than 25° (Fig. 14) were reported to hamper 17% of activities of daily living, and 59% of patients complained of contracture-associated hindrance of at least one daily activity.[568] Contractures are also felt to detract from appearance.

Like leg contractures, therefore, arm contractures should be prevented. However, there has been no attempt at studying the effects of ROM therapy, positioning, bracing, or surgery. At this time it may be most appropriate to recommend arm and hand along with leg ROM and stretching exercises several times a day. The use of resting splints for the wrists and fingers is warranted to maintain comfort and safety for people who have little or no remaining hand function (Fig. 15). The fact that a multidisciplinary approach including physical therapy, splinting, and surgery has been effective in ameliorating lower-limb contractures implies that effective treatment strategies may be possible for upper-limb contractures as well. A dynamic Orthoplast splint has been used to provide ROM and function for patients with motor neuron disease who have weak upper-limb extensors but functional flexors.[599] One group is working on developing a functional, body-powered exoskeletal upper-limb orthosis for patients with limited arm strength.[600] An overhead sling arm support system has been devised to facilitate function for sidelying children with SMA type 1 (twinscs@aol.com).

Likewise, although tendon transfers have been useful for normalizing lower-limb ROM and facilitating walking, there has only been one report of selective upper-extremity tendon transfers performed for one patient with SMA type 4. This 25-year-old patient with weak deltoids and wrist and finger extensors underwent the following transfers: flexor digitorum superficialis III to extensor pollicis longus, flexor digitorum superficialis IV to extensor digitorum communis II-V, flexor carpi radialis to extensor carpi radialis longus, extensor carpi ulnaris to extensor carpi radialis brevis, palmaris longus to abductor pollicis longus and extensor pollicis brevis, and triceps to biceps tendons. A long arm cast was applied for 5 weeks from the fifth postoperative day and was

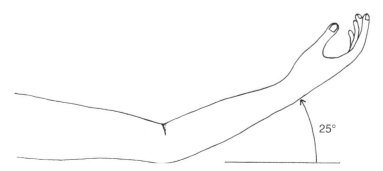

Figure 14. Elbow flexion contracture of 25°.

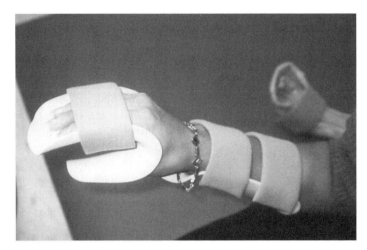

Figure 15. Hand-resting splint.

then replaced with a dynamic Orthoplast splint. Intensive physical and occupational therapy was instituted for muscle re-education and resulted in increased functional ability. Four months later the patient was able to hold utensils, feed herself, write, dress herself, and drive. The improvements have lasted for at least a 2-year follow-up period.[601]

Lungs and Chest Wall

All patients and their families come to understand what is meant by limb ROM and how it applies to stretching tight soft tissues and preventing joint contractures. However, the lungs and chest walls also need ROM mobilization to grow and stay compliant and healthy. Although, on occasion, people with NMDs require such therapy while they are still able to walk, for the great majority of patients it becomes a consideration during the stage of wheelchair use. Lung and chest wall ROM mobilization is discussed in Chapter 7.

Stage 2: Stage of Loss of Ambulation

I am not confined to a wheelchair, I am mobilized by one. I am not ventilator-dependent, I am a happy consumer of a lung-expanding, breathing device which allows me to continue doing the things I love.[602]

·◉· The Honorable Justice Sam Filer, using a computer-activated communication system

Stage 2, Loss of Ambulation, begins when the patient can no longer walk safely and a wheelchair or scooter is needed. The goals of this stage are as follows:

1. Optimize nutrition (Chapter 3)
2. Prevent back deformity
3. Maintain activities of daily living (ADL)
4. Monitor and prevent cardiac complications (Chapter 5)
5. Maintain pulmonary compliance (Chapter 10)
6. Prevent nocturnal alveolar hypoventilation (Chapter 8)

Early Prevention or Correction of Spinal Deformity

The paraspinal muscles support the spine, and the spine, in turn, supports the rib cage and chest muscles. This system is much like the rigging that fixes the mast of a ship so that the mast can support the ship's sails. When the rigging is weak, the mast and sails collapse. Likewise, weak paraspinal muscles result in collapse of the spinal column and deformity of the rib cage and chest wall. Scoliosis is the lateral displacement and rotation of the spine, whereas kyphosis is the forward collapse of the spine. Most people with neuromuscular disease (NMD) develop both. Some develop three lateral curves or an "S" curve. In the great majority of cases, at least for Duchenne muscular dystrophy (DMD), the major convexity seems to develop on the side of the dominant hand.[603] There is also a tendency for the convexity to develop on the side with the tighter iliotibial band (Fig. 1). In one study, the natural course of back deformity was classified into three types for DMD: unremitting progression of scoliosis with kyphosis (21 patients), transition from kyphosis to lordosis before 15 years of age (18 patients), and less deformity without prominent longitudinal changes (7 patients).[604] Age at loss of ambulation did not correlate with extent of subsequent scoliosis.

For children with NMDs, spinal deformities can develop in infancy and progress rapidly during puberty, especially when the child becomes wheelchair-dependent. Like joint contractures, neuromuscular scoliosis is a result of muscle weakness and strength imbalance across joints. In the case of spinal muscular atrophy (SMA), children with type 2 develop more severe scoliosis than children with type 1. Because children with

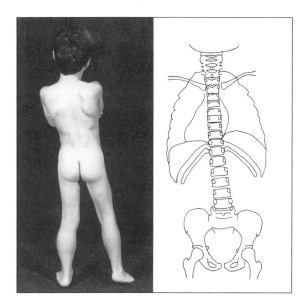

Figure 1. The tighter left iliotibial band rotates the pelvis down on the left, and the spine tends to curve to the left on leaving the pelvis. (Courtesy of Dr. Yves Rideau.)

type 1 are weaker, have less strength imbalance, and sit for shorter periods, the role of gravitational forces is less significant.

About 15% of patients with DMD begin to develop scoliosis while still ambulatory. In one study of 105 patients with DMD, however, scoliosis developed and progressed rapidly in 95% of patients after the loss of ambulation.[605] Left untreated, the collapsing spine not infrequently results in severe scoliotic curves over 100°. If surgery is delayed until the scoliosis has entered its rapidly progressive phase, the loss of breathing function (vital capacity [VC]) discourages physicians from performing surgery. Furthermore, the greater the degree of curvature and the longer its duration, the less it is reversible by surgery. Thus, early, essentially prophylactic surgery is the best and often the only means to prevent serious spinal deformities for many children with NMD.

Infants with NMD require thoracic supports for stroller (see Fig. 17 in Chapter 1) or wheelchair seating to keep them symmetric and to prevent slouching. For children who do not attain independent ambulation and who have scoliosis by 15 months of age but are not yet 6 years old, thoracolumbar bracing or a body jacket is fabricated. The jacket must not restrict abdominal expansion and breathing as monitored by VC or cry VC. The brace is worn whenever the child is seated. It may retard or at least keep the progressing curve a little more flexible and correctable by surgery. No evidence indicates that thoracolumbar bracing causes harm. For patients with SMA who walk but may lose the ability to walk if they undergo scoliosis surgery, the use of bracing during ambulation may retard scoliosis progression.[606] Therefore, bracing is reasonable, at least until age 6 years, to "buy time" for growth of the spine. Surgical intervention is first justified to prevent severe back deformity at this point.[44,607,608]

While waiting for curves to exceed 40°, many clinicians recommend back bracing even for children over age 6 years.[577] For people with normal muscle strength, however, the brace acts as a reminder to use the paraspinal muscles to straighten the back, an option that a child with NMD does not have. Physical therapy, manipulation, and bracing do not affect the ultimate degree of kyphoscoliotic curvature (Fig. 2).[605,609,610] Bracing essentially delays effective surgical intervention, often to the point that the patient has severely diminished pulmonary function.[610] Because surgical correction of scoliosis usually does not result in much more than a 40° correction in the curvature and because it is important to prevent scoliosis, it is better to intervene earlier rather than later.

One study showed that the strongest predictor for scoliosis in DMD was the VC at 10 years of age rather than the age at which ambulation ceased, the curve pattern, or the Cobb angle.[611] The plateau VC is the maximum VC ever attained. Although the VC normally plateaus at age 19 then decreases by 1–1.2% per year, for children with DMD the plateau occurs between ages 9 and 16 years; it can occur at any time before age 19 for children with SMA and other NMDs. For children with DMD whose plateau never exceeds about 1500 ml of air, the incidence of scoliosis approaches 100%. If the scoliosis is left untreated, back deformity becomes quite severe and progresses throughout life. On the other hand, when the plateau exceeds 3000 ml, up to 25% of children with DMD do not develop severe scoliosis and do not require surgical intervention.[610] For children in this group, it is safe to wait to intervene surgically until the curve reaches 40°.

When the standard criterion of 40° for surgical intervention for idiopathic scoliosis is used for DMD, patients with relatively low plateau VCs may have less than 30% of predicted normal VC at the time of intervention (Fig. 3).[610] This value greatly increases the risk of pulmonary complications in most centers, and the treating physicians may not offer surgery or may request an otherwise unnecessary tracheotomy before spinal instrumentation. Many physicians also reject surgical options for patients with very low VCs, thinking that the child with little VC has little hope of long-term survival. Therefore, VC is evaluated every 6 months, and surgical intervention is recommended for patients with low plateau VC, even though they may have only pelvic obliquity or mild curves.[610,612–614]

With use of noninvasive respiratory muscle aids, even patients with little or no VC or ability to breathe can safely undergo spinal surgery without a tracheostomy. Because

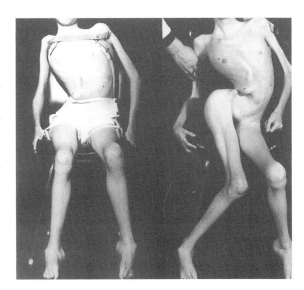

Figure 2. Thoracolumbar bracing for patient with Duchenne muscular dystrophy since age 10 has no apparent effect on preventing scoliosis. (From Duport G, Gayet E, Pries P, et al: Spinal deformities and wheelchair seating in Duchenne muscular dystrophy: Twenty years of research and clinical experience. Semin Neurol 1995;15:29–37, with permission.)

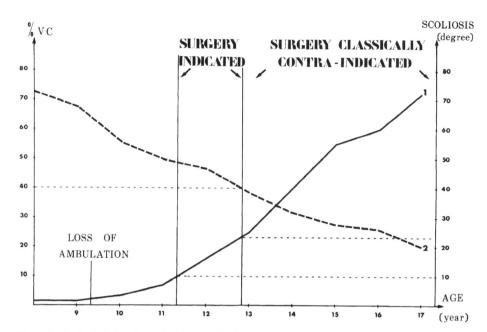

Figure 3. Optimal window for surgical intervention for scoliosis for patients with Duchenne muscular dystrophy. (From Rideau Y, Glorion B, Delaubier A, et al: Treatment of scoliosis in Duchenne muscular dystrophy. Muscle Nerve 1984;7:281–286, with permission.)

most physicians are unfamiliar with these methods and because patients and parents almost always refuse tracheostomy, in most NMD clinics the scoliosis is left to progress and results in the problems noted below.[615] Some investigators have recommended prophylactic spinal instrumentation for all patients.[614] We recommend that patients with DMD whose VC plateaus below 1500 ml undergo surgical intervention as soon as they are wheelchair-dependent and have any curve or pelvic obliquity. With plateaus between 1500 ml and 1800 ml, a curvature of 20–40° is an indication for intervention. With plateaus of greater than 1800 ml, intervention can usually be delayed until the curve exceeds 40°.

Surgical intervention to diminish or correct back curvature involves the placement of rods alongside the spine and linking the spinal bodies to the rods. Usually in the United States the spinal column is also fused so that the fixation becomes solid and permanent. The most common approach was described in 1977 by Luque (Fig. 4). Correction of 40–50° is usually possible. After surgical intervention the patient is discharged from the hospital within 4 or 5 days, provided that no complications develop (Fig. 5). Although the most common complications are respiratory, they are usually preventable with effective use of respiratory muscle aids. Other possible complications include blood loss, infection, cardiac and hardware complications, and reactions to the anesthetics. Major and minor complications were reported in 27% and 16% of 30 patients with DMD at one center.[616] We have had no mortality and no respiratory complications in over 30 patients with DMD undergoing scoliosis prevention surgery, although some patients who were temporarily unweanable from ventilator support had to be extubated to continuous

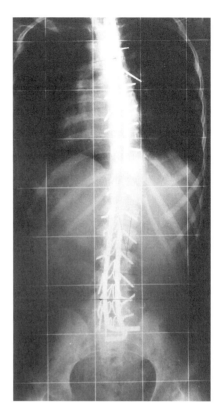

Figure 4. Luque rods are surgically implanted to correct and prevent further scoliosis. (From Duport G, Gayet E, Pries P, et al: Spinal deformities and wheelchair seating in Duchenne muscular dystrophy: Twenty years of research and clinical experience. Semin Neurol 1995;15:29–37, with permission.)

noninvasive IPPV. At any rate, it is so important to prevent scoliosis in NMD that any risk might well be considered acceptable, considering the tragic nature of scoliosis-associated complications.

The worst complication of severe scoliosis is descent of the ribs into the abdomen so that the person can no longer sit. The inability to sit hampers the ability to operate a motorized wheelchair or robot arm, and the unfortunate person must remain permanently in a bed or stretcher. The other complications can be equally disabling. Even for those who continue to be able to sit in wheelchairs, the loss of sitting balance can necessitate highly complicated and expensive seating support systems and much time for positioning to achieve acceptable comfort. Scoliosis can also restrict cardiac function. It can result in intolerable buttock pressure under an ischial tuberosity as well as back and leg pain due to radicular lumbar neural compression. In addition, scoliosis can render ineffective otherwise practical methods of inspiratory muscle assistance, such as use of an intermittent abdominal pressure ventilator for ventilatory support.

In a study of 40 patients with SMA who underwent posterior spinal fusion with Harrington rod instrumentation or Luque rods at a mean of 12 years of age, the average postsurgical correction was 42° with either method, although the complication rate was lower (16% vs. 35%) with the Luque method.[607] However, spine flexibility was decreased. Sitting tolerance was maintained after fusion, but additional use of mobile arm supports, lapboards, and reaching aids was necessary for all patients. Personal care needs

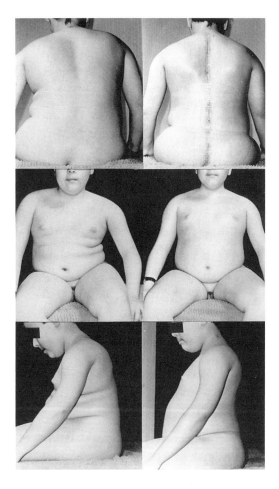

Figure 5. Patient with Duchenne muscular dystrophy before (*right*) and after (*left*) spinal instrumentation with Luque rods. (Courtesy of Dr. Yves Rideau.)

increased in the 2 years postoperatively, improved by 5 years, but never approached preoperative skill levels.[607]

In a study of 19 patients with SMA undergoing spinal instrumentation for scoliosis with comparable improvements in curvature, preoperative VC mean of 1033 ml was noted to decrease to 860 ml 7 years later.[617] Another report suggested that VC might be increased by 40% after surgery to correct scoliosis in patients with SMA.[618] However, VC can increase simply by using a thoracolumbar spinal orthosis to hold the spine more erect before surgery. It is unlikely that fixing the rib cage by spinal fusion will result in an increase in VC.

Other interventions include instrumentation with or without partial spinal fusion,[582,619] and unit rod segmental spinal instrumentation.[620] A study was done of 37 patients with DMD undergoing Luque instrumentation at 12 years of age with a mean preoperative Cobb angle of 19°. The surgery included the insertion of a pedicular screwing system in the lumbosacral area and transverse attachments with steel threads at the thoracic level. A sublaminar fastening was placed at L1. Bone bank arthrodesis was performed only at the lumbosacral level to maintain flexibility in the thoracic part of the spine and to enable growth. After a mean follow-up of 57 months, the Cobb angle, which had been decreased by surgery to 5.2°, was 9.5°. Pelvic balancing was correct, and VC decreased by 3.6% per year.[619] Thus, there appear to be considerable advantages to early intervention with no fusion of the thoracic spine. New and safer surgical methods and hardware are under development to decrease the incidence of rod breakage and other postoperative complications.[621]

Besides posterior instrumentation and fusion, a second intervention for anterior fusion with Dwyer instrumentation is required for patients with severe scoliosis or kyphosis. When spinal deformities are accompanied by severe pelvic obliquity, Luque segmental instrumentation with Galveston pelvic fixation can be used. Sacral screws can be placed in each S1 pedicle, along with a device for transverse traction between the caudal right-angle bends of the L-rods.[622] The use of posterior fusion with pelvic fixation using an iliosacral screw has been reported to correct scoliosis Cobb angles by 53–84° and pelvic obliquity by 60–84% with minimal loss of correction subsequently.[623] The further loss of flexibility by pelvic fixation can further decrease function, however. Fusion from T2 or T3 to L5 without pelvic fixation has yielded good results, provided that the curve is not severe and pelvic obliquity is minimal at the time of surgery.[624] On the other hand, in one study of 48 patients with DMD, 38 with a spinal curvature of less than 40° and with less than 10° between a line tangential to the superior margins of both iliac crests and a line perpendicular to the spinous processes of L4 and L5 were fused to L5. Ten patients not meeting these criteria were fused to the sacrum. Spinal and sitting obliquity increased in patients fused to L5 rather than to the sacrum, but the severity of the worsening obliquity was significantly greater in patients in whom the apex of the curve was below L1. Two of the 10 patients fused to the sacrum required surgical revision procedures for worsening obliquity. Thus, it was recommended to fuse to the sacrum for DMD-associated scoliosis, especially in patients with an apex to the curve below L1.[625]

In summary, scoliosis reduction surgery has a positive effect on function, self-image, cosmesis, pain, patient care, quality of life for at least 2–12 years after surgery,[626] and probably cardiac function, but not necessarily respiratory function. VC usually decreases by 10–20% as a result of spinal fusion fixing the rib cage, but, in a controlled study of DMD, the subsequent rate of loss of VC was the same with or without surgical correction.[627] One article reported a postfusion improvement in VC for 3 of 8 patients with DMD whose preoperative curves ranged from 50° to 80°.[628] Prevention of severe scoliosis greatly facilitates lung insufflation and assisted coughing.

Facilitation of Activities of Daily Living

Far from rendering me "disabled," the ventilator, the wheelchair, the computer, have empowered me, to a level of ability not previously considered, given the constraints imposed by ALS. They allow me to maximize my abilities, rather than focus on my disabilities.[602]

⋅❧⋅ Justice Sam Filer

Upper-limb Assistive Devices

Numerous appliances and assistive technologies are available to control the environment and facilitate mobility, ADL, and communication. Patient and care provider creativity and ingenuity are also essential for developing practical substitution methods that can compensate for physical limitations.

For people with some limb function who have the potential to feed themselves with assistance, correct positioning and table height are important. Rather than bring the head forward to the food, the table surface can be raised so that the hand is closer to the mouth. Using a raised tray avoids having the table too high for other family members. Adaptive utensils can be helpful (Fig. 6). A Universal cuff permits the use of utensils without finger or hand function (Fig. 7). A swivel spoon or fork can be used for people who cannot rotate the wrist. These devices maintain the spoon or fork surface in a horizontal position, regardless of the orientation of the wrist. Light-weight utensils are often helpful. Plastic drinking cups and straws can be useful. Built-up plate rims can be used to help guide food onto the fork or spoon and to help prevent spills.

Specialized clothing catalogues with practical, yet fashionable and inconspicuous solutions are available. Velcro closures are convenient on shoes and bras and as a substitute for buttons and button-holes on shirt cuffs. Bras can also be hooked in front. Shirts and socks one size too large are easier to don. A zipper can be operated more easily if it has a ring pull. The steel hook of a button helper can facilitate buttoning for people with limited hand mobility. Long-handle sock aids and shoehorns, dressing sticks, reachers, and elastic shoe laces can be used. Grooming aids can include large lipstick tubes, long-handled hair brushes, electric toothbrushes, hands-free hair dryer holders, and easy-spray deodorant handles.

Many assistive devices are available to make cooking easier for the physically challenged. An under-the-counter jar opener permits jar opening with less effort. An all-purpose utility knob fits over most knobs, is easy to hold, and, because of its long handle, increases leverage for turning on/off stoves, televisions, and radios. Doorknob extenders can make door opening easier. A reacher can help some people who are restricted to wheelchair use. A light extension switch fits over any wall switch for easy on-off accessibility from a wheelchair.

Upper-limb assistive devices include an overhead sling (Fig. 8), a counterweight and motorized system of arm suspension, and a ball-bearing forearm orthosis or mobile arm support (Fig. 9).[581] These devices can be useful for self-feeding and other activities. Some shoulder and elbow flexor strength is needed to use the latter. In a long-term study of 29 patients who had been fitted with mobile arm supports, spinal fusion increased the percentage of successful users. Successful use declined with muscle grades below poor in elbow flexors. The incidence of success was greater when self-feeding, driving a motorized

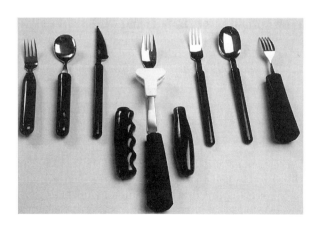

Figure 6. Adaptive utensils. From left to right: rocker knife, button loop, pen holder, adaptive spoon.

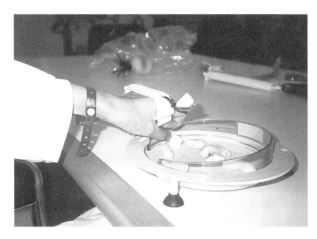

Figure 7. Universal cuff.

wheelchair, and performing leisure activities could be accomplished only with the support.[629] A harness designed for a patient with ALS permitted relatively strong elbow extensors in one upper limb to assist the weak contralateral elbow flexors to bring the hand to the mouth for feeding.[630] When the use of these mechanical devices is not adequate for self-feeding, finger excursion can be used to operate wheelchair-mountable, programmable robotic arms (Figs. 10–12) as well as computers, environmental control systems (see below), and motorized wheelchairs. Robot arms can be inexpensive and fairly simple or expensive and sophisticated. Examples include the Magpie, $1500 (Oxford Orthopedic Engineering Center, Headington, Oxford, England), and the Manus, $13,000 (Exact Dynamics, Zevenaar, Holland). Voice-activated systems are also available, such as The DeVar (Independence Works, Inc., Stanford, CA).

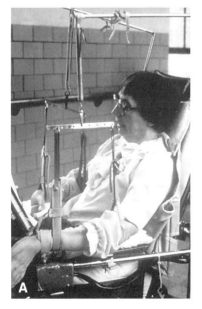

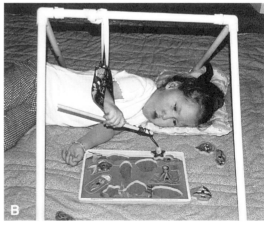

Figure 8. *A*, Wheelchair-mountable overhead sling supports the forearm to permit hand function for a patient with muscular dystrophy. *B*, Overhead sling supports the forearm to permit a 6-year-old girl with spinal muscular atrophy type 1 to fish with a magnet puzzle.

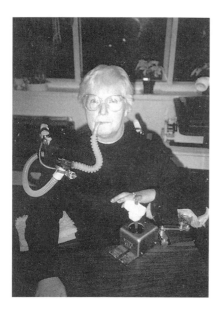

Figure 9. A balanced forearm orthosis for a noninvasive ventilation user postpoliomyelitis.

Mobility

Strollers

Adapted strollers are available for children who are unable or too young to walk or to propel a wheelchair and who require postural support to be positioned somewhat upright or when reclining (Figs. 13 and 14; see also Fig. 17 in Chapter 1). Seat depth, height, and width must be adjustable, and the distance from seat to foot rest must be extendible.

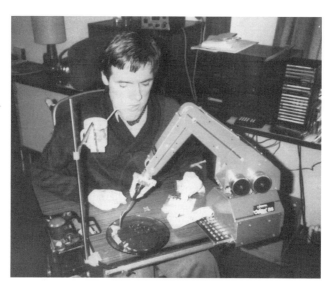

Figure 10. Man with Duchenne muscular dystrophy using a programmable, wheelchair-mountable robot arm to feed himself.

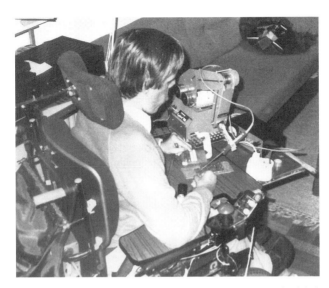

Figure 11. Man with Duchenne muscular dystrophy using a programmable, wheelchair-mountable robot arm to construct a circuit board.

Strollers are lighter than wheelchairs and easily folded for storage. Their complexity can vary greatly. Like wheelchairs, the bases can have a Tilt-in-Space option (see below) that allows the parent to rotate the sitting child from vertical to horizontal position for rest. The wheelchair lifts of city buses can also be used by strollers.

As for wheelchairs, seating systems that provide stability for the child while sitting are available for strollers (Chapter 7). Head rests, lateral trunk supports, guides for hip

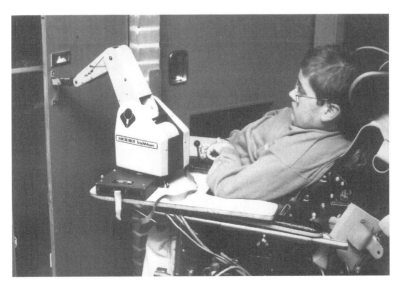

Figure 12. Boy with Duchenne muscular dystrophy using a programmable, wheelchair-mountable robot arm to open a door.

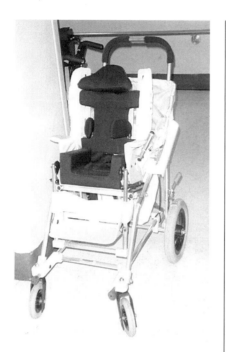

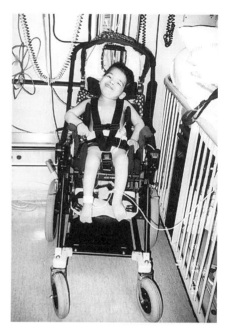

Figure 14. Adapted stroller seat with thoracic support and head rest.

Figure 13. Adapted stroller.

placement, foot rests, seat cushions, and harness systems can be used. Trays can also be mounted onto many strollers to carry ventilators and other items. Strollers should not be used as a substitute for motorized wheelchairs for children over 18 months old.

Unfortunately, there are few appropriately adapted car seats for small children with NMD. The Snug Seat Car Bed (Snug Seat, Inc., Mathews, NC) provides maximum security for infants. Car seats with lateral head and thoracic supports are also available (Gorilla and Snug Seat 2, Snug Seat Inc.) for children from 20–70 lb, but the seats are too vertical and have insufficient anterior-posterior head support for fragile children with SMA type 1 as well as many other children. Velcro forehead straps can be added to increase support. Some stroller seats with good supports have also been custom-designed so that they can be detached from the stroller and used as car seats.

Standard Wheelchairs

Depending on individual lifestyle, a standard wheelchair is usually ordered for anyone who has a serious risk of falling or who cannot walk for at least several blocks. It can be useful at shopping malls, at school, at work, or for transport over uneven terrain. The user should not spend any more time in the wheelchair than is necessary. For such part-time use the ideal wheelchair is usually a light folding type for ease of transfer into an automobile (Fig. 15). A more substantial standard wheelchair is needed when the person is no longer able to ambulate independently.

Detachable arm rests and swingaway and detachable leg rests with heel straps are recommended. Off-set foot plates and heel and toe loops are used for people with severe ankle and foot deformities. The feet are maintained flat on the plates to impede further

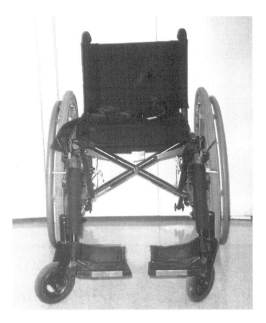

Figure 15. Folding-frame wheelchair.

deformity. Elevating footrests often increase the turning radius of the wheelchair and should be used in conjunction with a reclining back when lower-limb swelling, difficulty in maintaining blood pressure when sitting, and skin pressure relief are considerations (Fig. 16). Most people with neuromuscular weakness should have a reclining seat or Tilt-in-Space (Versitilt Inc., Portland, OR) (see below) because it is difficult to transfer them into and out of chairs for rest periods. The ability to recline with extended knees may also reduce the tendency to develop flexion contractures of the knees and

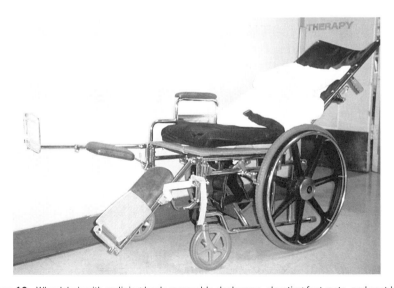

Figure 16. Wheelchair with reclining back, removable desk arms, elevating foot rests, and seat belt.

hips. Invacare Inc. (Edison, NJ) and Permobil Inc. (Woburn, MA) make both standard and motorized wheelchairs that permit automatic Tilt-in-Space and full reclining and leg elevation. Fixed partially reclining backs are rarely necessary because users always prefer to lean forward to optimize arm and hand functioning.

The user has the option of full-length wheelchair arms or desk arms. Desk arms are usually preferred because they permit the user to approach and use desks and tables. Full-length arms may be useful to support a lap tray. A lap tray can facilitate the performance of school work, gainful employment, and recreational activities. Elevating arms are rarely required, but the arms must be removable to facilitate transfers.

For proper fit, with the user sitting upright and against the wheelchair back with the feet squarely on the foot plates, it should be possible to put 3 fingers between the undersurface of the knee and the seat. It should also be possible to place the palm of the hand between the user's thighs and the side of the chair. The hips, knees, and ankles should rest at approximately a 90° angle. Proper seating also allows enough room for wearing a coat and using braces when applicable. Wider, more heavily constructed chairs can be made for obese users. One report of 18 limb fractures (13 of the distal femur, 2 of the proximal humerus, and 3 of the distal tibia) in 11 patients with DMD, one with BMD, and one with SMA resulting from falling from a wheelchair emphasizes the necessity of a seat belt for users with poor sitting balance or weak trunk musculature.[195] Severely disabled patients may require additional support for the head, neck, trunk, and limbs. Low sling backs, sling seats, nonremovable static leg rests, and large frames should be avoided.[631]

The E-fix (Ulrich Alber Co., www.ulrich-alber.com) converts standard wheelchairs into power wheelchairs. Electric motors are added to the hubs of the drive wheels, and a joy stick control is typically used to operate the chair. They are gearless, brushless, and have no moving parts. The drive wheels are the heaviest part of the chair, weighing 19 lb (over 40 lb lighter than the heaviest sections of most standard motorized chairs). The batteries can also be disengaged (interchangeable) and the wheelchair propelled manually. Quick and easy wheel removal permits the otherwise standard chair to be folded and stored in the trunk of most cars, eliminating the need for a van in many cases. The E-motion reduces the effort of propelling a manual chair by up to 80%, thereby facilitating long-distance as well as both uphill and downhill travel. The pushrims of the standard wheels turn on the E-motion motors. Sensors automatically determine the energy and length of support necessary (Ulrich Alber Co., www.ulrich-alber.com). The two E-motion, active drive wheels provide a range of up to 6 miles with one battery charge. A Canadian company, Medbloc, Inc., of Toronto, has also developed the capacity to convert some Invacare (Edison, NJ) motorized wheelchairs into chairs that can tilt and stand patients and permit them to operate while standing.

Rigid Frame Wheelchairs

Light-weight wheelchairs can have rigid or nonrigid frames. A rigid frame refers to a solid axis connecting one wheel to the other (Fig. 17). These durable chairs are well suited for carrying heavy loads and for rugged use. They also provide more stability and a smoother ride. A disadvantage of the rigid frame wheelchair is that it cannot be folded and put into a car without first removing the wheels. "Quick-release" wheels, with a pin and a lock configuration, can facilitate transport.

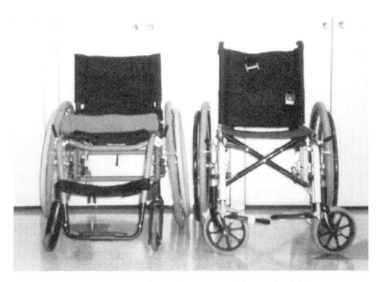

Figure 17. Rigid (*left*) and folding (*right*) frame wheelchairs.

Nonrigid Frame Wheelchairs

The nonrigid frame wheelchairs have a foldable crossbar connecting one side of the wheelchair to the other (Fig. 17). This feature greatly facilitates transport, permits the chair to "grow" with a young user, and facilitates storage of the chair in cars. The crossframe, however, wears out with use, compromising the integrity and stability of the wheelchair. The user should be able to try both frame styles before choosing.

Seating Systems

Special seating modifications are often useful for people with muscle weakness or contractures. Proper positioning enhances comfort and optimizes arm function and, at least for small children, may decrease the rate of development of irreversible back and other deformities. Seating systems range from simple wheelchair cushions (Fig. 18) to custom-molded seats (Fig. 19). Commonly used cushions include the Roho (Roho, Inc., Belleville, IL), Jay (Jay Medical Ltd., Boulder, CO), and Avanti (Invacare, Inc., Elyria,

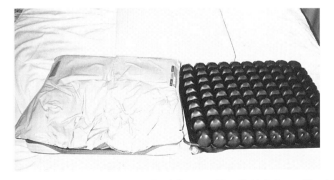

Figure 18. Adaptive seating: J-cushion (*top*), foam cushion (*left*), Roho cushion (*right*).

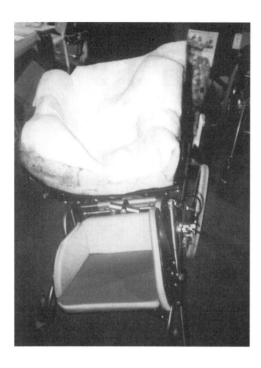

Figure 19. Pressure-relief custom-molded seat.

OH) systems. These cushions provide excellent pressure relief. The StimuLITE Honeycomb cushion (Supracor Systems, Inc., Sunnyvale, CA) has a sophisticated architecture in the form of a honeycomb that is 90% air and 10% thermoplastic polyether urethane; it also has antifungal and antibacterial properties. The average size weighs less than 3 pounds. It remains cool in warm weather, absorbs moisture, resists odor, and is machine-washable. It is ideal for patients in warm climates and patients who have problems with skin maceration. All potential users should have the opportunity to try more than one seating system before choosing.

Wedges that separate the legs can be useful. Both wedges and straps can be used to bring the thighs closer together for proper body alignment. Other inserts and supports can also be used to support the trunk, neck, or head. Neck rests with a forehead strap provide total support for the head and neck. The lower sections of head supports can be extended forward along the neck and under the mandible to the chin. People with severe deformities may best benefit from a fully contoured seat and head rest.

The Tilt-in-Space seating mobility system rotates the user and the wheelchair seat and back simultaneously up to 55° between vertical and horizontal planes, thus changing the seating orientation and shifting skin pressures. This system assists with transfers and varies skin contact pressures. It can be operated independently.

Motorized Wheelchairs

Motorized wheelchairs are recommended for patients who cannot propel a standard chair or for whom the energy required to propel a manual chair is excessive or contraindicated. They are prescribed for children from the age of 18 months so that they can explore their environments like children without disabilities.

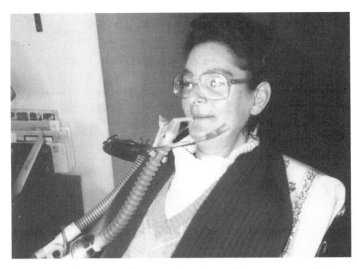

Figure 20. Woman dependent on continuous noninvasive positive-pressure ventilatory support since 1954 receiving mouthpiece IPPV via a mouthpiece fixed adjacent to sip-and-puff controls for her motorized wheelchair.

Most people with NMD operate motorized wheelchairs by joystick controls. When hand function is absent, sip-and-puff (Fig. 20), chin (Fig. 21), scanning, and proximity sensing systems can be used. Proportional or nonproportional input switches can be electronic, fiberoptic, pneumatic (Adaption Switch Lab, Inc., Austin, TX), and multiple. Several of our ventilator users operate their wheelchairs and computers by leg or toe movements (Fig. 22).

Other motorized wheelchair considerations include the chair's style; adjustability of the control box for sensitivity of operation, speed, acceleration, and turning radius; noise; brake efficiency; tire treads and suspension system; curb jumping ability; range on a battery charge; durability; warranty; and price. Front-wheel drive facilitates maneuverability in the confined spaces of the home, whereas rear-wheel drive grips the ground better to facilitate outdoor use. Some motorized wheelchairs permit the user to come to

Figure 21. Woman dependent on continuous noninvasive positive-pressure ventilatory support since 1953 receiving mouthpiece IPPV via a mouthpiece fixed adjacent to chin controls for her motorized wheelchair.

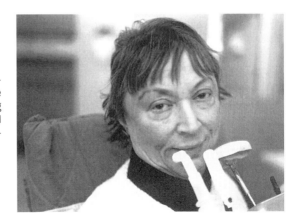

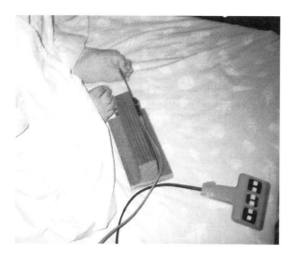

Figure 22. Toe switch used to operate computer software and environmental control system of a patient with Duchenne muscular dystrophy who has had no ventilator-free breathing ability since beginning to use mouthpiece IPPV 23 years ago.

a standing position and to operate the chair while standing (Chairman Stander, Chairman Corpus, Chairman Vertical, Permobil, Inc., Woburn, MA; Standing D, Davismade, Inc., Burton, MI, www.standingdani.com; Levomobil LCMTM, Levo, Ltd., Dottikon, Switzerland, www.levo.ch; and the Lifestand Compact Electric Standing Wheelchair, Life Stand-Independence Providers, Inc., Pleasantville, NY, www.lifestandusa.com) (Fig. 23). The Lifestand chair provides up to full tilt and full recline as well as operation from a standing position with firm lower-limb and thoracic support.

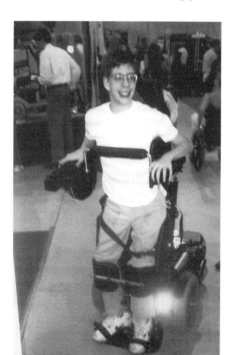

Figure 23. Motorized wheelchair that permits the user to sit or stand.

Although some of these chairs have been withdrawn from the American market because of liability concerns, they can help to maintain bone integrity, limit leg contractures and skin pressures, improve circulation and reduce edema, build endurance, reduce the risk of renal system infections and stasis, improve bowel regularity and function, and promote important psychological benefits. Contraindications are cardiac orthostasis, systemic orthopedic disorders, and hip and knee flexion contractures greater than 20°.

Today children with SMA type 1 and type 2 and other children with severe NMDs are surviving. They often require the most support. They may require head and neck support as well as lateral thoracic supports and Tilt-in-Space and full-reclining options. Stealth Products, Inc. (www.stealthproducts.com) has a number of seating options for such patients as they transition from adapted strollers to standard and motorized wheelchairs.

The Permolock permits the user to lock the Chairman Stander wheelchair at the van controls for hand operation of a van. It has been especially designed for the Chryslar Voyager IMS but can be used with many vans. It can be used as a driver's or passenger's seat. The Playman Miniflex and Koala Miniflex permit children to raise their seats several feet so that they can be on eye level with others who are standing. Permobil chairs (Permobil, Inc., Woburn, MA) and the Skwirrel (Huka Mobile, Enschede, Holland) also permit users to stand supported to operate their chairs.

Scooters

Other options for people with limited mobility are three- and four-wheel motorized scooters (Fig. 24). Scooters can have a maximum speed of 10 miles per hour, ascend a grade of 30°, and go about 20 miles on one battery charge. They have swivel seats and

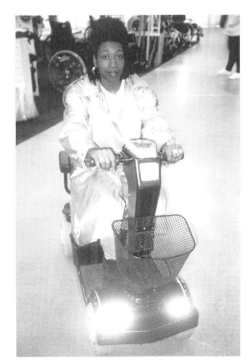

Figure 24. Motorized scooter (Shoprider, Shoprider, Inc., Rosemont, PA).

may have elevating seats to assist transfers. Although scooters have seat belts, trunk and upper limbs must be functional to operate them. A wire basket is attached to the frame of the scooter for transporting objects. A ventilator tray can be attached to the frame of the scooter. Scooters are often most useful for people with poor endurance and fatigue and limited lower-limb function. They tend to be most useful for people with milder NMDs such as SMA type 3 or type 4 and mild myopathies, especially in middle age. The Quickie Kid Cart (Sunrise Medical, Inc., Arleta, CA) is a scooter specifically designed for children. Likewise, Trikes (Triaid Rehabilitation Products, Cumberland, MD) are tricycles that support patients with inadequate sitting balance. They are built to accommodate growth.

A new booklet, "Scooter vs. Power Chair: Which One Is Right For Me," (SFC, Inc., Victoria, BC, Canada) is designed to help patients decide which would be most appropriate. It offers key points about various chairs and scooters (www.changing.ca).

Transferring and Lifting

Care providers need early, thorough, and ongoing instructions in the most efficient and safe way to transfer patients. Important guidelines include the following:[632]

1. Use proper biomechanics to prevent back strain. Lifting is done with the back straight and with a wide base of support to emphasize that the power comes from the legs.
2. Optimize conditions for transfers. This goal may require equalizing the height of the transfer surfaces.
3. Have the patient assist in the transfers as much as possible. The patient should also be comfortable with instructing in and directing the transfers.
4. Evaluate the use of transfer boards (Fig. 25) to facilitate transfers and minimize the risk for falls.

Portable lifts and mechanical hoists include the Hoyer lift (Fig. 26) and Translift or Institutional Lift (Guardian Sunrise Medical, Arleta, CA), Barrier Free Lift (Barrier Free Lifts, Inc., Manassas, VA), and EasyPivot Lift (Rand-Scott Corp., Fort Collins, CO).

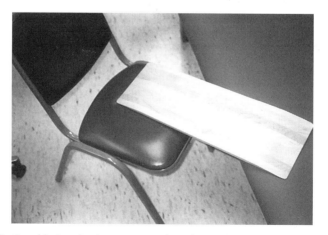

Figure 25. Sliding board for transfers between two surfaces for people with good upper body but poor lower body strength. The person slides the hips along the board.

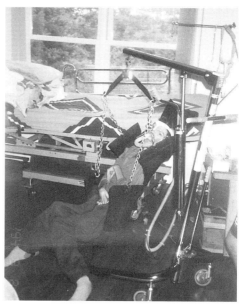

Figure 26. Use of Hoyer lift to transfer from bed to commode a 39-year-old patient with Duchenne muscular dystrophy who has used continuous noninvasive IPPV since 23 years of age. Using a Hoyer lift, with feet on the ground, thighs applying pressure to the abdomen, and buttocks in optimal dependent position over the commode, bowel movements are initiated and rapidly completed.

The EasyPivot Lift requires less space for transfers. Ceiling lifts (Barrier Free Lifts, Inc., Manassas, VA) have the advantages of multidirectional user transport and optional battery operation; they can be used independently. The Meyland-Carlift (Access Unlimited, Binghamton, NY) can be fixed onto a car door, in a bathroom area, or elsewhere to lift the user into and out of a car, onto a toilet seat, and so on. Turning Automotive Seating (Bruno Independent Living Aids, Inc., Oconomowoc, WI) is a car seat that rotates and exits the car to permit easy wheelchair transfers. Ordinary car seats can be replaced by motorized car seats (Fig. 27). Sunrise Medical, Inc. also makes a Poolift.

Stair glides enable ascent and descent of stairs. Some glides accommodate wheelchairs. Vertical platform lifts are options that may necessitate home remodeling.

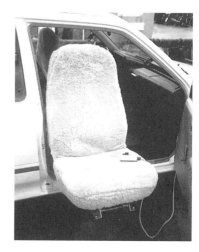

Figure 27. Motorized car seat to facilitate car transfers. (Merlin 360 Degrees, Medgroup, Inc., Newbury Park, CA.)

Portable folding and telescoping ramps can be custom-made to bypass stairs. Remote-controlled door systems can facilitate wheelchair accessibility (Open Sesame, Inc., San Leandro, CA; Gentleman Door Co., Yorklyn, DE). The home visit of an occupational therapist can aid in the identification of useful devices and other modifications.

For patients who have some leg movement but insufficient trunk or limb function to use canes, 4-legged "quad" canes, Lofstran crutches, ceiling-mounted hoists (Fig. 28) (Guldmann, Inc., Atlanta), and hoists supported by a lift can be used to facilitate walking about or treadmill use (Lite-Gait and Walk-Able, Mobility Research, Inc., lite-gait.com). Lifts can also be used to put heavy objects such as scooters and wheelchairs into a van. One example is the Curb-Sider Super XL3 (Bruno Independent Living Aids, Inc., Oconomowoc, WI). Although these hoists generally need to be bolted into the vehicle, 2004 General Motors vans, minivans, and sport utility vehicles with removable back seats have the capacity to be fitted with a removable hoist that permits entry of scooters and motorized wheelchairs up to 300 lb. The cost of the hoist is $3000.

Beds and Mattresses

People normally move about a great deal during sleep. Those who are too weak to change position during sleep often awaken and ask to be turned. Often turning is needed every hour or two. However, various beds and mattress surfaces are available to disperse pressure over large areas and to decrease or eliminate the need for turning assistance. Choosing the most comfortable bed and mattress is an empirical process; users should have the opportunity to try them for a few nights before making a final choice.

Common mattress choices are egg-crate, water, and air. The egg-crate mattress is convenient and inexpensive, but the foam can deform with time, causing skin pressure build-up in some areas. Air and water mattresses disperse pressure and moderate body

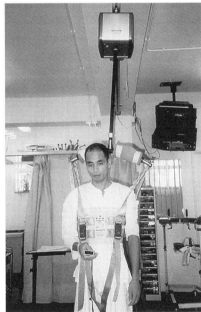

Figure 28. Ceiling rails suspend a thoracic support system that permits ambulation without personal assistance.

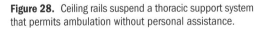

temperature. However, activities such as dressing, grooming, and eating can be more difficult to perform on a water mattress; transfers are more difficult; and water leakage can occur. Contact with sharp or angular surfaces must be avoided. Thus, one must be especially careful while wearing splints or using equipment in bed.

A motorized hospital bed can facilitate comfort and transfers. Although the operation systems are usually at the foot of the bed, push-button or touch-control, sip-and-puff, and other systems can be installed for independent operation. Bed rails and an overhead trapeze can also facilitate turning and mobility. Alternating pressure pad air mattresses can decrease the need for assisted turning. Lengthwise sections of this mattress inflate and deflate in a wave-like activity that constantly changes skin pressures.

"Rotating" mattresses are also available from Kinetics Concepts, Inc., Texas (Triadyne system); Invacare, Inc., Edison, NJ (Turn-Q Plus); Span America, Inc., Greenville, SC (Pressure Guard Turn Select); Progressive Medical, Inc., Overland Park, KS (Sapphire Sure Turn); and the Air Prism Multi-Functional Portable Rotation System from Plexus, plexusmed.com. The Plexus mattress has optional contour cushions that facilitate patient centering and leg abduction. These mattresses turn the patient by the alternate inflation of long pneumatic panels. The ProAire Portable Rotation System (Bio Clinic, Inc.) provides full-body rotation in a single unit. It has microprocessor circuitry that automatically controls the inflation of a five-zone upper mattress to customize pressure relief and comfort. These mattresses can be used on standard hospital beds. Rotational beds such as the RotoRest (Kinetic Concepts, Inc., Texas) can also be used but are more expensive. A laterally rotating bed, the Motion Bed, can be ideal to eliminate assisted turning. It was less expensive but is no longer commercially available (J. H. Emerson Company, Cambridge, MA). Some patients still use it.

Bathing and Toileting

High bath and shower chairs and tub benches can be fitted with seat belts. These devices make it feasible for people with limited muscle strength to wash in a tub or shower. Some, like the Tub Slide Shower Chair, permit the user to slide onto the chair or over the tub or under the shower from either side. The Tub Slide Shower Chair has a padded seat and backrest. It can also roll over a standard height commode (R.D. Equipment, Inc., www.takegoodcare.com). Some chairs also feature a Tilt-In-Space option (Tilt-In-Space Slider Bathing System, Assistive Technology, Inc., New Buffalo, MI; www.pvcdme.com). Seats with a hole in the center can facilitate bathing the perineum, but transfer off the seat can be difficult (Fig. 29). Bathtub or wall-mounted rails and shower-tub transfer seats can also be quite useful. The Swivel-Bather is a versatile shower-tub seat that swivels to facilitate transfers (Assistive Technology, Inc., New Buffalo, MI). It can transfer the user into and out of the shower. When the bathroom can be remodeled, a roll-in shower permits a rolling chair or commode chair to be wheeled into the shower.

Portable lifts can also be used for bathing heavy or severely disabled people. A water-powered bath chair (Bath Mate, Inc., Ontario, CA) can lower the user to within 2 inches of the bottom of the tub. A shampoo tray can be used to help wash hair while sitting in the wheelchair. Bathrooms need to be evaluated to determine whether there is enough room for such devices. Other equipment that at times may be helpful includes long-handled combs, brushes, sponges, dressing sticks, toilet paper holders, shoe horns, and flexible shower hoses and adapters.

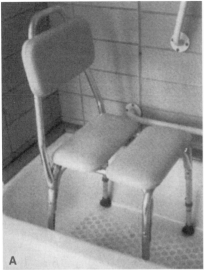

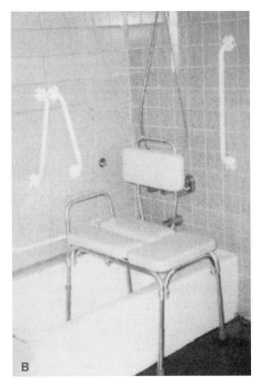

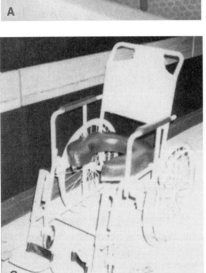

Figure 29. Bath chair (*A*), bath bench (*B*), and rolling shower chair (*C*).

Specially adapted potty chairs provide support and positioning for children. They vary from sophisticated systems to support the head, trunk, and pelvis to minimal systems consisting of a ring encircling the user's waist and a seatbelt. Some potty chairs can be placed onto the toilet, whereas others are used only on the floor. These systems have adjustable parts that accommodate growth of the child. Equipment should be chosen with practicality, adaptability, and durability in mind.

Commode chairs can be used at bedside or placed over a toilet or in some other convenient location. In general, commode chairs are narrower than wheelchairs and available on wheels; they more readily fit through doors for easier access to the bathroom. Some are rolled into a shower. Commode chairs on wheels can also have seat belts, foot rests, and removable arm rests.

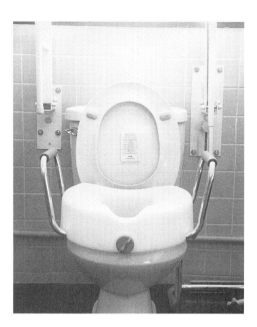

Figure 30. An elevated toilet seat makes it much easier to sit and get up.

A raised toilet seat and grab bars attached to the wall or to the toilet seat can assist with toilet transfers (Fig. 30). The bars can be removable or fixed. Some can be suction-cupped to surfaces.

Male wheelchair users can conduct daily affairs much more independently without need for personal assistance for urinating by using a condom catheter urinary drainage system (Fig. 31). The catheter drains into a collection bag strapped around the lower leg. Some women use an internal (Foley) catheter for this purpose. Because the catheter passes through the urethra into the bladder, it renders the user susceptible to urinary tract infections.

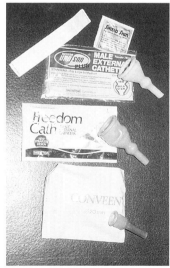

Figure 31. Condom catheter urinary drainage system.

Communication and Computer Environmental Control

Bulbar muscle weakness commonly results in dysarthria in bulbar-type ALS and occasionally in SMA type 1 and FSH. Dysarthria results from hypophonia or insufficient air volume for audible speech or from problems with articulation or vocal cords. Hypophonic patients can receive deep insufflations by mouthpiece IPPV to increase speech volumes and audibility (Chapter 11). For patients with nonbulbar ALS, speech is often the initial reason for ventilator use and placement of a ventilator on a wheelchair tray. Typically patients with SMA type 1 are hypophonic but have too little lip muscle strength to grab a mouthpiece for insufflation therapy, and it is not practical to wear a nasal interface all day for the sole reason of increasing speech volume. Such patients should have a microphone adjacent to their mouths to amplify speech.

Dysarthria is often accompanied by dysphagia (Chapter 3). Nasal regurgitation and nasal speech are associated with velopharyngeal incompetence. This problem often can be improved by surgical pharyngeal flap elevation.[633] Other possible surgical interventions include Teflon inverted question mark injections and obturator fitting.[634] A palatal lift/augmentation prosthesis can also be constructed and used successfully, provided that the patient's gag reflex does not interfere.[635] In one study, 21 of 25 patients with this prosthesis demonstrated improvement in dysarthria, with 19 reporting at least moderate benefit for over 6 months. Of 10 treated with a combination palatal lift and augmentation prosthesis, 6 had improved articulation with less effort required for speaking.[636]

When word articulation is difficult, maintaining eye contact is emphasized. Practice in slowing speech, overarticulating, and optimizing word-phrase groupings can help. Speech production computer systems can facilitate communication. The ability to type or use touch-sensitive controls permits the use of the Tablet, Handheld, and Palmtop portable impact devices (Enkidu Research, www.enkidu.net/enkidu); Crespeaker Maxx II (Crestwood Communication Aids, Inc., www.communicationaids.com); and small portable computers such as the NEC MobilePro 780 to provide voice synthesis and operate printers.

Averbal patients who retain at least one reliable muscle movement, such as eye blink or finger excursion, can use computers for communication and environmental control. Blinking can operate an eye switch activated by infrared reflection off the eye. This device enables communication with the use of a speech-generating device (Words+ Software, Inc., Sunnyvale, CA). The family of one patient with ALS installed computer augmentative communication software, formerly known as "SpeakEasy," on the Internet, as version 5.0 (www.etriloquist.com). Like Words+, this software makes use of on-screen keyboards, scanners, word-predictors, single-switch input, and other assistive input devices such as Virtual On-Screen Keyboard (MiloSoft, Inc.), SofType (Origin Instruments Inc.), WiViKTM (Prentke Romich Company), or My-T-Mouse (IMG, Inc.), among others. Assistive input devices can work all Windows programs. This software handles word groupings up to the size of a book that can be spoken or printed with the blink of an eye. Prerecorded phrases in the user's own voice can be prepared, or the voices of friends can be used. The voice synthesis can also produce voices of different pitches, genders, and age groupings. Communication Independence for the Neurologically Impaired, Inc. (www.cini.org/), Dynavox, Inc. (www.dynavoxsys.com), and Gus Communications, Inc. (www.gusinc.com) have websites devoted to many of these options and information about how to obtain them.

Other activation methods include the use of eye movements to trigger electrical impulses.[637] The user simply gazes at the desired letter or word on the computer screen for a fraction of a second (Fig. 32). Users are able to create about 6–10 words per minute; store and quickly reproduce complex phrases, sentences, and paragraphs; and initiate communication. Many other augmentative communication devices are also available (www.augcominc.com), including the possibility of activating computers without visible muscle movement by the use of surface electromyographic and electroencephalographic electrodes (Technos America, LTD, Bailey CO, www.mctos.com). A thought translation device has also been described for brain-computer communication. After several months of training, 3 locked-in patients with ALS learned to control their slow cortical potentials in a 2-second rhythm, producing either cortical negativity or positivity according to the task requirement. The slow cortical potential differences were transformed into vertical or horizontal cursor movements on a computer screen. Seventy to 80% accuracy was achieved for 2 of the 3 patients.[638] Cyberlink(GSTS Design, Inc., Madison, NC) is a computer interface that allows control of the computer by means of a headband equipped with sensors that detect muscle and brain activity (www.alsa.org).

Phone systems can be programmed with automatic dialing functions initiated by striking a key, sip-and-puff, finger switch, joystick, or voice activation (Temasek Telephone, Inc., San Francisco, CA) (Fig. 33). A typical voice-activated speaker phone answers automatically once the user says hello after the second ring and also disconnects by itself. A sip-and-puff can connect to the operator, who can place the call. Voice-activated phones can also be used with sip-and-puff dialing. Voice amplification is another option. A vast network of on-line services, including food and clothes shopping, can increase independence. Because voice, finger switch, eye movement, and blink activation computer control can permit environmental control of doors and all electrical appliances

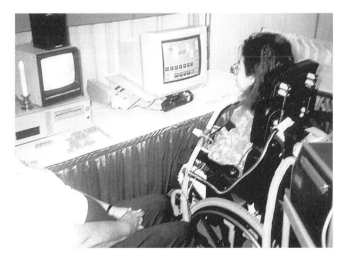

Figure 32. Eyegaze systems use a low-power, infrared light-emitting diode mounted in the center of a video camera lens. This system illuminates the eye and provides a bright image of the pupil and a bright spot reflecting off the cornea. Image-processing software computes where on a control monitor screen the user is looking and enables the user to activate rapidly keys as small as five-eighths of a square inch (Eyegaze system, LC Technologies, Inc., Fairfax, VA).

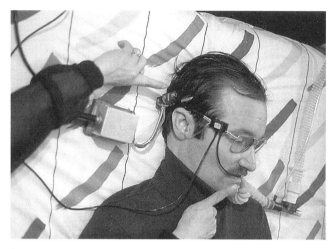

Figure 33. Ventilator user with no volitional movement below the neck, using an adapted telephone head set. Head rotation activates the system and contacts the operator. The speaker is in his ear, and the small mouthpiece microphone is kept just over his lip and adjacent to the mouthpiece for ventilatory support.

in the home,[581] patients can achieve interpersonal, instrumental, and professional goals despite severe disability and continuous ventilatory support.

Service Animals

Service dogs can provide an extra pair of arms and legs (Fig. 34). The dogs undergo about 15 months of training to learn 60 commands. The Americans with Disabilities Act mandates that service dogs be granted access virtually everywhere. A recent study

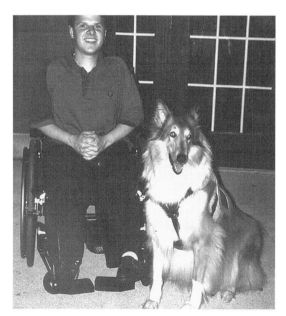

Figure 34. Young man with muscular dystrophy and his service dog.

showed that people with service dogs required an average of 72% fewer hours of human personal assistance.[577] The service animals can retrieve items dropped on the floor or objects from high counters. They can operate wall switches, open and close doors, and go for help when needed. Trained dogs can also help with dressing by pulling garments up over the legs. They are used to power standard wheelchairs, thus delaying or eliminating the need for a motorized wheelchair until daytime ventilator use is required. The Delta society (Renton, WA) publishes a Service Dog Directory that lists 70 or so training programs, including Canine Assistants, Inc. (Alpharetta, GA) and Canine Companions for Independence, Inc. Fees are about $12,000. The cost of maintaining the dog is about $1,000 a year, including food, grooming, veterinary care, and equipment. Insurance or federal rehabilitation service programs may subsidize the cost.

Service chimpanzees can be more versatile than dogs because their fine hand motor skills permit them to operate finer environmental controls and to manipulate small objects. For example, they can position a mouth stick, install a cassette, and feed the companion. Chimpanzees have most often served patients with high-level spinal cord injury. At this time it is unclear whether anyone is continuing to train them.

Transportation

Mass transit is not always possible to use. Motorized vehicles can be modified for operation by upper-limb activity alone. As a rule, a sedan is less expensive to purchase, modify, and drive than a van. However, if the user cannot be transferred efficiently into an automobile, a van is the vehicle of choice. A wheelchair-accessible van is particularly important for the transport of people with heavy motorized wheelchairs. With a lowered floor-accessible minivan, the touch of a button opens a sliding door, causes a folded ramp to descend, and lowers the rear suspension by approximately 5 inches to decrease the ramp angle for easier access (National Mobility Corporation, Elkhartz, IN) (Fig. 35).

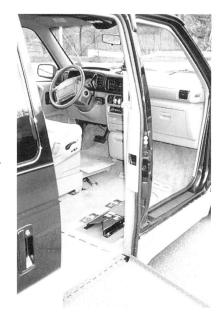

Figure 35. Adapted van.

Accessible vans can be rented in at least 37 states (Wheelchair Getaways, www.wheelchair-getaways.com).

Resources

Organizations with periodicals that provide information about options to facilitate ADL include the following:

- Muscular Dystrophy Association, Tuscon, AZ
- Families of SMA, Highland Park, IL
- Living SMArt, Milwaukee, WI
- National Easter Seal Society, Chicago, IL
- Polio Society, Washington, DC
- International Polio Network, St. Louis, MO (Its publication Gazette International Network Incorporated is enormously useful for ventilator users with any diagnosis.)
- ALS Association, Sherman Oaks, CA
- Myasthenia Gravis Foundation, Chicago, IL
- Charcot-Marie-Tooth Association, Upland, PA
- National Support Group for Myositis, Cooperstown, NY
- Guillain-Barré Syndrome Foundation International, Wynnewood, PA
- Malignant Hyperthermia Association of the United States, Westport, CN
- ALS Interest Group (ALS Digest, available at bro@huey.met.fsu.edu)
- Parent Project for Muscular Dystrophy Research, Middletown, OH

Other resources of interest include:

- New Mobility, a magazine designed for people with spinal cord injury (North Hollywood, CA)
- www.RehabInfo.net, a government-funded site with information about NMDs
- Living For Today, NIVNetwork.com, operated by Richard Clingman, Webmaster for DoctorBach.com

Chapter 8

Conventional "End-stage" Management

With contributions by Mr. Ira Holland

Tradition nicht anders sei als Schlamperei.
Tradition is nothing other than negligence.

• ☞ • Gustav Mahler

The conventional approaches to managing patients with NMDs involve the following:
- Monitoring sleep for sleep-disordered breathing
- Treatment with continuous positive airway pressure (CPAP) or low-span bilevel PAP with the least expensive CPAP interfaces and without giving the patient a choice of interfaces (Fig. 1)
- When acute ventilatory/respiratory failure is triggered by supplemental oxygen administration or an intercurrent chest cold, intubation followed by extubation in a manner more appropriate for patients with respiratory rather than ventilatory impairment
- Once extubation fails, reintubation and resort to tracheotomy
- No treatment or oxygen and morphine to hasten death

Tracheostomy Tubes

After surgical placement of a tracheostomy site, a tracheostomy tube is inserted through the stoma (Fig. 2). Tracheostomy tubes are placed to facilitate mucus removal from the airways, to provide supplemental oxygen, to maintain patency of the upper airway, and to allow invasive mechanical ventilation. The tubes are made of plastic or metal and may have cuffs or be cuffless. They have the common features seen in Figure 3.

The outer cannula is inserted through the stoma to keep the lower airway open to the atmosphere and to keep the stoma from closing. The obturator is used when inserting the outer cannula into the stoma (Fig. 4). Its tip is lubricated, and it is inserted into the outer cannula. The obturator provides a blunt separation of tissue to guide the outer cannula down the stomal tract. Any inner cannula must be removed when the obturator is used. Some tubes have only an outer cannula. It may be fenestrated and have a cuff or be cuffless. Single-cannula tubes are most often used by patients who require tubes for the long term without needing a ventilator (e.g., patients with laryngeal cancer after laryngectomy).

The inner cannula has a Universal connector that can lock it into the outer cannula. It is slid into the outer cannula and can be connected to ventilator circuitry. It is removed to facilitate cleaning and when the tube is changed. Nondisposable inner cannulas are

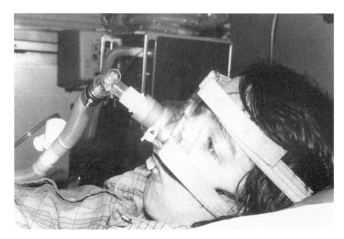

Figure 1. Woman with spinal muscular atrophy and chronic respiratory muscle insufficiency who was born in 1959. She used nasal IPPV via a standard CPAP mask for nocturnal ventilatory assistance from 1971 until March 1988, when she ill-advisedly underwent tracheotomy during hospitalization for a respiratory tract infection. She died from pneumonia in April 1990.

cleaned once or twice daily. The skin around the stoma is also inspected, cleaned, and covered to avert skin irritation and infection. For patients with disposable inner cannulas, the inner cannula is simply discarded and replaced with a new one.

The cuff can be inflated with air via the cuff inflation line. The pilot balloon on the cuff inflation line helps to regulate the air pressure inside the cuff. The pilot balloon inflates when air is inserted into the cuff. The cuff is attached to the outside of the outer cannula. For patients with even minimal bulbar muscle function, such as that adequate for comprehensible speech, cuff use is usually unnecessary to guarantee adequate ventilatory

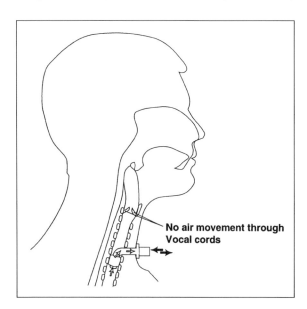

No air movement through Vocal cords

Figure 2. Tracheostomy tube inserted into airway with inflated cuff cutting off any airflow via the upper airway.

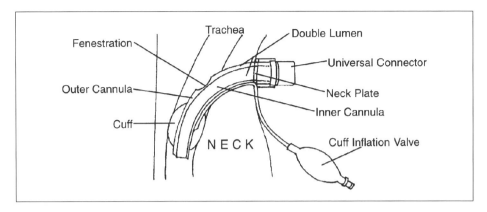

Figure 3. Fenestrated tracheostomy tube with an inflated cuff.

support,[639] but in such cases the tube itself is also unnecessary. Nevertheless, the cuff is conventionally left inflated when a patient receives tracheostomy IPPV, particularly during sleep. Inflation of the cuff enables the ventilator to deliver IPPV to the patient without insufflation air leakage out of the upper airway. Although leakage and speech decrease air delivery to the lungs, this decrease can almost always be compensated by increasing ventilator-delivered volumes.

There are many types of cuffs. Some require that the air pressure inside the cuff be regulated manually, and some are self-regulating. Although cuffs are usually filled with air, some are filled with a foam sponge to modulate cuff pressures. Most cuffs have a high residual volume of air inside the cuff to maintain low pressure against the tracheal wall and thus minimize pressure damage (trachiectasis) and tracheal wall ischemia. When the cuff is inflated, it conforms to the shape of the trachea, sealing off the space between the trachea and the outer cannula. This seal can also limit the aspiration of food and upper airway secretions (see Fig. 2).

The cuff is inflated by a syringe connected to the pilot balloon. Although 5–7 ml of air is usually adequate initially, with time and the gradual destruction of the tracheal wall, more air (often 10–15 m) is usually required. An air pressure manometer can be attached to the pilot balloon after inflation to indicate air pressure in the cuff. One attempts to maintain pressures of 18–22 cmH$_2$O in the cuff to prevent tissue ischemia, but patients often demand higher cuff volumes and pressures.[640]

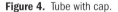

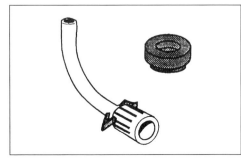

Figure 4. Tube with cap.

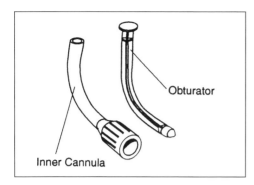

Figure 5. Obturator.

A fenestrated tracheostomy tube has a hole in the outer cannula. When the inner cannula is removed, this hole decreases the tube's obstruction of air flow via the upper airway, thus facilitating spontaneous breathing via the upper airway and the use of noninvasive IPPV. Likewise, it facilitates exhalation via the vocal cords and upper airway. Some fenestrated tubes also have a fenestrated inner cannula, allowing more air to pass through the upper airway during tracheostomy IPPV. Phonation and the ability to cough can be enhanced by the fenestration, but the fenestration can also irritate and possibly damage local mucus membranes and facilitate the formation of granulation tissue.

Fenestrated tubes come with caps (Fig. 5) that can seal the tubes to permit spontaneous breathing and noninvasive IPPV via the upper airway. To utilize the fenestration, one must deflate the cuff (if present), remove the inner cannula (if nonfenestrated), and lock the cap onto the outer cannula (Fig. 6). The cap is used when the patient is not receiving IPPV via the tube. With the fenestration open (the inner cannula removed) the patient breathes through the upper airway or uses noninvasive IPPV. Spontaneous phonation and coughing are then possible.

Tracheostomy phonation valves facilitate verbalization for patients with tracheostomy tubes (see below). Phonation valves (Passy-Muir, Inc., Irvine, CA) can be attached to open tracheostomy tubes for use during spontaneous breathing, or they can be used

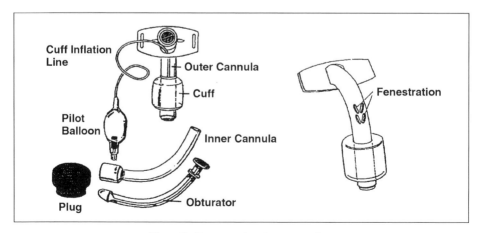

Figure 6. Fenestrated tracheostomy tube.

during tracheostomy IPPV with the cuff, if present, deflated. The valve opens during in-spiration to allow air to go through the tube and into the lungs. It closes during expira-tion and forces air up through the vocal cords to create speech. The swallowing ability of patients also often improves with the use of these valves. Patients may have a decrease in secretions, which results in less patient suctioning. Because of direct air flow through the mouth and nose, the patient's sense of smell and ability to cough up secretions for ex-pectoration are improved.

The Talking Trach is designed for use during tracheostomy IPPV with an inflated cuff. Air, injected via a conduit attached to the outer cannula, is expelled above the tube in the trachea so that it can traverse the vocal cords and provide some verbalization. This device generally works poorly and, ironically, there should rarely be any need for it be-cause patients who can speak should not require cuff inflation or tracheostomy tubes. Nevertheless, conventionally managed patients with tracheostomy tubes who are unable to find any clinician willing to remove them may suffer the clinician's clumsy attempts at these methods.

Intubation and Tracheostomy Paradigm Paralysis

Paradigm paralysis is the failure to learn new and superior approaches because they differ radically from the generally used methods in which one has invested time and energy.[641] It is the terminal disease of misplaced certainty.[642]

Most patients with NMD visit physicians who do not understand the concept of aiding respiratory muscles. Even pulmonologists rarely think in terms of assisting in-spiratory and expiratory muscle function because they see mostly patients with lung diseases rather than muscle weakness. Furthermore, physicians learn as medical stu-dents and residents that the airway must be "controlled" and that respiratory insuffi-ciency must be treated with translaryngeal intubation and tracheotomy. The use of noninvasive methods is contrary to the treatment paradigms and invasive high tech-nology that physicians spent so much time learning. Thus, most physicians suffer from intubation and tracheostomy paradigm paralysis. They often tell patients that trache-otomy is the only option when they cannot be weaned from ventilator use. Even when the patient is entirely weaned from ventilator use, the tracheostomy may still not be closed because the physician is unfamiliar with effective noninvasive ways to clear airway secretions.

As a result of paradigm paralysis, patients with progressive neuromuscular weakness are often warned that the day will come when a crisis decision must be made—whether to "go on a respirator [undergo tracheostomy] for the rest of your life" or die. This warning often leaves patients and families feeling hopeless and depressed. To make matters worse, physicians usually mistakenly believe that people with NMDs have poor quality of life and are dissatisfied with life;[643] physicians also tend to be biased against the use of respi-ratory support via indwelling tracheostomy tubes.[643] As a result, many patients and fam-ilies are convinced by physicians to "refuse respirator use." Because patients are not told about noninvasive options, this practice in fact means to refuse tracheotomy and die.

Conventional respiratory management strategies are invasive and reactive rather than noninvasive and proactive. They essentially ignore the problem until the inevitable oc-currence of respiratory failure causes the patient to seek help in a local emergency de-partment or die before getting there.

Thus, many clinicians consider NMDs to be terminal because they know of no way to prevent morbidity and mortality from respiratory failure and feel justified by the inevitably fatal results of nihilistic conventional approaches.[63,644] Instead of helping to keep patients alive in anticipation of possible medical treatments and cures, they more often transmit hopelessness, provide "palliative care" that only expedites death, and make no valid effort to prevent respiratory morbidity. Thus, patients either die from acute cardiopulmonary failure or undergo tracheotomy during a usually preventable episode of acute respiratory failure. Tracheostomies can prolong survival, but many if not most patients with tracheostomies eventually die from related complications, and tracheostomies adversely affect quality of life (see below).

The Most Common Evaluation Errors

Misinterpretation of Symptoms

The symptoms of hypoxia due to lung disease can include shortness of breath, difficulty with thinking, and anxiety. There are many more symptoms of hypercapnia (Table 1), yet hypercapnia is often ignored. Even underventilating (hypercapnic) patients themselves often do not recognize early symptoms. Many people have few or no symptoms when sitting but require the use of 3 or 4 pillows to sleep because they cannot breathe for very long when lying down. This problem is often due to diaphragm dysfunction out of proportion to weakness of other inspiratory muscles. Sometimes it takes a trial of nocturnal use of inspiratory muscle aids before the user feels more energy and less fatigue and has more restful sleep.

Although people with either ventilatory impairment or lung disease with oxygenation impairment often complain of shortness of breath when walking, wheelchair users with ventilation impairment rarely complain of shortness of breath despite severe hypercapnia and impending respiratory failure. Instead, they complain of anxiety and inability to

Table 1. Symptoms of Chronic Alveolar Hypoventilation and Sleep-disordered Breathing*	
Fatigue	Lower extremity edema
Dyspnea (particularly in patients capable of ambulation)	Irritability
	Anxiety
Morning or continuous headaches	Nocturnal urinary frequency
Multiple nocturnal awakenings with dyspnea/tachycardia	Polycythemia
	Impaired intellectual function
Difficult arousals	Depression
Hypersomnolence	Decreased libido
Difficulty with concentration	Weight loss or gain
Frequent nightmares	Muscle aches
Nightmares about breathing difficulties (e.g., suffocation, drowning)	Memory impairment
	Poor control of airway secretions
Congestive heart failure	
* In order of appearance.[567]	

fall asleep. Unfortunately, these symptoms are often treated as though they are due to oxygenation impairment until decompensation results in death or translaryngeal intubation. Ventilatory failure can also cause the syndrome of inappropriate secretion of antidiuretic hormone.[645]

For small children with NMD, the initial signs of nocturnal underventilation may be frequent arousals from sleep and episodic perspiration, flushing, and tachycardia. If recognized at all, such symptoms may be mistaken for the simple need to be turned. Certainly, any small child with NMD who was once sleeping most or all of the night without arousals and then requires increasingly more frequent turns, especially the child with paradoxical breathing who awakens frequently despite using a bed that continuously turns him or her, is quite likely to have nocturnal hypoventilation.

Inadequate Pulmonary Function Studies

People with neuromuscular conditions are routinely sent to pulmonary function laboratories, where they undergo a comprehensive and expensive battery of tests designed for people with lung disease. These tests include spirometry (i.e., the measurement of forced expiratory volumes and flows to evaluate for airway obstruction), studies to test the integrity of the respiratory exchange membrane, diffusion studies, and, often, painful and inaccurate arterial blood gas analyses (see below). However, because people with neuromuscular conditions do not usually have a long history of cigarette smoking or asthma, all of these tests except for spirometry are unnecessary. Furthermore, because lung underventilation begins during sleep, spirometry or simple determination of vital capacity (VC) is best done with the person lying down. For people with many diagnoses, the VC in the supine position is often much less than in the sitting position. There can also be a great difference in VC when the patient is lying on one side or the other and when the patient is wearing or not wearing a back brace or body jacket. A well-fitting body jacket can increase the VC, whereas a poorly fitting body jacket can decrease VC. Unfortunately, pulmonary function laboratories do not measure the VC in various positions or situations, and if the physician knew enough to ask the lab to do so, he or she would perform the tests with a simple hand-held spirometer.

Although they are the most important tests of all, pulmonary function laboratories do not measure assisted cough peak flows (see Manually Assisted Coughing) or maximum insufflation capacities and are rarely equipped for or asked to measure end-tidal carbon dioxide levels.

Failure to Monitor Sleep Appropriately

Either the ability to breathe supine or during sleep is entirely ignored, or expensive and unnecessary polysomnography is ordered to diagnose sleep-disordered breathing (Chapter 10). To perform polysomnography, patients are usually asked to sleep in the hospital and are observed for at least one night. Electroencephalography, plethysmographic measurement of chest and abdomen movement, air flow at the nose, and SpO_2 are typically monitored. It can be difficult to sleep under these circumstances. The test attributes symptoms to central or obstructive apneas; it does not attribute them to underventilation secondary to inspiratory muscle weakness and, therefore, has little relevance to people with NMDs. Furthermore, once the polysomnographer has the interpretation of central or obstructive apneas, almost invariably he or she inappropriately prescribes oxygen therapy, CPAP, or bilevel PAP at insufficient levels to fully rest or adequately assist the inspiratory muscles during sleep or otherwise (see below). In reality, the only tests needed to monitor sleep are oximetry and end-tidal carbon dioxide. Polysomnography is warranted to evaluate symptoms only when the VC and maximum inspiratory pressures are essentially normal and nocturnal $EtCO_2$ and SpO_2 are unremarkable despite symptoms.

Overreliance on Arterial Blood Gases

Arterial blood gas analyses are not needed for medically stable people with NMDs (Chapter 11). Pain from the arterial stick causes hyperventilation and can cause falsely low carbon dioxide tensions 30% of the time.[646] Furthermore, unlike the use of end-tidal carbon dioxide and oximetry (which are practical and painless methods of blood oxygen and carbon dioxide analysis), an arterial blood gas analysis gives only a one-point rather than a continuous look at the body's gas exchange. Without hospitalization and the painful and hazardous placement of an arterial catheter, invasive blood gas analyses cannot be monitored during sleep, the most important time of all.

The Most Common Conventional Treatment Approaches

1. "Palliation" with narcotics, sedatives, and supplemental oxygen to lighten and hasten death while obtaining "advanced directives" or "informed consent" interdicting the use of "heroic measures," generally intubation or tracheotomy.
2. Treating ventilatory insufficiency and episodes of acute ventilatory failure as though they were respiratory insufficiency—with some combination of oxygen, bronchodilators, chest physical therapy, airway suctioning, and, ultimately, intubation and tracheostomy.
3. "Prophylactic" tracheotomy.
4. Using nocturnal bilevel PAP at low inspiratory and expiratory pressure spans that are ultimately inadequate to avert ventilatory failure, intubation, and tracheotomy.

Easing and Hastening Death or "Not-so-benign Neglect"

Prescribing oxygen therapy with or without morphine is an especially popular approach with clinicians who do not offer noninvasive respiratory aids and who preach "therapeutic nihilism."[644] This approach, commonly used for amyotrophic lateral sclerosis (ALS) and motor neuron disease (MND), decreases dyspnea while hastening hypercapnic narcosis and death.[647,648] Eighty-two percent of patients with ALS die while receiving morphine, and 64% receive benzodiazepines; few if any are provided with noninvasive aids in Great Britain.[649] Often, without consulting the patient, the physician judges the patient's quality of life as unacceptable and the disease as terminal, ignores options that prevent respiratory complications, and biases the family against any ventilator use, which the physician usually associates with tracheostomy.[643] This approach emphasizes "palliation" but results in hopelessness and mental anguish. Patients die from carbon dioxide narcosis, aspiration of airway secretions, or an intercurrent chest cold that results in pneumonia and acute respiratory failure.[14,650] If morphine levels are not high enough to obtund the patients and they become short of breath, they often change their minds and ask for intubation and tracheotomy.

Treating Ventilatory Insufficiency Like Respiratory Insufficiency

Conventional approaches to managing ventilatory insufficiency are identical to those for respiratory insufficiency and include supplemental oxygen administration, bronchodilators, and chest physical therapy, as is typical for chronic obstructive pulmonary disease (COPD). The goals of medical therapy can be to increase diaphragm contractility, to dilate the airways and facilitate airway secretion clearance, to improve ventilatory drive, and to improve oxygenation without exacerbating hypercapnia. Unfortunately, no medical therapy has been shown to be effective and safe for any of these goals for patients with NMD.[651] It has also been suggested that tricyclic antidepressants or monoamine oxidase inhibitors (e.g., safrazine hydrochloride) can be used to suppress rapid-eye-movement (REM) sleep to correct nocturnal hypoxemia in patients with DMD.[652] Nocturnal REM hypoxemia, however, is often the first sign of nocturnal hypoventilation and is rarely symptomatic until it progresses to cause long periods of nocturnal oxyhemoglobin desaturation (dSpO$_2$) and hypercapnia. When patients become symptomatic, noninvasive ventilatory assistance is appropriate rather than further sleep disruption.

Bronchodilators, although often helpful for mobilizing peripheral airway secretions during intercurrent upper respiratory infections, are too often used on a routine long-term basis with no subjective or objective benefits. Bronchodilators often cause anxiety and, by increasing heart rate, can exacerbate cardiac dysfunction in patients with cardiomyopathies. Bronchodilators can even increase production of airway secretions.

Oxygen therapy became widely accepted for treating hypoxia in the mid-1960s. It has been demonstrated to improve survival significantly for patients with COPD.[653] This success and general familiarity with oxygen therapy have led to its use for treating hypoxia due to ventilatory impairment. However, considering the pathophysiology of ventilatory impairment (Chapter 9), such patients fare poorly because hypercapnia is exacerbated. Oxygen supplementation for such patients results in a significantly higher incidence of pneumonia, hospitalization, and hospitalization days than for untreated patients or when respiratory muscle aids are used.[14] In addition, because of its relatively high pressure gradient for absorption by comparison with nitrogen, supplemental oxygen can cause and help to maintain atelectasis.[654] Most patients with NMD who become comatose from carbon dioxide narcosis do so while receiving oxygen supplementation rather than assisted ventilation. Oxygen should not be used for people with NMDs other than for acute resuscitation, unless they are hospitalized in intensive care and monitored intently for intubation.

Although most conventionally managed patients avoid carbon dioxide narcosis, they inevitably undergo tracheotomy or die from retention of airway secretions during chest infections because of failure to teach and equip them to use mechanically assisted coughing (MAC).[655] Attempts to suction patients' airways via the nose or mouth are rarely effective and can further impair breathing. There is even less chance to enter the left main stem bronchus in this manner than with suctioning via a tube. Lung suctioning via the upper airway should rarely if ever be required or used as an alternative to MAC.

Prophylactic Tracheotomy

Because a higher rate of complications is associated with emergency rather than elective tracheotomy, and because respiratory failure is inevitable for conventionally managed patients, physicians unfamiliar with respiratory muscle aids or the indications for tracheostomy[656] may recommend it prophylactically.[657] Most often, however, this option is appropriately refused by the patient. Prophylactic tracheotomy is appropriate only for patients with severe bulbar ALS or other patients with minimal assisted CPF and baseline SpO_2 less than 95% (Chapter 11).

Low-span Positive Inspiratory Pressure Plus PEEP or Bilevel Positive Airway Pressure

As the widespread prevalence of obstructive sleep apnea syndrome (OSAS) became appreciated in the 1980s, CPAP was used to maintain upper airway patency. CPAP pneumatically splints open the airway and increases functional residual capacity. It is in-effective, however, for patients whose hypercapnia is based on inspiratory muscle weakness or excessive load because it does not directly assist inspiratory muscle function. Although this point may appear to be obvious, a recent study of pressure support venti-lation vs. CPAP confirmed its validity.[658]

In pressure support ventilation, the ventilator delivers a preset inspiratory pressure to assist spontaneous breathing efforts. Many ventilators permit patient-triggering with a set back-up rate. With pressure control ventilation as delivered by BiPAP-ST (Respironics, Inc.), for example, time-cycled preset inspiratory and expiratory pressures are delivered at a controlled rate with adjustable inspiratory-expiratory ratios. Ven-tilators can cycle to expiration when they sense a fall in inspiratory flow below a thresh-old value or at a preset time. Flow triggering of inspiratory cycling, which is often available on pressure-cycled machines, is generally more sensitive than the pressure trig-gering of many volume-cycled ventilators.[659]

The BiPAP machine was developed because of the frequent ineffectiveness of CPAP and the difficulties that patients have in tolerating high CPAP levels. The pressure-cycled ventilators' light weight, inspiratory pressures to greater than 20 cmH_2O, PEEP (equivalent to EPAP) capabilities, similarity to CPAP (CPAP plus additional inspiratory positive airway pressure [IPAP]), and relatively low cost compared with volume-cycled ventilators led to quick acceptance and widespread use.

The BiPAP-ST, the Synchrony, and the BiPAP Harmony (Respironics, Inc.); the PB335 Respiratory Support System and the Quantom (Mallincrodt-Puritan-Bennett, Inc., Pleasanton, CA); the ResMed VPAP-STII (ResMed, Inc., San Diego, CA), and other similar units are essentially pressure-cycled blowers up to pressures of 22–40 cmH_2O with delivered volumes plateauing at the higher pressures. The IPAP and the EPAP are adjusted manually, and the ventilator delivers air flows to achieve the set pressures.

The inspiratory pressure minus the PEEP (IPAP-EPAP difference) or pressure span is essentially the amount of inspiratory muscle assistance that the patient receives. The fail-ure of all of the ventilator-delivered air to enter the lungs from any style of ventilation (i.e., insufflation leakage) is due to any combination of mask leakage and leakage out of the nose for mouthpiece ventilation or out of the mouth for nasal ventilation. Pressure-cycled ventilators, at least in part, compensate for leakage, whereas increased airway re-sistance (e.g., from mucus plugging) results in a decrease in delivered volumes. Excessive mask leakage can impair the expiratory trigger cycling mechanism and result in pro-longed duration of the inspiratory phase, auto-PEEP, and patient-ventilator dyssyn-chrony. In the presence of air leaks, time-cycled expiratory triggers facilitate better patient-machine synchrony than flow-cycled expiratory triggers.[660]

Nocturnal low-span bilevel PAP has become part of the conventional management of patients with NMD. A recent survey of NMD clinic directors indicated that nocturnal low-span bilevel PAP was used for patients in about 80% of the clinics.[647,661,662] Nocturnal-only delivery of bilevel PAP at low spans (IPAP minus EPAP less than 10 cmH$_2$O) using commonly available, inexpensive, generic CPAP masks as patient-ventilator interfaces provides a small pressure boost to assist inspiratory effort (see Fig. 1). It is widely used even in the absence of diurnal hypercapnia or symptoms of ventilatory insufficiency. Although it can be helpful during early stages, low spans of typically 5–7 cmH$_2$O inadequately rest respiratory muscles and insufficiently assist inspiratory muscle function to sustain patients as inspiratory muscle weakness progresses.

Increasing the EPAP without increasing the IPAP decreases the span. EPAP is conventionally used, even though it does not benefit patients with predominantly inspiratory muscle impairment. The greater the level of EPAP, the greater the IPAP that must be used to provide the same level of inspiratory assistance and the greater the resulting intrathoracic pressure. It has been shown that increases in intrathoracic pressure cause dose-dependent decreases in cardiac stroke volume and cardiac output.[663] Such decreases can be hazardous for ventilator users with cardiomyopathies.

Even the maximum spans of most commonly used machines generally deliver less than 1200-ml volumes to patients with normal lung impedance. These volumes do not permit the cough volumes or flows needed to clear airway secretions or optimally raise voice volumes. When lung impedance is increased, even adequate ventilation may not be achieved. Thus, the fact that pressure-cycled ventilators are widely used at suboptimal spans plays a large role in patients with neuromuscular weakness who develop ventilatory failure or respiratory failure during intercurrent chest infections.[615]

As noted previously, in many centers patients with weak respiratory muscles, with or without symptoms, are treated on the basis of polysomnographic findings interpreted as central or obstructive apneas rather than inspiratory muscle weakness.[664] Use of CPAP or low-span bilevel PAP results from the inability of polysomnography to evaluate respiratory muscle dysfunction, failure to appreciate the need for respiratory muscle rest, unjustified fear of barotrauma (Chapter 10), and physicians' much greater familiarity with CPAP, OSAS, and lung disease than with neuromuscular weakness in patients with essentially normal lung tissues.

Nocturnal-only Nasal Ventilation

Ventilatory insufficiency progresses insidiously. Patients with symptoms of ventilatory insufficiency and hypoxia can benefit from nocturnal nasal ventilation whether it be provided as bilevel PAP or IPPV.[14] Nasal ventilation typically relieves fatigue and other symptoms of which patients may have been unaware. When such patients feel better the day after using nocturnal nasal ventilation, they rarely need to be prompted to continue use.

A consensus conference in 1991 suggested the following indications and considerations for instituting nocturnal nasal ventilation for stable patients with DMD: rapid speed of disease progression, presence of hypercapnia or end-tidal carbon dioxide exceeding 50 mmHg during sleep, nocturnal mean SpO$_2$ less than 95%, and symptoms of ventilatory insufficiency. In addition, it was agreed that in the absence of symptoms, nocturnal nasal ventilation is indicated for patients with DMD when PaCO$_2$ exceeds 45 mmHg and/or

PaO_2 is less than 60 mmHg in blood gas samples taken early in the morning, late in the day, or during periods of $dSpO_2$.[665] Another consensus conference in 1999 determined that for patients with NMD and chest wall deformities the indications for nocturnal nasal ventilation were symptomatic hypoventilation, $PaCO_2$ greater than 45 mmHg, nocturnal SpO_2 less than 89% for at least 5 consecutive minutes, or maximal inspiratory pressures less than 60 cmH_2O or FVC less than 50% of predicted.[666]

Numerous other opinions have been offered with various criteria, especially VC, for patients with ALS and other neuromuscular diseases. The American Thoracic Society has recommended institution of bilevel PAP once the patient with ALS is symptomatic or the FVC is noted to be below 50%. Third-party payors often demand quantifiable indications involving criteria concerning maximum inspiratory pressures, FVC, CO_2 levels, and SpO_2. However, in one ALS study, symptomatic hypoventilation occurred at greatly varying levels for these parameters (e.g., with normal SpO_2 and with FVC from 16–111% of normal). Some patients with ALS are asymptomatic despite VCs as low as 40%.[667] Another study of 20 patients with ALS also found that FVC% correlated poorly with respiratory symptoms.[668] Although symptomatic nocturnal hypoventilation is a valid indication, patients do not always realize that they are symptomatic until they have a treatment trial. It has also been suggested that MIP and nocturnal oximetry are sensitive measures of early ventilatory insufficiency and can serve as indicators for introduction of nocturnal nasal ventilation.[668] However, 23 of 29 patients with at least two symptoms of hypoventilation had only about 1 minute or so of SpO_2 below 90% during sleep.[667] There is also no correlation between VC and nocturnal $dSpO_2$s or mean SpO_2.[667,669]

Thus, it should be appreciated that some "indications" (e.g., speed of progression) are irrelevant and others are draconian. The only true indication is relief of symptoms although before treatment VC is usually less than 100% of normal, MIPs are reduced, nocturnal mean SpO_2 is usually less than the normal 96.5%,[670] and episodes of nocturnal $dSpO_2$ occur with increased frequency.[667]

Patients tend to become symptomatic when diurnal hypercapnia causes the SpO_2 to decrease below 95%. When diurnal SpO_2 is normal, even when untreated, many patients can tolerate hypercapnia for years or until they have an intercurrent chest cold. Although nocturnal low-span bilevel PAP can benefit mildly affected patients, instead of increasing the spans or switching to the use of volume-cycled ventilators for daytime IPPV via a mouthpiece when low-span pressure assistance is no longer adequate, clinicians conventionally prescribe oxygen or recommend tracheotomy.[665,671] Once the patient is intubated or a tracheostomy tube is placed, the patient then receives appropriate tidal volumes at adequate peak inspiratory pressures (usually 20–25 cmH_2O) to maintain normal lung ventilation and facilitate coughing. Ironically, if these pressures had been provided noninvasively, the patient would not have progressed to invasive management.

Along with suboptimal bilevel PAP spans, conventional management includes medical interventions, chest physical therapy, and occasionally IPPB for inadequate periods and at inadequate pressures to fully expand the lungs and chest walls or to support or rest inspiratory muscles. These therapeutic measures do not address the fundamental need to support inspiratory muscles and increase cough flows. Failure to assist the cough must inevitably result in respiratory failure for patients with NMD. Even now, airway mucus accumulation tends to be considered a "complication" of the use of noninvasive ventilation rather than the failure of the clinician to institute insufflation therapy and MAC.[672]

A recent review of nocturnal (conventional) nasal ventilation inadvertently provided an excellent example of common errors and misunderstandings.[673] The review notes that "patients with severe neuromuscular weakness, prominent pulmonary secretions, or significant bulbar dysfunction" may require tracheostomy. This review ignored the fact that patients with no measurable VC successfully use noninvasive IPPV; it failed to consider assisted coughing to clear secretions; and it failed to quantitate bulbar muscle dysfunction (Chapter 11). The review arbitrarily recommended normalizing end-tidal carbon dioxide by "no more than 15 mmHg." It advised that ventilatory assistance be initiated in a monitored environment, even though we have instituted noninvasive IPPV for hundreds of patients, many eventual 24-hour users, in the outpatient clinic and home settings. The review also noted that polysomnography is necessary and supplemental oxygen required when bilevel PAP does not increase SpO_2 to greater than 90%. Both suggestions are harmful and dangerous for patients with primarily ventilatory impairment.

Okay, Maybe It's Not Sexy

With a mask on my nose
   Or a mask on my face
With black straps and Velcro
   To hold it in place

With tubes from the floor
   Tubes over my head
With air hissing out
   From the vent by my bed

With this strange contraption
   What a sight I must be
But breathing more deeply
   Is better for me

The headaches are gone
   During the day I'm awake
I'm eating much better
   At my lunchtime break

Though strange it may look
   And strange it may feel
I don't wear this mask
   For its sex appeal

The breath of life
   By night I am given
My NIV system
   Is a gift straight from heaven!

Rich Clingman

Volume-cycled Ventilators

The expiratory volume alarm of intensive care volume ventilators makes them impractical to use for delivery of noninvasive IPPV, and they are usually not sufficiently portable for home use. Nasal ventilation was initially and has been most frequently described using portable volume-cycled ventilators (Table 2).[674–677] Nonetheless, in the United States, portable volume-cycled ventilator use is conventionally limited to providing long-term tracheostomy rather than noninvasive IPPV.

Volume-cycled ventilators—such as the PLV-100 (Respironics, Inc.); LP-10, LP-20, and Achieva (Puritan-Bennett, Inc.); LTV-900 (Pulmonetic Systems, Inc., Colton, CA); I-Vent (Versa-Med, Inc., Rochelle Park, NJ); and Newport HT50 (Newport NMI, Inc., Newport Beach, CA)—can also be pressure-cycled and deliver volumes up to 2500 ml. Typically, control, assist-control, and synchronized intermittent mandatory ventilation (SIMV) modes can be used. The Eole 3 portable ventilator (Vivisol, Inc., Monza, Italy)

Table 2. **Pressure Assist vs. Portable Volume Ventilators**

Advantages of volume ventilators
1. Can deliver higher volumes and pressures as needed for patients with poor lung compliance
2. Can adjust flow rates for comfort
3. Use 3–8 times less electricity for comparable air delivery, permitting greater patient mobility
4. Operate more quietly
5. Generate less mean thoracic pressures with less untoward hemodynamic effects on cardiac preload
6. Permit air-stacking to maximum insufflations
7. Can be used to operate intermittent abdominal pressure ventilators as well as for noninvasive IPPV
8. Have alarm systems that can facilitate effective nocturnal use of noninvasive IPPV

Disadvantages of volume ventilators
1. Heavier
2. Have more annoying alarms
3. Needlessly complicated (ventilators with fewer modes should be available)

Advantages of bilevel PAP devices
1. Have fewer or no annoying alarms
2. Light-weight
3. Cost less
4. Can compensate to some extent for insufflation leaks

Disadvantages of bievel PAP devices
1. Cannot be used for air-stacking
2. Have fixed, high initial flow rates that can cause mouth drying, gagging (especially with insufflation leakage), and arousals from sleep
3. High power utilization limits patient mobility
4. Have inadequate pressure generation capabilities to ventilate some patients
5. Create discomfort and increased thoracic pressures from unnecessary expiratory positive airway pressure
6. Pressure gauges are less useful for feedback concerning insufflation leakages
7. No alarms to facilitate effective nocturnal IPPV (useful for some patients)
8. Noisier
9. EPAP is unnecessary for most patients but cannot be turned off
10. Cause significant rebreathing of carbon dioxide that can be corrected by using a nonrebreathing valve at the cost of greater expiratory resistance[758]
11. EPAP can make eating difficult or hazardous for 24-hour ventilator users

---

is not practical for noninvasive ventilation because tidal volumes are limited to 1550 ml; in addition, it has expiratory volume and minute ventilation alarms that sound unnecessarily when noninvasive ventilation is used. The LTV, which weights 12 lb and is the size of a laptop computer, and Newport machines (15 lb) are small but relatively noisy and expensive. The Newport, however, can operate 10 hours on its internal battery. The I-Vent is relatively large and expensive. The LTV-900 has had relatively frequent technical glitches. This and other small units, however, can be ideal for patients who are able to walk despite ventilator dependence (see Chapter 13 and Case 2 of Chapter 15 of reference 103) as well as for others who need small, light units to optimize mobility.[677]

The most commonly used mode for home noninvasive ventilation is assist-control. With this mode, set volumes of air are delivered, triggered by the patient's inspiratory effort. A back-up rate provides air delivery in the absence of effort. For volume-cycled ventilators, once set, the volume to be delivered to the ventilator circuit remains constant regardless of the insufflation leakage, pulmonary compliance, and airway resistance. However, since insufflation leakage can change from breath to breath, the volumes delivered to the lungs change from breath to breath. The volumes delivered to the lungs correlate with ventilator gauge pressures. Thus, the pressures indicated on the volume ventilator pressure gauge vary depending on ventilator-delivered volumes, insufflation leakage, and lung impedance. There are also low- and high-pressure alarms, sensitivity controls that permit the patient to trigger ventilator-delivered breaths, and flow-rate adjustments. These ventilators can be pressure-cycled like pressure-cycled ventilators by increasing the delivered volumes and lowering the high-pressure alarm.

Volume- vs. Pressure-cycled Ventilators

A number of studies have attempted to compare the efficacy of ventilatory assistance using bilevel PAP vs. noninvasive IPPV from volume-cycled ventilators in both acute and long-term settings and for both daytime and overnight use. In a review of these studies, no clear advantage can be appreciated using either system. Hill concluded that "the choice between the two comes down to clinician preference and a consideration of the particular advantages and disadvantages."[678] This conclusion, however, is true only for patients who cannot air-stack.

Advantages and disadvantages of using volume-cycled and pressure-cycled ventilators are listed in Table 2. Because the currently available pressure-cycled units are limited to pressures of less than 40 cmH$_2$O, they may be inadequate for managing conditions characterized by poor pulmonary compliance or high work of breathing, such as severe scoliosis or obesity. On the other hand, bilevel PAP can be useful for managing COPD and sleep-disordered breathing. Even low-span bilevel PAP can effectively assist inspiratory muscle function for emphysematous patients with hypercompliant lungs. The positive pressures can also stabilize the airway in the event of concurrent obstructive sleep apneas or bulbar muscle dysfunction with airway collapse, and PEEP can decrease the work of breathing by relieving the effort required of patients with COPD to reverse the expiratory flows associated with air trapping, thus countering auto-PEEP. However, few patients with NMD have COPD. In general, depending on settings, work of breathing can be equally decreased during pressure-cycled and volume-cycled ventilation.[679] Because patients cannot air-stack when using the former, the long-term use of pressure-cycled ventilators for patients with NMD who are capable of air-stacking is suboptimal unless the patient is equipped with the means to expand the lungs and assist the cough.

Currently available pressure-cycled ventilators can weigh as little as 5.5 lb. They are becoming lighter, smaller, and quieter. The Harmony, for example, weighs only 2.5 kg, is quiet, and can provide IPAP up to 30 cmH$_2$O. It uses only 10% more amperage than typical portable volume-cycled ventilators and can now operate most of the day on a fully charged external battery. The ResMed VPAP-STII is 1 kg heavier but provides IPAP up to 40 cmH_2O and, therefore, can be more useful for deep insufflation therapy for patients who do not have Cough-Assist devices or volume-cycled ventilators and who are unable to air-stack via a manual resuscitator (Chapter 10). These machines are useful for air delivery without high- and low-pressure alarms. This feature can be an advantage or a disadvantage, depending on the particular patient. These devices do not have internal batteries. They also use more electricity than volume-cycled ventilators and, therefore, run for shorter periods on an external battery source when they are equipped to do so.

Air-stacking to facilitate coughing, to increase voice volume, and to expand the lungs optimally is not possible with pressure-cycled ventilators. Depending on the unit and lung impedance characteristics, most patients cannot obtain the minimum 1.5-L insufflation volumes generally needed for an effective assisted cough.[265] In addition, despite increases in minute ventilation and reductions in respiratory effort, bilevel PAP does not always reduce $PaCO_2$. It has been suggested that this finding is due to the rebreathing of carbon dioxide inherent with the standard exhalation device, the fixed-resistance exhalation Whisper-Swivel (Respironics, Inc.), The patient rebreathes air exhaled into the ventilator tubing, and dead space ventilation is increased.[680] A completely unacceptable EPAP level of 8 cmH_2O would be required to eliminate the rebreathing. The problem can be eliminated by using non-rebreather valves and exhalation plateau valves. However, the former can malfunction if valve materials stiffen or secretions become impacted within it, and the latter is not yet commercially available. A generally better alternative is to switch to volume-cycled ventilation at appropriate settings. The use of bilevel PAP by clinicians with little experience in noninvasive aids almost invariably leads to failure to intervene appropriately during intercurrent chest infections.

Ventilator Capabilities and Battery Operation

All ventilators can operate on direct current from external batteries. In addition, all volume-cycled ventilators have internal batteries that can power the ventilator for periods of 45 minutes to up to 10 hours (Newport ventilator). The ventilator continues to operate from an external battery until the battery is depleted, at which point the ventilator switches to the internal battery. The internal battery comes equipped with a charger that is built into the ventilator. It must be used from time to time, or else it may not function when needed.

Although the primary external battery types are lead-acid batteries, no-maintenance sealed batteries and deep-cycle, gel-cell batteries, all batteries used with portable ventilators should be the marine-type, deep-cycle gel-cell batteries because of their safety and power. Although the gel cells contain acid, it is in a gel form; the battery is completely sealed and can be operated in almost any position. Airlines and other transport vehicles always require the use of deep-cycle gel cells. The most reliable deep-cycle, gel-cell battery manufactures are Interstate, Inc.; MK, Inc.; and Sears, Inc.

MK deep-cycle, gel-cell batteries of the 12-volt type are generally available in three sizes: the group-22 supplies approximately 35 amp hours; the group-24 supplies approximately 72 amp hours; and the group-28 supplies approximately 98 amp hours. The group-24 is the most often used battery for portable ventilators. It permits sufficient operating time and usually has good reserve.

Ventilators have varying power demands, and patients use ventilators at different power utilization rates (volumes, pressures, and cycling rates). The greater the volume/pressure delivery and the higher the ventilator rate, the greater the ventilator's amperage utilization and the shorter the utilization time of the battery. Portable ventilators can use 2–6 amps per hour, depending on ventilator characteristics. With normal use, the batteries that come with the PVL100 and PVL102 are capable of supplying power for approximately 16–20 hours. An IAPV often requires volumes of at least 1600 ml, pressures of at least 40 cmH$_2$O, and breath rates of at least 22 bpm. Consequently, the demand on the battery is very high.

All ventilators are not created equally. Although the Respironics PLV series is ideal for sleeping purposes using noninvasive ventilation or ventilation via tracheostomy, it is not powerful enough to operate an IAPV. The LP10, LP20 (now discontinued), and Achieva series are more suitable for the high operating demands of the IAPV. Whereas all other ventilators on the market today were designed to operate on a 12-volt DC system, the Achieva series is the only portable ventilator that requires a 24-volt DC operating system for optimal performance. The clinical manual repeatedly notes that "although the ventilator will operate on a 12-volt battery, it will not deliver optimal performance at higher settings." One IAPV user with no respiratory muscle function used the Achieva with the small 12-amp, 24-volt external battery that was delivered with it. His IAPV required high volumes of 1700 ml and pressures of at least 40 cmH$_2$O at rates of about 22 per minute with an I/E ratio of 1:1.2. This setting provided the patient with 330-ml tidal volumes that were supplemented by GPB to maintain normal alveolar ventilation throughout the day. When 12-volt DC operation batteries (MK group-24, 72-amp hour battery) or the 12-amp, 24-volt CarGo battery was used to operate the IAPV, IAPV use was limited to under 9 hours. CarGo Battery International, Inc. (Colorado) constructed a group-28 24-volt battery that fit nicely on a wheelchair and was able to operate the IAPV at the high settings for over 25 hours. It should be emphasized that routine use of noninvasive or tracheostomy IPPV does not require such powerful batteries because even the most active ventilator users can recharge batteries while sleeping overnight.

Battery chargers for the gel cells have automatic tapers and automatic shut-off systems. The chargers automatically provide a boost every few hours so that the battery is kept fully charged. When a battery is recharged, it should be detached from the ventilator and the charger attached to the terminals before plugging in the charger. Otherwise, a severe shock or short circuit may occur. To optimize the "memory" of the battery, all new batteries should initially be charged only as recommended by the manufacturer.

Conventional Intensive Care and Extubation

Intubation is a clinical decision based on the assessment of need for invasive respiratory support and secretion management. For children and others with NMD without access to respiratory muscle aids, it is often dangerously delayed for fear of inability to extubate the patient successfully. As a result, some patients remain in peril, unable to expel airway secretions effectively, and lingering for weeks in intensive care. This scenario occurs because approaches to avoid intubation and conventional approaches to extubation are inappropriate for patients with primarily ventilatory impairment.

Vocal cord paralysis, scarring and narrowing of the voice box and dysfunction of its muscles, and airway collapse can also result from endotracheal intubation. Sometimes an endotracheal tube is passed into a bronchus, causing a pneumothorax. Because acute respiratory failure is almost always avoidable for patients with NMD other than infants with SMA type 1, intubation and its complications are usually avoidable. However, when respiratory aids are not used, acute respiratory failure and intubation can become inevitable.

Typically, like any patient presenting to the emergency department with respiratory distress, patients with NMD receive supplemental oxygen along with bronchodilators, mucolytics, chest physical therapy, and, possibly, sedation. Oxygen therapy and sedation often cause respiratory arrest. Once the patient is intubated, ventilator weaning parameters are often used to guide subsequent extubation. They include resting minute ventilation, maximum voluntary ventilation, tidal volume, VC, maximum inspiratory force, arterial-alveolar oxygen gradient on 100% oxygen, ratio of dead space to tidal volume, and functional residual capacity. There are so many parameters because none of them are very sensitive; most are related to inspiratory rather than expiratory function. Most physicians believe that intubated patients need to be weaned from ventilator use before they can be extubated, whereas we routinely extubate patients with little or no measurable VC. We have demonstrated that post-extubation CPF is the most sensitive parameter to predict successful extubation for patients with primarily ventilatory impairment.[656] Pre-extubation generation of peak expiratory flows, a measure of expiratory muscle function, has also been shown to be quite important in predicting success in extubating patients with primarily respiratory impairment.[681]

Whether the patient is intubated or has a tracheostomy tube, attempts at ventilator weaning are conventionally done by using some combination of assist-control ventilation, SIMV, pressure support, PEEP, and supplemental oxygen. Occasionally, periods of ventilator-free breathing are tried with the patient receiving CPAP or oxygen and humidification by T-piece. With these approaches, "weaning schedules" are imposed on the patient. The schedule either causes anxiety because the patient is not ready to breathe autonomously, or the schedule is too conservative, delaying respiratory muscle reconditioning. Furthermore, the use of pulse oximetry, which can signal the presence of airway mucus encumberment as well as its elimination with treatment, is lost with oxygen administration, and ventilatory drive is also depressed. The supplemental oxygen therapy becomes tantamount to putting a "Bandaid on a cancer," with the "cancer" being some combination of hypoventilation and airway mucus.

Because SpO_2 from 90% to 95% is considered acceptable for most patients with lung disease, patients with neuromuscular weakness are often extubated without concern for their ability to maintain normal SpO_2 in ambient air. However, when the SpO_2 in ambient air is not greater than 94%, it is invariably because of hypoventilation, airway mucus, or residual lung disease. Desaturations are often managed by increasing oxygen delivery rather than by clearing airway secretions. Thus, when such patients are extubated without normal SpO_2 in ambient air, they are expected to be ventilator-weaned and able to clear airway secretions despite some combination of hypercapnia, residual airway mucus encumberment, and lung disease. Furthermore, they are often extubated to CPAP, to inappropriately low-span bilevel PAP, or simply to breathing on their own. Cough aids are not used. This approach effectively puts them in a "sink-or-swim" situation and often results in re-intubation.

Intubated ventilator-supported patients can develop hypo- or hypercapnia, decreases in pulmonary function because of airway mucus, and inspiratory muscle deconditioning. A study of normal rats demonstrated a daily decrease in diaphragm weight and contractile properties after just 48 hours of mechanical ventilation.[682] These factors, along with laryngeal edema or airway damage, can make post-extubation CPF ineffective. In addition, the patients' mucociliary elevators are impaired by intubation. Thus, mucus accumulation can greatly hamper ventilator weaning and the ability to remain extubated and is the main reason that patients require intubation and reintubation.[656] These effects are exacerbated by the tendency of intubated patients to be undernourished (Chapter 4). Thus, it is not surprising that conventional extubation of patients with NMD is successful significantly less often compared with extubation using respiratory muscle aids (Chapter 12).

Complications of Invasive Management

Whether performed under emergency or elective circumstances, and despite the proliferation of ventilation modes that include proportional assist, pressure support, jet, SIMV, and assist-control ventilation as well as PEEP and precise oxygen delivery systems, the hospital survival rates of intubated and tracheostomy IPPV users have not improved over the past 20 years.[683] Numerous complications of invasive support have been described.[684] They include infection and destruction of airway cilia[685–688] associated with pathogenic bacterial colonization of the airway, chronic purulent bronchitis, granuloma formation, and sepsis from paranasal sinusitis.[689,690] Indeed, in 2002 the Surgeon General reported that over 100,000 Americans die each year from nosocomial infections, many (if not most) of which are engendered by the use of invasive airway tubes. Sudden death is common from mucus plugging,[691–693] cardiac arrhythmias,[694–696] accidental disconnections, and other causes also related to the presence of an indwelling tube, including tracheomalacia, tracheal ulcers, perforation, and hemorrhage.[697,698] A not uncommon autopsy report in patients with a tracheostomy tube who die suddenly reads as follows: "Approximately 17 cm from the ostomy there is a 0.8 mm mucosal ulceration on the tracheal wall. When probed it is found to communicate with the right common carotid artery that is 'pulled' at this level towards the trachea by the soft scar and granulation tissue of the tracheal ulcer bed. The lungs have extensive areas of parenchymal blood imbibition."

There is an 8%[699] to 65%[700] incidence of tracheal stenosis,[701] tracheoesophageal fistula,[702,703] tracheopulmonary-subcutaneous fistula associated with anaerobic subcutaneous abscess, painful hemorrhagic tube changes, aspiration of upper airway secretions and food,[704] and psychosocial difficulties. Vocal cord paralysis, laryngeal strictures, hypopharyngeal muscle dysfunction, and airway collapse can also result from invasive ventilation.[705,706] Tracheotomy was shown to exacerbate endotracheal tube-associated laryngeal damage and to increase the risk of laryngeal stenosis.[707] In fact, because the incidence of laryngotracheal stenosis is higher after tracheotomy of intubated patients than in either patients intubated for several weeks or patients undergoing tracheotomy without prior intubation, it appears preferable to maintain intubation longer in the hope of successful extubation than to resort to tracheotomy for intubated patients with any potential for extubation without tracheostomy.[708] The airway obstruction of laryngeal stenosis decreases cough flows and, thus, can ultimately prevent removal of the tracheostomy tube.[546]

Once the patient undergoes tracheotomy, the tube cuff is conventionally left inflated and verbal communication is lost (see Case 2 of Chapter 11). Patients also experience the morbidity, swallowing difficulties (Chapter 4), and higher mortality risk associated with prolonged cuff inflation.[14] The tube and cuff disrupt mucociliary transport.[709] Four hours of tracheostomy cuff inflation was shown to affect ciliary appearance and function for 3 days.[710] Cuff pressure causes tracheal wall ischemia, necrosis, and ulceration that scars and leads to stenosis or malacia and tracheal collapse during inspiration or expiration. In a study of 37 tracheostomy IPPV users who failed to wean from the ventilator, had tracheal obstruction, and required high peak airway pressures when ventilated, insertion of a longer tracheal tube became necessary for 34 patients to bypass the obstruction and re-establish the airway; 3 patients required stenting.[711] Tracheobronchomalacia has been defined by observing greater than a 50% narrowing of the distal trachea and mainstem bronchi on expiration during spontaneous breathing.[712] This condition can close the upper airway so that the tracheostomy tube can never be removed.

In addition, patients receiving tracheostomy rather than noninvasive IPPV tend to become continuously ventilator-dependent for the reasons discussed in Chapter 10. Often, hypercapnic patients who never before used ventilatory assistance and nocturnal-only noninvasive IPPV users become ventilator-dependent for 24 hours/day immediately after tracheotomy (Chapter 12).[713] Adequate expiratory flows cannot be generated by coughing or assisted coughing methods because of leakage out of or around the walls of the tube. The presence of the tube, suctioning, and bacterial colonization result in loss of physiologic coughing, chronic inflammation, denuding, ulceration, and scarring of the mucociliary elevator,[714–716] especially when suction catheters are inserted until resistance is met.[717,718] Deep suctioning, in general, is associated with greater necrosis and inflammation and greater loss of cilia and increased mucus than is shallow suctioning.[719] Thus, physiologic and assisted airway secretion elimination methods are incapacitated by intubation or tracheostomy.

Even though indications for airway suctioning have not been determined, patients with tracheostomy tubes are routinely suctioned an average of 8 times per day and 30 or more times per day when they have chest infections.[14] In a survey of intensive care nurse managers, the indications for suctioning, in order of decreasing frequency, were as follows: time from last suctioning, coughing, rhonchi, increased work of breathing, mucus visible in tube, dyspnea, patient request, before extubation, increased peak inspiratory pressures, decreased breath sounds, before drawing of blood gases, and other.[720] At best, suctioning can clear only superficial airway secretions. Suctioning misses mucus adherent between the tube and the tracheal wall, and routine suctioning misses the left mainstem bronchus in 54-92% of cases.[721] The result is a high incidence of left lung pneumonias,[721] potentially fatal mucus plugging, and perceived need for bronchoscopies. Airway suctioning is also often accompanied by discomfort, dyspnea, and severe hypoxia.[722]

An indwelling tracheostomy tube necessitates regular cleaning of the site and tube as well as tube and tubing changes and supplemental humidification. Appetite is decreased for reasons noted in Chapter 4. The chronic hypocapnia often associated with long-term tracheostomy IPPV may also result in bone decalcification.[723–725] In addition, in many states tracheostomy is considered an "open wound." This classification can prevent community living without prohibitively expensive nursing care for suctioning and stomal care (Chapter 13) and can restrict access to schools, places of employment, and recreational facilities such as swimming sites.

Optimal Use of Tracheostomy Tubes

Although tracheostomy tubes are rarely needed, their optimal use should be discussed. If speech and swallowing are possible, the cuff is deflated and the ventilator volumes increased to compensate for the leakage of air around the deflated cuff. The ventilator user and care provider know that alveolar ventilation remains adequate when (1) the patient remains asymptomatic and (2) the pressure on the ventilator's peak pressure gauge is the same with the cuff deflated as it was when the cuff was inflated. The air that leaks up and around the cuff traverses the vocal cords and is used for speech. Although normally speech occurs while one is exhaling, during tracheostomy IPPV speech occurs during the ventilator's inspiratory cycle. Typically ventilator-delivered volumes may need to be doubled to 1200–2000 ml to compensate for this leakage and to permit enough volume for effective ventilation and speech. If increasing the delivered volume to over 2000 ml cannot provide adequate lung volumes and pressures, the tracheostomy tube is too narrow or trachiectasis is severe. A wider-gauge tracheostomy tube is placed. On the other hand, if without changing delivered volumes the ventilator gauge pressures are about the same with the cuff inflated or deflated and speech is inaudible because of inadequate leak past the vocal cords, and if increasing the delivered volumes results in hyperventilation and increases in peak pressures over those when the cuff was inflated without permitting audible speech, the tracheostomy tube is too wide. In this case, one should first change to a tracheostomy tube without a cuff. If this change does not solve the problem, a narrower-gauge tracheostomy tube is placed. Ideally, there should be enough air leakage through the vocal cords to permit functional speech yet enough air entering the lungs to maintain normal lung ventilation.

Once the right tracheostomy tube gauge is determined and the user can speak effectively with the cuff deflated or removed, consideration can be given to using a one-way valve to extend the ability to speak throughout the breathing cycle, that is, to permit continuous speech. The simplest and cheapest way to accomplish this goal is by capping the expiratory valve of the ventilator tubing. The same goal can be accomplished by attaching a one-way valve—for example, a Passy-Muir valve (Irvine, CA)—between the tracheostomy tube and the ventilator tubing. When the expiratory valve is capped or a Passy-Muir valve is used, exhaled air must traverse the vocal cords and upper airway. A cuff must not be left inflated when the expiratory valve is capped or a one-way valve is used because it would prevent any exhalation and the lungs would continue to inflate, a potentially fatal situation.

Financial Liabilities of Mismanagement

Besides being unpleasant at the very least, conventional patient evaluation and management are also expensive. Referral to a pulmonary function laboratory, blood gas sampling, and polysomnography can cost over $4000. Failure to educate and equip the patient to prevent respiratory complications also results in needless and expensive hospitalizations and intensive care. In a recent study, the average length of hospitalization when tracheostomy tubes were placed for patients with NMD was 72 days,[14] most of which was spent in intensive care at $5000–$6000 per day. In Japan the average duration of ventilator care for patients with tracheostomy tubes was reported as 823 days.[726] However, the use of noninvasive IPPV, especially when required around the clock, was associated with significantly fewer hospitalizations and hospitalization days than use of tracheostomy IPPV.

We introduce noninvasive IPPV in outpatient clinics and in patients' homes.[14] We have many 24-hour noninvasive ventilation users who have never been hospitalized, intubated, or subjected to tracheotomy, in some cases for over 50 years. Quality of life is optimized and fortunes are saved when physicians learn to treat people with neuromuscular weakness to maintain lung ventilation and increase cough flows rather than for the lung diseases that they fail to teach them to avoid.

Summary of Outcomes with Conventional Management

Outcomes with conventional management have been thoroughly reviewed elsewhere.[651] All conventional approaches—oxygen therapy, CPAP, low-span bilevel PAP, and tracheotomy—lead to unnecessarily high hospitalization rates[14] and premature death for people with NMD.

Management by Tracheostomy

Although long-term tracheostomy for IPPV can greatly prolong survival, survival is often limited by complications associated with the tube itself.[97] A review of the largest series of conventional management with tracheostomy is instructive. For DMD, 90% of conventionally managed patients without tracheostomy die from pulmonary complications between 16.2 and 19 years of age and uncommonly after age 25.[5,15] Gatin reported 8 patients using tracheostomy IPPV. Two patients died 36 and 30 days after tracheotomy, one from accidental decannulation and the other from massive tracheal hemorrhage.[657] The other 6 patients survived at least 38 months. None required more than 16 hours per day of IPPV. They experienced a total of four cases of pneumonia, two cases of near-respiratory arrests from tracheobronchial mucus plugging, and adverse events such as tracheal stenosis, granulation, and pseudopolyp formation.[657] Baydur et al. reported 7 patients with DMD who received full-time tracheostomy IPPV for 18.2, 4.2, 3, 4.2, 6.3, 3.5, and 3.2 years, respectively, from the mean age of 22.3 ± 6.5 years (range = 17–36 years) to 28.5 ± 8.1 years (range = 20.5–42.3 years). Two of the 7 died from pneumonia, and 5 of the 7 were reported as having had pneumonia or recurrent pneumonia.[727] Soudon reported a 3.6-year mean survival rate for 23 tracheostomy IPPV users, most of whom had DMD.[728] Eagle et al. reported the survival times of 200 patients with DMD as 19.5 years for those untreated and 24.8 years for those receiving tracheostomy IPPV.[729] Cardiomyopathy was the cause of death for 7.4% of untreated patients but for 36.8% of ventilator users. Bach et al. reported 7 patients who received tracheostomy IPPV for a mean of 7.1 years from 21.1 ± 3.8 to 28.1 ± 4.5 years of age. Two of the 7 patients were still alive.[730] Complications were not reported. The Baydur and Bach patients who had survived long enough after episodes of acute respiratory failure to be referred to rehabilitation centers had mean prolongations of survival of 6.2 and a bit more than 7.1 years, respectively, by tracheostomy IPPV.

Noninvasive IPPV and suctioning via 4.5-mm diameter minitracheostomy tubes has been reported to avert intubation for patients with NMD in acute hypercapnic failure.[731] Of course, if these patients had been using noninvasive IPPV and cough aids properly at home, they would not have developed hypercapnic failure in the first place. Use of 4.5-mm minitracheostomy tubes by patients with DMD is consistent with the paradigm that a tracheostomy tube is needed for ventilatory support and airway secretion management. It ultimately condemns patients with NMD to using normal-sized tubes of 5 mm or more. Along with the usual tracheostomy sizes, minitracheostomy necessitates hospitalization for surgery. The tubes block the upper airway and, even when capped, diminish the generation of thoracoabdominal pressures needed for effective coughing. Minitracheostomy can also prevent glossopharyngeal breathing for breathing tolerance. The misguided patients with minitracheostomy in one center used nocturnal-only, low-span bilevel PAP and were, thereby, unable to "air-stack" deep volumes to facilitate coughing.[732] They were ventilated at inadequate volumes, both by nasal interface and by minitracheostomy. As a result of suboptimal assisted ventilation and secretion elimination, 6 of 10 patients with DMD received oxygen therapy. At least one of the 10 patients died in 1 year and others shortly thereafter. The patients were never introduced to mouthpiece interfaces for daytime IPPV, nor were they trained in the maximal insufflations or manual or mechanical cough assistance methods. With such limitations it is not surprising that the outcomes were so poor. More recently at the same center, the 5-year survival rate was reported to be only 50% for 89 patients with muscular dystrophy, including 51 with DMD.[733]

Tonoyama National Hospital in Osaka also reported its experience from 1984 to 1998.[734] Nocturnal nasal IPPV was used for 61 patients with NMD, of whom 46 had DMD. The indications were arbitrarily set at pCO_2 greater than 60 mmHg, regardless of symptoms, for all patients with NMD except those with ALS, for whom the pCO_2 had to be only greater than 50 mmHg because "ALS is more rapidly progressive." Eight patients underwent tracheotomy after 39.9 months (range = 8.5–73 months) of nocturnal-only nasal IPPV because "they wanted to be tracheostomized"! Thirteen used low-span bilevel PAP, and the others used volume-cycled ventilators at the low volumes associated with equally poor assisted ventilation. Eight patients who never underwent tracheotomy died after an average of 46.8 months: three from pneumonia, two from presumed CHF (circumstances not given), and three from "suffocation"! Sixty-two patients with NMD underwent tracheotomy without being introduced to noninvasive IPPV. Twenty-seven died, including 19 of 25 patients with DMD, after using tracheostomy IPPV for an undisclosed period. Causes of death were not reported. Nineteen additional patients with DMD who received supplemental oxygen instead of using ventilatory assistance had pCO_2 greater than 60 mmHg and died after a mean of 6 months (range = up to 1.5 years) of oxygen therapy at age 20!

In 1994, while visiting this hospital in Osaka, I observed patients with ALS and DMD, most of whom were confined to bed; all of the patients with DMD had severe scoliosis from failure to intervene surgically. All had indwelling cuffless tracheostomy tubes and were severely hypercapnic. Ventilator-delivered volumes were typically 250 ml. Despite the cuffless tubes, they had inadequate air delivery for speech. When I increased the delivered volumes for one patient from 250 to 350 ml, he complained of chest pain. This pain was most likely due to intercostal muscle stretching on the ipsilateral side of the scoliotic convexity. These patients received no "sighs," nor, in many cases, had their tidal volumes varied for years. Perhaps a more humane approach to limit the duration of suffocation would be simply to hang the patient once the pCO_2 reaches 70 mmHg! Unfortunately, this approach is not atypical for conventional management elsewhere.

In reviewing the outcomes of programs offering ventilatory support for patients with ALS from the standpoint of undergoing tracheotomy, a mortality rate of 76% was reported by 12 months for 24 IPPV users,[735] 20 months for 18 users,[736] 15 months (range = 3–48 months) for 12 users,[737] 26.6 months for 4 users,[738] 2.3 years for 3 users,[739] and 7 months for 3 users.[740] In a large study, 89 ventilator users with ALS survived using 24-hour assistance for a mean of 4.4 ± 3.9 years (range = 1 month to 26.5 years), with 37 of the patients still alive at the time of the report. Thirteen of the 89 patients had used only noninvasive methods of ventilatory support. The 76 ventilator users who ultimately received tracheostomy IPPV survived using ventilatory support for a mean of 4.5 ± 4.0 years (range = 1 month to 26.3 years). Six patients survived using tracheostomy IPPV for over 10 years, including 3 patients for over 14 years (Fig. 7). The 52 deceased patients used ventilatory support for a mean of 3.8 ± 2.9 years (range = 3 months to 14.5 years), including 4.1 ± 2.9 years (range = 1 month to 14.5 years) of tracheostomy IPPV for the 45 deceased patients who ultimately underwent tracheotomy. In this study of 89 patients with ALS, 74 with rapidly progressive disease and 15 with a slower form, 42 of the former (57%) and 11 of the latter (73%) were managed predominantly in the community.[97]

In another study of 362 patients with ALS, 194 were managed without respiratory intervention, 84 with noninvasive IPPV, and 84 with tracheostomy IPPV. Postdiagnosis survival was 19.4 months for the untreated group, 42.9 months for the noninvasive

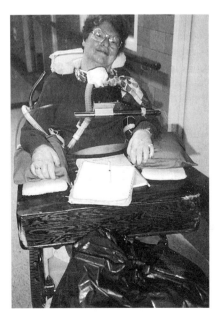

Figure 7. Woman with onset of motor neuron disease at age 23. She had been wheelchair-dependent since age 27 and a 24-hour ventilator user of tracheostomy IPPV with no residual upper extremity function since age 47. She died from complications of anemia and pneumonia at age 68. She was selling clothing (in the dark sack below her lap tray) and, with assistance, kept her own accounts (open account book on her lap tray).

IPPV users, and 87.9 months for the tracheostomy IPPV users.[95] Once bulbar dysfunction precludes use of noninvasive IPPV, survival can be further prolonged by tracheostomy. However, deterioration in physical functioning and in the ability to communicate,[97] limited family resources, and, most importantly, lack of a national personal attendant care policy (Chapter 13) often make it impractical for patients with ALS to be managed in the community. In addition, many of the sudden deaths after tracheotomy may be due to autonomic dysfunction as well as airway mucus plugging.[539] About 10–30% of patients with ALS who use tracheostomy IPPV over the long term eventually lose the ability to blink and, therefore, become blind and cannot operate augmentative communication systems.[97] Communication can also be lost when patients are placed in nursing facilities where their communication systems may not be set up or may be ignored. Cognitive impairment can also develop and progress after tracheotomy and institutionalization and can result in severe isolation and the loss of any meaningful social interaction. Understanding the family's commitment to the patient, therefore, is essential before considering tracheotomy.

In regard to SMA, Gilgoff et al. reported 15 patients who received tracheostomy IPPV for an average of 8 years and 10 months (range = 5 months to 23 years 10 months) from the average age of 12 years 5 months (range = 5 months to 18 years 10 months).[741] Three patients required 24-hour support from the point of undergoing tracheotomy. The other 12 used nocturnal-only assistance for an average of 8 years 7 months. All patients had VCs under 20% of predicted normal when using IPPV. Six patients underwent tracheotomy to clear airway secretions before requiring continuous ventilator use, and most of the patients had had multiple pneumonias before and while having tracheostomies. All patients had uncuffed tracheostomy tubes and could speak. Two patients died after 5 and 14 years of support, respectively; one weaned; and 9 were still using nocturnal support at the time of the report. One patient was institutionalized.

In another study, 6 patients with SMA survived using IPPV continuously via indwelling tracheostomy tubes for a mean of 11.7 ± 17.7 years despite frequent episodes of mucus plugging and pneumonia.[64] Four of the patients also received all nutrition via indwelling gastrostomy tubes because of bulbar muscle weakness. Four patients used tracheostomy IPPV with the tracheostomy cuffs deflated and could communicate verbally. Five of the 6 patients remained institutionalized from the onset of ventilator use. Two patients survived for 15 and 4 years, respectively, despite need for ventilatory support since infancy. All 4 ventilator users who could communicate remained socially active and one was gainfully employed.

Although these series do not take into account patients with SMA who died suddenly during initial episodes of respiratory failure and the reports tend to ignore the more severe forms of infantile SMA that are considered in Chapter 12, clearly, as for patients with other NMDs, the survival of many patients with SMA, with or without severe bulbar muscle involvement, can be prolonged by ventilatory support via indwelling tracheostomy tubes. Interestingly, however, even though bulbar muscle dysfunction was not so severe as to necessitate enteral nutrition or preclude verbal communication for most patients, the incidence of pneumonia and bronchial mucus plugging in these tracheostomy IPPV users was very high compared with the incidence in noninvasive IPPV users in a large national survey[14] or in our patients with SMA type 1 who are managed noninvasively.[742]

Management by Part-time Nasal Ventilation

In 80% of NMD clinics in the U.S., with and sometimes without any sleep-related or hypoventilation symptoms, patients are offered nocturnal-only, low-span bilevel PAP on the basis of polysomnograms.[743] Many such patients are found to have nocturnal desaturations and frequent hypopneas. The hypopneas tend to be associated with reduced chest wall movement or with chest wall paradox, suggesting a noncentral origin (that is, inspiratory muscle weakness), but clinicians typically fail to increase bilevel PAP spans or to offer daytime noninvasive IPPV.

In a series of patients with NMD limited to nocturnal-only nasal ventilation, Simonds et al. began the technique for 23 patients with DMD at 20.3 ± 3.4 years of age with mean VC of 306 ± 146 ml. The 1-year survival rate was 85%; the 2-year survival rate was 73%; and the 5-year survival rate was less than 40%, with at least 5 deaths due to respiratory failure.[744] Another series limiting 70 patients with DMD to nocturnal-only nasal ventilation demonstrated no benefit and is discussed in Chapter 8.[745] Many other examples of poor outcomes are listed in Table 3. Indeed, conventional management can be so inadequate that patients "asphyxiate" or even "ask to undergo tracheotomy"! Other reports of suboptimal to tragic outcomes of conventional management for patients with non-Duchenne myopathies, including mitochondrial myopathies, nemaline myopathies, and acid maltase deficiency, have been reviewed elsewhere.[651]

In a recent survey, 1.2% of 2357 patients with ALS from 48 centers were using CPAP, 49% were currently on do-not-resuscitate status or refusing "mechanical ventilation," 1.5% were using IPPB, 15% (360) were using low-span bilevel PAP, and 2.8% had tracheostomies.[746] Thus, although only a small percentage of patients with ALS undergo tracheotomy, many more are now receiving nocturnal bilevel PAP. The following goals were suggested: detection of early respiratory failure, early intervention if it develops, prevention of complications, avoidance of tracheostomy ventilation, standardization of respiratory care, and improvement in survival and quality of life. Unfortunately, support of respiratory muscle function for assisted ventilation and coughing was not a goal.

Many studies have reported statistical prolongation of survival by 2 to 13 months with the use of generally low-span bilevel PAP as ventilatory assistance during sleep (Table 3).[661,662,747,748] At times, control groups consisted of similar patients with ALS treated with supplemental oxygen. Thus, some of the apparently positive outcomes from ventilatory assistance were probably due to the untoward effects of oxygen therapy on alveolar ventilation and airway secretion management in the controls.[661] Most studies did not take the extent of bulbar muscle involvement into account when considering the benefits to patients with ALS who tolerated the use of bilevel PAP.[662] Regardless of the possible minimal benefits for survival, however, many studies have demonstrated improvements in quality of life by reversing the symptoms of sleep-disordered breathing with nocturnal ventilatory assistance.[749] Although it is not surprising that minimal ventilatory assistance offers minimal benefit to patients with mild-to-moderate inspiratory muscle weakness who have not yet developed respiratory failure from airway secretion encumberment, the difference between outcomes in these studies and patients benefiting from respiratory muscle aids is striking (see Section 3).[750]

Use of nocturnal-only noninvasive IPPV has been demonstrated to improve daytime blood gases, to relieve symptoms of sleep-disordered breathing and hypoventilation, and

Table 3.	**Nocturnal Nasal Ventilation: Results in Neuromuscular Ventilatory Impairment***				
Year	First Author	Ventilator[a]	Users	Diagnoses	Results[b]
1987	Kerby[676]	Volume	5	NMD	> 3 mo
1987	DiMarco[759]	Pressure	1	Scoliosis	NR[f]
1988	Ellis[760]	Volume	5	Scoliosis	> 3 mo
1988	Carroll[761]	Volume	6	Various	> 3–9 mo
1989	Guille[762]	Volume	1	OSAS	NR[f]
1990	Heckmatt[763]	Volume	14	NMD	2–34 mo
1991	Goldstein[764]	Volume	6	NMD/scoliosis	> 14 mo
1991	Gay[765]	Volume	21	NMD	Up to 39 mo
1991	Laier[766]	Volume	23	Restrictive[c]	Up to 33 mo
1991	Thommi[767]	Pressure	1	OSAS	NR[f]
1992	Hill[768]	Pressure	6	DMD/scoliosis[d]	> 12.7 mo
1992	Waldhorn[769]	Pressure	8	Restrictive	> 3 mo
1993	Paulus[770]	Volume	34	NMD	> 3.0 yr
1993	Delguste[771]	Volume	9	NMD	NR[f]
1993	Barois[772]	Volume	46	NMD	g
1993	Chetty[773]	Pressure	1	Phrenic neuropathy	NR[f]
1993	Sekino[774]	Volume	6	Ventilatory impairment	NR[f]
1994	van Kesteren[775]	Pressure	64	NMD, polio, scoliosis	NR[f]
1994	Vianello[776]	Volume	5	DMD	> 2 yr
1994	Leger[777]	Volume	279	e	> 2 yr
1994	Piper[778]	Volume	13	OSAS	NR[f]
1994	Raphael[745]	Volume	70	DMD	No benefit
1994	Robertson[779]	Pressure	2	LGMD	NR[f]
1995	Pinto[661]	Pressure	10	ALS	Up to 36 mo
1996	Piper[673]	Volume/pressure	14	NMD	NR[f]
1996	Yasuma[780]	Unknown	27	DMD	10.3 yr
1997	Aboussouan[747]	Volume/pressure	39	ALS	13 mo
1998	Simonds[744]	Volume/pressure	23	DMD	< 40% 5-yr survival
1998	Escarrabill[781]	Pressure	6	MND	NR[f]
1998	Schlamp[782]	Pressure	24	ALS	17/24 NR[f]
1998	Guilleminault[783]	Pressure	20	NMD	NR[f]
1999	Polkey[647]	Unknown	25	ALS	None
1999	Jardine[784]	Unknown	103	78% NMD	NR[f]
1999	Kleopa[662]	Pressure	38	ALS	7–11 mo

(Cont'd. on next page)

Table 3.	Nocturnal Nasal Ventilation: Results in Neuromuscular Ventilatory Impairment*				
Year	First Author	Ventilator[a]	Users	Diagnoses	Results[b]
1999	Annane[785]	Pressure	20	NMD	None
1999	Schucher[786]	Volume	87	Ventilatory impairment	NR[f]
1999	Bullemer[787]	Volume/pressure	277	NMD/scoliosis	NR[f]
2000	Kang[734]	Pressure	13	DMD	8 died/2 yr
2000	Hukins[788]	Unknown	19	DMD	None
2000	Ohi[789]	Unknown	51	Hypercapnia	None
2000	Baydur[757]	Volume/pressure	73/79	Various	See text
2001	Masa[753]	Unknown	36	Scoliosis/obesity	NR[f]

Settings were either not noted (in 15 studies), low spans of bilevel PAP, or set to titrate improvements in carbon dioxide or AHI. In general, in the studies in which volume-cycled ventilators were used, the settings were more appropriate to rest inspiratory muscles.

NMD, neuromuscular diseases/weakness; OSAS, obstructive sleep apnea syndrome; DMD, Duchenne muscular dystrophy; ALS, amyotrophic lateral sclerosis; COPD, chronic obstructive pulmonary disease.

* In these studies, the indications for nocturnal nasal IPPV included symptomatic alveolar hypoventilation. Symptoms were alleviated, and arterial blood gases improved with treatment.
[a] Volume-cycled (volume), bilevel positive airway pressure, or other pressure-cycled (pressure).
[b] Time in years of clinical improvement and delay in resort to tracheostomy or death.
[c] Four with kyphoscoliosis and 2 with muscular dystrophy.
[d] Restrictive pulmonary syndromes, including 3 patients with OSAS.
[e] Diagnoses: scoliosis, 56; tuberculosis, 52; DMD, 75; COPD 49; and bronchiectasis, 49.
[f] Tracheostomy was delayed for greater than 2 years for 183 patients, and 54 patients underwent tracheostomy or died in less than 2 years. The treatment populations included 155 patients with intrinsic lung diseases.
[g] Successful for ameliorating symptoms and arterial blood gases, but duration of benefit not reported.
[h] In this study of patients with congenital myopathies, congenital muscular dystrophy, and spinal muscular atrophy, at least 14 patients underwent tracheostomy after periods of nocturnal nasal IPPV for up to over 3 years, and several patients died from cardiomyopathies.

to avert tracheostomy for patients with scoliosis and thoracic wall deformity as well as for patients with obesity-related hypoventilation (Table 3).[751–753] Very advanced patients can deteriorate to the point of requiring continuous ventilatory assistance, but rather than being offered noninvasive means, they are conventionally told that the only option is tracheotomy.

Nocturnal-only ventilatory assistance of any kind,[745,754] especially low-span bilevel PAP, must eventually fail for patients with progressive disease, as observed in all of the reports cited in Table 3. Failure of nocturnal-only nasal IPPV and need for resort to tracheotomy have been described as occurring when symptoms and signs of hypoventilation persist or recur or when its use becomes necessary over 15 hours a day.[665,755,756] In reality, failure occurs when the contraindications for using noninvasive IPPV are not respected, when insufficient effort is made to find or fabricate comfortable IPPV interfaces, when only low-pressure spans are used, when inadequate attention is given to clearing airway secretions, and when mouthpiece IPPV is not used for air-stacking or daytime aid. Thus, nocturnal-only nasal ventilation can at best prolong life or delay respiratory failure only marginally for patients with NMD.[745]

Management by Tracheostomy and Nocturnal-only Ventilation

A recent study reported a "46-year experience" in noninvasive ventilation involving 73 (of 79) patients with primarily ventilatory impairment. Included were 45 post-polio and 15 DMD ventilator users; 48 patients who used mouthpiece or nasal ventilation; and 31 who used body ventilators. Fourteen of 25 body ventilator users with polio, 10 of 15 noninvasive IPPV users with DMD, and 5 others with NMD underwent tracheotomies "because of progressive disease and hypercarbia which could not be controlled by noninvasive ventilation; the remaining nine were placed because of bulbar dysfunction." Despite these figures, the authors reported that "the difference in the number of patients eventually receiving tracheostomies between the body ventilator and positive pressure ventilation groups was fairly high (56% versus 5% [1], p < 0.001)." Certainly, however, most if not all of the tracheotomies could have been safely avoided. Examples of suboptimal noninvasive management were the fact that 56% of the body ventilator users, mostly post-polio patients with more than adequate bulbar muscle function, underwent tracheotomy rather than be switched to using more effective noninvasive IPPV and assisted coughing strategies, and the patients with DMD underwent tracheotomies with mean FVCs of 530 ml and daytime hypercapnia.[757] Thus, the tracheostomy tubes must have been placed as a result of episodes of respiratory failure triggered by chest infection, as is the case 90% of the time.[14] Indeed, most of our patients and the patients of others[744] with VCs of this level do not even require nocturnal nasal ventilation between chest colds. "One patient [with DMD] whose FVC declined to an unmeasurable value over five years was adamantly opposed to a tracheostomy and was able to sustain himself using a face mask/IPPV device 24 hours a day." This unfortunate patient had to be "adamantly opposed" to the clinicians' efforts to pressure him into undergoing tracheotomy. If he been born in northern New Jersey, tracheostomy would never have been a consideration. Thus, instead of being trained and equipped to maintain normal daytime ventilation and, more importantly, to maintain normal SpO_2 during intercurrent chest infections, these patients were ill advisedly counseled to undergo tracheotomy.

...la prudencia requiere que lo que se puede hacer por las buenas, no se haga por las malas.

⋯❦⋯ Don Quijote de La Mancha

THE STAGE OF PROLONGED QUALITY SURVIVAL (STAGE 3)

Nonintervention in fatal illness becomes a self-fulfilling prophecy.

❦

Because there are no effective medical treatments or cures for any neuromuscular disease (NMD) at present and because the great majority of morbidity and mortality is due to respiratory complications of muscle weakness, pulmonary management is the most critical aspect of treating NMDs. It has also been the most ignored aspect of NMD management.

Goals for Stage 3
1. Encouragement for self-direction and direction of care providers (Chapter 13)
2. Facilitation of activities of daily living (Chapter 7)
3. Use of respiratory muscle aids to prevent respiratory morbidity and mortality (to prolong life without detracting from quality of life by resorting to tracheotomy)
4. Prevention of cardiac morbidity and mortality (Chapter 5)

Chapter 9

The Physiologic Basis of Aiding Respiratory Muscles

With contributions by Cees van der Schans, Ph.D.

There is just one point I would like to mention, which has just come along which, I think, makes it [noninvasive positive-pressure ventilation] even more feasible. It is so simple that why it wasn't thought of long ago I don't know. Actually, some of our physical therapists, in struggling with the patients, noticed that they could simply take the positive pressure attachment, apply a small plastic mouthpiece..., and allow that to hang in the patient's mouth. You can take him to the Hubbard tank by such means and you can do any nursing procedure, if the patient is on the rocking bed and has a zero vital capacity, if you want to stop the bed for any reason, or if you want to change him from the tank respirator to the bed, or put the cuirass respirator on, or anything to stop the equipment, you can simply attach this, hang it by the patient, he grips it by his lips, and thus it allows for the excess to blow off which he doesn't want.

It works very well. We even had one patient who has no breathing ability who has fallen asleep and been adequately ventilated by this procedure, so that it appears to work very well, and I think does away with a lot of complications of difficulty of using positive pressure. You just hang it by the patients and they grip it with their lips, when they want it, and when they don't want it, they let go of it.

It is just too simple.[790]

> •☞• Dr. John Affeldt, Round Table Conference on Poliomyelitis Equipment, Roosevelt Hotel, New York City, Sponsored by the National Foundation for Infantile Paralysis, Inc., May 28-29, 1953.

Respiratory Muscle Dysfunction

Ventilatory impairment is due to either central hypoventilation or respiratory muscle dysfunction in NMD. Dysfunction results most commonly from weakness, contracture, or myotonia. As for the skeletal muscles, it is the combination of weakness and contractures that results in dysfunction and causes respiratory morbidity and mortality when untreated.[487]

The rib cage and abdomen are separated by the diaphragm. The diaphragm and abdominal muscles contract against essentially incompressible abdominal contents. As the diaphragm contracts, it displaces the abdominal wall forward. Because its downward movement is resisted by the abdominal contents, diaphragm contraction also results in upward movement of the ribs to a more horizontal position and in anterior and lateral expansion of the lower chest wall. Thus, the muscles that raise the ribs are primarily inspiratory in nature. Downward rib motion results in contraction of the chest wall and expiration. The muscles that lower the ribs are primarily expiratory in nature. The diaphragm is innervated by the phrenic nerve.

The parasternal, intercostal, and scalene muscles elevate the ribs and lift and expand the rib cage. These muscles are normally active when the diaphragm contracts. Their activity is essential during normal inspiration to prevent paradoxical inward movement of the chest and to increase thoracic volumes.

The internal and external intercostal muscles run at right angles to each other. It is commonly thought that the external intercostals have an inspiratory function and that the internal intercostals have an expiratory function.

The accessory muscles of inspiration are quiet during normal tidal breathing but can increase tidal volumes in times of need. Chest and shoulder girdle muscles, including the pectorals, trapezii, serrati, parasternal, and sternocleidomastoid muscles, run from the shoulder girdle to the spine or rib cage and elevate the ribs. These muscles and the latissimus dorsi can also aid in expiration by decreasing chest diameter and assisting coughing, especially in the sitting position. In this position the trapezius can raise the shoulders. The dropping back of the shoulders into place provides an expiratory pulse or cough assist. This mechanism is particularly useful for tetraplegic patients with spinal cord injury and little expiratory reserve volume.

The muscles of the pharynx and larynx are innervated by the lower cranial (bulbar) nerves. The pharyngeal dilator muscles, including the genioglossus, contract to decrease upper airway resistance and prevent pharyngeal collapse. Their contraction is synchronized with contraction of the diaphragm and intercostal muscles. Supralaryngeal resistance is increased during sleep, whereas laryngeal and pulmonary resistances remain unchanged.[791] The pharyngeal and laryngeal muscles can also be considered accessory muscles of inspiration when they are used for glossopharyngeal breathing (GPB). In the absence of any other inspiratory or expiratory muscle function, GPB can be used to provide normal tidal volumes and normal minute ventilation or deep inspiratory volumes, often to 3 liters or more.[792] Weakness or dysfunction of bulbar musculature and decreased pulmonary compliance decrease the capacity for GPB (Chapter 10).

Typically, patients with childhood-onset myopathies or spinal muscle atrophy (SMA) have very weak intercostal muscles and breathe predominantly with the diaphragm. Their chest wall volumes decrease during inspiration,[793] and vital capacity (VC) in the sitting position is less than or equal to VC in the supine position. On the other hand, patients with paralyzed diaphragms who breathe to a large degree with accessory breathing or abdominal muscles and patients whose diaphragms are too weak in the supine position to move the abdominal contents to ventilate the lungs can have much lower VCs and less breathing tolerance when supine. They may also occasionally have chest expansion with abdominal retractions during inspiration.

In a recent study, a cutoff of supine VC that was less than 75% of predicted was 100% sensitive and specific for predicting an abnormally low transdiaphragmatic pressure (Pdi). Both accessory muscle use and abdominal paradox had a significant negative association with Pdi, and the presence of accessory muscle use had a sensitivity of 84% and a specificity of 100% for detecting a low Pdi.[794]

Abdominal muscle contraction increases intra-abdominal pressure and retracts the abdominal wall. This action displaces the relaxed diaphragm into the thoracic cavity for expiration and coughing. The abdominal muscles also pull the lower ribs downward and inward. Some patients ventilate their lungs by using this action of abdominal muscles to passively elevate the diaphragm. Such is the case for patients with diaphragm and chest wall paralysis (e.g., post-polio patients). Some wheelchair users who have seat belts rock forward into the belt to compress the abdominal contents and elevate the diaphragm. This is also the mechanism of action of the intermittent abdominal pressure ventilator (Chapter 10). After the diaphragm is elevated by the abdominal muscles' contractions or applied pressure, air enters the lungs as gravity causes the abdominal contents and diaphragm to redescend.

Ventilation vs. Oxygenation Impairment

Most patients with impairment of pulmonary function can be differentiated into two categories: (1) those who have primarily oxygenation impairment with hypoxia due to predominantly intrinsic lung/airways disease, for whom hypercapnia is an end-stage event, and (2)those with lung ventilation impairment on the basis of respiratory muscle weakness, for whom hypercapnia causes hypoxia. This distinction is important because, although many patients in the former category have been described to benefit from non-invasive ventilation in the acute care setting, long-term use is more controversial. Patients with primarily ventilatory impairment, on the other hand, can benefit from the use of both inspiratory and expiratory muscle aids, often avoid episodes of respiratory failure despite total respiratory muscle paralysis, do not require tracheostomy, and have excellent prognoses with long-term home mechanical ventilation.

It is useful to define terms that can distinguish between the natural courses of these two patient populations. Whereas patients with oxygenation impairment can develop respiratory insufficiency or respiratory failure, ventilatory impairment can be characterized as ventilatory insufficiency or ventilatory muscle failure. Ventilatory insufficiency is defined by hypercapnia in the presence of a normal arterial-alveolar (A-a) gradient. The hypercapnia is not caused by intrinsic lung disease or irreversible airway obstruction. The ventilatory insufficiency can be due to inspiratory muscle dysfunction or central hypoventilation. When due to inspiratory muscle dysfunction, hypoventilation is a teleologic unloading of hypofunctional respiratory muscles. Patients with ventilatory insufficiency secondary to respiratory muscle dysfunction can have airway obstruction from bronchial mucus plugging. This obstruction causes an elevated A-a gradient. However, because the mucus plugging is reversible with the use of respiratory muscle aids, such patients still fall into the category of having primarily ventilation impairment.

A typical example of ventilatory insufficiency is the hypercapnic patient with Duchenne muscular dystrophy (DMD) who has normal SpO_2 when awake and who is minimally symptomatic with little or no ventilator use. Patients symptomatic from ventilatory insufficiency most often have dips in SpO_2 below 95%. Symptomatic hypercapnic patients benefit from the use of noninvasive ventilation for at least part of the day, most often overnight. With progressive ventilatory muscle weakness, withdrawal of periods of daily or nightly aid for these patients eventually results in ventilatory failure.

Ventilatory muscle failure is defined by the inability of the inspiratory and expiratory muscles to sustain respiration without resort to ventilator use. Patients with ventilatory muscle failure do not have unlimited breathing tolerance and require "ventilatory support." Ventilatory insufficiency leading to failure can be nocturnal-only and may result from diaphragm failure (with the patient unable to breathe when supine), a lack of central ventilatory drive (as seen with congenital central hypoventilation), or severe generalized respiratory muscle dysfunction.

This issue deserves further elucidation. Many patients with ventilatory insufficiency survive for years without ventilator use at the cost of increasingly severe hypercapnia, its associated symptoms and dangers, and a compensatory metabolic alkalosis that depresses the hypoxic and hypercapnic central ventilatory drive. The alkalosis allows the brain to accommodate to hypercapnia without overt symptoms of acute ventilatory failure. The respiratory acidosis and metabolic alkalosis can be corrected by using noninvasive IPPV, permitting the kidneys to excrete excessive bicarbonate ions. However, once drive is normalized, because of the need to take bigger breaths to maintain normal $PaCO_2$ and blood pH levels, the ventilator user becomes intolerably short of breath when ventilator use is discontinued and, at least temporarily, loses any significant breathing tolerance. Breathing tolerance can be lost in supine, sitting, side-lying, or all positions. Thus, without ventilator use, the untreated patient with severe ventilatory muscle dysfunction develops increasingly severe hypercapnia that can eventually result in coma due to carbon dioxide narcosis or ventilatory ("respiratory") arrest, despite the absence of intrinsic lung disease. With ventilator use, patients with ventilatory muscle dysfunction and little or no measurable VC can maintain normal alveolar ventilation, in some cases by using only nocturnal aid and relying on GPB to ventilate their lungs during daytime hours. Thus, untreated respiratory muscle failure results in ventilatory failure but not necessarily respiratory failure.

Patients with primarily oxygenation impairment, on the other hand, have an increased A-a gradient with or without hypercapnia. The A-a gradient increases whenever there is decreased diffusion or increased blood flow. The increased blood flow that occurs with increased physical activity can exacerbate the A-a oxygen gradient and cause or exacerbate dyspnea. Arterial pO_2 decreases before there is an observed rise in $PaCO_2$ because of the greater rate of carbon dioxide diffusion. Thus, hypoxia in the presence of eucapnia or hypocapnia is characteristic of intrinsic lung diseases, such as emphysema, pulmonary fibrosis, and pneumonia, and is characteristic of either respiratory insufficiency or failure. Unlike patients with ventilation impairment due to respiratory muscle dysfunction, when patients with oxygenation impairment are hypercapnic and hypoxic, the hypoxia cannot be reversed by assisted ventilation or elimination of airway secretions by noninvasive means. The typical patient in this category is the NMD patient with pneumonia who has a normal pH and whose hypoxia can be alleviated only by supplemental oxygen administration.

The term *respiratory failure* is reserved for acute decompensation in pulmonary function due to intrinsic lung or airways disease with deterioration in arterial blood gases and a decrease in blood pH to less than 7.25. Like patients with primarily ventilatory impairment, those with respiratory insufficiency (such as that due to chronic obstructive pulmonary disease [COPD]) often develop acute respiratory failure during pulmonary infections. Respiratory muscles can fatigue, and mucus accumulation, which cannot be adequately relieved by noninvasive means, worsens. Pulmonary vascular resistance increases in the presence of generalized or local ventilation-perfusion mismatching or pulmonary tissue hypoxia. This problem is especially common in the presence of the acidosis that results from local or generalized hypercapnia. The severe hypoxia, hypercapnia, and acidosis that occur during acute respiratory failure can lead to pulmonary artery hypertension and right ventricular failure. Although such patients require ventilator use, their hypoxia cannot be simply resolved by ventilator use or assisted coughing.

For patients with primarily ventilatory impairment, respiratory morbidity and mortality are a direct result of failing to assist inspiratory and expiratory muscle function as needed. For patients with primarily oxygenation impairment, the respiratory muscles, although not primarily involved, can be placed at a mechanical disadvantage by the development of lung and chest wall deformities, weakened by malnutrition and overuse, and strained to their limits by the need to ventilate stiff, noncompliant, diseased lungs or irreversibly obstructed airways. Overwork, relative or absolute, can eventually lead to secondary respiratory muscle dysfunction and overt respiratory failure. In patients with primarily ventilatory impairment who also have bulbar muscle dysfunction so severe that maximum assisted CPF are less than 160 L/min, upper airway obstruction is essentially irreversible. Such patients develop hypoxia without hypercapnia and, functionally speaking, have primarily oxygenation impairment.

Lung Physiology and Pathophysiology

Gas Exchange

The respiratory exchange membrane is the gas exchange surface of the lungs. It is the membrane between the alveolar air and capillary blood.[795] Gas exchange depends on alveolar ventilation, capillary blood perfusion, and diffusion of gases across the respiratory exchange membrane. The quantity of oxygen and carbon dioxide that diffuses across the membrane depends on the oxygen and carbon dioxide partial pressure differentials across the membrane and its total surface area and is an inverse function of membrane thickness. Exchange normally takes place in one-third of the pulmonary capillary blood transit time. It is effective in maintaining arterial blood gases within normal range over a 20-fold range of metabolic demand. The gas exchange membrane is reduced in patients with intrinsic lung disease of any etiology. Alveolar ventilation, capillary blood perfusion, and diffusion of gases across the respiratory exchange membrane are also commonly affected in intrinsic lung diseases.

Gas exchange in the lung depends on the matching of lung ventilation with capillary blood perfusion and the gas diffusion capabilities of the gas exchange membrane. Even in normal lungs, the distribution of ventilation is not uniform. During inspiration this lack of uniformity is caused by (1) the shape of the thoracic cage and the movement of the ribs, which increase volume proportionately more at the bases of the lungs than at the apices; (2) the descent of the hemidiaphragms, which expand the lower lobes of the lungs more than the upper lobes; (3) the expansion of the peripheral lung more than the deeper tissues (in the upright position); and (4) the lesser degree of inflation of the lower lung regions because the degree of stretch of the lungs at any level is related to the transpulmonary pressure at that level.

Lung and chest wall pathology exaggerates physiologic causes of nonuniform ventilation. Regional elasticity changes and intrathoracic fluid accumulation decrease local compliance and, thus, local lung inflation. Lung restriction, regional airway obstruction, variations in breathing rate, excision of lung tissue, and body positioning in patients with asymmetric lung disease can also decrease local ventilation.

Despite nonuniformity of distribution and mismatching of ventilation and perfusion, the efficiency of gas exchange is normally 97–98% of the theoretic maximum value for both oxygen and carbon diozide.[796] In people with ventilatory or respiratory impairment, mild normocapnic hypoxemia is common, however.[797] It is often due to decreased total oxygen diffusion across a diminished or blocked respiratory exchange membrane from microatelectasis, bronchial mucus accumulation, or, occasionally, the scarring that results from recurrent pneumonic infiltrations. In the absence of intrinsic lung disease or severe sudden bronchial mucus plugging, PaO_2 to levels under 55 mmHg are uncommon without concomitant hypercapnia.

SpO_2 depends on lung ventilation perfusion relationships. Increasing temperature, pCO_2, hydrogen ion concentration, and 2,3-diphosphoglycerate levels decrease hemoglobin affinity for oxygen and, therefore, SpO_2. A decrease in these levels and carbon monoxide poisoning increase hemoglobin affinity for oxygen.[798] Thus, provided that supplemental oxygen administration is avoided, decreases in SpO_2 are a result of hypoventilation or fever, the ventilation perfusion mismatching caused by bronchial mucus plugging or intrinsic lung disease, or perfusion impairment caused by vascular disease.

Lung Growth and Mechanics

The trachea divides into left and right mainstem bronchi. Normally, the mainstem bronchi then divide 26 more times, and all of the walled bronchi and bronchioles, down to the terminal bronchioles, are formed in the prenatal period.[799] There are about 20,000,000 alveoli at birth, but subsequently the respiratory bronchioles and alveoli multiply, with the latter ultimately reaching the adult total of 300,000,000 by age 8 years. Interestingly, until the age of 7 or 8 years, the diameter of the alveoli decreases and afterward increases, suggesting a much more rapid increase in number than in size until that time.[800] Interference with lung development before birth affects airways development, whereas interference after birth affects alveolar development.[801]

Adults generally have 4 liters of alveolar volume. The respiratory exchange membrane grows, reaching 85 m^2, the equivalent surface area of a tennis court, by late adolescence.[795] Lung growth peaks with the plateauing of VC at 19 years of age. After the plateau, the VC then decreases by 1–1.2% or about 30 ml per year throughout life.[802]

Sixty to 70% of VC and tidal volumes are provided by the diaphragm. The percentage of the tidal volumes provided by the diaphragm usually increases greatly in patients with NMD. However, when the diaphragm is weak or the work of breathing is increased, the accessory muscles expand the upper chest to increase tidal volumes. With severe or advanced NMD and intercostal muscle weakness, upper thoracic volumes can decrease during inspiration (paradoxical breathing).[793] For infants with NMD, this process can result in underdevelopment of the lungs and chest wall and in pectus excavatum.

Although expiration is passive in nonexercising normal people, with bronchospasm or during exercise the abdominal muscles contract to generate high thoracoabdominal pressures that elevate the diaphragm and become the principal muscles of expiration.

The Oxygen Cost of Breathing and Hypoventilation

The oxygen cost of breathing is normally approximately 2.5 ml/min or 1–2% of total body oxygen consumption. This cost increases to 30 ml/min or more, or over 15% of total oxygen consumption,[803] at the high levels of ventilation that accompany pneumonia, other lung diseases, and disorders of the chest wall such as obesity and kyphoscoliosis. In inactive patients with NMD and generalized muscle weakness in whom overall oxygen consumption is decreased, energy expenditure for breathing can exceed 15% of overall consumption.

Fatigue has been described as "failure to maintain the required or expected force."[804] Increasing the work of breathing, in absolute terms or relative to respiratory muscle strength and mechanical factors, can result in respiratory muscle decompensation. Because this decompensation can lead to an acute decrease in blood pH and possibly death, respiratory muscle fatigue must be avoided. To accomplish this goal, the brain's set point for control of ventilation changes to permit shallow breathing. This change eases the load on the respiratory muscles at the expense of hypercapnia and diffuse lung hypoventilation.[567] It explains the hypercapnia seen in patients with neuromuscular muscle weakness, severe vertebral or chest wall deformities, or advanced respiratory impairment. Hypercapnia is insidiously progressive with disease progression or, in patients with "static" NMDs, with age.[805] Thus, hypercapnia results directly from the resort to shallow breathing to avoid overloading respiratory muscles.[806] Although hypercapnia is not considered a sign of respiratory muscle fatigue but rather a sign of minimal functional reserve, resting inspiratory muscles by using ventilatory assistance on a daily and, most often, nightly basis can greatly improve diurnal blood gases without necessarily improving pulmonary function or muscle strength.

Pulmonary Defense Mechanisms and Cough Peak Flows

Pulmonary defense mechanisms include alveolar phagocytosis and lymphatic clearance, the mucociliary elevator, proteolytic enzymes and immunoglobins, and cough. Phagocytosis and ciliary action keep the normal lower respiratory tract almost sterile. One of the most important lung defense mechanisms to clear the airways and maintain lung sterility is the production of airway mucus. Mucus continuously transports debris from the peripheral to the central airways and eventually to the oropharynx. Airway mucus is a heterogeneous fluid that consists of about 95% water and 5% electrolytes, amino acids, sugars, and macromolecules.[807–812] It is produced throughout the bronchial tree, more peripherally than centrally, because airway area decreases centrally. The total amount of mucus that reaches the trachea is normally about 10–100 ml/day.[808,813] The parasympathetic nervous system increases mucus production. Accumulation of mucus in the central airways is normally countered by the higher mucus transport rate centrally than peripherally[814,815] (Fig. 1) and possibly by a greater reabsorption of watery constituents centrally.[816,817] Sputum formation arises from a mixture of mucus, inflammatory cells, cellular debris, and sometimes bacteria. Hypersecretion can be caused by inhalation of smoke, antigens, or other airway irritants that trigger inflammation or by mechanical stimulation of the upper airways (e.g., from the presence of a tracheostomy tube).[818,819] In healthy subjects mucus transport is decreased during sleep.[820]

The most important transport mechanism of mucus in the bronchial tree is mucociliary transport, which takes place by coordinated activity of cilia that cover the bronchial surface of the airways to the terminal bronchioles.[821] Each cell contains about 200 cilia,[822–824] all of which end in little claws.[825] The cilia beat in the direction of the oropharynx at 8–15 Hz, moving the mucus at 1 mm/min in smaller airways and at up to 2 cm/min in the trachea[826] (Fig. 2).

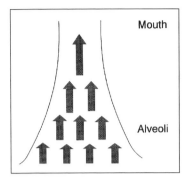

Figure 1. The total airway diameter decreases from the peripheral to the central airways. Consequently, air flows increase from the peripheral to the central airways.

Normally the upper airway warms, humidifies, and filters inspired air. Two-thirds of this process is done by the nose so that by the time the air reaches the nasopharynx, gas temperature is about 30°C and relative humidity is 95%. At the level of the main bronchi, air is fully saturated with water and at body temperature. Numerous studies have demonstrated that air conditioned to core body temperature and 100% relative humidity promotes optimal mucociliary transport velocity.[827] With decreasing humidity mucus thickens, mucociliary transport velocity slows and ultimately stops, cilia stop, and with severe dehydration cells are damaged and atelectasis occurs.[827] On the other hand, if inspired gas is warmer than 37°C and is 100% saturated, condensation occurs, causing reduced mucus viscosity and increased pericellular fluid depth. As a result, cilia lose contact with the mucus, which may be too liquid to be properly engaged by the cilial tips, again decreasing mucociliary transport velocity. Excessive heat may also cause cell damage. Exposure time to suboptimal conditions is also a factor. Optimal humidity helps prevent pooling of mucus, an ideal environment for pathogen replication.

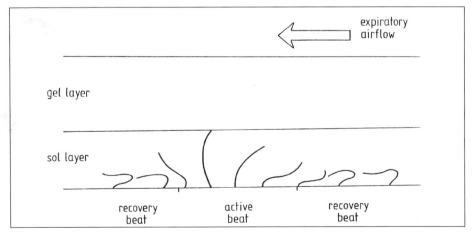

Figure 2. Respiratory secretions in the airways are separated into two layers: a sol layer and a gel layer. Respiratory cilia have an effective beat in the direction of the trachea (to the left) and a recovery beat in the direction of the bronchiole (to the right). (Modified from Sleigh MA: The nature and action of respiratory tract cilia. In Brain JD, Proctor DF, Reid LM (eds): Respiratory Defense Mechanisms. New York, Marcel Dekker, 1977, p. 247.)

In healthy people, the amount of mucus in the bronchial tree is small and readily mobilized by the mucociliary elevator. Mucociliary clearance can be overwhelmed, and stasis of secretions can occur when mucus is produced during chest infections or the airway is encumbered by aspirated material and the cough is ineffective. Mucociliary clearance is also decreased by hyperoxia, hypoxia, drying, smoke and other pollutants,[828] ciliary-inhibitory factors seen in certain disease states, anticholinergic medications, and bacterial colonization and airway trauma associated with the presence of an indwelling tracheostomy tube. It is, at times, increased by adrenergic bronchodilitation and can be increased by the generation of high cough flows. Mucus retention can cause pathologic changes in the lungs[829] and greatly increases the risk of pneumonia, lung collapse, and acute respiratory failure for patients with respiratory or ventilatory impairment.

A normal cough requires that the arytenoid cartilages and vocal folds enlarge airway diameter to permit a pre-cough inspiration to about 85–90% of total lung capacity.[830] Then there is a rapid and firm closure of the glottis, reinforced by the closure of the ventricular folds and epiglottis for about 0.2 sec. Both glottic opening and closure require gross muscular movements, including active intentional movements of the intrinsic laryngeal muscles. Contraction of abdominal and intercostal muscles results in intrapleural pressures of up to 140 mmHg. Upon glottic opening this pressure causes an explosive decompression that generates transient CPF of 6–20 L/sec. The expiratory flow is facilitated by active gradual abduction of the vocal cords.[831] The rapid air flows cause vibration of the soft structures of the larynx. The transient high and more prolonged lower flow rates traverse the partially collapsed trachea and other airways, reaching the mucus layer adhering to the airway walls, and transfer some energy as momentum to decrease viscosity. This shearing force causes acceleration of the fluid layer, leading to transport of the accumulated secretions.[832] Thus, diminished inspiratory and expiratory muscle function can result in decreased cough flows as well as decreased mucociliary clearance due to the reduced mechanical movement of the lungs and the reduction in airflows.[833]

Perhaps the most important variable in the clearing of mucus and foreign bodies from the airways is the peak velocity of the gas stream.[834] The peak velocity is the flow of the center of the stream, which may be much greater than the flow of the entire stream. Hand-held peak flow meters may be insensitive to the rapid flow transients of a true cough peak flow. Although the CPF of children might not be considered functional for adults, the peak velocities can result in effective coughs.

Total expiratory volume during normal coughing is 2.3 ± 0.5 L.[830] It has been demonstrated that, regardless of expiratory muscle function, CPFs are decreased for patients whose inspiratory muscles cannot generate tidal volumes over 1500 ml.[265] Thus, to optimize CPF for patients with low VCs, particularly for those with VCs below 1000 ml, coughing needs to be preceded by the delivery of maximal insufflations or maximum air stacking (Chapter 11). The delivered air should approach the maximum insufflation capacity (MIC) which, even when not greater than 1500 ml, can greatly increase the pressure of the lung's recoil once the glottis is opened during the cough. This process can dramatically increase CPF even without applying an abdominal thrust to augment the flows manually[265] (Fig. 3).

Maximum inspiratory and maximum expiratory pressures are direct measures of inspiratory and expiratory muscle strength. For patients with primarily ventilatory impairment,

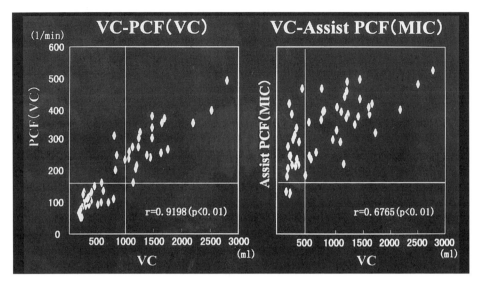

Figure 3. A comparison of peak cough flows (PCF) generated by patients after taking a deep breath, essentially from their vital capacities (VCs), vs. PCF generated by the same patients from lung volumes increased by maximal air stacking, essentially to maximum insufflation capacities (MICs).

expiratory muscles are usually weaker than inspiratory muscles.[805,835,836] Expiratory muscle weakness decreases not only peak expiratory flows but also CPF. Routine pulmonary function testing includes the measurement of maximum expiratory pressures and peak expiratory flow rates but not CPF. This approach is ironic because the importance of CPF has been recognized for quite some time.[830] Although expiratory flow rates are important for patients with bronchospasm, expiratory pressures can be useless if they do not translate into effective cough flows to clear the airways. Normal peak expiratory flows range from 6 to 14 L/sec for adults and from 2.5 to 14 L/sec for children and adolescents, depending on gender, age, and height.[837,838] CPF are usually greater than peak expiratory flows (PEF) in healthy people as well as in patients with DMD.[839] When equal to CPF, PEF may or may not be as effective at expulsing airway debris, keeping in mind that it is not the expiratory flow measured at the mouth that best correlates with cough effectiveness but the velocity of airflow in the airways themselves.[834] The velocity is further increased by the narrowing of airways during coughing. In patients with severe bulbar ALS, however, CPF may not be measurable because of inability to close the glottis. When CPFs are under 160 L/m (2.7 L/sec), they are insufficient to eliminate secretions and debris from the airways.[656] Despite their importance, CPFs have not yet been standardized.

Besides inspiratory and expiratory muscle weakness, CPFs are also decreased by bulbar muscle dysfunction that impairs glottic retention of an optimal breath, glottic patency, vocal cord movement, and glottic and pharyngeal dilator function and leads to aspiration of food or saliva and inspiratory and/or expiratory stridor. The extent of maximum assisted CPF is the best indication of the functional integrity of bulbar musculature. CPFs are also decreased by upper or lower airway obstruction, whether it be anatomic or functional.

Excessive functional collapse of the upper airway during coughing or exsufflation, caused by weakness or spasticity, can also render cough flows ineffective. After the glottis opens during the cough cycle, the intrathoracic pressure remains momentarily higher than intraluminal pressure, causing the normal decrease in the caliber of the airways. Mild narrowing serves to increase cough flows, thereby making them more effective. A greater-than-50% decrease in the cross-sectional lumen of the upper airways during coughing is considered abnormal and results in ineffective coughing.[840] Airways can collapse in the mediastinum (i.e., in the trachea, right mainstem bronchus, and part of the left mainstem bronchus) and in proximal and distal subpleural and intrapulmonary bronchi. The degree of bronchial collapse varies with the extent of pulmonary disease, with all locations collapsing in severe disease. Tracheal collapse is usually caused by invagination of the posterior membrane. When tracheal collapse is complete, collapse of the airways below this level does not occur because of the increase in luminal pressure.

The alveolar pressure, which is the sum of the elastic recoil pressure and the pleural pressure, is the driving force to produce expiratory flow. During the cough the pressure in the bronchi decreases from the peripheral airways to the mouth because of loss of frictional pressure and convective acceleration pressure.[841] Coughing is mainly effective in the central airways to about the sixth division.[842] There exists a point within the airways at which the intrabronchial pressure equals the pleural pressure. This point is called the equal pressure point (EPP) (Fig. 4). Upstream, in the direction of the alveoli, bronchial pressure is higher than pleural pressure, and no compression takes place. Downstream, in the direction of the mouth, the surrounding pleural pressure is higher than the bronchial pressure, and compression of the airways can take place, depending on the stiffness of the airway wall.[843] In the event of severe obstruction to airflow, the frictional pressure loss in the bronchi is higher and results in a shift of the EPP in the direction of the alveoli. A lower elastic recoil pressure (as seen in pulmonary emphysema), forced expiration from a lower lung volume, and higher pleural pressures due to higher expiratory forces lead to an upstream shift of the EPP. Less obstruction to airflow, higher elastic recoil pressure, and lower pleural pressures lead to a shift of the EPP downstream, in the direction of the mouth. The degree of compression is related to the compliance of the airway wall. The more compliant the peripheral airways by comparison with the central

Figure 4. During a forced expiration there is a point in the airways where bronchial pressure (Pbr) equals pleural pressure (Ppl). This point is called the equal pressure point (EPP). Downstream from the EPP, compression of the airways can take place and lead to high linear airflow velocities.

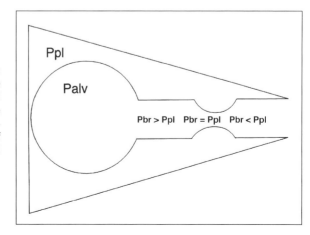

airways, the greater will be the degree of compression when the EPP is located more upstream. Dynamic compression contributes to the development of local high airflow velocities in these airways. Experimental animal models have shown that cough-induced mucus transport is much greater when airways are constricted[844,845] (Fig. 5). This finding supports the hypothesis that dynamic compression of the airways can be used to assist mucus clearance during chest percussion and that maneuvers that attempt to maintain maximal airway patency may reduce cough effectiveness.

Airway obstruction can be considered reversible or irreversible, depending on whether it can be alleviated by the use of respiratory muscle aids or bronchodilators. Essentially irreversible upper airway obstruction is most often due to tracheal stenosis, pharyngeal and laryngeal muscle dysfunction, or postintubation vocal cord adhesions or paralysis. Tracheomalacia, a frequent complication of tracheostomy tubes, especially those with

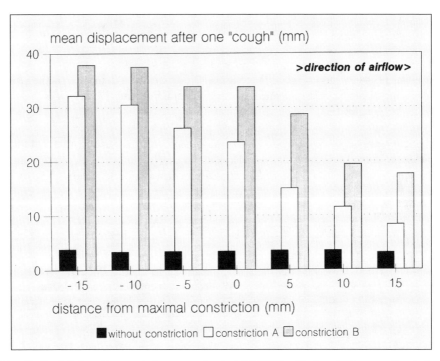

Figure 5. Cough-induced transport of a mucus simulant gel (MSG), with viscoelastic properties similar to human sputum, was measured in an artificial trachea. A constriction with a length of 73 mm and a maximal diameter of 7.5 mm (constriction A) and a constriction with a length of 87 mm and a maximal diameter of 10 mm (constriction B) were used. MSG samples of 40 μl were spread linearly over the width of the trachea under the point of maximal constriction and 5, 10, and 15 mm both upstream and downstream from the maximal constriction point. Measurements without the constriction were made at the same positions. Displacement of the MSG was measured after a single simulated cough. The application of the constrictive elements significantly increased mucus displacement (ANOVA p < 0.001). The position of the MSG relative to the point of maximal airway constriction significantly influenced cough displacement with constriction A (ANOVA p < 0.001) and constriction B (ANOVA p < 0.001). The displacement was higher in the upstream positions than in the downstream positions. Without constriction the displacement was unrelated to the position of the MSG (ANOVA p > 0.2). (From van der Schans CP, Ramirez OE, Postma DS, et al: Effect of airway constriction on the cough transportability of mucus. Am J Respir Crit Care Med 1994;149:A1023, with permission.)

inflated cuffs, not infrequently causes excessive airway collapse and stridorous breathing. Essentially irreversible lower airway obstruction is most often caused by COPD. Reversible airway obstruction is a result of acute bronchospasm, airway mucus accumulation, or the presence of a foreign body or granulation tissue in the airways of any patient without irreversible airway obstruction. Airway obstruction can vary from inspiration to expiration.

We demonstrated that CPF exceeding 160 L/min is the most important parameter for predicting successful extubation.[656] In patients whose spontaneous or assisted CPF cannot exceed 270–300 L/min when they are well,[655] there is a high risk that expiratory muscles will generate 10–15 cmH$_2$O less pressure and CPF will decrease below 160 L/min during chest colds or after general anesthesia because of fatigue, temporary weakening of both inspiratory and expiratory muscles[75] (due to direct injury mediated by oxygen-derived free radicals), abnormalities in neuromuscular transmission, changes in the supply of magnesium and phosphate because of anorexia,[74] and bronchial mucus accumulation. It has been demonstrated that, for patients with NMD, VC and maximum inspiratory and expiratory pressures often decrease by 10–25% and PaCO$_2$ increases by 10% during the first day after onset of cold symptoms.[650] Concomitant weakness of oropharyngeal muscles exacerbates the problem. The attainment of adequate CPF is critical for preventing pneumonia and respiratory failure in these patients.[655,656,846] Even in otherwise healthy elderly patients, the inability to generate adequate expiratory[847] or cough flows[848] is a most important indicator of 5-year mortality. For patients with NMD whose assisted CPFs are less than 160 L/min even when they are well, airway collapse can prevent manual assistance and MAC from reversing airway mucus-associated dSpO$_2$ and preventing pneumonia and acute respiratory failure. Such patients often require translaryngeal intubation, particularly during chest infections.[849]

Long-term aspiration of upper airway secretions and failure to eliminate airway mucus can lead to chronic ventilation perfusion imbalance, atelectasis, and lobar or segmental collapse. Bronchial mucus can also cause reversible obstructive emphysema.[692] Other potential problems include lung collapse, loss of lung compliance with pulmonary infiltrates and subsequent scarring, ventilatory decompensation, and cor pulmonale and eventually cardiopulmonary arrest. Mucus plugging can simulate pulmonary emboli. Sudden, severe hypoxia, dSaO$_2$, dyspnea, and chest pain can occur in the presence of normal chest radiographs, whereas perfusion scintiscans show diminished or absent perfusion of the involved portions of the lungs.[691] Flow-volume curves have also been used to detect airway secretions in ventilator users.[850] Airway mucus accumulation is particularly dangerous when it causes SpO$_2$ to decrease suddenly below 95%. With irreversible airway obstruction and chronic aspiration of upper airway secretions that causes the SpO$_2$ baseline to remain below 95% in the absence of hypercapnia and despite aggressive MAC, tracheostomy is needed. It should not need to be considered unless assisted CPF also cannot exceed 160 L/min in the long term.[545,655,656]

Because the cough reflex is suppressed during sleep, mucus accumulation is more likely to cause sudden hypoxia and acute respiratory failure overnight, especially if the patient receives supplemental oxygen or sedatives. Many patients with myopathic disease have varying degrees of cardiomyopathy that render them particularly susceptible to mucus-associated, hypoxia-triggered arrhythmias and cardiac decompensation.

Regulation of Pulmonary Ventilation and Sleep

Hypoxia, hypercapnia, and changes in blood pH affect lung ventilation. Peripheral chemoreceptors in the aortic and carotid bodies sense pCO_2 and pH but are primarily sensitive to pO_2 levels. Chemodenervation of the peripheral chemoreceptors can result in a 12–20% reduction in ventilation with an increase in $PaCO_2$ of 5–10 mmHg.[851] Gamma-afferents from the intercostal muscles, diaphragm, and pulmonary stretch receptors are also involved in regulating the timing and depth of breathing. Central receptors located on the surface of the medulla respond to the pCO_2 and hydrogen levels of the central spinal fluid and play an important role in regulating overall lung ventilation.[796] The controller in the brainstem generates the respiratory rhythm and integrates input from the peripheral receptors and other parts of the CNS; its output is to the respiratory muscles. Emotional states can also alter ventilation. With the change in the set point of the control of ventilation to avoid fatigue for patients with respiratory muscle dysfunction, chronic hypercapnia results in the development of a compensatory metabolic alkalosis with retention of bicarbonate ions in both peripheral blood and cerebrospinal fluid (CSF). High bicarbonate levels in CSF decrease the ventilatory response to hypercapnia and the effectiveness of nocturnal noninvasive ventilation.[852] Hypercapnia can also result from compensation for metabolic alkalosis of any cause (e.g., secondary to furosemide therapy). Other factors that decrease the ventilatory response to hypercapnia are sedative and narcotic medications, heavy mechanical loads, oxygen administration, and sleep.

Ventilatory drive is assessed by instantaneously occluding the mouth during the onset of inspiration. Except for patients with very weak inspiratory muscles, the decrease in pressure during the 100 milliseconds of occlusion at the outset of inspiration is thought to reflect the level of neural drive that was present at the outset of the previous unoccluded breath.[853] Ventilatory drive generally appears to be intact for hypercapnic patients with NMD. A second measure of ventilator drive derives from expressing minute ventilation as the product of the mean inspiratory flow rate (tidal volume/inspiratory time) and the fractional duration of inspiration (inspiratory time/inspiratory plus expiratory time). The first term reflects neural drive to the inspiratory muscles, whereas the second term reflects timing. Minute ventilation can be altered by changes in either variable alone or, as is usually the case, by changes in both drive and timing.

The anatomic proximity of respiratory centers to the pontobulbar control system provides a foundation for central anatomic and functional connections between respiratory centers and sleep state-related neuronal systems. Reticular activating system stimulation that results in or heightens alertness also stimulates phrenic nerve activity;[854] and neuronal discharge rates of the rostral pontine pneumotaxic center and the respiratory neurons of the ventral part of the medulla are diminished during non-REM sleep and even more so during REM sleep.[855,856] Decreased rate of discharge of these respiratory centers during non-REM sleep may largely explain the ventilatory changes that occur during non-REM sleep.

The maintenance of normal arterial blood gas levels depends on automatic and behavioral systems. The former depends on communication between dorsal and ventral groups of respiratory neurons in the brainstem. Input to these neurons comes from medullary and peripheral chemoreceptors as well as from stretch, irritant, and juxtacapillary receptors in the lungs via the vagus nerve and from chest wall receptors via the spinal nerves. These factors modulate breathing during non-REM sleep, whereas the behavioral system modulates breathing through inputs to the brainstem from cortical or subcortical neurons.

During sleep, there are decreases in ventilatory drive, cough reflex, accessory inspiratory muscle recruitment, minute ventilation, functional residual capacity, and PaO_2, whereas upper airway resistance and $PaCO_2$ increase.[857] The set point for $PaCO_2$ at which ventilation begins to increase is higher than during wakefulness, and sensitivity to hypercapnia is decreased. In addition, the ventilatory response to carbon dioxide during tonic REM sleep is equal to that during non-REM sleep, but during phasic REM sleep the ventilatory response to hypercapnia is virtually abolished. Thus, neural rather than metabolic factors maintain ventilation. During non-REM sleep the ventilatory response to hypoxia depends primarily on peripheral chemoreceptors, whereas during REM sleep the response is significantly decreased. Hypercapnia to 55–60 mmHg arouses normal subjects from non-REM sleep, but up to 66 mmHg is required for arousal from REM sleep. Oxyhemoglobin desaturations also result in brief arousals.

During REM sleep tonic automatic activity of intercostal muscles and the diaphragm is abolished, and phasic activity of the intercostals is diminished. Phasic diaphragm activity is preserved, and the diaphragm normally increases its contribution to tidal volume to compensate for decrease or loss of accessory and intercostal muscle activity. When the diaphragm is distorted or involved in the primary NMD process, it may be unable to increase its contribution. The result is underventilation. The decrease in rib cage and accessory muscle tone during REM sleep may further reduce the FRC and, along with the common problem of airway secretion retention, can increase ventilation perfusion mismatching. Indeed, nocturnal hypoventilation and hypoxia can be due to any combination of cardiopulmonary disease with diminished diffusion, shunting, and ventilation perfusion inhomogeneities, respiratory muscle dysfunction, decreased lung compliance, central and obstructive apneas,[858] and bronchial mucus accumulation as well as to normal changes with sleep.

Arnulf et al. reported that as diaphragm weakness progresses, REM sleep diminishes, even though apneas and hypopneas are rare for patients with ALS.[859] Until recently, however, it was thought that only the diaphragm functioned effectively during REM sleep. However, phasic inspiratory sternocleidomastoid activation during REM appears to permit REM sleep for some patients with ALS.[859] Another study recently suggested that 70% of patients with NMD can have accessory muscle activity during REM and slow-wave sleep.[860]

Hypoxic patients with intact respiratory musculature hyperventilate in an effort to normalize blood oxygen levels. Oxygen administration, therefore, can decrease ventilation, relieve respiratory muscle strain, ease tachypnea, ease shortness of breath and other symptoms of hypoxia and respiratory distress, and decrease pulmonary hypertension and the tendency to cor pulmonale. For hypercapnic patients, however, oxygen administration exacerbates hypoventilation and its symptoms. It also further impairs respiratory muscle function[861] and leads to carbon dioxide narcosis and ventilatory arrest. For patients having nocturnal SpO_2 between 70% and 80% and transcutaneous carbon dioxide of 72 mmHg, supplemental oxygen that increases SpO_2 to 90% has been reported to increase $PaCO_2$ levels to over 95 mmHg.[862] Thus, whereas oxygen must be given with great care to hypercapnic patients with primarily oxygenation impairment, it must not be administered to patients with primarily ventilatory impairment until every effort has been made to normalize SpO_2 by normalizing alveolar ventilation and eliminating airway secretions by MAC. When oxygen is administered, the patient must be continuously monitored and prepared for imminent intubation.

The first blood gas abnormalities in people with primarily ventilatory impairment occur during REM sleep as short periods of hypoxemia and later as hypercapnia.[863] Sleep hypoventilation commonly results in decreases in baseline SpO_2.[864] Hypercapnia and hypoxemia generally extend throughout most of sleep before hypercapnia occurs with the patient awake.[865,866] Awake hypercapnia tends to occur when the VC decreases below 40%[805] of predicted normal. Likewise, a FEV_1 below 40% and $PaCO_2$ greater than 45 mmHg are 91% sensitive for indicating sleep hypoventilation.[864] Base excess greater than 4 mmol/L was 100% specific but 55% sensitive for signaling nocturnal hypoventilation[864] (Chapter 8).

Decreases in FRC and total lung volume also correlate with nocturnal desaturations. For the same decrement in PaO_2, patients who already have reduced daytime PaO_2 experience more profound desaturation because they are operating on the steeper portion of the oxyhemoglobin dissociation curve. Once daytime hypercapnia is present, a further reduction in ventilation during sleep greatly exacerbates desaturation. This effect occurs because with the inverse hyperbolic relationship between alveolar ventilation and $PaCO_2$, a small decrease in ventilation in an already hypercapnic patient can result in a greater change in carbon dioxide tension than a comparable decrease in ventilation in eucapnic subjects. For patients who have a $PaCO_2$ greater than 50 mmHg when awake, nocturnal periods of SpO_2 below 85% are common.[867] The rapid, shallow, irregular breathing of normal REM sleep also exacerbates dead space ventilation and further reduces effective alveolar ventilation. Because the ventilatory responses to hypoxia and hypercapnia are diminished with hypercapnia[14] and the threshold for arousal is lower to hypoxia and higher to hypercapnia, more severe and prolonged blood gas alterations occur without arousing the patient. Increasing $PaCO_2$ and decreasing PaO_2 levels cross at about 60 mmHg, a point at which it is tempting, but ill-advised, to provide supplemental oxygen.

Medications such as calcium channel blockers, aminoglycosides, steroids, and benzodiazepines can reduce the ventilatory response to hypercapnia and hypoxia and exacerbate hypoventilation, especially during sleep. Beta blockers can increase airway resistance. Malnutrition, acidosis, electrolyte disturbances, cachexia, infection, fatigue, and muscle disuse or overuse can exacerbate ventilatory insufficiency. Hypokalemia, a common problem in these patients with small muscle potassium reserves, especially during intercurrent upper respiratory infections, can cause weakness, constipation, and abdominal distention and thereby exacerbate inspiratory muscle dysfunction.[192] The hypophosphatemia that commonly occurs during episodes of acute respiratory failure also decreases diaphragm contractility.[181] The risk of long-term pulmonary complications is also increased by oxygen administration[14] used to give the patient with ventilatory insufficiency "a comfortable night's rest."[866] Oxygen therapy has also been shown to prolong hypopneas and apneas by 33% during REM sleep and otherwise by 19% in patients with DMD who still have good ventilatory function (average VC of 1.4 L).[868] It also appears to suppress the CNS-mediated reflex muscular activity needed to support ventilation overnight by noninvasive IPPV methods.[567,751]

The muscle weakness that often results in chronic hypercapnia for most patients with NMD cannot explain the chronic hypercapnia seen in many patients with myotonic dystrophy, myasthenia gravis, and other conditions when supine VC is greater than 60% and respiratory muscle weakness is not severe. Such cases are explained by the presence of primary central hypoventilation, disordered afferents from diseased muscle, upper airway instability, abnormal muscle tone such as myotonia, upper motor neuron dysfunction, and increased work of breathing caused by decreased pulmonary compliance.

Sleep-disordered Breathing

Sleep-disordered breathing is a common entity in the general population that can develop into or exacerbate ventilatory insufficiency. It refers to the occurrence of central, obstructive, or mixed apneas, hypopneas, or both during sleep. Sleep apneas, hypopneas, and hypoventilation are pathophysiologically distinct. Apneas and hypopneas are associated with disturbed sleep architecture and recurrent arousals. The obstructive apneas are most commonly due to hypopharyngeal collapse from a translumenal pressure gradient across the airway during inspiration and failure of airway dilator muscles that are normally reflexively activated at the onset of inspiration. Obstructive apneas are often accompanied by central apneas. There may be an etiological association between the two. It is conceivable that for some patients with severe obstructive sleep apnea syndrome (OSAS), central apneas result at least in part from CNS desensitivity to hypoxia. This desensitivity also occurs in the presence of chronic respiratory muscle weakness. Patients with generalized neuromuscular weakness and especially patients with bulbar neuromuscular weakness are particularly susceptible to the development of sleep-disordered breathing.[869,870] Many investigators now believe not only that obstructive apneas associated with snoring and increased upper airway resistance can cause arousals but also that obstructive apneas can be triggered by arousals and result from disturbed sleep architecture.[858]

For subjects over 62 years of age, Carskadon and Dement found that 37.5% had apneas or hypopneas.[871] Apneas were defined as cessation of airflow for 10 seconds or more, and hypopneas were defined as reductions in normal tidal volumes by greater than 30%. Many apneas and hypopneas were associated with $dSpO_2$ of 4% or greater.[872] At least 3% of the general population is symptomatic for this condition and has an average of 5 or more episodes of apnea and hypopnea per hour (apnea/hypopnea index [AHI]).[872] OSAS is diagnosed when symptomatic people have an AHI of 10 or more.[872,873] Symptoms, which include hypersomnolence, morning headaches, fatigue, frequent nocturnal arousals with gasping or tachycardia, and nightmares, are similar to those of simple ventilatory insufficiency.[874] Uncomplicated sleep-disordered breathing can result in nocturnal hypercapnia, hypoxia, right ventricular strain, systemic hypertension, and, when severe, neuropsychiatric disturbances, cardiac arrhythmias, and acute cardiopulmonary failure.[875–877]

The risk of symptomatic sleep-disordered breathing is higher in males and increases with age, androgen therapy, obesity, brainstem or spinal cord lesions, hypothyroidism, generalized NMDs, and any conditions that obstruct the airway.[878,879] Pharyngeal cross-sectional area decreases with age, particularly for men, increasing susceptibility to OSAS.[880] Sleep-disordered breathing also occurs in most patients who use negative-pressure body ventilators[875,881] or electrophrenic nerve pacing.[882] Patients with NMD may have a higher incidence of sleep-disordered breathing because of a higher incidence of bulbar muscle weakness and obesity.[270,883] Kimura et al. have suggested that the incidence of sleep-disordered breathing increases with bulbar and diaphragm weakness in patients with ALS.[884] Bulbar dysfunction can increase susceptibility to hypopharyngeal collapse and, therefore, obstructive apneas during sleep.[270,869] Patients with spinal cord injury also appear to have a high incidence of sleep-disordered breathing.[878,885,886]

CPAP is usually effective in treating sleep-disordered breathing that is uncomplicated by scoliosis, obesity, muscle weakness, or predominantly central alveolar hypoventilation, but often the condition can be treated by a dental appliance that moves the mandible forward (Fig. 6). Less often and as a last resort, uvulopalatopharyngoplasty can benefit a minority of patients.[887] Recently, cardiac pacing with atrial synchronous ventricular pacemakers has been reported to decrease central and obstructive sleep apneas.[888]

Congenital central alveolar hypoventilation is a congenital but apparently not genetically determined[889] disorder of impaired control of ventilation of unknown etiology. Typically, patients maintain adequate ventilation when awake but hypoventilate severely during sleep and have absent or depressed ventilatory responses to hypercapnia and hypoxia when awake or asleep.[890] A similar ventilatory drive insensitivity to hypoxia and hypercapnia is seen in patients with familial dysautonomia or Down's syndrome, some patients with diabetic microangiopathy, and patients with diseases of the mid-brain or certain NMDs.[891] The extent of central alveolar hypoventilation and sleep-disordered breathing and their effects on patients with respiratory muscle compromise have not been adequately studied.

Airway Resistance Syndrome

Airway resistance syndrome is characterized by repeated increases in upper airway resistance to airflow that result in symptoms of sleep-disordered breathing and often in systemic hypertension. Patients complain of fatigue, insomnia and frequent arousals as well as daytime drowsiness. Women account for 56% of patients and have an incidence greater than that seen in OSAS.[892] Such patients have a narrow posterior airway space

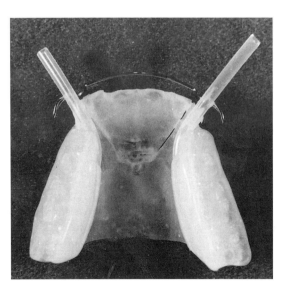

Figure 6. An intra-oral appliance used to bring forward the jaw and open the airway in the treatment of obstructive sleep apneas. (Courtesy of John R. Haze, D.D.S., Montville, NJ).

behind the base of the tongue.[893] The condition is diagnosed when nocturnal esophageal pressure monitoring indicates crescendo changes in intrathoracic pressures followed by arousals.[894] Because of the invasive nature of this procedure, the diagnosis is often made indirectly on the basis of clinical symptoms and polysomnographic evidence of sleep disruption.

Airway resistance syndrome is on a continuum of upper airway collapsibility during sleep between normal people and patients with OSAS. Considering the pharyngeal critical pressure for airway collapse (Pcrit), such patients have been reported to have a mean Pcrit of -4 ± 2.1 cmH$_2$O, whereas this figure is -15 ± 6.1 in normal people, -1.6 ± 2.6 for patients with sleep-disordered breathing characterized predominantly by hypopneas (AHI > 10 and < 40), and 2.4 ± 2.8 for patients with severe OSAS (AHI > 40). For these patients the AHI may be slightly increased but is usually less than 5.[895] Mean CPAP levels of 6.9 ± 1.7 cmH$_2$O are required to treat this disorder as opposed to mean levels of 7.9 ± 1.9 for moderate OSAS and 10.5 ± 2.4 cmH$_2$O for severe OSAS.[892]

In some cases, sleep quality can be improved and fatigue, hypersomnolence, and AHI can be reduced by wearing an oral appliance, as noted above. Some users experience temporary masticatory muscle or temporomandibular joint discomfort.[895]

Pulmonary Function of Patients with Ventilatory Muscle Impairment

Patients with ventilatory impairment develop a restrictive pulmonary syndrome with a reduction in total lung volumes, VC (Fig. 7), expiratory reserve volume, and, in most

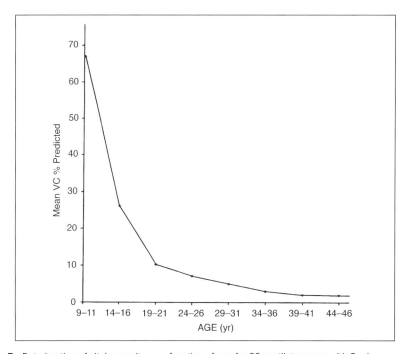

Figure 7. Deterioration of vital capacity as a function of age for 29 ventilator users with Duchenne muscular dystrophy. (From Bach J, Alba A, Pilkington LA, Lee M: Long-term rehabilitation in advanced stage of childhood onset, rapidly progressive muscular dystrophy. Arch Phys Med Rehabil 1981;62:328–331, with permission.)

cases, FRC. When diaphragm weakness predominates, supine posture can often result in loss of breathing tolerance because of loss of effective accessory muscle use and the inability of the diaphragm to move the abdominal contents in the supine position. When the patient is erect, the abdominal contents exert hydrostatic pressure to displace the diaphragm caudally at end-expiration. This action opposes the tendency of the intercostal muscles to suck the diaphragm upward into the chest. When the patient is supine, the opposite action takes place. The hydrostatic forces displace the paralyzed diaphragm cranially, thereby working in conjunction with the action of the intercostal muscles and tending to decrease pulmonary volumes. In a study of 8 patients with severely paretic diaphragms, VC was 30–65% of normal when patients were sitting and fell by half when they were supine.[896] The weaker the diaphragm by comparison with the chest and abdominal muscles, the higher the VC will be when the patient first develops hypercapnia or breathing intolerance. The stronger the diaphragm by comparison with the chest and abdominal muscles, the lower the VC will be when the patient first develops hypercapnia or breathing intolerance. In addition, decreases in VC to 50% over a short period are likely to result in loss of breathing tolerance, whereas greater losses over longer periods are likely to result in good breathing tolerance in the face of increasing hypercapnia.[897]

In studying patients with ALS, we found that in 368 VC evaluations the mean VC was 1749 ± 327 ml in the sitting position and 1475 ± 298 ml in the supine position. In some cases the VC values in the sitting position were as much as twice the VC values in the supine position, and patients without difficulty breathing when erect or sitting had no breathing tolerance when supine. In 647 measurements of VC in patients with NMD old enough to cooperate with spirometry, the mean VC was 1808.7 ml in the sitting position and 1582.8 ml in the supine position. In a small study of 24 patients with NMD (15 with muscular dystrophy, 8 with other myopathies, and 1 with polyradiculoneuritis), 11 of the 14 patients with clinically apparent paradoxical diaphragm movements had a greater than 25% drop-off in VC when changing from the sitting to the supine position. The drop-off was less than 25% for 9 of the 10 patients without paradoxical diaphragm movement. The extent of the drop-off was also associated with decrease in mouth pressure generated during a maximum static inspiratory effort and, thus, with diaphragm weakness.[898]

Pulmonary compliance is a measure of the distensibility of the chest and lungs. Restriction and decreased compliance are due to any combination of respiratory muscle weakness, paralysis, and mechanical factors that stiffen the chest wall and lungs. As the VCs of patients with NMD become inadequate or diminish with time, the patients lose the ability to attain their predicted inspiratory capacities. There are similarities between the development of extremity joint contractures and rib cage contractures with loss of maximum insufflation capacity (MIC).[487,682] The use of air-stacking and maximal insufflations via oral, nasal, or oral-nasal interfaces can provide respiratory muscle and rib cage range of motion (ROM) to maintain or increase MIC in much the same way that ROM applied passively to skeletal articulations benefits ROM and articular integrity.[487]

The chronic hyperventilation associated with long-term dependence on IPPV via indwelling tracheostomy tubes does not result in improved pulmonary compliance. In fact, a contrary effect results, charcterized by a decrease in total compliance of the respiratory apparatus, a sharp increase in bronchial resistance during inspiration and expiration, and a reduction in nonelastic resistance of the chest.[725] The decreased compliance is due to the constant-depth tidal volumes and failure to provide intermittent insufflations to predicted inspiratory capacities (Chapter 8). Likewise, long-term isocapnic, high-tidal, volume-increased dead space ventilation results in loss rather than increases in compliance by depleting lung surfactant (Chapter 10).

Measurement of transpulmonary pressure, the difference between intrapleural and alveolar pressures, is needed to determine lung compliance. Dynamic compliance is reflected by the extent of lung volume change with changes in intrapleural pressure from the end of expiration to the end of inspiration. In a study of hypoventilated animals supine for as little as 2 hours, overperfusion of dependent portions of the lungs resulted in fluid accumulation and microatelectasis. When the animals were intermittently given insufflations to 40 cmH$_2$O, this adverse effect did not occur.[899]

When human patients with diminished VCs do not receive maximal insufflations, they, too, develop a rapid, shallow breathing pattern and microatelectasis, along with areas of compensatory emphysema. These changes are often not seen on plain radiographs of the chest.[899] Microatelectasis can develop in 1 hour when tidal volumes cannot be increased.[900] Decreases in pulmonary compliance by 300% or more can occur in less than 3 months after loss of the ability to take deep breaths.[899] For children, chronic underinflation results in underdevelopment of lung tissues as well as decreased chest wall elasticity[901,902] and static pulmonary compliance.[868,903,904] Diseases that destroy the lung's connective tissue (e.g., emphysema) pathologically increase compliance.

Mechanical problems associated with ventilatory impairment include obesity, the use of improperly fitting thoracolumbar orthoses, sleep-associated hypopharyngeal collapse or other upper airway narrowing, and thoracic deformities.[567] Hypoxia and hypercapnia are exacerbated when intrinsic lung disease and concomitant mechanical conditions complicate inspiratory muscle weakness. Ultimately, right ventricular strain and serum acid-base imbalance result, but they can be reversed by the effective use of inspiratory muscle aids.[905]

Kyphoscoliosis and Ventilatory Dysfunction

Idiopathic kyphoscoliosis reduces VC and respiratory reserve independently of any concomitant muscle weakness. Scoliosis can exacerbate the loss of pulmonary compliance, which, in turn, increases the work of breathing. This is not the case, however, for patients with scoliosis due to NMD, in whom decreases in VC and respiratory reserve are due entirely to respiratory muscle weakness and failure to provide deep insufflations. This point is clear because surgery to correct scoliosis generally decreases rather than increases VC, and no improvement occurs in the subsequent rate of loss of VC (Chapter 7). Patients with kyphoscoliosis also develop ventilation-perfusion mismatching and have a higher incidence of obstructive sleep apneas when the skeletal deformities involve the upper cervical region and, therefore, the hypopharynx.

Pulmonary Function of Patients with Respiratory Impairment

Older patients with NMD can have concomitant COPD. This condition is characterized by low expiratory flow rates, normal or increased lung compliance, abnormal rib cage-abdominal motion from asynchronous breathing, rib cage-abdomen time lag, paradoxical breathing, and overuse of accessory muscles. Patients hyperventilate and have an increased oxygen cost of breathing. Forced expiratory volume in 1 second is decreased and maximum mid-expiratory times are increased.

The COPD results in air trapping and collapse of airways as patients use active expiratory muscle contraction in an attempt to exhale more completely. The greater thoracoabdominal pressures resulting from the expiratory muscle activity exacerbate airway collapse and air trapping. This process essentially causes irreversible peripheral airway obstruction. Respiratory exchange membrane is blocked by airway collapse and obstruction, and hypoxia results in greater work of breathing to increase lung ventilation in an attempt to normalize blood oxygen levels. With advanced disease, inadequate respiratory exchange membrane is ventilated to maintain normal carbon dioxide levels, and hypercapnia develops.[805] Exacerbations of COPD are caused by trapping of airway secretions in peripheral airways, just as episodes of acute respiratory failure in NMDs are caused by pneumonias due to trapping of secretions because of an ineffective cough.

As with pure, untreated ventilatory insufficiency,[797,906] hypercapnia is associated with increased morbidity and mortality in patients with COPD.[881] There is also a strong physiologic rationale to rest[835] the respiratory muscles of hypercapnic patients and normalize carbon dioxide levels.[907] The effect of hypoxia on causing right ventricular decompensation is greatly diminished when acidosis is minimized by maintaining more normal $PaCO_2$ levels[905] (Fig. 8). Although the use of noninvasive ventilation can relieve hypercapnia and rest inspiratory muscles in COPD, it can also increase air trapping.

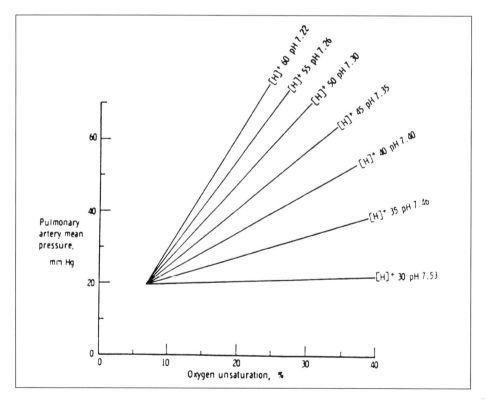

Figure 8. Relationship among pulmonary artery mean pressure, oxyhemoglobin unsaturation, and hydrogen ion concentration. (From Enson Y, Giuntini C, Lewis ML, et al: The influence of hydrogen ion concentration and hypoxia on the pulmonary circulation. J Clin Invest 1964;43:1146–1162, with permission.)

Respiratory Insufficiency in Patients with Bulbar Muscle Dysfunction

Patients with severe bulbar muscle dysfunction who have a long-term decrease in SpO_2 baseline below 95% because of chronic aspiration of upper airway secretions tend to have primarily respiratory rather than ventilatory insufficiency with hypoxia in the presence of eucapnia or hypocapnia because of irreversible airway secretion encumberment. Such patients also have assisted CPF less than 160 L/min and inevitably develop pneumonia and acute respiratory failure, usually before developing chronic hypercapnia, unless they undergo tracheotomy. Since patients are averbal at this point, they can benefit from laryngeal diversion (Chapter 4). This situation is rarely seen in patients other than those with severe bulbar-type ALS.

The art of medicine lies in keeping the patient alive while nature cures the disease.

⋅⟨☞⟩⋅ Voltaire

Noninvasive Respiratory Muscle Aids: Intervention Goals and Mechanisms of Action

With contributions by Barbara Rogers and Angela King, B.S.

Comprendre...
C'est comme un mur que l'on traverse
C'est la brume qui se disperse
Une promesse encore plus belle
La connaissance universelle

·❦· Apprendre by Yves Duteil

What are Physical Medicine Respiratory Muscle Aids?

Inspiratory and expiratory muscle aids are devices and techniques that involve the manual or mechanical application of forces to the body or intermittent pressure changes to the airway to assist inspiratory or expiratory muscle function. The devices that act on the body include negative-pressure body ventilators (NPBVs) and oscillators that create atmospheric pressure changes around the thorax and abdomen as well as body ventilators and exsufflation devices that apply force directly to the body to mechanically displace respiratory muscles. Negative pressure applied to the airway during expiration or coughing assists the expiratory muscles via forced exsufflation just as positive pressure applied to the airway during inhalation (noninvasive ventilation) assists the inspiratory muscles.

Certain positive-pressure ventilators or blowers have the capacity to deliver continuous positive airway pressure (CPAP). Likewise, certain negative-pressure generators or ventilators used to power NPBVs can create continuous negative expiratory pressure (CNEP). CPAP and CNEP, both first described in the 1870s,[908] act as pneumatic splints to help maintain airway and alveolar patency and to increase functional residual capacity (FRC). They do not directly assist respiratory muscle activity, are rarely indicated for patients with primarily ventilatory muscle weakness, and will not be considered examples of "noninvasive ventilation."

Intervention Objectives

The three major goals of intervention are as follows:
1. To maintain lung and chest wall elasticity and to promote normal lung and chest wall growth for children through the use of lung and chest wall mobilization (range of motion [ROM])
2. To maintain normal alveolar ventilation around the clock
3. To facilitate airway clearance

The long-term goals are to avert episodes of acute respiratory failure during intercurrent chest infections, to avoid hospitalizations, and to prolong survival without resort to tracheotomy. All goals can be attained by evaluating, training, and equipping patients in the outpatient setting and at home.

Goal One: Maintenance of Pulmonary Compliance, Lung Growth, and Chest Wall Mobility

The reasons for loss of pulmonary compliance are discussed in Chapter 9. As the vital capacity (VC) decreases markedly, the largest breath that one can take can expand only a small portion of the lungs. Use of incentive spirometry or deep breathing can expand the lungs no greater than the VC. Although possibly useful, manual chest wall stretching and rocking the pelvis onto the chest to decrease costovertebral tightness[899] have not been shown to increase lung volumes. Like limb articulations and other soft tissues, the lungs and chest wall require regular ROM to prevent chest wall contractures and lung restriction. As recognized since at least 1952, this goal can be achieved only by air stacking, providing deep insufflations (via the upper airway or via sighs for patients using invasive mechanical ventilation), or nocturnal noninvasive ventilation for patients who cannot cooperate with air stacking or insufflation therapy.[899]

Maximum insufflation capacity (MIC) is determined by measuring spirometrically the largest volume of air that a patient can hold with a closed glottis. The patient air-stacks via a mouthpiece consecutively delivered volumes from a volume-cycled ventilator or manual resuscitator. This technique is performed multiple times 3 times daily. The patient stacks the consecutively delivered volumes with a closed glottis until the lungs are maximally expanded. If the lips or cheeks are too weak to permit air-stacking, stacking is done via a nasal interface or lipseal. Patients who learn GPB can often air-stack, without mechanical assistance, consecutive GPB gulps to or beyond the MIC obtained by mechanical air-stacking. This value is known as the glossopharyngeal breathing maximum single-breath capacity (GPmaxSBC).[792] The extent to which the MIC or GPmaxSBC is greater than the VC predicts the patient's capacity to be maintained by noninvasive rather than tracheostomy ventilatory support.[545] The MIC-VC difference, like the extent of assisted CPF, is a function of bulbar muscle integrity. For most patients with NMD, the VC decreases with time, but the MIC increases for years before declining.[910] If the facial muscles or glottis is too weak for effective air-stacking, single deep insufflations are provided via a Cough-Assist at 40–70 cmH_2O 3 times daily. These volumes are measured spirometrically. Lung mobilization for small children is discussed in Chapter 12.

The primary objectives in using air-stacking or in providing maximum insufflations as lung and chest wall ROM are to increase the MIC (Fig. 1), to maximize CPF (Fig. 2), to

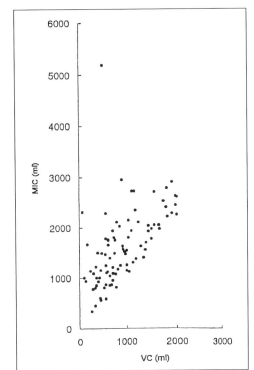

Figure 1. Relationship between vital capacity (VC) and maximum insufflation capacity (MIC) for patients with neuromuscular disease and sufficient glottic function to air-stack.

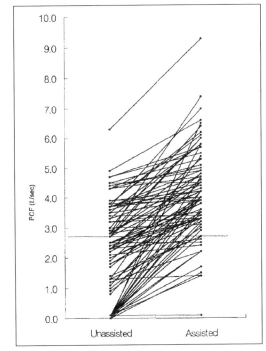

Figure 2. Relationship between unassisted and assisted cough peak flows for patients with neuromuscular disease and sufficient glottic function to air-stack.

maintain or improve pulmonary compliance, to prevent or eliminate atelectasis, and to master noninvasive IPPV. Patients who can air-stack can use noninvasive IPPV and be extubated without tracheotomy.

Air-stacking may not only help maintain static lung compliance; it also improves dynamic pulmonary compliance, at least temporarily.[911] The only studies in humans that have explored the effects of regimens of deep insufflations on static pulmonary compliance were instituted only after patients had developed severe pulmonary restriction (VCs less than 50% of predicted normal), involved the use of insufflation pressures under 30 cmH$_2$O (which are grossly inadequate to fully expand even normally compliant lungs), and called for the use of insufflations for only minutes each day. No evidence indicates that static pulmonary compliance was maintained or improved by such regimens.[912] On the other hand, it has been shown that the MIC can be increased with the use of regimens designed to expand the lungs.[910,913] In 278 spirometry evaluations of patients with NMD old enough and able to air-stack, we found mean VC to be 1190.5 ml in the sitting position and 974.9 ml in the supine position, whereas the MIC was 1820.7 ml. The higher volumes increase both unassisted and manually assisted CPF and permit the patient to raise voice volume as desired.

Lung ROM in this manner can also promote lung growth in children (Chapter 9). Positioning of the patient to reduce pulmonary stress, avoidance of prolonged singular positioning, and use of optimal trunk support when sitting have also been suggested as methods to help improve chest wall structure and reduce pectus.[914]

Any patient who can air-stack is also able to use noninvasive IPPV. Therefore, if such a patient loses breathing tolerance during chest colds or when intubated for respiratory failure, he or she can use noninvasive IPPV or be extubated directly to continuous noninvasive IPPV, whether or not any breathing tolerance has been regained (Chapter 11). This principle is extremely important for eliminating the need to resort to tracheostomy because such patients are extubated without being ventilator-weaned. Extubation of a patient with little or no breathing tolerance who has not been trained in air-stacking and noninvasive IPPV can result in panic, massive insufflation leakage, glottic closure, ventilator dyssynchrony, asphyxia, and possible reintubation.

Before VC decreases to 70% of predicted normal, patients are instructed to air-stack 10–15 times at least two or three times daily. Thus, the first respiratory equipment that is prescribed for patients with ventilatory impairment is often a manual resuscitator. In general, because of the importance of air-stacking, patients without air trapping who have diminished VCs use volume-cycled ventilators rather than pressure-cycled ventilators, which cannot be used for air-stacking. Use of an abdominal binder or palm pressure to the abdomen during maximal insufflations facilitates chest expansion for patients with paradoxical chest wall retraction.[915]

Just as the ongoing use of nocturnal high-span bilevel PAP prevents pectus and promotes lung growth and chest wall development for infants and small children with NMD, it has been suggested that the use of nocturnal nasal IPPV can decrease the rate of loss of VC following the VC plateau in patients with Duchenne muscular dystrophy (DMD).[916] Attempts to maintain pulmonary compliance in this manner may slightly benefit VC for some populations. However, since the authors did not avoid tracheotomy for their patients, the benefits achieved by using only nocturnal noninvasive ventilation were relatively minimal compared with the benefits of using respiratory muscle aids to avoid tracheotomy (Chapter 10).

Goal Two: Continuous Maintenance of Normal Alveolar Ventilation by Assisting Inspiratory Muscles as Needed

Inspiratory Muscle Aids for Sleep

Negative-pressure Body Ventilators and the Rocking Bed

Currently available negative-pressure body ventilators (NPBVs) include the iron lung (Coppa Biella C-900, Biella, Italy), Porta-Lung (Fig. 3), chest shell ventilator (Fig. 4), and various wrap style ventilators (Respironics, Inc.) (Fig. 5). They assist inspiratory muscles by creating negative pressure around the chest wall so that air enters the lungs via the upper airway. They are practical only for use during sleep.

NPBVs have been used to ventilate the lungs of patients with little or no VC for decades, despite frequent transient episodes of dSpO$_2$ due to apparent episodes of airway collapse.[881] With aging and decreasing pulmonary compliance or airway stability, NPBVs can become ineffective and may be associated with the development of systemic hypertension. Such patients[752,874,917,918] benefit from switching to the more effective noninvasive IPPV.[285] Furthermore, except for the iron lung and Porta-Lung, NPBVs are generally not useful for patients with severe scoliosis or weight extremes.

Although NPBVs continue to be used in a few centers, including ours, as a bridge to noninvasive IPPV during extubation of unweanable patients previously untrained in air-stacking or noninvasive ventilation,[919,920] their long-term use is rarely if ever warranted.

One of two body ventilators that apply force directly to the body to allow gravity to move the abdominal contents and diaphragm is the rocking bed ventilator (J. H. Emerson Company, Cambridge, MA) (see Fig. 12 of Chapter 3 of reference 1113). Although it is still in use[921] and can provide tidal volumes as high as 1000 ml for some patients with no

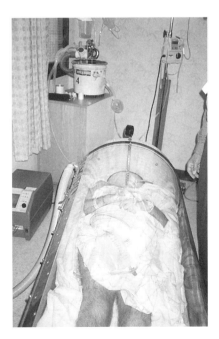

Figure 3. Porta-Lung, a "portable" iron lung available from Respironics, Inc., used temporarily for ventilatory support by a continuously ventilator-dependent patient with Duchenne muscular dystrophy for tracheostomy tube de-cannulation and training and transition to noninvasive IPPV.

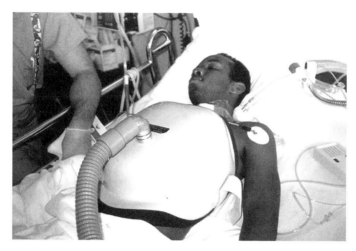

Figure 4. The chest-shell ventilator used during and immediately after tracheostomy tube decannulation for ventilatory support during training and transition to noninvasive IPPV.

measurable VC, like NPBVs, it is predominantly of historical interest. It is usually less effective than NPBVs,[922] but many patients like it for other reasons (Chapter 13).[923]

Noninvasive IPPV

IPPV can be noninvasively delivered via mouthpieces, nasal interfaces, and oral-nasal interfaces for ventilatory support during sleep. Although for acutely ill patients noninvasive ventilation is usually introduced in the hospital setting, the great majority of users can be introduced to noninvasive IPPV in the outpatient and home setting.

Mouthpiece IPPV

Many patients who have little or no measurable VC and no upper extremity function have used ventilators without alarms, kept simple 15- or 22-mm angled mouthpieces (Reference 4-730-00, Puritan-Bennett, Inc.) between their teeth (see Figs. 20 and 21 in

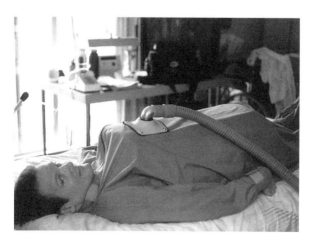

Figure 5. "Wrap"-style ventilator used for nocturnal ventilatory assistance for a patient with ventilatory muscle failure who complements its nocturnal use with daytime mouthpiece IPPV.

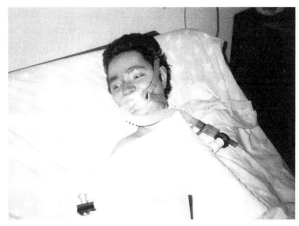

Figure 6. Thirty-four-year-old man with Duchenne muscular dystrophy dependent on continuous noninvasive IPPV since age 14 using a lipseal (seen here) for nocturnal support and a simple, angled mouth piece for daytime support.

Chapter 7), and received mouthpiece IPPV for continuous ventilatory support (even during sleep) for years without losing the mouthpiece and dying from asphyxia. However, such patients invariably have disturbed sleep architecture and many episodes of nocturnal dSpO$_2$. When mouthpiece IPPV is used during sleep, a Lipseal retention system with two cloth straps and Velcro closures is strongly recommended (Fig. 6). The retention straps of an Adam circuit (Puritan-Bennett) can be substituted for the cloth straps.

The Lipseal can provide an essentially closed system of noninvasive ventilatory support. Mouthpiece IPPV with lipseal retention (see Fig. 6) is delivered during sleep with little insufflation leakage from the mouth and with virtually no risk of the mouthpiece falling out of the mouth. A strapless lipseal system called the Oracle is also available. Yet another newly available lipseal is made of transparent silicon. It has no intra-oral mouthpiece but a similar strap retention system (Masque Buccal, Metamed, France).[924] Orthodontic bite plates for use with custom-fabricated acrylic oronasal (Fig. 7), oral,

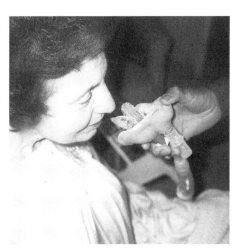
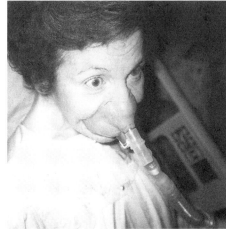

Figure 7. Post-poliomyelitis patient who has used mouthpiece IPPV during the day and IPPV via a strapless oral-nasal interface (seen here) nocturnally since 1984.

and nasal (Fig. 8) interfaces can also increase comfort and efficacy and eliminate the orthodontic deformity that otherwise may occur in some long-term users of continuous mouthpiece IPPV (Fig. 9).

Generally, symptoms from nasal insufflation leakage during nocturnal lipseal IPPV remain subclinical because the typically used high ventilator insufflation volumes of 1000–2000 ml compensate, at least in part, for nasal leakage. Whether using nocturnal nasal or lipseal IPPV in a regimen of 24-hour noninvasive IPPV, and despite the maintenance of normal daytime alveolar ventilation, some patients with no breathing tolerance[752] have symptomatic arousals due to episodes of insufflation leakage and dSpO$_2$ during sleep. Such patients may also complain of recurrence of morning headaches, fatigue, and perhaps nightmares and anxiety. The nasal ventilation user can be switched to oronasal or lipseal IPPV. Lipseal systems can be "closed" by using nostril clips or by plugging the nostrils with cotton and covering them with a Bandaid during sleep (Fig. 10). Covering the nostrils was found to be necessary for 5 of 163 nocturnal mouthpiece IPPV users with little or no breathing tolerance.[752] Another practical solution is to set the ventilator's low pressure alarm at a level that, by its sounding, stimulates the patient sufficiently to shorten periods of excessive insufflation leakage during sleep. A low-pressure alarm setting of 10–20 cmH$_2$O is used for this purpose, and the patient develops conditioned reflexes to prevent prolonged, excessive leak-associated episodes of dSpO$_2$ and hypoventilation.

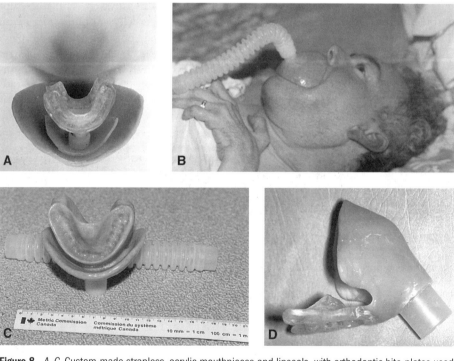

Figure 8. *A–C,* Custom-made strapless, acrylic mouthpieces and lipseals with orthodontic bite-plates used by a patient with no ventilator-free breathing tolerance since 1955. *D,* A custom-made acrylic nasal interface with bite-plate retention. (A-C courtesy of G. McPherson.)

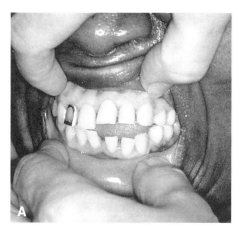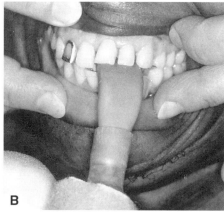

Figure 9. *A* and *B*, Orthodontic deformity caused by 15 years of 24-hour use of mouthpiece IPPV without a custom bite-plate. (Courtesy of Dr. Augusta Alba.)

Nasal IPPV

Nasal ventilation is preferred over lipseal ventilation by more than 2 of 3 patients who use noninvasive ventilation only for sleep.[567] Nasal ventilation can be provided as bilevel PAP or as nasal IPPV with or without positive end-expiratory pressure (PEEP) by using volume-cycled ventilators. Numerous nasal interfaces (CPAP masks) are now commercially available (Table 1). Each interface design applies pressure differently to the paranasal area. One cannot predict which model will be most effective and preferred by any particular patient (Fig. 11). Nasal bridge pressure and insufflation leakage into the eyes are common complaints with several of these generic models. Such difficulties resulted in the fabrication of interfaces that mold themselves to facial tissues and in custom-molded interface designs[567,774,925-927] (Fig. 12). Creative interface designs include a retention system that provides the air delivery (Fig. 13). A newly available nasal interface, called the Nasal-Aire (InnoMed Technologies, Boca Raton, FL), comes in 5 sizes

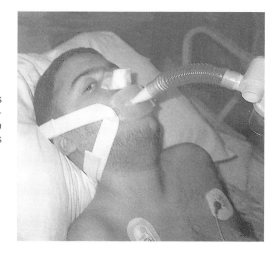

Figure 10. Thirty-three-year-old continuous noninvasive IPPV user with Duchenne muscular dystrophy using lipseal IPPV during sleep with the nostrils sealed by cotton pledgets and a Bandaid.

Table 1. Interfaces

Manufacturer	Interface Model	Headgear Mode	Interface Sizes	Headgear Sizes	Interface Material in Contact with Patient	Customizeable Features	Facial Coverage	Comments
AirSep	Ultimate Nasal Mask	Y type or Polynet type	S, M, L	S, M, L	Translucent silicone rubber Optional Gel Ultimate Seal	Malleable nose strap, optional Ultimate Seal (gel interface)	Small nasal mask	
Fisher Paykel	Aclaim	Aclaim		Comes with mask	Silicone rubber		Oronasal	
Fisher Paykel	Oracle	No headgear is needed	One size	NA	Silicone rubber		Oral	
Hans Rudolph	Nasal CPAP Mask	Meshnet headgear or strap-only	S, M, L	S, M, L	Silicone rubber	Nose strap, Comfort Seal, Ultimate Seal, chin strap	Small nasal mask	
Hans Rudolph	Face Mask	Meshnet	Premie, neonate, infant, Ped S, Ped L, Adult S, M,L	4 sizes	Silicone rubber	Comfort Seal, Ultimate Seal	Covers mouth, nose, and chin	Ultimate Seal (hydrogel material) Comfort Seal (soft foam) has sound healing properties Single piece, molded design–no bonded pieces Can wash in dishwasher
Mallincrodt-Puritan Bennett	Lipseal	2 Velcro straps			Plastic		Covers mouth	
Metamed	Masque buccal	Straps	Silicone				Mouth and lips	

Manufacturer	Mask	Headgear	Sizes	Spacer	Material	Adjustments	Mask coverage	Notes
ResMed	Full Face Mirage	Full Face Headgear	S, M, L	Comes with mask	Silicone Rubber	Adjustable arms so nasal cushions can sit closer or further from face	Standard nasal with forehead assembly	Mask may be disinfected or sterilized. Mask may be purchased with or without nasal partition (making it a mouth breathing mask only); can wash in dishwasher
ResMed	Sullivan Mirage oronasal mask	Mirage headgear	Standard, Large	Comes with mask	Silicone Rubber	Angle of forehead pads can be adjusted	Standard nasal with forehead assembly	Standard, large, shallow (lower nasal bridge, e.g., Japanese customers) or very high nasal bridge (e.g., American Indian and mustaches and patients who take dentures out at night)
						None noted	Covers mouth, nose, and parts of cheeks	The instructions say the mask must be disassembled for cleaning. It is difficult to separate the elbow from the mask
ResMed	Ultra Mirage Nasal	Ultra Mirage Headgear	Standard, large, shallow	Comes with mask	Silicone Rubber	Removable gel spacer	Standard nasal mask with 1 forehead pad	Includes antiasphyxia valve in case flow generator stops. Valve membrane must be changed every 6 months. Also has "quick-release" tab to quickly remove mask in case of emergency

(Cont'd.)

Table 1. Interfaces *(Continued)*

Manufacturer	Interface Model	Headgear Mode	Interface Sizes	Headgear Sizes	Interface Material in Contact with Patient	Customizeable Features	Facial Coverage	Comments
Respironics	Contour Deluxe	Any 4-point attachment headgear	S, M, L		Silicone rubber	Spacers, support ring, chin strap, comfort flap (gel interface)	Standard nasal mask	The exhalation port is included in the mask
Respironics	Reusable Contour	Any 4-point attachment headgear	P, S, M/S, M, M/W, L, L/N		Silicone rubber			Must also purchase exhalation port
Respironics	Mini Monarch and Monarch		1 size each	1 size fits all	Silicone rubber	Spacers, support ring, and mask may be boiled to adjust to facial contours	Standard nasal mask	
Respironics	Angled mouthpiece		15 mm; 22 mm		Silicone rubber		Mouthpiece	
Respironics	Profile Lite	Any 4-point attachment	P, S, M/S, M, MW,		Soft polyurethane film over pliable	Hose may be worn up or down, comes with stability clip	Small nasal	
Respironics	Simplicity	Simplicity nasal mask	S, M	1 size fits all	Silicone rubber	Forehead pad and comfort flap (optional, included)	Covers mouth and nose and some of the chin	Stability clip is provided for attaching hose to maskstrap or bed clothing to relieve tension on hose. The exhalation port is included in the mask

Respironics	Soft Series	Any 4-point attachment headgear	Ped, S, M, MW, MN, L, LN	Silicone rubber	None noted	Covers entire face	Must also purchase an exhalation port Mask includes a Fresh Air Entrainment valve in case blower unit fails; the patient can draw in room air An NG tube sealing pad is an optional accessory to maintain mask seal when NG tube is in place
Respironics	Spectrum Reusable Full Face Mask	Convertible Headgear, Softcap,	P, S, M, L	Silicone rubber		Oronasal	The system pressure and oxygen therapy must be modified for the mask vs. standard nasal interfaces Fresh air entrainment valve contains a magnet, so do not use near MRI
Respironics	Total Face Mask	Total Face Mask Headgear	1 size	Silicone rubber		Oronasal	
SleepNet	Phantom	Phantom Headgear	1 size (comes with 2 strap lengths)	Soft polyurethane film over pliable gel material	Nose clip, strap length; design allows tubing to attach to either side	Standard nasal plus covers part of cheeks	
Sunrise Medical	DeVilbiss Serenity	Strap-Style or Cap-Style	S, MS, M, L	Silicone rubber		Standard nasal	
Tiara	AirPilot Nasal Mask	AirPilot Headgear	1 size	Silicone rubber	Forehead pad height adjustment	Standard nasal mask plus forehead assembly	

(Cont'd.)

Table 1.   Interfaces (*Continued*)

Manufacturer	Interface Model	Headgear Mode	Interface Sizes	Headgear Sizes	Interface Material in Contact with Patient	Customizeable Features	Facial Coverage	Comments
Tiara	CoolCap	Blue Horizon Headgear	1 size	S, M, L, XL	Soft polyurethane film over pliable gel material	Nose clip, and strap length; designs allow tubing to attach to either side	Standard nasal	Standard nasal plus covers part of cheeks
Tiara	Comfort System Mask	CoolCap		S, M, L, XL	Silicone rubber	Pliable ring molded into flexible shell; tubing can be worn up or down	Standard nasal	
Tiara	IQ	CoolCap	1 size	S, M, L, XL	Soft polyurethane film over pliable gel material	Optional spacer pad	Standard nasal	
Tyco	Adam Ciruit (nasal pillows)	SnugFit	Pillows come in S, M, L, XL; dilator pillows come in S, M, L	1 size	Pillows are silicone rubber	Different pillow sizes	Nostrils	
Tyco	Breeze Sleepgear with Nasal Pillows Assembly	Breeze Sleepgear	Pillows come in S, M, L, XL; dilator pillows come in S, M, L	1 size	Pillows are silicone rubber	Straps can be adjusted to various configurations (height, length, and angle of the headgear)	Nostrils	

Tyco	Breeze Sleepgear with Dreamseal Assembly	Breeze Sleepgear	1 size	Silicone gear	1 size	Standard nasal mask	Straps can be adjusted to various configurations (height, length and angle of the headgear)
Tyco	Companion Vinyl Mask	Snugfit	S, M, L	Vinyl	1 size	Standard nasal	Foam forehead pads and forehead clip (used to hold pad)
Tyco	SoftFit	Snugfit	SN, S, SW, M, MW,		1 size	Standard nasal	Foam forehead pads and forehead clip (used to hold pad)
Tyco	Lipseal (Mouth Seal)	Strap Assembly	1 size		1 size	Covers lips only	None noted

S = small, M = medium, L = large, P = pediatric, Ped S = pediatric small, Ped L = pediatric large, NA = not applicable, SW = small wide, MW = medium wide, MN = medium narrow, LN = large narrow, XL = extra large, NG = nasogastric, MRI = magnetic resonance imaging.

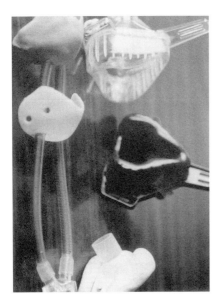

Figure 11. Various nasal interfaces.

from extra large to extra small. Because of its comfortable, light-weight, and practical air delivery system, it has the potential to become the most popular interface on the market (see Fig. 13C). The nose piece requires minimal pressures on the retention tubes to seal the nostrils to prevent insufflation leakage. It is also an ideal interface for patients who require noninvasive ventilation continuously because it does not interfere with the user's vision. Smaller sizes are needed, however, for infants and small children.

Because everyone's face—especially the nose (Fig. 14)—has different anatomy, one cannot predict which interface will provide the best seal with the least insufflation leakage or which interface a particular patient will find most comfortable. Therefore, no patient

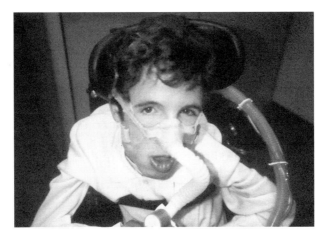

Figure 12. Patient with Duchenne muscular dystrophy who required continuous noninvasive ventilatory support for 7 years but whose facial muscles were too weak to permit mouthpiece use. He had 4 or 5 low-profile, custom-molded acrylic nasal interfaces that he alternated daily for around-the-clock use.

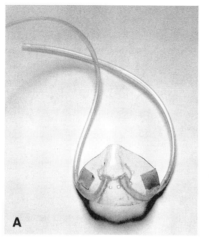
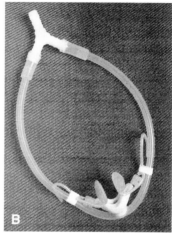
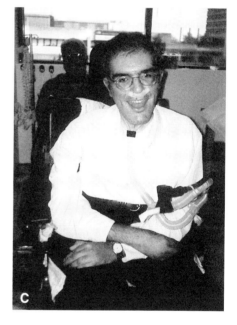

Figure 13. *A* and *B,* Custom-made interfaces with the retention systems also serving as conduits for air delivery. *C,* The Nasal-Aire nasal interface, which consists of a soft nosepiece with exhaust ports for potential use with bilevel PAP machines and two soft silicone nasal cannulas for fitting into the nostrils. Connected on each side of the nosepiece is the air-delivery tubing that also serves to retain the interface. The two lengths of tubing are joined at the opposite ends by a Y-shaped coupling, forming a loop with the nosepiece at one end and the Y coupling at the other. At the base of the coupling is a rigid port for connection to the ventilator circuit. The user is a 26-year-old second-year law student with Duchenne muscular dystrophy. He requires continuous ventilator use, alternating between mouthpiece (also seen here) and nasal IPPV.

should be offered and expected to use only one nasal interface any more than a patient should be offered only lipseal or a single oronasal interface. Alternating interfaces nightly varies skin pressure sites and minimizes discomfort and therefore should be encouraged.

Excessive insufflation leakage via the mouth is prevented by keeping ventilatory drive intact by maintaining normal daytime carbon dioxide and avoiding supplemental oxygen and sedatives. However, in the presence of daytime hypercapnia and excessive episodes of nocturnal $dSpO_2$ and bothersome arousals, for patients not wishing to switch to lipseal IPPV, a chin strap (Fig. 15) or plugged lipseal (Fig. 16) without mouthpiece can be used to decrease oral leakage. In the presence of nasal congestion, patients may use decongestants

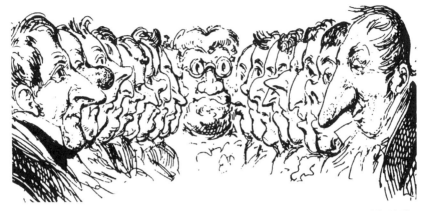

Figure 14. Different style noses for interface fit. (Drawing by George Cruikshank, 1792–1878.)

to permit nasal IPPV, switch to lipseal ventilation, or, on rare occasions, use a body ventilator. Most often the patient continues nasal IPPV and uses decongestants.

Oral-nasal Interfaces

Oral-nasal interfaces can have strap retention systems like those for mouthpiece or nasal IPPV. Respironics, Inc. and HealthDyne (Minneapolis, MN) produce comfortable strap-retained oronasal interfaces (Fig. 17). Respironics, Inc. manufactures a transparent full-face mask with an inner gasket that creates a hermetic seal around the nose and mouth. It was reported in one center to be more comfortable and to provide a better seal than commonly available nasal interfaces.[928] Custom-prepared strap-retained oral-nasal interfaces are also available.[929,930] These delivery systems can be comfortable alternatives

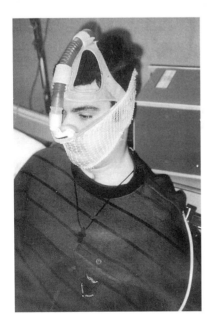

Figure 15. This patient was switched from continuous tracheostomy IPPV to daytime mouth piece and nocturnal nasal IPPV in 1992 and continues to require continuous noninvasive IPPV. He feels that strapping the mouth closed in this fashion helps to decrease nocturnal oral insufflation leakage.

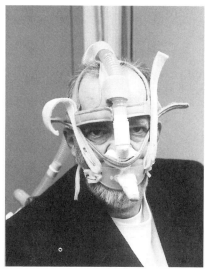

Figure 16. Patient with Milroy's disease who has been a continuous noninvasive ventilator user for 17 years. He uses daytime mouthpiece IPPV and nocturnal nasal IPPV with the mouth sealed by a plugged lipseal to eliminate insufflation leakage.

to lipseal or nasal IPPV. However, because effective ventilatory support can usually be provided by either nasal or mouthpiece/lipseal IPPV, strap-retained oral-nasal interfaces have been used for long-term ventilatory assistance in few centers. They are used more frequently in the intensive care setting.[931]

Strapless acrylic oral-nasal interfaces (SONIs) with bite-plate retention may require 10 hours or more to construct. However, they provide a more air-tight seal for the delivery of IPPV and can be expelled by simple tongue thrust. They also permit better speech than lipseal use.[932] The bite-plate retention is important for patients living alone who are unable to don straps independently (see Fig. 7). Adequate and stable dentition is necessary to use them.

Mouthpiece IPPV and nasal IPPV are usually used as open systems, and the user relies on CNS reflexes to prevent excessive insufflation leakage during sleep.[933] However,

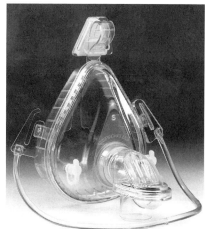

Figure 17. Respironics Full Face Mask with strap retention.

essentially closed noninvasive IPPV systems include lipseal with nasal pledgets (see Fig. 10), strap-retained oral-nasal interfaces (Fig. 18), and SONIs (see Fig. 7). A small study comparing a generic nasal "mask" with nasal prongs and full-face interface reported significantly higher minute ventilation and greater decreases in $PaCO_2$ with the full-face interface. For an essentially leakless system using a SONI, however, the user needs to be observed during sleep, and the final touches should be applied to the acrylic shell and bite-plate to eliminate any insufflation leakage created by loosening of the interface seal as facial soft tissues shift during sleep.[926]

Choice of Interface

Patients should be offered a variety of interfaces and, to a large degree, allowed to choose. One study found no differences in tolerance to ventilation, blood gases, or breathing patterns whether assist control or pressure-assist modes were used. The study concluded that, regardless of the underlying pathology, the type of interface affects the outcome of noninvasive ventilation more than the ventilatory mode.[934]

Daytime Inspiratory Muscle Aids

Intermittent Abdominal Pressure Ventilator and Chest Shell Ventilator

The chest shell ventilator (see Fig. 4) is cumbersome, inconvenient, and often not very effective when the user is seated. The IAPV, on the other hand, can be highly effective. It involves the intermittent inflation of an elastic air sac that is contained in a corset or belt worn beneath the patient's outer clothing (Fig. 19). The sac is cyclically inflated by a positive-pressure ventilator. Bladder inflation moves the diaphragm upward. During bladder deflation gravity causes the abdominal contents and diaphragm to return to the resting position, and inspiration occurs passively. A trunk angle of 30° or more from the horizontal is necessary for the belt to be effective. It requires a powerful ventilator (pump) to fill the air sac. Currently, the best portable pump on the market for this purpose appears

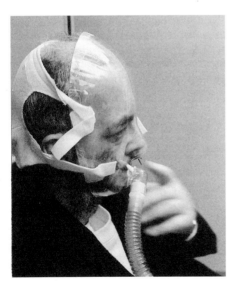

Figure 18. Continuous noninvasive IPPV user with strap-retained oral-nasal interface for nocturnal use.

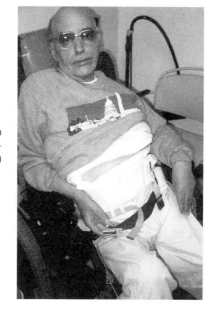

Figure 19. A 51-year-old man with muscular dystrophy who has been a 24-hour ventilator user. He has used the intermittent abdominal pressure ventilator (Exsufflation Belt) during daytime hours and lipseal IPPV nightly since 1979.

to be the Achieva series (Tyco-Puritan-Bennett, Pleasanton, CA) (Chapter 8). If the patient has any inspiratory capacity or is capable of GPB, he or she can autonomously add volumes of air to those taken in mechanically. The IAPV generally augments tidal volumes by about 300 ml, but volumes as high as 1200 ml can be obtained.[935] Patients with less than one hour of breathing tolerance usually prefer to use the IAPV rather than noninvasive IPPV during daytime hours.[935] The IAPV is less effective in the presence of scoliosis or obesity. Recently, a pediatric IAPV was created from two blood pressure cuffs,[936] and IAPVs are being custom-made in southern France (Chapter 12).

Mouthpiece IPPV

Mouthpiece IPPV is the most important method of daytime ventilatory support for patients who need ventilatory support continuously and after extubation of patients who are unable to breathe autonomously. Most commonly, simple, flexed mouthpieces are grabbed by the patient's lips and teeth for deep insufflations as needed (Fig. 20; also see Figs. 21 and 22 of Chapter 8). Some patients keep the mouthpiece between their teeth all day (Fig. 21). Most patients prefer to have the mouthpiece held near the mouth. A metal clamp attached to a wheelchair can be used for this purpose (Fig. 22), or the mouthpiece can be fixed onto motorized wheelchair controls, most often sip-and-puff, chin (see Figs. 20 and 21 of Chapter 8), or tongue (Fig. 23) controls. The ventilator is set for large tidal volumes, often 1000-2000 ml. The patient grabs the mouthpiece with the mouth, thereby supplementing or substituting for inadequate autonomous breath volumes. Some patients prefer the comfort of custom-made orthotic mouthpieces (Fig. 24). The patient varies the volume of air taken from ventilator cycle to ventilator cycle and breath to breath to alter tidal volume, speech volume, and cough flows as well as to air-stack for full expansion of the lungs to maintain lung and chest wall compliance.

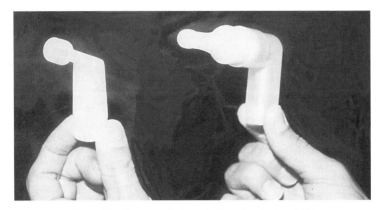

Figure 20. Simple angled mouthpieces for daytime IPPV.

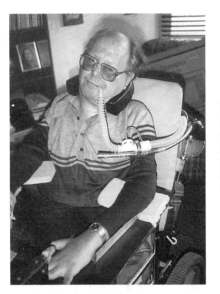

Figure 21. Patient with post-poliomyelitis syndrome who used 24-hour mouthpiece IPPV from 1958 until 1995, when he died from leukemia. He kept the small, flexed mouthpiece in his mouth without any other retention device despite the fact that he had no upper limb function.

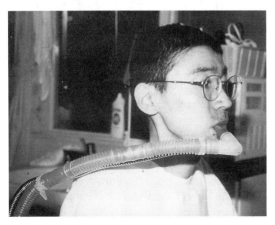

Figure 22. Patient with Duchenne muscular dystrophy using mouthpiece IPPV with mouthpiece supported by "gooseneck clamp" within reach of the patient's lips.

Figure 23. Patient with Duchenne muscular dystrophy who has used 24-hour mouthpiece IPPV for 22 years. He now has less than 1 minute of breathing tolerance. The mouthpiece is fixed adjacent to the chin controls of his motorized wheelchair.

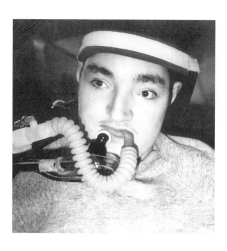

To use mouthpiece IPPV effectively and conveniently, adequate neck rotation and oral motor function are necessary to grab the mouthpiece and receive IPPV without insufflation leakage. To prevent insufflation leakage, the soft palate must move posterocaudally to seal off the nasopharynx. In addition, the patient must open the glottis and vocal cords, dilate the hypopharynx, and maintain airway patency to receive the air. These normally reflexive movements may require a few minutes to relearn for patients who have been receiving IPPV via an indwelling tube, especially one with an inflated cuff, because reflexive abduction of the hypopharynx and glottis is lost during invasive IPPV. Often patients are thought to have tracheal stenosis or other reasons for upper airway obstruction before they learn to reopen the glottis to permit IPPV. Patients, especially children, may fail extubation to noninvasive IPPV because of upper airway obstruction due to laryngeal edema. This problem can often be avoided by glucocorticoid therapy before extubation.

Since the low-pressure alarms of volume-cycled ventilators often cannot be turned off, a flexed 15-mm mouthpiece (see Fig. 20) for IPPV or an in-line regenerative humidifier

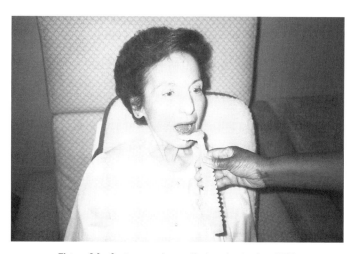

Figure 24. Custom-made mouthpiece for daytime IPPV.

can be used to prevent sounding of the alarm during routine daytime IPPV when not every delivered volume is received by the patient. These options create a back pressure of 2–3 cmH$_2$O, which is adequate to prevent sounding of the low-pressure alarm.

Nasal IPPV

Because patients prefer to use mouthpiece IPPV or the IAPV for daytime use,[567,935] nasal IPPV is most practical only for nocturnal use. Daytime nasal IPPV is indicated for infants and for patients who cannot grab or retain a mouthpiece because of oral muscle weakness, inadequate jaw opening, or insufficient neck movement. Twenty-four-hour nasal IPPV is, therefore, a viable and desirable alternative to tracheostomy for some patients with severe lip and oropharyngeal muscle weakness[567] (see Fig. 12). Nasal IPPV users learn to close their mouth or seal off the oropharynx with the soft palate and tongue to prevent oral insufflation leakage.

Effects of Noninvasive Ventilation on Muscle Endurance, Lung Compliance, Chemotaxic Sensitivity, and Hemodynamics

Any combination of respiratory muscle weakness and increased elastic load can modulate central respiratory output and result in shallow breathing or neuroventilatory uncoupling of the ventilatory pump.[937] The shallow breathing pattern avoids inspiratory muscle fatigue[938] but results in hypercapnia and is an indication of limited inspiratory reserve. Blood gas improvements for patients with acute exacerbations of COPD induced by noninvasive ventilation were largely the result of re-establishing an efficient breathing pattern rather than providing high inspiratory pressures.[939] However, for patients with primarily ventilatory impairment, inspiratory muscle rest and the increased tidal volumes permitted by using noninvasive IPPV or high- rather than low-span bilevel PAP relieve nocturnal hypoventilation and, thus, are important means for improving daytime symptoms and gas exchange.[768,940] Indeed, the improvements in daytime PaCO$_2$ with the use of nocturnal noninvasive IPPV appear to be dose-related because equal improvements have been observed with equivalent duration of use of noninvasive IPPV during daytime hours.[941,942] In addition, the rest afforded respiratory muscles may result in increased inspiratory muscle strength. Furthermore, with ongoing nocturnal nasal IPPV, decreases in mouth occlusion pressures (PO.1) with carbon dioxide stimulation have been observed. This decrease may be due to an increase in tidal volume, which allows a reduction in respiratory rate.[943]

In the awake patient, diaphragm and accessory muscle activity has been shown to decrease when patients are ventilated by body ventilators[944] or nasal IPPV.[945] Body ventilator use and noninvasive IPPV[938] also decrease inspiratory muscle use during sleep. Nasal IPPV, which improves blood gases during sleep,[567] also suppresses phasic respiratory drive via thoracic afferent inhibition and, therefore, effectively unloads the ventilatory pump and permits a decrease in respiratory muscle activity during sleep. Although the carbon dioxide threshold is increased in hypercapnic patients to minimize load, it is restored by the increase in alveolar ventilation. This effect maintains more normal carbon dioxide tensions and blood pH during sleep and decreases or reverses any hypercapnia-associated compensatory metabolic alkalosis. Such results are very important because elevated bicarbonate levels blunt central respiratory sensitivity to carbon dioxide tensions, permit worsening hypercapnia, and appear to decrease the effectiveness of noninvasive ventilation during sleep.

Annane et al. found that with nocturnal noninvasive IPPV, daytime PaO_2 increases, $PaCO_2$ and bicarbonate decrease, the apnea-hypopnea index and SpO_2 time spent below 90% during sleep decrease, sleep efficiency and mean SpO_2 increase, and the ventilatory response to carbon dioxide increases significantly.[785] Patients can deteriorate rapidly when, with discontinuance of nocturnal nasal IPPV, nocturnal SpO_2 levels decrease each night,[768,946] carbon dioxide levels increase each night, and symptoms return.

Noninvasive IPPV has also been shown to reverse cor pulmonale without concomitant oxygen therapy.[947,948] Eleven patients with edema and recent hypercapnic and hypoxic worsening of chronic ventilatory insufficiency were shown to have normalization of carbon dioxide, improvement in oxygenation, complete relief of edema, a decrease in body weight of 4 kg, and decreases in systolic and mean pulmonary arterial pressures.[947,948] They also had a long-term increase in the right without a change in the left ventricular ejection fraction and normalization of neuroendocrine levels (Chapter 5).[947]

In addition, nocturnal nasal ventilation has been reported to increase maximum inspiratory pressures[764] and may transiently increase or stabilize VC for patients with ventilatory insufficiency.[776] FRC and dynamic lung compliance may also be increased by IPPV.[764,949,950] This effect may reduce the work of breathing and further improve daytime ventilation. Thus, nocturnal noninvasive ventilation may improve daytime pulmonary function for some patients.[567,764] It can also reduce the airway closure caused by the supine position, and in this way it may maintain more advantageous lung volume-pressure relationships. The benefits, therefore, appear to be due to some combination of respiratory muscle rest, increases in tidal volumes and alveolar ventilation, improvements in blood gases, lung compliance, and chemotaxic sensitivity, and, possibly, improved ventilation/perfusion matching by reduction of atelectasis and small airway closure.

What Can Be Learned from Closed-system Ventilation

If a patient is going to be left a respirator cripple with a very low VC, a tracheotomy may be a great disadvantage. It is very difficult to get rid of a tracheotomy tube when the VC is only 500 or 600 cc and there is no power of coughing, whereas, as we all know, a patient who has been treated in a respirator [NPBV] from the first can survive and get out of all mechanical devices with a VC of that figure.[883]

In 1980, hypocapnia was described for tracheostomy IPPV users with ALS, post-polio syndrome, and myasthenia.[725] In 1989, Banzett et al. described chronic hypocapnia in a patient with high-level spinal cord injury receiving IPPV 24 hours/day via a tracheostomy tube.[951] In 1992 Manning et al. reported severe hypocapnia in five tracheostomized, IPPV-supported patients with traumatic spinal cord injury and VCs less than 90 ml.[952] Bach et al. described chronic hyperventilation in 33 tracheostomized ventilator users with a variety of paralytic/restrictive conditions[723] (Fig. 25). Watt, Oo, and Silva reported hypocapnia in 30 tracheostomized IPPV users with high-level tetraplegia.[724] Patterson et al. reported similarly severe hypocapnia in a tracheostomized patient with poliomyelitis and less than 30 ml of VC; the patient was supported by an iron lung.[953] Patterson suggested that the patient "was unable to increase the magnitude of the volley of impulses from the stretch receptors of the lung, or the frequency of these volleys [and was therefore] unable to increase by the Hering-Breuer mechanism the inhibition

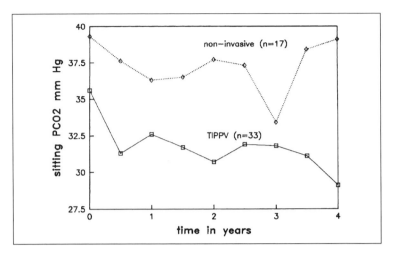

Figure 25. Plot of end-tidal PCO_2 recorded with the ventilator users in the sitting position. The data were summarized into 6-month intervals. The noninvasive IPPV users were significantly less hypocapnic than the tracheostomy IPPV users.

of inspiratory cell discharge in the respiratory center." Earlier Wright suggested that loss of such inhibition might play a central role in the production of breathlessness and demands for ever-increasing minute ventilation and hypocapnia.[954] All of the hypocapnic ventilator users in these reports were unable to trigger their ventilators and had received the same ventilator-delivered volumes for extended periods. Thus, the absence of control over inspiratory effort may be related in some way to the increased inspiratory cell activity in the production of breathlessness at hypocapnic levels.

Air satiety is governed by $PaCO_2$ and maintenance of normal blood pH.[955] In healthy people, any acute increase in $PaCO_2$ from baseline that decreases pH causes an increase in alveolar ventilation.[956] The chronic hypocapnia and metabolic acidosis of tracheostomized IPPV users greatly hampers breathing tolerance since patients with 500 ml or so of VC cannot autonomously ventilate their lungs sufficiently to maintain the low carbon dioxide level needed for acid-base homeostasis in the chronically hyperventilated state. Often breathing tolerance is regained only when the tracheostomy tube is removed, the patient is switched to noninvasive IPPV, and the carbon dioxide levels drift back upward to normal.[713]

During an attempt to reverse chronic hypocapnia without decannulation, tracheostomy IPPV users experienced severe dyspnea when the addition of carbon dioxide to inspired gases led to an 18-mmHg increase in $PaCO_2$ (to 38 mmHg).[956] In another study of hypocapnic tracheostomy IPPV users, elevations of $PaCO_2$ by only 10 mmHg created air hunger.[951] When IPPV tidal volumes were decreased to reverse hypocapnia, dyspnea began at a $PaCO_2$ of 26 mmHg.[956] When supplemental oxygen was given, breath-holding could be maintained to an increase of 16 mmHg; however, the increased tolerance to $PaCO_2$ was dependent on continued oxygen supplementation.[957] Gradual reductions in tidal volume also created intolerable air hunger in tracheostomy IPPV users with spinal cord injury whose $PaCO_2$ and PaO_2 were maintained at a constant level by control of the inspired gas mixture concentrations.[952] The severe $dSpO_2$ immediately following acute hyperventilation[958] and the dSpO$_2$, dyspnea, and increases in PaCO$_2$ that can accompany discontinuation of noninvasive IPPV, especially discontinuation of nocturnal ventilator use, illustrate the difficulties that can occur on resumption of autonomous breathing when lung ventilation is artificially maintained.[958]

As opposed to tracheostomy IPPV with an inflated cuff, which provides a closed system of ventilatory support in which alveolar ventilation is supported passively, carbon dioxide levels can also be maintained within normal limits by open systems of noninvasive ventilation. As seen later in this chapter, successful use of open noninvasive IPPV systems appears to depend largely on the intactness of ventilatory drive.

As noninvasive IPPV users sleep, ventilator-delivered (insufflation) volumes leak out of the nose or mouth rather than go entirely into the lungs. Higher ventilator-delivered volumes than those typically used during conventional tracheostomy IPPV compensate in part for variable air delivery leakage (insufflation leakage) during noninvasive ventilation.[959] Pressure-limiting the air delivery of volume-cycled ventilators or using pressure-cycled ventilators such as BiPAP-ST machines can also help compensate for insufflation leakage,[956] although the increase in flows can disturb sleep. As seen below, in addition to these passive mechanisms, chemotaxic-mediated reflex muscular activity intermittently decreases or eliminates insufflation leakage to normalize SpO$_2$ and avert excessive hypoxia and hypoventilation during sleep.[751]

In the 1950s it was common knowledge that patients with 200–500 ml of VC using body ventilators overnight could breathe autonomously during daytime hours; once they underwent tracheotomy, however, they became ventilator-dependent 24 hours/day with no breathing tolerance.[883] Resort to tracheostomy for IPPV results in increased production of airway secretions,[14] impaired mechanisms for clearance of airway secretions,[682] respiratory muscle deconditioning,[682] and chronic hyperventilation and hypocapnia.[713] Pulmonary function (VC) also decreases because of the presence of airway mucus and impaired mucociliary clearance caused by the tube. Thus, it should not be surprising that many 24-hour tracheostomy IPPV users with DMD, ALS, spinal cord injury, and other conditions whom we have decannulated and switched to noninvasive IPPV have progressed from having no breathing tolerance to nocturnal-only use of noninvasive IPPV (Chapter 11).[752,917,918]

Why Does Noninvasive IPPV Work During Sleep for People with No Breathing Tolerance?

Although most physicians mistakenly continue to think that intubation or tracheostomy is needed when patients have no ability to breathe, open systems of noninvasive IPPV have been used for continuous ventilatory support since 1964 by patients with little or no measurable VC or breathing tolerance. When mouthpiece IPPV is used during sleep, why doesn't the insufflated air leak out of the nose to the extent that the patient asphyxiates? Likewise, when a patient with no inspiratory muscle function uses nasal IPPV, why doesn't too much air leak out of the mouth during sleep? Excessive insufflation leakage limiting the effectiveness of noninvasive IPPV is surprisingly uncommon in patients with primarily neuromuscular ventilatory failure.[960] This section explores the answers to these questions.

The following criteria have been described as necessary for effective long-term use of noninvasive IPPV in patients with little or no breathing tolerance: absence of a history of substance abuse, absence of acute pulmonary or intrinsic lung disease that warrants oxygen therapy, and absence of seizure activity.[960] Narcotics, sedatives,[961] and oxygen administration depress ventilatory drive, leading the sleeping brain of patients with inspiratory muscle dysfunction to permit excessive insufflation leakage and hypercapnia. Seizure activity and postictal CNS depression also interfere with ventilatory drive, volitional access to a mouthpiece for noninvasive IPPV, and movements required to limit insufflation leakage during sleep.[567] Indeed, in the author's experience the only patients who have had no breathing tolerance and who have died during sleep using noninvasive IPPV either received narcotics, sedatives, or supplemental oxygen or consumed excessive alcohol. Thus, all of these nocturnal deaths had in common the suppression of ventilatory drive.

Patterns of Insufflation Leakage

In one report, four patterns of ventilator insufflation air leakage were observed in 36 patients using nocturnal nasal IPPV:

1. Minimal insufflation leakage and no significant dSpO$_2$ (Fig. 26). The lips remained closed or were plugged by tongue movement with each breath, or oral leakage was blocked by the passive mechanical effect of nasal IPPV sealing the soft palate against the tongue. For the patients who plugged lip opening with the tip of the tongue with each breath, the floor of the mouth moved upward and outward with each insufflation. This movement may have been a passive mechanical effect because the one patient who had electromyographic (EMG) monitoring of the genioglossus while using nasal IPPV during sleep demonstrated no increase in electrical activity.

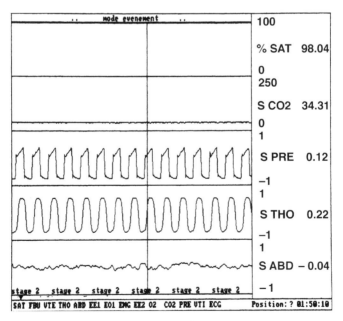

Figure 26. A minimal or no leakage pattern during stage 2 sleep. The monitored parameters are oxyhemoglobin saturation (SAT), end-tidal PCO$_2$ (CO$_2$), nasal interface pressure (PRE), and thoracoabdominal movement (THO and ABD). The SAT and CO$_2$ are normal, the airway pressures increase steadily and smoothly with the air delivered by the ventilator, and thorax movements are full and smooth.[751]

2. Continual, limited leakage from the mouth, creating a snoring effect with the lips vibrating (Fig. 27). Insufflation pressures dropped, with resulting periods of mild hypercapnia and dSpO$_2$.

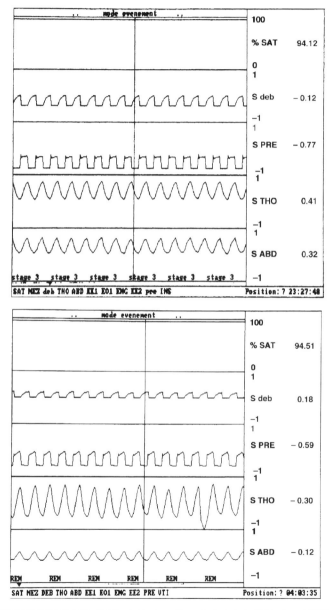

Figure 27. A minimal or partial insufflation leakage pattern during stage 3 (*top*) and REM (*bottom*) sleep associated with lip vibration and mild oxyhemoglobin desaturation to 94.1–94.5%. The monitored parameters are oxyhemoglobin saturation (SAT), exhaled air volume through the nose (DEB), nasal interface pressure (PRE), and thoracoabdominal movement (THO and ABD). The airway pressures tend to be flat by comparison with those of Figure 26, but thoracoabdominal movements are still good.[751]

3. Intermittent leakage with the mouth open and episodes of $dSpO_2$ of 4% or more over 20- to 60-second intervals (Fig. 28). Oropharyngeal movements occurred at the nadir of the $dSpO_2$s and diminished insufflation leakage. They appeared to be CNS-triggered reflexive tongue and pharyngeal movements and usually were associated with brief arousals or lightening of sleep stage. As the movements eliminated leakage, the SpO_2 returned to baseline before the next leak episode. These insufflation leakages and the leak elimination movements that they triggered at SpO_2 nadirs resulted in a "sawtooth" pattern of $dSpO_2$.

4. Prolonged insufflation leakage. Nocturnal noninvasive IPPV users who are hypercapnic during daytime hours but who do not use daytime noninvasive IPPV tend to

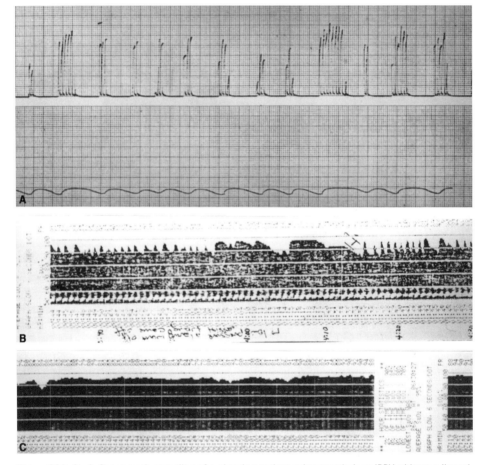

Figure 28A–C. *A,* Capnograph recording of a sleeping patient using mouthpiece IPPV without a lipseal. Although the mouthpiece remains in the mouth, insufflation leakage occurs until oxyhemoglobin desaturation develops. This episode triggers the patient to grasp the mouthpiece firmly for several deep insufflations that once again normalize the SpO_2 until the next leak episode. *B,* Sawtooth pattern of oxyhemoglobin desaturation common in patients with sleep-disordered breathing as well as during use of nasal ventilation or mouthpiece ventilation without lipseal retention. *C,* Severe desaturations can be eliminated by using lipseal retention for nocturnal IPPV.

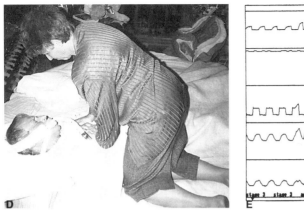
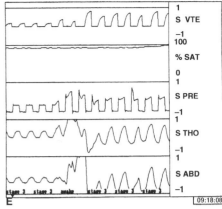

Figure 28D–E. *D*, The severe desaturations are eliminated for a post-polio patient by using lipseal retention for nocturnal mouthpiece IPPV. The patient's wife is applying a tussive thrust to the chest to assist his cough. *E*, The abrupt termination of a run of 147 leaky insufflations by reflex muscle activity during a brief arousal. The exhalation flows (VTE), airway pressure pattern (PRE), and thoracoabdominal movements (THO and ABD) are characteristic of a variable insufflation leakage pattern. Nevertheless, this scenario results in an increase in oxyhemoglobin saturation (SAT) to about 99%. The initial sharp upward inflection of the airway pressure wave form (PRE) of the 5th, 6th, 7th and 10th breaths indicates an initial obstruction to the ventilator-delivered volume of air. It may be due to passive airway closure related to the pressure or flow wave in the upper airway or to active contraction of the upper airway muscles. A decrease in the air delivery to the lungs can be seen in the decrease in air flow exhaled at the nose (VTE) and less thoracoabdominal movement (THO and ABD).[751]

have more severe nocturnal insufflation leakage, along with prolonged, severe episodes of nocturnal dSpO$_2$ (Fig. 29).[567]

Leak-limiting Measures and Sleep

Whether using simple mouthpiece IPPV, bite-plates without firm lipseal retention, or nasal IPPV during sleep, patients with or without breathing tolerance usually develop a sawtooth pattern of dSpO$_2$ and often have mean nocturnal SpO$_2$ slightly under 95%.[567,960] When mouthpiece IPPV users (without lipseals), for example, loosen their grip on the mouthpiece during sleep, it does not fall from the mouth. A loosened grip, however, does result in insufflation air leakage and dSpO$_2$. At the nadir of the dSpO$_2$, the user invariably regrips the mouthpiece firmly with teeth and oral musculature to eliminate leakage until SpO$_2$ increases to the preleakage baseline. Thus, insufflation leakage is stopped or markedly decreased and SpO$_2$ is normalized during the oropharyngeal muscular activity associated with and perhaps triggered by dSpO$_2$s or associated increases in carbon dioxide, changes in airflow sensation, or other factors (Figs. 29C and 30). One recent study suggested that arousals and decreased insufflation leakage were caused not by decreases in SpO$_2$ but rather by the increased effort of inspiratory muscles and hypercapnia.[962]

Excessive nocturnal hypercapnia and dSpO$_2$, therefore, are avoided by neurophysiologic mechanisms that include intermittent mechanical sealing of the oropharynx by the soft palate or lip closure during nasal IPPV and sealing off of the nasopharynx by the soft palate during mouthpiece IPPV. Although at times a passive mechanical seal operates to a certain degree, we found that the sawtooth pattern of dSpO$_2$ seen in most nasal

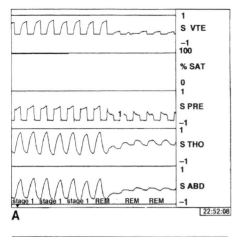

A

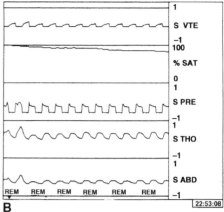

B

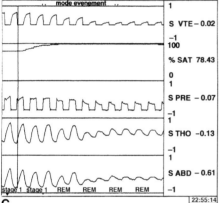

C

Figure 29. A patient who is hypercapnic during daytime hours receives effective assisted insufflations during stage 1 sleep (*A*), as indicated by high mask pressures (PRE), adequate expiratory flows recorded at the nose (VTE), and good thoracoabdominal movement (THO and ABD). On entering REM sleep, all parameters indicate massive insufflation leakage. His alveolar ventilation is inadequate because virtually all of the ventilator-delivered air leaks out of the mouth and oxyhemoglobin saturation (SAT) decreases to 78% in 3 minutes (*B*). On reaching the SAT nadir, he returns to sleep stage 1 and completely terminates insufflation leakage. His SAT returns to 98% (*C*). Insufflation leakage once again began as soon as he entered REM sleep. This time, once the SAT decreased to 87%, he had a brief arousal of which he was unaware and again returned insufflation parameters and SAT to normal levels.[751]

and simple mouthpiece IPPV users during sleep is also reversed by active muscle activity associated with brief arousal in 71% of cases or lightening of sleep stage or arousal in 76% of cases (see Figs. 28E and 29C); in about 24% of cases, electroencephalography shows no apparent sleep stage change[751] (see Fig. 30A). Since brief arousals may not be found during electroencephalography and are sometimes detectable only by monitoring of the autonomic nervous system,[858] it is possible that all termination of insufflation leakage is associated with arousals. However, if this were the case, it would be difficult to explain why—after a brief, undetectable arousal that terminates insufflation leakage—the patient returns to the same sleep stage. On rare occasions, dSpO$_2$s and insufflation leakage were reversed at the point of entering a deeper stage of sleep (see Fig. 30B).

With or without sleep stage changes we reported that all recoveries in SpO$_2$ were accompanied by changes in the configuration of the pneumotachograph flows or mask pressure patterns that indicated decreased insufflation leakage. This finding can be explained by a dSpO$_2$-triggered adjustment in body position or initiation of specific oromotor and pharyngeal movements to decrease or eliminate leakage. Adjustment in body position was not seen and indeed, for many patients, would be impossible, whereas specific oromotor and pharyngeal movements were clearly observed at the nadir of most

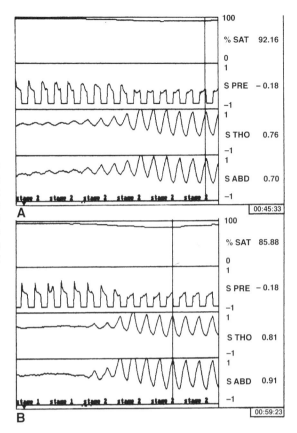

Figure 30. Normalization of tidal volumes and oxyhemoglobin saturation with reduction of insufflation leakage without apparent sleep stage change (*A*) and with deepening in sleep to stage 2 (*B*). The parameters include oxyhemoglobin saturation (SAT), nasal interface pressure (PRE), and thoracoabdominal movement (THO and ABD).[751]

dSpO$_2$s, resulting in the characteristic sawtooth pattern.[751] The importance of soft palate movements can be seen in the fact that patients who have undergone uvulopharyngoplasties and patients with advanced bulbar ALS and no residual bulbar muscle function experience excessive insufflation leakage through the mouth when using nasal CPAP[963] or nasal ventilation.

The results of increasing ventilatory stimulation in 8 normal men during sleep were studied to determine whether arousals would result from increased inspiratory effort. Electroencephalography, electromyography, electrooculography, minute ventilation, end-tidal carbon dioxide, SpO$_2$, and esophageal (balloon) pressure were measured during induction of arousal from non-REM sleep by using added resistive loads, progressive hypoxia, and progressive hyperoxic hypercapnia. The extent of increasing inspiratory effort was determined by measuring esophageal pressures to estimate pleural pressures. All subjects were eventually aroused by the added load of 30 cmH$_2$O/L/sec and during progressive hypercapnia. However, only six of eight were aroused when the SpO$_2$ was reduced to a minimum permissible 70%. For each stimulus, arousal occurred at very different levels of ventilation, carbon dioxide, and SpO$_2$. However, the ventilatory effort was similar at the point of arousal, regardless of the stimulus. The peak-negative esophageal pressure was 16.8 ± 1.4 cmH$_2$O for the single inspiration preceding arousal, 14.7 ± 2.1 cmH$_2$O for hypercapnia, and 15.0 ± 2.4 cmH$_2$O for hypoxia; two of the 8 men were not aroused by $dSpO_2$ to 70%.[962] It makes sense that arousals would be induced by increasing inspiratory effort, but it is interesting to speculate about how this parameter would be assessed in patients who have severe inspiratory muscle weakness and are unable to make any measurable inspiratory effort (e.g., 24-hour noninvasive IPPV users with no measurable VC). Although $dSpO_2$ (see Fig. 28B) was common, 24-hour mouthpiece IPPV (without lipseal retention) had been used by patients with no VC for years[752] before lipseals became available in 1968. Thus, an important question remains: are arousals caused by the effect of added inspiratory muscle effort or by some central drive that attempts to increase inspiratory muscle effort?

In a polysomnography study of nasal bilevel PAP insufflation leakage during sleep in 6 hypercapnic patients with chest wall disease or NMD, the mean FEV_1 was 1 ± 0.2 L; all six patients had oral insufflation leakage for the majority of sleep. Sleep quality was diminished because of poor sleep efficiency and reduced percentages of slow-wave and REM sleep. Oral leakage was associated with frequent arousals during stages 1 and 2 and REM sleep that contributed to sleep fragmentation, but arousals were infrequent during slow-wave sleep despite leakage. Thus, the threshold for arousals seems to increase during slow-wave sleep. Sixty to 99% of arousals occurred toward the end of a period of leakage, bringing about a temporary cessation of leak. Patients used a combination of passive and active mechanisms to control air leaking. When no leak was detectable the submental EMG showed absent upper airway muscle activity consistent with a passive leak control mechanism. Once leaking occurred, patients repositioned the mandible and performed "what appeared to be a swallowing maneuver associated with an increase in submental EMG activity and no other perceptible body movements. Air leaking through the mouth would then cease and assisted breathing would continue without leaking until, after a few minutes, the lips would part again and the cycle would repeat itself."[964]

A study of CPAP use noted similarly absent genioglossus EMG activity with an essentially passive sealing off of the oropharynx until insufflation leakage increased, causing the lips to part and flutter and eventually leading to the submental EMG activity and swallowing-like motion that temporarily terminated the leakage.[965] In the 6 nasal ventilation patients in the above study,[964] there was only a slight drop-off in tidal volumes during insufflation leakage, probably because the lowest FVC of any of the 5 successful users was 870 ml. Oxygenation was also well maintained with a mean nocturnal SpO_2 of 94% in all but one patient, whose FVC was only 560 ml, who was also receiving supplemental oxygen, and who was the most severely hypercapnic during daytime hours both before and during treatment. This patient, who had restrictive disease secondary to tuberculosis and obesity, refused an oral-nasal interface and tracheotomy, was never offered a lipseal or daytime support, and died a few weeks after the sleep study.[964]

The patients who had 4% or less REM sleep had six times more leak-associated arousals per hour than those with greater than 10% REM sleep, even though the same amount of time was spent with air leakage in stages 1 and 2 sleep. These patients may have had innately higher arousal thresholds than those with lower REM percentages; alternatively, they may have accommodated to leaks by raising their arousal thresholds in a process resembling adaptation of the arousal threshold for noise, which has been demonstrated experimentally.[964] Insufflation leakage, therefore, is associated with frequent arousals during lighter stages of sleep that interfere with progression to REM and deeper stages, compromising sleep quality. However, sleep quality is unquestionably better with nasal ventilation than without it. The patients in this study could not sleep without it, and we and others have shown daily deterioration in sleep quality with withdrawal of nocturnal nasal ventilation.[768,946]

The obese patient with tuberculosis merits further discussion. For many patients who are hypercapnic during daytime hours but who use only nocturnal noninvasive IPPV, nocturnal hypercapnia and $dSpO_2$ persist and nasal ventilation is less successful. In such cases, extending ventilator use into daytime hours reverses the compensatory metabolic alkalosis that suppresses the chemotaxic response to insufflation leakage and $dSpO_2$. In one study, 16 patients with less than 400 ml of supine VC and less than 15 minutes of breathing tolerance maintained normal alveolar ventilation by using noninvasive IPPV up to 24 hours per day; they had a mean nocturnal SpO_2 of 95.9 ± 2.6% using nasal IPPV. In contrast, 17 other patients who were hypercapnic during daytime hours and used only nocturnal nasal IPPV did not normalize nocturnal SpO_2.[933] Thus, nocturnal use of open systems of noninvasive IPPV may not be adequate. Either closing the system by using mouthpiece IPPV with a lipseal and, possibly, nasal plugs or extending ventilatory assistance into daytime hours may become necessary.[752] Ventilator patients who use daytime as well as nocturnal assisted ventilation and thus maintain intact chemotaxic drive may use nasal or mouthpiece IPPV during sleep with few $dSpO_2$s, whereas patients with daytime hypercapnia have less improvement in nocturnal ventilation by nasal IPPV.[567,752]

No simple passive methods appear to be effective by themselves for mechanically preventing excessive oral air leakage during nocturnal nasal IPPV. Taping the mouth closed (Fig. 31) and stuffing the mouth with a bite-plate (Fig. 32) or other object are rarely effective. Strapping the chin to keep the mouth closed (see Fig. 9) can be helpful but does not compensate for suboptimal daytime ventilation or a suboptimal interface for nocturnal aid. Often, switching from nasal to lipseal IPPV (Fig. 33) is effective when oral leakage results in severe nocturnal $dSpO_2$s.

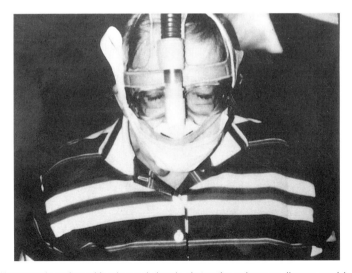

Figure 31. Hypercapnic patient with advanced chronic obstructive pulmonary disease receiving continuous supplemental oxygen therapy and nasal ventilation. The clinician attempts to decrease oral insufflation leakage by taping the mouth shut, an effective technique if one is prepared to replace the tape every 15 minutes.

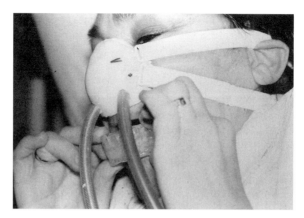

Figure 32. Severely kyphoscoliotic nocturnal nasal IPPV user who remains hypercapnic during daytime hours and attempts to decrease oral insufflation leakage by wearing a bite-plate.

When nasal congestion precludes the effective use of nasal IPPV, we have routinely switched patients to lipseal IPPV. Mouthpiece IPPV with lipseal retention passively seals the lips and mouth. This seal, along with an increase in ventilator-delivered volumes, compensates for insufflation leakage from the nose and can change a sawtooth $dSpO_2$ pattern into a normal one (see Fig. 28C). Thus, nocturnal lipseal IPPV, with or without nasal plugging, can normalize mean nocturnal SpO_2[752] by possibly reducing insufflation leakage and, thereby, the need to resort to centrally mediated mechanisms for effective alveolar ventilation. It can also probably improve sleep quality since arousals are often necessary to reverse desaturations.[933]

In one study of patients using nocturnal mouthpiece IPPV with lipseal retention, expiratory passage of air through the nose occurred during an average of only 33% ± 27%

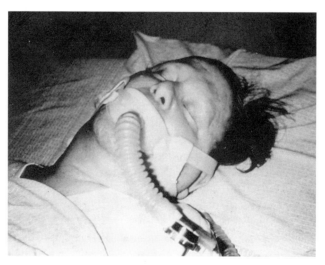

Figure 33. Post-polio continuous mouthpiece IPPV user, including nocturnal use with lipseal retention (seen here), from 1955 until succumbing to leukemia in 1995.

of the total sleep time. Despite the fact that only three of the 27 lipseal IPPV users had sufficient VC for 10 minutes of breathing tolerance when supine and only one used supplemental oxygen, all slept in the supine position, 22 (82%) of the nocturnal oximetry studies yielded normal (greater than 95%) mean SpO_2, and 12 of 15 had maximum end-tidal carbon dioxide levels under 45 mmHg. The lowest mean nocturnal SpO_2 for any patient using nocturnal lipseal IPPV was 92%. The smoothing out of the sawtooth pattern of $dSpO_2$ and the normalization of mean nocturnal SpO_2 imply that lipseal IPPV normalizes nocturnal ventilation by creating at least a partially closed system to ventilate the lungs with less need for arousal or reflex elimination of insufflation leakage. For 13 nocturnal mouthpiece/lipseal IPPV users undergoing inpatient polysomnography, the time periods in the deeper sleep stages tended to be normal as a percentage of total sleep time.[933] Ten had normal and three had increased duration of stage 3 and 4 sleep. Eight had normal and five decreased REM sleep duration as a percentage of total sleep time. Only five had mean SpO_2 less than 95% for 1 hour or more, SpO_2 less than 90% for 6% or more of the recording time, and numerous transient $dSpO_2$s. Three of these five used mouthpiece IPPV without a lipseal or with a lipseal with inadequate retention. All three were also symptomatic with hypoventilation during daytime hours but did not use daytime ventilatory assistance.[933]

Just as we have noted nocturnal nasal IPPV to be ineffective in ventilator users receiving heavy sedation or narcotics, evidence also indicates that nasal IPPV is less effective in the acute setting for ventilator users requiring high oxygen supplementation, particularly during sleep.[752,966] We speculate that this finding can be explained in large part by failure of centrally mediated activity to decrease insufflation leakage when SpO_2 is maintained artificially (by supplemental oxygen).

Periods of insufflation leakage and $dSpO_2$ alternate with effective insufflations during all sleep stages. Indeed, the SpO_2 pattern can oscillate between 94% and 95% (Fig. 34). Perhaps the most interesting pattern is that of effective assisted ventilation and insufflation leakage alternating with every breath (Fig. 35). These findings may also represent activation of central neural mechanisms. The highest percentage of $dSpO_2$ per unit time occurs during REM sleep, despite the fact that effective insufflation patterns are often maintained during REM sleep for prolonged periods (Fig. 36). As for patients with obstructive sleep apnea syndrome,[967] lesser frequencies of $dSpO_2$s and arousals are observed in the deeper stages than in stages 1, 2, and REM sleep.

During use of mouthpiece IPPV without a lipseal, the CNS, probably through chemotaxic sensitivity, reflexively triggers the muscular activity needed to prevent potentially life-threatening air leakage and $dSpO_2$. This finding is not surprising since it is extremely unlikely that open systems of ventilatory support, such as nasal or simple mouthpiece IPPV, could sustain patients with little or no VC 24 hours per day by postural or passive mechanisms alone. The centrally triggered activity occurs at the nadir of the $dSpO_2$s, or possibly at nadirs of PaO_2, with sensitivity to $dSpO_2$ differing in all sleep stages. Other centrally mediated responses to the need to increase alveolar ventilation may also play a role. The improvements in nocturnal SpO_2 are in large part due to the deeper lung insufflations that are fostered by arousal-triggered oromotor movements to decrease insufflation leakage. Respiratory muscle recruitment can not explain the maintenance of nocturnal ventilation for patients with no measurable VC who use noninvasive IPPV.[567,674,752] Such patients could not have tolerated 147 severely leaky insufflations (see Fig. 28E)

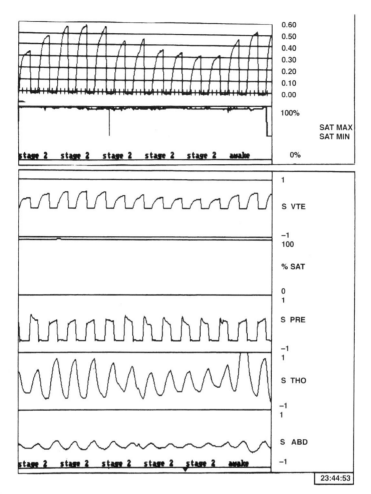

Figure 34. Alternating optimal insufflations with variable insufflation leakage as oxyhemoglobin saturation oscillates in 8 breath cycles between 94% and 95% in stage 2 sleep. This pattern may represent intermittent activation of central neural mechanisms. Parameters include expired flow (VTE), oxyhemoglobin saturation (SAT), nasal mask pressure (PRE), and thoracoabdominal movement (THO and ABD).

before eliminating excessive leaking. The fact that patients with little or no measurable VC can often tolerate periods of limited insufflation leakage without significant changes in SpO$_2$ during all sleep stages implies that passive mechanisms such as lip plugging by the tongue or apposition of the tongue and soft palate are also likely to be at work to prevent excessive insufflation leakage.[567,674]

Upper Airway Movements to Obstruct Air Delivery

Figure 28E demonstrates initial inspiratory cycle obstruction to ventilator-delivered volumes first during an arousal after a long period of insufflation leakage and later during stage 3 sleep. For nasal IPPV users with DMD, leakage can occur in association with downward movements of the soft palate and tongue that narrow the pharynx

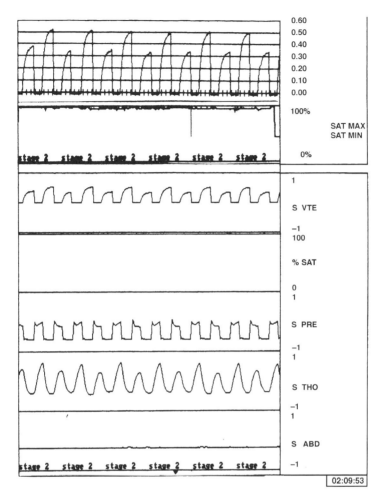

Figure 35. Another example of alternating optimal insufflations with variable insufflation leakage as oxyhemoglobin saturation oscillates between 94% and 95% in stage 2 sleep. This time, however, the cycles are two breaths. Parameters include expired flow (VTE), oxyhemoglobin saturation (SAT), nasal mask pressure (PRE), and thoracoabdominal movement (THO and ABD).[751]

during REM sleep and apparently result in dSpO$_2$s.[968] Glottic movements and the compliance of the upper airways modulate ventilator-delivered volumes entering the lungs. Obstructions to airflow can increase insufflation leakage and may be centrally triggered events to prevent hyperventilation.

Jounieux et al. found that during sleep the glottic aperture narrows and delivered tidal volumes fall during lighter stages of sleep, but the aperture widens, permitting more ventilation, during the deeper stages. If minute ventilation is increased excessively, the aperture narrows as a function of decreased carbon dioxide levels.[969] Parreira et al. reported that such changes occur more often with control-mode assisted ventilation than with bilevel PAP in spontaneous mode.[970,971] Delguste et al. observed apnea for up to 1 minute in association with hypocapnia caused by passive nasal IPPV in 3 of 4 patients during

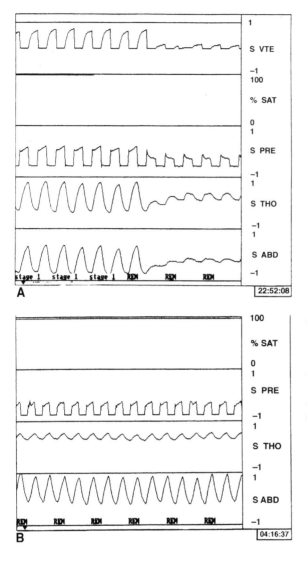

Figure 36. *A*, Assisted insufflations in stage 1 sleep indicated by high mask pressures (PRE) and expiratory flows (VTE) and good thoracoabdominal movement (THO and ABD). With change into REM sleep, all parameters indicate massive insufflation leakage. Once the oxyhemoglobin saturation (SAT) decreased to 87%, the patient had a brief arousal of which he was unaware; insufflation parameters and SpO₂ returned to normal levels. (From Bach JR, Robert D, Leger P, Langevin B: Sleep fragmentation in kyphoscoliotic individuals with alveolar hypoventilation treated by nasal IPPV. Chest 1995; 107:1552-58, with permission of the American College of Chest Physicians.[751]) *B*, Maintenance of effective ventilation during REM sleep. The monitored parameters are oxyhemoglobin saturation (SAT), nasal interface pressure (PRE), and thoracoabdominal movement (THO and ABD).[751]

sleep.[972] The apneas seemed to be caused by complete upper airways obstruction. This finding, too, suggests that active glottic closure occurred to avoid excessive hypocapnia during nocturnal noninvasive IPPV.

Besides narrowing or obstructing the airway to prevent hyperventilation during nocturnal noninvasive ventilation, obstructive apneas can result in frequent arousals and disturbed sleep architecture during noninvasive IPPV and thus cause severe dSpO₂s, as they do in patients with sleep-disordered breathing.[858] Obstruction can be due to pharyngeal wall instability and collapse. Indeed, airway muscles are normally activated during both inspiration and expiration to preserve an open upper airway.[973] Patients with neuromuscular weakness or OSAS may have excessive upper airway collapsibility, which, when observed and measured by applying negative pressure to the airway in awake patients, predicts airway collapsibility during sleep. In one study, pharyngeal collapse occurred in response to pressures of −17 to −40 cmH_2O.[974] Collapse may be due to loss of protective reflexes and decreased dilator muscle activation as well as the pressure gradient. Inspiratory resistive loading correlated with negative-pressure pulses in predicting airway collapse. This finding explains in large part the high incidence of OSAS in obese patients. Likewise, pharyngeal collapsibility can be so severe in patients with NMD, especially those with bulbar ALS and occasionally those with myotonic dystrophy,[975] that it can make cough flows unmeasurable and cause both inspiratory and expiratory stridor (see Chapter 4).

Obstructions can decrease with extension of the head and neck, use of a collar, and modification of ventilator settings to improve patient coordination with the ventilator. As for obstructive sleep apneas that may cause and, at times, be caused by arousals and continuous activation of the sympathetic nervous system[858] (see Fig. 28E), obstruction can appear at the end of a period of massive insufflation leakage as well as during brief arousals during which SpO_2 recovers. Thus, sleep stage, bulbar muscle function, and the amount of ventilatory assistance influence glottic and upper airway aperture, an important determinant of the efficacy of noninvasive ventilation.

Complications of Noninvasive IPPV and Barotrauma

In addition to orthodontic deformities and skin pressure from the interface, other potential difficulties include allergy to the plastic lipseal or silicone interfaces (13% vs. 5% for nonsilicone interfaces), dry mouth (65%), eye irritation from air leakage (about 24%), nasal congestion (25%) and dripping (35%), sinusitis (8%), nose bleeding (4–19%), gum discomfort (20%) and receding due to nasal interface or lipseal pressure, maxillary flattening in children, aerophagia,[927,976] and, as for invasive ventilation, barotrauma. In addition, occasional patients express claustrophobia. Proper interface selection eliminates or minimizes discomfort. RoEzit is a petroleum-free moisturizer that can be applied to the nasal passages and to the face when skin becomes dry due to mask usage.

Pressure drop-off through the narrow air passages of the nose is normally between 2 and 3 cmH_2O. Suboptimal humidification dries out and irritates nasal mucus membranes, causes sore throat, and results in vasodilatation and nasal congestion. Increased airflow resistance up to 8 cmH_2O can be caused by the loss of humidity due to unidirectional airflow with expiration via the mouth during nasal CPAP or ventilation.[977] This problem cannot be ameliorated by using a cold passover humidifier, but the increase in airway resistance can be reduced by 50% by warming the inspired air to body temperature and humidifying it with the use of a hot water bath humidifier.[977] Decongestants can also relieve sinus irritation and nasal congestion. Switching to lipseal IPPV can relieve most if not all difficulties associated with nasal IPPV. Lipseal IPPV also necessitates use of a hot water bath humidifier.

Abdominal distention tends to occur sporadically in noninvasive ventilation users. Normally the gastroesophageal sphincter can withstand peak air pressures up to 25 cmH_2O without stomach dilatation. Aerophagia can occur when ventilator-delivered volumes meet with airway obstruction, resulting in peak pressures over 25 cmH_2O or whatever pressure the particular sphincter cannot withstand. It may occur or be exacerbated when patients assume the supine position, especially when the patient reclines in the hour or so after meals.[978] Gastric insufflation can often be decreased or eliminated by decreasing the inspiratory pressure delivery of pressure-cycled ventilators, by pressure- limiting volume-cycled ventilators, or at times by switching from one ventilator style to the other.[979] When gastric insufflation occurs, the air usually passes as flatus once the patient gets up or is placed into a wheelchair. When severe, it can present as intestinal pseudo-obstruction with diminished bowel sounds and increased ventilator dependence (Chapter 4). Although we have never had to discontinue noninvasive ventilation for any patient because of aerophagia first observed after beginning noninvasive ventilation, aerophagia and severe abdominal distention that are present before institution of ventilatory assistance are usually exacerbated by noninvasive ventilation. For this reason, the patient often cannnot tolerate noninvasive ventilation unless a gastrostomy tube is placed to alleviate the problem. Patients with lower intestinal distention may require colostomy or fare better with a tracheostomy.

Barotrauma is essentially volutrauma. It is lung damage due to overexpansion of lung units. It can occur with invasive or noninvasive ventilation and results from rupture of the boundary between the alveoli and the bronchovascular sheath. Extra-alveolar air entering the lung parenchyma presents as interstitial emphysema and subpleural air cysts. Air can also rupture into the mediastinum and present as subcutaneous emphysema, pneumomediastinum, or pneumoperitoneum, or it can rupture through the fascial planes into the pleural space to result in hemodynamically significant pneumothoraces. Its incidence has been cited as 4–15% for ICU invasive ventilation users with primarily respiratory impairment,[980] but in a study of 139 patients it was reported in 60% of patients with acute respiratory distress syndrome and none of the patients with congestive heart failure (CHF) or neurologic disease.[981] Only one case of recurrent pneumothoraces has ever been reported—in a 26-year-old patient with unclassified NMD who had numerous subpleural blebs. He had no subsequent pneumothoraces following open pleurodesis.[982] Extra-alveolar air can also enter the systemic circulation of patients with a bronchovenous communication and an adequate pressure gradient. Systemic gas embolization is a well-recognized complication in neonatal respiratory distress syndrome.

Pneumothorax in a patient receiving positive-pressure ventilation impairs gas exchange and hemodynamics by increasing intrathoracic pressure, decreasing venous return, and increasing afterload to the right side of the heart. The decrease in cardiac output appears to correlate linearly with the volume of pneumothorax.[983] Blood gas alterations may not occur despite the presence of a large pneumothorax, but the airway pressures noted on the ventilator gauge usually increase before blood gas deterioration and acute cardiac decompensation. CT scans of the chest are sensitive in diagnosing pneumothoraces. The combination of lateral decubitus, erect, and supine radiographs can detect pneumothoraces as small as 50 ml. For patients with cardiomyopathies and low left ventricular ejection fractions, sudden evacuation of a pneumothorax can result in hemodynamic collapse.

Numerous investigators have demonstrated that diffuse lung edema, tissue histopathologic changes, and hypoxemia indistinguishable from that which occurs in acute respiratory distress syndrome can occur in normal animals ventilated with moderately high peak airway pressures of 30–50 cmH_2O.[980] Sheep ventilated at a pressure of 50 cmH_2O developed severely reduced static lung compliance, decreased FRC, hypoxemia, and grossly abnormal lungs within 35 hours.[984] Peak inspiratory pressures above 40 cmH_2O are associated with an increased risk of alveolar rupture during mechanical ventilation in humans, and the incidence of barotrauma exceeds 40% in patients exposed to pressures above 70 cmH_2O, albeit predominantly in those with lung disease.[985] However, high airway pressures can be applied to the respiratory system without injury if excessive lung inflation is prevented, as seen in obese patients or patients with decreased abdominal compliance. In such patients, a given change in lung volume is associated with a larger increase in pleural pressures; thus, a greater pressure change at the airway is necessary to inflate the respiratory system. However, the transmural pressure across the alveolus would be no different from that in patients with normal abdominal compliance, and the risk of lung injury is not increased.[986] Dreyfuss et al. avoided barotrauma in rats by strapping their chests.[987] He also induced barotrauma by using negative-pressure ventilation that created similar transalveolar pressures. Thus, injury from hyperinflation is due to the extent of the inflation rather than the pressure per se.

It appears that high pressures also may be used with little or no risk if exposures are very short, as with air-stacking, when lung tissues are essentially normal. We have had no barotrauma in hundreds of patients practicing air-stacking at pressures of 40–70 cmH_2O. On the other hand, the risk of barotrauma is greatly increased by tissue fragility, secretion retention that leads to overexpansion of unobstructed lung units, surfactant depletion, shear forces, and prolonged duration of ventilation or exposure to high pressures.[980] Patients ventilated over the long term by increasing dead space ventilation with high delivered volumes and pressures over 40 cmH_2O develop surfactant depletion, inflammation, and alveolar rupture associated with shear and alveolar distention similar to that seen in adult respiratory distress syndrome.[984,988]

The strategies for diminishing the risk of barotrauma in patients with primarily respiratory impairment include using pressure-cycled ventilation and lowering pressures while increasing rate, adding PEEP, and permitting hypercapnia. However, the lungs of patients with COPD may be hypercompliant and require low IPAPs for assisted ventilation. In addition, PEEP can counter the effects of air trapping, hypercapnia may be necessary for ventilator weaning, ventilator use may only increase air trapping, and the prognosis is generally poor. For patients with primarily ventilatory impairment, on the other hand, this approach is inappropriate. Permitting hypercapnia in such patients increases the risk of morbidity and mortality.[14] Air trapping is not a problem for them. PEEP only decreases the extent of respiratory muscle rest (lowering the IPAP-EPAP span) and increases discomfort. We have not observed barotrauma in patients who air-stack regularly, and there have been very few pneumothoraces in our over 800 ventilator users, many of whom have been using noninvasive IPPV at airway pressures of 30–45 cmH_2O for over 50 years. No increased incidence of barotrauma has been reported with the use of volume- rather than pressure-cycled ventilators. Limiting ventilation volumes at the cost of increasing breathing rate and hypercapnia and avoiding lung and chest wall ROM result in increasing pulmonary and chest wall restriction and work of breathing (Chapter 9).

Inspissated secretions are often considered a "life-threatening" complication of noninvasive ventilation.[672,989] However, except for patients who have an ineffective assisted CPF less than 160 L/min and essentially respiratory rather than ventilatory impairment, secretion encumberment is more a complication of the clinician's failure to teach assisted coughing than it is a complication of noninvasive ventilation. It should be recalled that there are 1012–1017 bacteria per milliliter of saliva.[990] Chronic aspiration of saliva to the extent of lowering baseline SpO_2 can overwhelm normally sterile airways and lead to pneumonia,[991] tracheitis, bronchitis,[992] and chronic lung disease.[991] Thus, the only respiratory indication for tracheostomy is assisted CPF less than 160 L/min and SpO_2 baseline less than 95% due to chronic airway secretion aspiration. Relative contraindications to the long-term use of noninvasive inspiratory muscle aids are listed in Table 2.[285] There was also a single report of a unilateral orbital herniation following initiation of noninvasive ventilation for OSAS diagnosed after an intracranial hemorrhage.[993]

Goal Three: Facilitate Airway Clearance

Facilitation of Peripheral Mucus Clearance

Approaches to preventing retention of peripheral airway secretions in patients with NMD include the use of medications to reduce mucus hypersecretion or to liquefy secretions and facilitation of mucus mobilization. Mucus mobilization can be facilitated by manual or mechanical chest percussion or vibration, direct oscillation of the air column, and postural drainage. The goal is to transport mucus from the peripheral to the central airways, from which it can be eliminated more easily by assisted coughing and MAC.

Postural Drainage and Vibration

Gravitational forces can enhance mucus transport when bronchi are vertically positioned. Postural drainage is the facilitation of airway drainage by having the patient assume gravity-assisted positions. It is probably most effective in patients with relatively large quantities of mucus with low adhesiveness. Nine postural positions have been described for draining the large bronchi (Fig. 37).[994] Localization of airway mucus is essential. The object is to position vertically the secretion-encumbered bronchi for a sufficient period, generally about 20 minutes, to allow drainage. The time required probably depends on the quantity of mucus, its viscoelasticity and adhesiveness, and the effectiveness of concomitant use of chest percussion or vibration. If the patient can tolerate it, he or she sleeps in a postural drainage position.

Chest percussion is the manual application of rhythmic clapping to the ventral, lateral, and dorsal side of the thorax at about 3–6 Hz. It is often prescribed and used for 10- to 20-minute treatment sessions in patients with auscultatory or oximetry evidence of airway secretion retention. As for other vibration and oscillation techniques, its efficacy may be due to its effect on decreasing mucus viscosity and inducing small coughs or

Table 2.	Situations That Can Decrease the Efficacy of Noninvasive Ventilation
1. Use of sedation or narcotics	
2. Oxygen therapy	
3. SpO_2 not maintained above 94% due to encumberment or obstruction of airway secretions	
4. Substance abuse or uncontrollable seizures	
5. Unassisted or assisted CPFs that cannot exceed 2.7 L/sec	
7. Conditions that interfere with the use of ventilation interfaces (i.e., facial fractures, inadequate bite for mouthpiece entry, presence of beards that hamper airtight interface seal)	

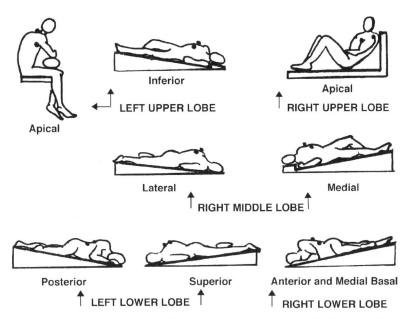

Figure 37. The nine positions for drainage of large airways. Percussion and vibration are applied to areas demarcated by the points.

resonance with ciliary action.[995] It facilitates the proximal migration of airway secretions but at the cost of acutely increasing metabolic rate, oxygen consumption (by 40–50%), heart rate, blood pressure, intracranial pressures, plasma catecholamine concentrations, hypoxia, and gastrointestinal reflux in infants.[996,997] Patients receiving chest physical therapy who are able to increase minute ventilation do so by about 35%, and those who are not able to do so require ventilatory assistance to the same extent.[996]

Vibration can be applied externally to the chest wall or abdomen by rapidly oscillating pressure changes in a vest (e.g., the ThAIRapy Vest, American Biosystems, Inc., St. Paul, MN); by cycling oscillating pressures under a chest shell (e.g., the Hayek oscillator, Breasy Medical Equipment, Inc., Stamford, CN); or by using chest vibrators (Fig. 38). The ThAIRapy Vest provides oscillation at 5–25 Hz. Mechanical vibration is performed at frequencies up to 40 Hz. Vibration is applied during the entire breathing cycle or during expiration only. The adjustable I/E ratio of the Hayek oscillator permits asymmetric inspiratory and expiratory pressure changes (for example, +3 to –6 cmH$_2$O), which favor higher exsufflation flow velocities to mobilize secretions. Baseline pressures can be set at negative, atmospheric, or positive values, thus commencing oscillation above, at, or below the functional residual capacity (FRC).

Oscillations up to 16 Hz or greater can also be applied at the mouth by high-frequency positive-pressure ventilation or jet ventilation. One such air column oscillator based on high-frequency jet ventilation was developed by the Bird Corporation (Exeter, UK). This hand-held device delivers 30 ml sine wave oscillations through a mouthpiece at 20 Hz. Lower-frequency air column oscillators are the Intrapulmonary Percussive Ventilator, Percussionator, Impulsator, and Spanker Respirators (Percussionaire Corp., Sandpoint, ID). They can deliver aerosolized medications while providing intrapulmonary percussive

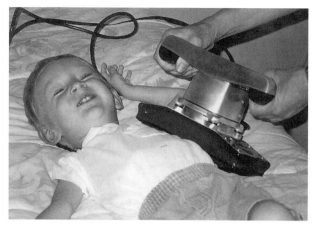

Figure 38. Use of a Jeanie Rub Vibrator M69-315A (Morfam, Inc., Mishawaka, IN) by a 5.5-year-old boy with spinal muscular atrophy type 2.

ventilation—that is, high-flow mini-bursts of air to the lungs—at a rate of 2–7 Hz[998] (Fig. 39). Although numerous publications attest to the usefulness of this device for patients with cystic fibrosis, there is one report of its helping to clear persistent pulmonary consolidation refractory to conventional therapies for 3 patients with NMDs. The patients had clinical and radiographic improvement within 48 hours after onset of therapy.[999]

It has been reported that high-frequency oscillations act like a physical mucolytic, reducing both the spinnability and viscoelasticity of mucus and enhancing cough-clearability.[1000] The effect of combining rhDNase medications with oscillation may be complementary.[1001] An in vitro study also suggested that shearing at the air-mucus interface may also be a factor in the enhanced tracheal mucus clearance during high-frequency chest wall oscillation.[1002] Hansen et al. suggested that mucus transport is enhanced in three ways: by altering cross-linkage density of mucus glycoproteins, by creating a cough-like expiratory flow bias, and by increasing the strength of ciliary beat through resonance.[995]

Contraindications for high-frequency oscillation are listed in Table 3. In addition, in some publications the following have been listed as relative contraindications for chest wall oscillation: pulmonary edema due to CHF, esophageal surgery, recent epidural spinal infusion, spinal surgery, spinal anesthesia or acute spinal injury, presence of a transvenous

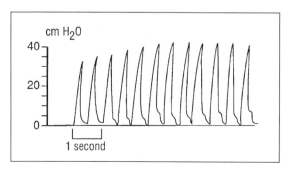

Figure 39. Pressure delivery pattern of the Intrapulmonary Percussive Ventilator (Percussionaire Corp., Sandpoint, ID).

Table 3.   **Contraindications for High-frequency Oscillation and Mechanical Insufflation-Exsufflation**

Absolute	Relative
Unstable head or neck injury	Pneumothorax
Active hemorrhage with hemodynamic instability	Pulmonary embolism
	Subcutaneous emphysema
Active or recent gross spontaneous hemoptysis	Bronchopleural fistula
	Suspected or confirmed pulmonary tuberculosis
	Bronchospasm
	Rib fracture or other severe chest wall trauma
	Lung contusion
	Chest wall pain

or subcutaneous pacemaker, increased intracranial pressures, uncontrolled hypertension, empyema or large pleural effusion, osteoporosis, osteomyelitis, coagulopathy, distended abdomen, thoracic burns, open wounds, infection, and recent skin graft.

Use of chest vibrators, such as the Jeannie Rub Percussor (Morfam Inc., Mishawaka, IN) (see Fig. 38) or the Neo-Cussor (General Physical Therapy, St. Louis, MO), may be most practical for chest percussion. They, too, can vibrate the chest at optimal frequencies but are small, light, easy to use, and inexpensive.

The use of chest percussion, vibration, oscillation, and similar techniques may be helpful to clear the airways during intercurrent URIs when cough is severely impaired or aspiration of saliva is chronic. The airways of patients with bulbar ALS, like those of people with COPD, collapse with the pressures generated by coughing or mechanical exsufflation; thus, inching secretions outward by these methods makes sense. However, a recent review of chest physical therapy concluded that there is no role for routine use in hospitalized patients, that there is little evidence of benefit from percussion and vibration compared with postural drainage alone, and that chest physical therapy is potentially harmful.[997]

People with NMD, however, usually have functional bulbar musculature and normally secretory airways. They just do not have adequate inspiratory and expiratory strength for sufficient cough flows. Thus, instead of overemphasizing the effort-intensive use of chest percussion, such patients primarily need to learn how to normalize cough flows by using inspiratory and expiratory muscle aids. Chest physical therapy should not be used routinely for well children or anyone without excessive airway secretions. Chest clapping also causes hypoxia, and at times supplemental oxygen needs to be administered.

Nasotracheal suctioning, the last resort, is considered for patients with fixed upper or lower airway obstruction but never for patients with predominantly ventilatory impairment who can use MAC effectively. Mucus is suctioned through a catheter passed via the nose or mouth into the trachea or a mainstem bronchus. It is much easier to enter the right than the left mainstem bronchus for anatomic reasons.[1003] During the procedure saline may be instilled through the suction catheter into the trachea to liquefy the mucus. Because of triggering the cough reflex, the instillations may reach only the trachea and, therefore, may not have any liquefying or diluting effect on mucus lower in the airway.[1004] The direct bronchoscopic aspiration of secretions can be preferable to endotracheal or nasotracheal suctioning because the bronchoscope permits visual inspection of the airway and direction of the suction pressure. Once airway secretions are mobilized peripherally, they are ideally eliminated by MAC.

Facilitation of Central Airway Clearance by Providing Functional Coughs by Assisting Expiratory Muscles

Why Are Expiratory Muscle Aids Needed?

Bulbar, inspiratory, and expiratory muscles are needed for effective coughing. The latter are predominantly the abdominal and intercostal muscles (Chapter 9). Clearing airway secretions and airway mucus can be a continual problem for patients with airway diseases, certain lung diseases, and generalized muscle weakness as well as for patients who cannot swallow saliva or food without aspiration. For patients with respiratory muscle dysfunction and functional bulbar musculature it becomes a problem during chest infections, after general anesthesia, and during any other periods of bronchial hypersecretion or excessive aspiration.

Manually Assisted Coughing

The importance of the use of manually assisted coughing to permit effective long-term use of noninvasive ventilation is being increasingly recognized by NMD clinic physicians and others[615,1005] (Fig. 40). CPFs are increased by manually assisted coughing.[910] If the VC is under 1.5 L, insufflating the patient to the MIC is especially important to optimize cough flows.[265] Once the patient takes a breath to at least 1.5 L, maximally air-stacks, or is maximally insufflated, an abdominal thrust is timed to glottic

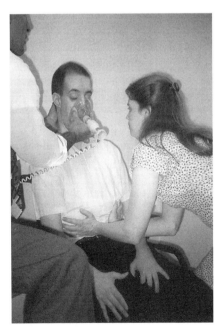

Figure 40. The hands are placed under the ribs for inward and upward abdominal thrusts to manually assist cough and augment cough flows. The patient's assisted cough flow is being measured by peak flow meter.

opening as the patient initiates the cough. It was recognized as early as 1966 that assisted CPF could be doubled and readily exceed 6 L/s in patients receiving maximal insufflations prior to manual thrusts.[1006] In 364 evaluations of our patients with NMD who were able to air-stack, the mean VC in the sitting position was 996.9 ml, the mean MIC was 1647.6 ml, and, even though CPFs were 2.3 L/sec (less than 2.7 L/sec or the minimum needed to eliminate airway secretions), mean assisted CPFs were 3.9 L/sec.

Although an optimal insufflation followed by an abdominal thrust provides the greatest increase in CPF, CPF can also be significantly increased by providing only a maximal insufflation or only an abdominal thrust without a preceding maximal insufflation. Interestingly, CPFs are increased significantly more by the maximal insufflation than by the abdominal thrust. According to data from Ishikawa's center in Hokkaido, 21 patients with DMD had unassisted CPF of 160 ± 88 L/min, CPF of 242 ± 92 L/min with an abdominal thrust, CPF of 274 ± 80 L/min from MIC, and CPF of 356 ± 88 L/min from MIC with an abdominal thrust (assisted CPF) (personal communication). Techniques of manually assisted coughing involve different hand and arm placements for expiratory cycle thrusts (Fig. 40). An epigastric thrust with one hand while the other arm and hand apply counterpressure across the chest to avoid paradoxical chest expansion further increases assisted CPF for 20% of patients.[265]

Manually assisted coughing requires a cooperative patient, good coordination between the patient and caregiver, and adequate physical effort and often frequent application by the caregiver. It is usually ineffective in the presence of severe scoliosis because of a combination of restricted lung capacity and the inability to effect diaphragm movement by abdominal thrusting because of severe rib cage and diaphragm deformity.

Abdominal compressions should not be used aggressively for 1–1.5 hours after a meal; however, chest compressions can be used to augment CPF (Fig. 41). Chest thrusting techniques must be performed with caution in the presence of an osteoporotic rib cage.

Unfortunately, because it is not widely taught to health care professionals,[1007] manually assisted coughing is underutilized.[1008] When cough is inadequate, especially when inadequacy is due to difficulty with air-stacking, the most effective alternative for generating optimal CPF and clearing airway secretions is the use of mechanical insufflation-exsufflation (MI-E).

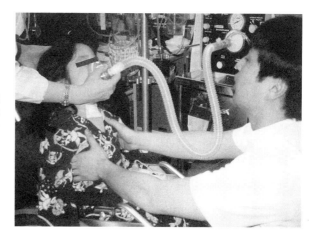

Figure 41. Tussive squeeze applied to the chest during the exsufflation cycle of mechanical insufflation-exsufflation.

The inability to generate over 2.7 L/sec or 160 L/min of assisted CPF despite having a VC or MIC greater than 1 L usually indicates fixed upper airway obstruction or severe bulbar muscle weakness and hypopharyngeal collapse during coughing attempts. Vocal cord adhesions or paralysis may have resulted from a previous translaryngeal intubation or tracheostomy.[708] Because some lesions, especially obstructing granulation tissue, can be corrected surgically, laryngoscopic examination is warranted.

Sir Patrick: Don't misunderstand me, my boy, I'm not belittling your discovery. Most discoveries are made regularly every fifteen years; and it's fully a hundred and fifty since yours was made last. That's something to be proud of...

••☞• George Bernard Shaw, *The Doctor's Dilemma*

Mechanical Insufflation-Exsufflation

Introduction of MI-E

Mechanical insufflator-exsufflators (Cough-Assists) deliver deep insufflations followed immediately by deep exsufflations (Fig. 42). The insufflation and exsufflation pressures and delivery times are independently adjustable. Insufflation to exsufflation pressures of +40 to –40 cmH_2O delivered via oronasal interface or normal adult tracheostomy tubes are usually the most effective and preferred by most patients. Lungs are insufflated until fully expanded and then immediately exsufflated until the lungs are fully emptied and the chest wall retracted. Normal cough and exsufflation volumes exceed 2 liters in adults.

Mechanical insufflation generates two flow notches. Onset of insufflation generates a flow peak (see Fig. 42). A second insufflation flow notch occurs when exsufflation terminates and is due to the reversal of air flow as air re-enters the lung and the lung volume returns to its functional residual capacity. Mechanical exsufflation also generates two (exsufflation) flow notches. One occurs when the insufflation pressure stops and is due to the elastic recoil of the lung. The second notch, a bit greater, is caused by the exsufflation pressure itself. Except after a meal, an abdominal thrust is applied in conjunction with the exsufflation. The combination of MI-E with an abdominal thrust is a mechanically assisted cough (MAC). MI-E can be provided via an oral-nasal mask, a simple mouthpiece, or a translaryngeal or tracheostomy tube. When delivered via a tracheostomy tube, the cuff, if present, should be inflated.

The Cough-Assist can be manually or automatically cycled. Manual cycling facilitates caregiver-patient coordination of inspiration and expiration with insufflation and exsufflation, respectively, but it requires hands to deliver an abdominal thrust, to hold the mask on the patient, and to cycle the machine. Although the Cough-Assist is currently the only commercially available device that performs MI-E, it is possible to devise less expensive systems. One such system devised in Israel is essentially a double cylinder valve mechanism simultaneously connecting a vacuum cleaner and a manual resuscitator to a face mask. A simple sliding mechanism operated by the caregiver or patient shifts between the vacuum cleaner and manual resuscitator (Eliezer Be'eri, Jerusalem).

One treatment consists of about five cycles of MI-E or MAC followed by a short period of normal breathing or ventilator use to avoid hyperventilation. Although insufflation and exsufflation pressures when used via the upper airway almost always range

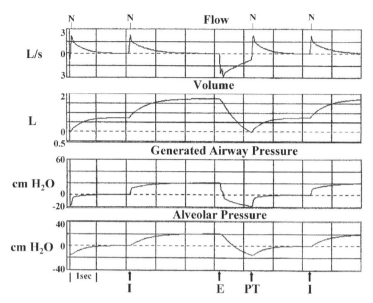

Figure 42. Pressure, volume, and flow relationships of mechanical insufflation-exsufflation for insufflation to exsufflation pressures of 20 to –20 cmH$_2$O, insufflation time 3 seconds, exsufflation time 1 second, pause time 2 seconds. I denotes onset of insufflation, E denotes onset of exsufflation, and PT denotes onset of pause between insufflation and exsufflation. N denotes flow notch.

from +35 to +60 cmH$_2$O to –35 to –60 cmH$_2$O, it must be kept in mind that the goal is rapid maximal chest expansion followed immediately by rapid lung emptying, both in about 1–3 seconds. The machine pressures required for this technique depend on the caliber of the interface between the machine tubing and the airways. Thus, the use of MI-E via narrow-gauge tubes may necessitate the application of pressures up to 70 cmH$_2$O (Chapter 12) until the endpoints are clinically observed. Most patients use pressures of 35–45 cmH$_2$O for insufflations and exsufflations via the upper airway or via wide-gauge, adult-sized tracheostomy or translaryngeal tubes. In experimental models, +40 to –40 cmH$_2$O pressures have been shown to provide maximum forced deflation VCs and flows.[1009] In a recent study in a lung model with normal human compliance, insufflation volumes exceeded 90% of predicted inspiratory capacity when insufflation times were over 5 seconds. In reality, because of lung inertial factors, pressures of 40 cmH$_2$O (via an interface with adequate caliber) can take a full minute to inflate lung tissues fully.[899]

When MI-E is used for airway secretion clearance, multiple treatments are given in one sitting until no further secretions are expulsed and any secretion- or mucus-induced dSpO$_2$s are reversed. Use can be required as frequently as every few minutes around the clock during severe chest infections. Although no medications are usually required for effective MI-E in neuromuscular ventilator users, liquefaction of sputum using heated aerosol treatments may facilitate mucus elimination when secretions are inspissated.

We routinely use MI-E via oronasal interfaces (especially in the immediate post-extubation period for respiratory failure) or via translaryngeal and tracheostomy tubes in children with SMA under 1 year of age. For infants and others who use MI-E via narrow-gauge pediatric tubes, even the maximum flow-pressure capabilities of the Cough-Assist are often inadequate to rapidly expand and empty the lungs. The severe pressure-flow drop-off across the narrow tubes greatly diminishes the efficacy of MI-E for expulsing airway secretions; more powerful units need to be developed. In addition to use for assisted coughing, the importance of using the Cough-Assist for the regular provision of full chest expansion for patients ineffective at air-stacking should not be underestimated.

A recent study measured flow-pressure relationships through endotracheal and tracheostomy tubes of various diameters.[1010] Although only positive pressures were used, drop-offs in pressures and flows with tube narrowing are comparable whether positive or negative pressures are used. Flows up to 200 L/min, only one-third of the maximum flows emanating from the Cough-Assist, were measured. Providing air pressure of 40 cmH$_2$O through a tracheostomy tube of 8.5-mm diameter resulted in flows of 170 L/min, whereas the same pressure via a 4.5-mm tube (size of a minitracheostomy tube, 0.5 mm smaller than a small adult tube) resulted in a flow of only about 65 L/min. The same 40-cmH$_2$O pressure via an 8.5-mm endotracheal tube achieved a flow of 200 L/min, whereas the resulting flow via a 5-mm tube was only 70 L/min and via a 4.5-mm tube only 55 L/min. Because infant tubes are even narrower, drop-offs would be even greater. In another study of pressure-volume relationships through variously sized tracheostomy tubes using a lung model, alveolar pressures and ventilated volumes via 4-, 4.5-, and 5-mm tubes were about 40%, 50%, and 60%, respectively, of the values via 8-mm endotracheal tubes in the absence of leakage. To obtain an insufflated volume of 500 ml, the inspiratory pressures needed were 40, 30, and 20 cmH$_2$O, respectively, for the 4-, 4.5-, and 5-mm tubes.[1011]

Whether via the upper airway or via indwelling airway tubes, routine airway suctioning misses the left mainstem bronchus about 90% of the time. MI-E, on the other hand, provides the same exsufflation flows in both left and right airways without the discomfort or airway trauma of tracheal suctioning—and it can be effective when suctioning is not (see Case 14, Chapter 15, of reference 1113). Patients almost invariably prefer MI-E to suctioning for comfort and effectiveness and find it less tiring.[1012] Deep suctioning, whether via airway tube or via the upper airway, can be discontinued for most patients with NMD.

Physiologic Effects of MI-E

Peripheral venous pressures as measured in the anterior cubital vein are slightly raised—that is, by 5.8 cmH$_2$O—during exsufflation. This is about one-third the increase seen during normal coughing. Blood pressure is increased by an average of 8 mmHg in systole and 4 mmHg in diastole. The pulse can increase or decrease during MI-E, and EKG changes reflect the rotation of the heart at peak inspiratory volumes. The increase in intragastric pressure is 26 mmHg during MI-E and 85 mmHg during normal coughing.[1013] With hyperinflation only, falls in cardiac output correlate with increases in tidal volume but not with increases in peak inspiratory pressure, and cardiac output can take up to 15 minutes to recover to baseline values.[1014] Physiologic effects of MI-E have been studied in depth and reported elsewhere.[1015,1016]

Indications for MI-E

Because MI-E has been on the market only since February of 1993, misinformation and confusion about its indications are still common. Of the three muscle groups required for effective coughing, MI-E can take the place only of the inspiratory and expiratory muscles. Thus, it cannot be used to avert tracheostomy for very long if bulbar function is inadequate to prevent airway collapse, as is often the case in advanced bulbar ALS. On the other hand, patients with completely intact bulbar muscle function, such as most ventilator users with traumatic tetraplegia, can usually air-stack to volumes of 3 liters or more, and, unless they are severely scoliotic or obese, a properly delivered abdominal thrust can often result in assisted CPF of 6–9 L/sec. Such flows should be more than adequate to clear the airways and prevent pneumonia and respiratory failure without need for MI-E. Thus, the patients who need MI-E the most are those whose bulbar muscle function can maintain adequate airway patency but is insufficient to permit optimal air-stacking for assisted CPF over 250–300 L/min. This scenario eventually occurs for most patients with NMD except for some with no measurable CPF due to bulbar ALS/MND. The most typical examples of patients who can consistently avoid hospitalization and respiratory failure by using MI-E during intercurrent chest infections are those with DMD and SMA. Patients with respiratory muscle weakness complicated by scoliosis and inability to manually displace the asymmetric diaphragm by abdominal thrusting also greatly benefit from MI-E. A recent study of 21 patients with SMA, DMD, post-polio syndrome, and congenital muscular dystrophy confirmed an earlier study[265] that demonstrated a significantly greater increase in cough flows by MI-E by comparison with unassisted coughing, manually assisted coughing, coughing after chest physiotherapy, or use of noninvasive IPPV alone.[1017] Its use in pediatrics is reviewed in Chapter 12.

Efficacy of MI-E

The efficacy of MI-E was demonstrated both clinically and in animal models.[1018] Flow generation can be adequate in both proximal and distal airways to effectively eliminate respiratory tract debris.[837,1019] VC, pulmonary flow rates, and SpO_2 (when abnormal) improve immediately with clearing of airway mucus and other debris by MI-E.[655,1000] An increase in VC of 15–42% was noted immediately after treatment in 67 patients with "obstructive dyspnea," and a 55% increase in VC was noted after MI-E in patients with NMDs.[1020] We have observed improvements ranging from 15% to 400% (200–800 ml) in VC and normalization of SpO_2 as MI-E eliminates airway mucus for ventilator-assisted NMD patients during chest infections.[265]

Significant increases in CPF were also demonstrated by use of MI-E in patients with poliomyelitis, bronchiectasis, asthma, and pulmonary emphysema.[1021] After instillation of a mucin-thorium dioxide suspension into the lungs of anesthetized dogs, bronchograms revealed virtually complete elimination of the suspension after 6 minutes of MI-E.[1018] The technique was shown to be equally effective in expelling bronchoscopically inserted foreign bodies.[1018] The use of MI-E through an indwelling tracheostomy tube was demonstrated to be effective in reversing acute atelectasis associated with productive airway secretions;[1022] however, CPFs were noted to be greater when MI-E was applied via a mask.[1023] Barach and Beck demonstrated clinical and radiographic improvement in 92 of 103 patients with upper respiratory infections with the use of MI-E.[1020] The group included 72 patients with bronchopulmonary disease and 27 with skeletal or neuromuscular conditions, including poliomyelitis.[1022] It was more effective for the latter than for the former.[1020]

MI-E has been noted to be effective in the elimination of tenacious sputum before bronchography and of contrast medium after bronchography in patients with bronchial asthma and bronchiectasis. It also has been suggested that MI-E may improve the results of bronchoscopy.[1020] Williams and Holaday reported that MI-E can effectively eliminate airway secretions and ventilate patients in the minutes following generalized anesthesia.[1024] They applied MI-E to both cooperative and unconscious patients and reported normalization of blood gases in all seven patients studied, including two with advanced pulmonary emphysema. In addition, improved breath sounds, increased percussion resonance, reduced respiratory rate, clearing of cyanosis, and reversal of right lower lobe collapse were reported for particular patients as a direct result of MI-E. Recent studies have reported that it was not only more effective by comparison with tracheal suctioning and chest physical therapy but also more comfortable and less expensive.[1012,1025,1026] In a group of 18 patients with spinal cord injury, its use made "the biggest impact on improving pulmonary status...and decreasing length of stay despite significant pulmonary problems on admission."[1026]

The use of MAC has consistently permitted us to extubate patients with NMD after general anesthesia despite their lack of any breathing tolerance and to manage them with noninvasive IPPV. It has also permitted us to avoid intubation or to quickly extubate patients with NMD in acute ventilatory failure with no breathing tolerance and profuse airway secretions due to intercurrent chest infections. The use of MAC in a protocol with oximetry feedback and home use of noninvasive IPPV effectively decreased hospitalizations and respiratory complications and mortality for patients with NMD[655] (Chapter 11). It may not be effective if the patient cannot cooperate sufficiently to keep the airway open or has a fixed upper or lower airway obstruction or collapsible airways upon exsufflation, such as occurs when assisted CPF in adults cannot exceed 160 L/min.[1027]

Safety of MI-E

Colebatch observed that applying negative pressure of 40–50 cmH$_2$O is unlikely to have any deleterious effects on pulmonary tissues.[1028] He noted that, because the negative pressure applied to the airways is analogous to positive pressure on the surface of the lungs during a normal cough, it is improbable that this negative pressure can be more detrimental to the lungs than the normal cough pressure gradient. Furthermore, because FEV$_1$ has been reported only to increase after MI-E, no sustained airway obstruction is caused by the exsufflation cycle of MI-E.[265] Bickerman found no evidence of parenchymal damage, hemorrhage, alveolar tears, or emphysematous blebs in the lungs of animals treated with MI-E.[1018] Barach and Beck reported no serious complications in 103 patients treated with over 2000 courses of MI-E, and for no patient did MI-E have to be discontinued.[1020] They noted that the initial transient appearance of blood-streaked sputum in a few patients probably originated from the bronchial wall sites of detachment of mucus plugs. Immediately after the initial elimination of blood-streaked sputum, the profuse outpouring of mucopurulent sputum indicated that "obstruction of the atelectatic area had been relieved." In one study, one of 19 patients complained of transient nausea associated with the initiation of MI-E. This symptom resolved with continued use.[1029] Patients with wounds of the abdomen or chest reported less wound pain during MI-E than during spontaneous coughing. No incidence of aspiration of gastric contents has been found either in humans[1024] or in anesthetized dogs.[1018] No reports of damaging side effects have been disclosed in more than 6000 treatments in over 400 patients using MI-E, most of whom had primarily lung disease.[1028,1030] There continue to be no publications contradicting the reports of effectiveness or describing significant complications of MI-E. Even when used after abdominal surgery and extensive chest wall surgery, no disruption of recently sutured wounds was noted.[1024]

We, too, have observed no serious complications of MI-E in thousands of applications for hundreds of patients with NMDs and other conditions, many of whom had regularly used MI-E for over 50 years either with the Cof-flators available since 1952 or with the In-exsufflators that came onto the market in February 1993. Interestingly, before 1993, patients unable to procure Cof-flators often air-stacked and then used vacuum cleaners for exsufflation. We have a number of patients who have depended on continuous noninvasive IPPV at inspiratory positive airway pressures of over 40 cmH_2O for over 45 years. Thus, the use of equivalent pressures for brief periods of MI-E are unlikely to cause any harm. A recent study using these pressures on baby monkeys also demonstrated no barotrauma.[1009] Borborygmus and abdominal distention are infrequent and can be eliminated by decreasing insufflation (not exsufflation) pressures.

As with tracheal suctioning, MI-E can be associated with bradycardias for patients with spinal cord injury in spinal shock and for occasional infants with SMA. Insufflation and exsufflation pressures are increased gradually for such patients. Premedication with anticholinergics can be helpful.

The use of high insufflation pressures can cause acute rib cage muscle pulls for patients with low VCs, especially those with severe scoliosis who have not routinely been air-stacking or receiving maximal insufflations. Insufflation pressures are increased gradually for such patients. Relative contraindications for the use of MI-E are listed in Table 3. We have used MI-E for many patients in CHF with pulmonary edema without untoward consequences.

Other Techniques That Assist Respiratory Muscle Effort

For patients with paralyzed abdominal musculature and relatively good diaphragm function, such as some patients with spinal cord injury or SMA, a thoracoabdominal corset limits the increase in FRC that occurs when the patient assumes the upright position. The resulting mild increase in VC can increase CPF in this position. The binder can also help to maintain blood pressure and trunk stability,[1006] decrease the subjective effort of breathing, relieve accessory neck and upper intercostal muscle use, decrease the respiratory rate, and increase tidal air with a lowering of the total pulmonary ventilation for patients with spinal cord injury and some patients with NMD or pulmonary emphysema.[1022]

A 4-inch wide abdominal belt with hand grips or handles has been designed as a postoperative coughing aid.[1031] When the patient needs to cough, he or she passes one handle through the other and pulls with both hands. This maneuver instantaneously applies pressure to the abdomen and facilitates a pain-free cough.

Glossopharyngeal Breathing

Both inspiratory and, indirectly, expiratory muscle function can be assisted by GPB.[792] GPB can safely provide a patient with weak inspiratory muscles and no VC or breathing tolerance with normal alveolar ventilation when a ventilator is not being used or in the event of sudden ventilator failure during the day or night.[792,917] The technique involves the use of the glottis to add to an inspiratory effort by projecting (gulping) boluses of air into the lungs. The glottis closes with each "gulp." One breath usually consists of 6–9 gulps of 40–200 ml each (Fig. 43). During the training period the efficiency of GPB can be monitored by spirometrically measuring the milliliters of air per gulp, gulps per breath, and breaths per minute. A training manual[1032] (Fig. 44) and numerous videos are available,[1033] the most detailed of which was produced in 1999.[1034]

Although severe oropharyngeal muscle weakness can limit the usefulness of GPB, Baydur et al.[727] reported two DMD ventilator users who were very successful using it. We have managed 11 ventilator users with DMD who had no breathing tolerance other than by GPB. Approximately 60% of ventilator users with no autonomous ability to breathe and good bulbar muscle function[917,918] can use GPB for autonomous breathing for periods ranging from minutes to all day. For those who cannot, it is usually because of inability to use the soft palate to seal off the nose. Although potentially extremely useful, GPB is rarely taught because few health care professionals are familiar with the technique. GPB is also rarely useful in the presence of an indwelling tracheostomy tube. It cannot be used when the tube is uncapped, as it is during tracheostomy IPPV; even when the tube is capped, the gulped air tends to leak around the outer walls of the tube and out the stoma as airway volumes and pressures increase during the GPB air-stacking process. The safety and versatility afforded by GPB are key reasons to eliminate tracheostomy in favor of noninvasive aids (Table 4).

Conclusion

Mechanisms by which nasal or mouthpiece/lipseal IPPV can improve the clinical picture include the following:

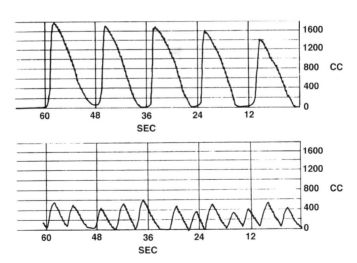

Figure 43. Top, Maximal GPB minute ventilation of 8.39 L/min. GPB inspirations average 1.67 L, 20 gulps, and 84 ml/gulp for each breath in a patient with no measurable vital capacity. Bottom, Same patient with regular GPB minute ventilation of 4.76 L/min, 12.5 breaths, average 8 gulps per breath, 47.5 ml/gulp performed over a 1-minute period. (Courtesy of the March of Dimes.)

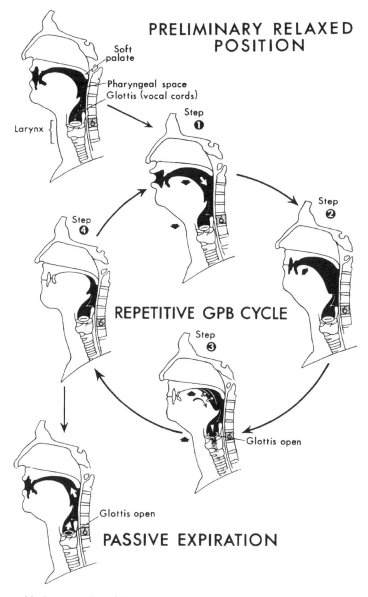

Figure 44. Demonstration of glossopharyngeal breathing from classic training manual.[1032]

- Resting respiratory muscles and decreasing metabolic demand
- Increasing tidal volumes and relieving hypercapnia
- Resetting chemoreceptors
- Opening atelectatic areas
- Maintaining airway patency
- Improving ventilation/perfusion matching
- Maintaining lung and chest wall range of motion and possibly compliance

Table 4.	**Uses of Glossopharyngeal Breathing**
Back-up in the event of ventilator failure when awake or asleep	
Ventilator-free breathing tolerance when awake	
Ventilatory support when transferring between methods of noninvasive ventilation	
To improve cough effectiveness	
To increase speech volume or shout	
To normalize speech rhythm	
To improve or maintain pulmonary compliance	
To prevent microatelectasis	

■ Improving mucociliary clearance

■ Most importantly, assisting, supporting, and substituting for inspiratory muscle function

Assisted lung ventilation and normal SpO_2 can be maintained indefinitely during sleep as well as during daytime hours for patients with little or no VC by using noninvasive IPPV (Chapter 11). Expiratory muscle aids such as MI-E permit patients to continue to use noninvasive ventilation despite intercurrent chest infections.

The Battle

by Jamys Moriarty (8/9/95)

Today I celebrate a victory, the joyous existence of life.
　For only four weeks ago, my body was burdened in strife.
It happened unexpectedly, and much to my chagrin;
　I was bitten by the Flu bug, and the battle did begin.
My lymphocytes assembled to bolster a strong defense;
　On the battlefield within lungs, the combat grew intense.
An army of antibiotics dispersed with a trumpeting call;
　Unrelenting were the invaders, affixed to my bronchial wall.
My chest muscle mechanics tried to expectorate those bugs;
　Still, germs swarmed my airways, building dams of mucus plugs!
Then I recalled reading in Quest, of Physiatrist John Bach;
　His creative understanding make him a most inventive Doc!
He's pioneered ventilation with a noninvasive technique,
　And re-established a coughing machine: The In-Exsufflator unique!
Now the battle still stormed, and my lungs began to tire.
　I had to take some action, as it was difficult to respire.
A trip to the hospital, was a journey I wanted to resist,
　Hence I dialed up Emerson, to ask if they'd assist.
It was to my advantage - a most fortunate quirk;
　That the person I spoke with was New England Rep. Kirk.
As a Respiratory Therapist, he knew I was in vital need;
　So he brought down the In-Exsufflator to me top speed!
The machine was a Wonder, I could cough and expel!
　My lungs breathed deeply as the virus bid fare-well!

Today I celebrate good health and pause for reflection,
    Many thanks to all who helped me Evict that infection!
        Conclusion
        No Need to fear.
        Should a virus adhere.
        My lungs will stay clear.
        With the In-Exsufflator near.

Dicen que hacerse poeta es enfermedad incurable y contagiosa.
They say that being a poet is a contagious and incurable disease.

                             La Sobrina de Quijote

Respiratory Muscle Aids: Patient Evaluation, Respiratory Aid Protocol, and Outcomes

Lorsque les chiens aboient, nous comprenons que nous allons au galop.
When the dogs bark, you know you're on your way.

Gustav Mahler, *Briefe*

Evaluation of Respiratory Muscle Dysfunction

The patient evaluation includes a survey for symptoms of chronic alveolar hypoventilation (see Table 1 of Chapter 8), physical examination, manual muscle testing, and four painless and simple pulmonary tests. Although severe diaphragm weakness and loss of the ability to breathe can occur without extremity weakness, Nathanson et al. reported that proximal upper limb weakness is a significant predictor of respiratory muscle dysfunction for patients with Charcot-Marie-Tooth disease.[1035] We have found this to be the case for patients with other NMDs as well.

The patient is also observed for paradoxical breathing and accessory respiratory muscle use. Lung auscultation, end-tidal carbon dioxide, oximetry, spirometry, and cough peak flow (CPF) are generally evaluated in this order. This order can be important because air-stacking and measurements of assisted CPF can hyperventilate the patient and render end-tidal carbon dioxide and oximetry measurement less accurate.

End-tidal carbon dioxide has been shown to be highly accurate and to correlate with lung underventilation, cardiac output, and lung perfusion pressures. It also correlates closely with $PaCO_2$ (r = 0.94–0.98) except in patients with severe concomitant lung or vascular disease with congestive heart failure (CHF) or impaired lung diffusion or perfusion.[1036,1037] End-tidal carbon dioxide approximates $PaCO_2$ when excessive physiologic dead space is not present.[1038] A recent decrease in end-tidal carbon dioxide without introduction of ventilator use often signals asymptomatic CHF and an early shock state. Measurements of end-tidal carbon dioxide are more accurate during full expiratory maneuvers than during tidal expiration. We always have patients exhale completely from deep breaths several times to see if this maneuver will increase end-tidal carbon dioxide readings or decrease them as a result of hyperventilation[1039] (Fig. 1). We record the maximum observed value.

For patients using nasal or mouthpiece IPPV, end-tidal carbon dioxide is measured via the hole normally used to monitor airway pressures in 15-mm tube adapters connected

271

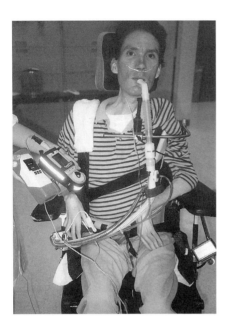

Figure 1. Measurement of end-tidal carbon dioxide with sensor at the nose and oxyhemoglobin saturation with pick-up electrode on the thumb for 24-hour noninvasive ventilation user.

between the mouthpiece/nasal interface and the ventilator tubing. Mouthpiece IPPV users can also be asked to exhale via the nose, and end-tidal carbon dioxide is measured at the nostrils as usual. The pick-up can also be slipped under triangular nasal interfaces for measurements of end-tidal carbon dioxide. For patients using tracheostomy IPPV, end-tidal carbon dioxide is measured at the hole of the 15-mm adapter between the tube and ventilator circuit, whereas it is measured via the tube opening as unaided patients breathe via open tubes.

SpO_2 is accurate to within 2% of arterial blood oxyhemoglobin saturation (SaO_2). It can be normal despite end-tidal carbon dioxide levels in the low 60s. However, once hypercapnia causes diurnal SpO_2 to decrease below 95%, patients tend to develop obvious symptoms of alveolar hypoventilation. If the SpO_2 baseline is found to be below 95%, the patient is asked to increase breathing effort. If this effort normalizes SpO_2, then the low baseline SpO_2 is likely to be entirely due to underventilation. If the patient is not strong enough to autonomously normalize alveolar ventilation and SpO_2 on his or her own, mouthpiece or nasal IPPV is used as needed to do so. When increasing and normalizing alveolar ventilation in this manner does not normalize SpO_2, severe ventilation-perfusion mismatching is present (Chapter 9).

Information about blood acid-base balance, if desired, can be obtained from a simple and less painful (than arterial) venous blood sampling of chloride and bicarbonate levels. Elevation of the latter indicates severe chronic hypercapnia and impending ventilatory failure, which, if not prevented by using assisted ventilation, often results in death within 5 months.[1040] We rarely need to resort to sampling arterial blood gases in the respiratory management of our patients.

A spirometer is used to measure vital capacity (VC) in sitting, recumbent, and side-lying positions and with a thoracolumbar brace on and off, when applicable. A well-constructed thoracolumbar brace can increase VC for scoliotic patients, whereas a

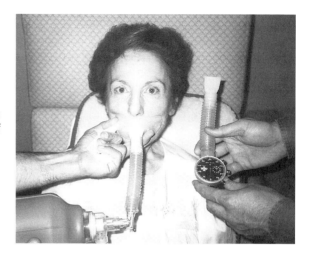

Figure 2. Patient air-stacking via lipseal for spirometric measurement of maximum insufflation capacity.

poorly prepared or poorly fitting one can decrease VC and impair breathing. The spirometer is also used to measure the MIC for patients with VCs less than predicted normal levels. Usually a manual resuscitator is used for the patient to air-stack (Chapter 10) via a mouthpiece for the MIC measurements. If the lips are too weak or the soft palate incompetent to seal off the nasopharynx and the patient cannot air-stack optimally via a mouthpiece, the patient air-stacks via a lipseal pressed against the lips (Fig. 2) or a nasal interface (Fig. 3). Many patients can air-stack beyond their MICs by glossopharyngeal breathing (GPB). Sometimes pinching the nostrils is necessary to permit maximum insufflation. An oronasal interface can also be used for patients with very weak buccal muscles, but MIC measurement may need to be done from volumes exhaled at the expiratory valve on the interface tubing without removing the interface.

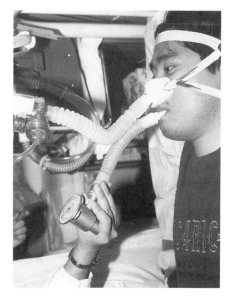

Figure 3. Patient air-stacking via nasal interface for spirometric measurement of maximum insufflation capacity.

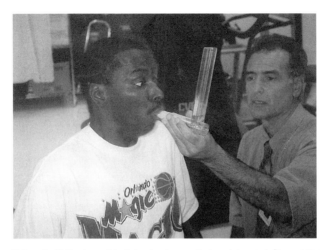

Figure 4. Patient coughing via simple mouthpiece into peak flow meter.

Sometimes patients can air-stack but not retain the volumes for accurate measurement because of buccal muscle insufficiency. Patients who cannot air-stack can still have maximal lung insufflation volumes delivered and measured via oronasal mask.

Unassisted CPF is measured by having the patient cough as hard as possible into a peak flow meter (Fig. 4). The CPF is then measured with the patient coughing from a maximally air-stacked volume (the MIC). If the patient's lips are too weak to firmly grab a mouthpiece or the soft palate is incompetent to prevent leakage from the nose, either the nose can be pinched for measurements via the mouth or the patient coughs via an oronasal interface (Fig. 5). Finally, fully assisted CPF is measured from the MIC with an abdominal thrust timed to glottic opening.[910] This is the most important CPF measurement because it is the manually assisted cough that the patient must often use to clear airway secretions to avoid respiratory failure and it is the best correlate of bulbar muscle

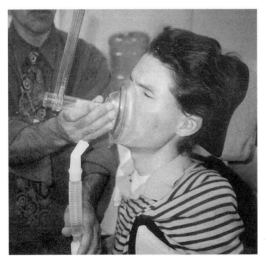

Figure 5. Patient with an incompetent soft palate who, after air-stacking to maximum insufflation, must cough via an oronasal interface into the peak flow meter. Concurrent abdominal thrust timed to cough permits the measurement of assisted cough peak flows.

function. It should be kept in mind that patients unable to close the glottis cannot cough but can have peak expiratory flow (PEF) increased by abdominal thrusting.

If the VC is at least 30% more in the sitting than in the supine position, symptoms of sleep-disordered breathing or chronic alveolar hypoventilation are present, the patient has dyspnea when supine, or daytime end-tidal carbon dioxide is greater than 45 mmHg, severe nocturnal hypoventilation is a strong possibility. In such cases, nocturnal SpO_2 and end-tidal carbon dioxide monitoring are performed. An Ohmeda oximeter (Louisville, KY) collates data by the hour and for the entire night and provides hourly means; percentages of time that the SpO_2 is less than 90%, 85%, 80%, and 70%; and hourly lows. Normal mean nocturnal SpO_2 is 96.5%,[670] and maximum end-tidal carbon dioxide should not exceed 47–50 mmHg. Quantifiable SpO_2 and end-tidal carbon dioxide data can be used to demonstrate objectively the need for nocturnal noninvasive IPPV and ameliorations with treatment. If the patient is symptomatic but has essentially normal VC and normal values for SpO_2 and end-tidal carbon dioxide both during the day and at night, polysomnography is used to evaluate for sleep-disordered breathing.

Besides SpO_2, oximetry also provides information about heart rate and, therefore, about the success of the use of certain cardiac medications, such as beta blockers. The pulse waveform also correlates significantly with systolic pressures and can be a sensitive indicator of hypovolemia.[1041] For patients susceptible to bradycardias, the oximeter indicates whether the bradycardias are primary and precede desaturation or whether they result from respiratory embarrassment, such as airway mucus plugging, that causes desaturation before bradycardia (Chapter 5).

Introduction of Respiratory Muscle Aids and Monitoring for Adolescents and Adults

Air-stacking, maximal insufflations, noninvasive ventilation, and assisted coughing are ideally introduced in the outpatient setting.[1042] Mouthpiece and nasal interfaces are introduced with the patient in any comfortable position. A variety of nasal and mouthpiece/lipseal interfaces and headgear can be tried and individually adapted (Chapter 10). Since all interface air leakage need not be eliminated and comfort and avoidance of excessive skin pressure are important, the straps need not be tightly applied unless ventilation pressures must be high (greater than 30 cmH_2O) because of poor lung compliance. If no ventilator is conveniently available, the interfaces and headgear can be tried, using a manual resuscitator. One or more interfaces are selected on the basis of fit, comfort, seal around the nostrils or mouth, and hours of daily use. Because we have found mouthpiece and nasal interfaces to be effective other than for patients with advanced bulbar incompetence, we have rarely used oronasal interfaces.

For hospitalized patients being switched from intubation to noninvasive ventilation using ventilators with expiratory volume alarms, the alarms can be set at the minimum of 10 ml; however, they will still sound during interface trials and noninvasive IPPV. Such patients must usually be switched to portable ventilators without expiratory volume alarms when noninvasive ventilation is attempted.

Selection of the ventilator is relatively easy. Volume-cycled ventilators are used for all patients except for the rare patient with recent or frequent history of barotrauma, patients whose MICs cannot exceed VCs because of glottic incompetence, and patients who are too small to cooperate with air-stacking. Patients need volume-cycled ventilators to air-stack to maximum insufflations independently as well as for eventual daytime IPPV. It is tempting to set delivered volumes according to some formula. However, because noninvasive ventilation is an open system and patients can take as much of the delivered air as they want, we generally initiate IPPV at the relatively high volumes of 600–1000 ml before quickly raising them to more effective levels of 800–1500 ml (see Mouthpiece IPPV in Chapter 7). Frequent sighs or air-stacking is also promoted.

Some patients may continue to use high-span bilevel PAP overnight and reserve volume-cycled ventilators for daytime use. When bilevel PAP is used, high spans with IPAP from 10 to 15 cmH_2O and EPAP of 2 cmH_2O are used initially. The IPAPs are increased to 15–20 cmH_2O or more as needed to maintain normal end-tidal carbon dioxide and provide more rest to inspiratory musculature during sleep. EPAPs are left at the minimum unless the patient has chronic obstructive pulmonary disease (COPD) and auto-PEEP or is being treated for documented obstructive sleep apneas. For patients without volume-cycled ventilators who use only nocturnal high-span bilevel PAP, air-stacking can be provided by manual resuscitators, or regular maximal insufflations can be provided by the Cough-Assist (J. H. Emerson Co., Cambridge, MA).

The first signs of successful use of noninvasive ventilation are decreased respiratory rate and accessory respiratory muscle use, increased chest expansion, triggering and breathing in synchrony with pressure-cycled ventilators or ventilator gauge pressures of 18–25 cmH_2O, normalization of end-tidal carbon dioxide and SpO_2, and relief of dyspnea and other symptoms. Because the initial primary goal is to rest respiratory muscles, whether pressure- or volume-cycled ventilators are used, lung insufflation volumes compatible with ventilatory support are used.

Supplemental oxygen is avoided for patients with primarily ventilatory impairment but may be beneficial for patients with lung disease or bulbar ALS whose SpO_2s cannot be normalized by improving alveolar ventilation and assisted coughing. Humidification must be considered (Chapter 12). Air leaks, interface retention, and strap tension are monitored periodically. Sedation is avoided or, at least, minimized. Noninvasive IPPV efficacy can be monitored when the patient is awake or asleep by end-tidal carbon dioxide, oximetry, observing ventilator gauge pressures, and monitoring expiratory volumes by attaching a spirometer to the expiratory valve when volume-cycled ventilation is used. Blood gas monitoring is unnecessary except to correlate end-tidal carbon dioxide with $PaCO_2$ for patients with primarily respiratory impairment who require supplemental oxygen or patients with suspected CHF.

For patients with chronic daytime as well as nocturnal hypercapnia and $dSpO_2$ who have not been using ventilatory support, introduction to and use of mouthpiece or nasal IPPV can be facilitated by oximetry feedback. Oximetry feedback serves as a guide to indicate how much noninvasive IPPV is required per day. Patients are instructed to normalize SpO_2 or end-tidal carbon dioxide by autonomously increasing lung ventilation—something they quickly find fatiguing. They are then taught to take mouthpiece-assisted breaths as necessary to normalize and maintain normal SpO_2. Initially, an oximetry alarm can be set to 94% to remind the patient to take assisted breaths (Fig. 6). The patient sees that taking slightly deeper or assisted breaths increases the SpO_2 above 94% within seconds. After a few weeks of maintaining normal SpO_2 by assisted ventilation more or less around the clock, the reversal of compensatory metabolic alkalosis, normalization of

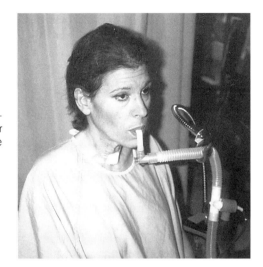

Figure 6. After decannulation this 24-hour ventilator-dependent hypercapnic patient with muscular dystrophy used oximetry as feedback to normalize alveolar ventilation with mouthpiece IPPV.

ventilatory drive, and respiratory muscle rest often result in the patient's ability to maintain normal SpO_2 and ventilation for most of, if not all of, the day without daytime assisted breathing. Over the passage of years, however, noninvasive IPPV use becomes continuous once again as autonomous breathing ability is lost with advancing weakness and age. The restoration of central ventilatory drive and normalization of daytime blood gases essentially guarantee the effectiveness of noninvasive IPPV during sleep (Chapter 10).

Once the maximum assisted CPF decrease below 270 L/min or 4.5 L/sec, risk of pneumonia is high during episodes of airway encumberment (Chapter 9), and the patient is trained in MAC. At this time, young or rapidly weakening patients are also prescribed an oximeter for home use and rapid access to MI-E and a portable volume ventilator to use during chest infections (if it is not already in daily use).[655] If the patient is told simply to call the physician when a cold develops to be equipped at that time, he or she often waits too long. The SpO_2 baseline will have often decreased below 80%, the VC may have decreased by 50–80% from baseline, and pneumonia may already be present. In this case there is often no recourse but hospitalization and translaryngeal intubation. For these reasons, an oximeter, along with a manual resuscitator for air-stacking, is prescribed when cough flows decrease. Thus, the patient and care providers are taught the outpatient oximetry feedback protocol (see below) before respiratory failure can develop.

A symptomatic patient with abnormal sleep SpO_2 (mean less than 96.5%) or elevated end-tidal carbon dioxide undergoes a trial of nocturnal noninvasive IPPV. Multiple episodes per hour of $dSpO_2$ of 4% or more and prolonged periods of SpO_2 less than 95% during sleep are often associated with symptomatic nocturnal hypoventilation. Once trying nocturnal noninvasive IPPV, patients often feel relief of fatigue and other symptoms that they did not know they had. The nocturnal oximetry and end-tidal carbon dioxide monitoring can be repeated with the patient using noninvasive IPPV. Typically, nocturnal SpO_2 means increase from lower levels to 94–95% with treatment. Often withdrawing nocturnal noninvasive IPPV from such patients results in nightly decreases in mean nocturnal SpO_2, increases in daytime symptoms, and worsening in blood gases[768,946] until nocturnal noninvasive IPPV is re-instituted or the patient stops breathing. If noninvasive IPPV leads to no improvement in symptoms or mean nocturnal SpO_2, no evidence indicates that benefit is derived from its nocturnal use.

Clinicians often fail to appreciate how and why noninvasive ventilation can be effective during sleep in the absence of any respiratory muscle function. Such clinicians are often tempted to monitor the efficacy of noninvasive IPPV by regular blood gas analyses, nocturnal end-tidal or transcutaneous carbon dioxide monitoring, chest radiographs, traditional pulmonary function analyses, measurements of minute ventilation during IPPV, and serial polysomnographs. However, because the efficacy of noninvasive IPPV depends on the intactness of central nervous system asphyxia-avoidance reflexes, there is no need for any of these measures for the asymptomatic patient who does not receive supplemental oxygen.

The consideration of insufflation pressures or pressure-volume curves of the lungs and thorax can be useful. Lung insufflation (ventilator gauge) pressures should usually be 18–25 cmH_2O. Increases in airway pressure without changes in ventilator settings can signal pulmonary edema, pneumonia, bronchospasm, intubation of a mainstem bronchus, atelectasis, and airway mucus accumulation or space-occupying lesions such as pneumothoraces. Pressure decreases, generally below 18 cmH_2O, signal inadequate ventilator-delivered volumes, interface leakage, or insufflation leakage to avoid hyperventilation or because of blunting of ventilatory drive. Electromyography of respiratory muscles during sleep has been used for optimizing inspiratory muscle rest by adjusting nocturnal noninvasive IPPV settings.[764]

The Oximetry Feedback Respiratory Aid Protocol

Headaches, fatigue, a little bit lazy...
Too much CO_2 can make me feel crazy

꧁꧂ Richard L. Clingman, Sr., Webmaster for DoctorBach.com

Because supplemental oxygen is avoided for patients with NMD, patients and care providers are instructed that, once artifact is ruled out,[1043] SpO_2 below 95% is due to one of three causes: hypercapnia (hypoventilation), airway encumberment (secretions), or, if these are not managed properly, intrinsic lung disease, usually gross atelectasis or pneumonia. The oximetry respiratory muscle aid protocol consists of using an oximeter for feedback to maintain SpO_2 greater than 94% by maintaining effective alveolar ventilation and airway secretion elimination.

The protocol is most important during respiratory tract infections and extubation of patients with little or no breathing tolerance. Because respiratory muscles are weakened and bronchial secretions are profuse during chest infections and after surgical general anesthesia,[75] patients often need to use noninvasive IPPV continuously at such times both to maintain alveolar ventilation and to increase CPF by air-stacking. If, when noninvasive IPPV is used at adequate delivered volumes, the SpO_2 is not above 94%, the desaturation is not due to hypoventilation but to airway mucus accumulation. Indeed, sudden $dSpO_2$s for ventilator users during chest infections are almost always due to mucus accumulation. Manually assisted coughing with air-stacking as needed and MAC are then used until the mucus is expulsed and SpO_2 returns to normal or to baseline levels.

If the baseline SpO_2 decreases below 95% despite ventilatory support and MAC, the outpatient then presents for a formal evaluation. A clear radiograph in the presence of a baseline SpO_2 of 92–94% can denote microscopic atelectasis. Radiographic evidence of pneumonia accompanied by $dSpO_2$ and ventilator dependence warrants admission and, when respiratory distress is present, possible intubation. Despite hyperpyrexia and elevated white blood cell counts, baseline SpO_2 often returns to normal and hospitalization can be avoided when patients use respiratory muscle aids with oximetry feedback.[655] As the SpO_2 baseline returns to normal, most patients gradually wean to nocturnal-only noninvasive IPPV or, at times, to no daily use of respiratory muscle aids until the next chest infection.

In the event of hospitalization, the patient's primary care providers are asked to continue to use MAC with oximetry feedback to eliminate airway secretions and avoid intubation. This protocol is recommended because we have found it impossible to expect nursing and respiratory therapy staff to perform the procedures as often as needed to avoid intubation, during intubation, or after extubation. It is most practical and efficacious to let the family and care providers administer the respiratory muscle aids up to every 5 minutes, if necessary, to expel secretions and return SpO_2 to normal, even when the patient is in intensive care. Overnight, provided that sedatives, narcotics, and oxygen therapy are avoided, heavy mucus accumulation will arouse the patient, and he or she will request MAC. The family or primary care providers quickly learn that, since they are doing most of the work anyway, the patients most often can be best and most safely cared for at home as long as baseline SpO_2 remains greater than 94%.

Intubation and Extubation

Noninvasive IPPV can be used to avoid intubation for patients with primarily respiratory impairment in about 70% of cases.[1044] The properly managed, cooperative patient with primarily ventilatory impairment, however, should rarely if ever require intubation for ventilatory or respiratory failure in the first place. However, we are often called to manage such patients who are intubated because they have never been trained to use noninvasive respiratory aids or the oximetry feedback protocol. Some who use only nocturnal nasal IPPV develop respiratory failure because of lack of knowledge of daytime assisted ventilation or assisted coughing or because of inadequate home care to help them with these techniques. In addition, some patients have mixed ventilatory and respiratory impairment due to severe bulbar dysfunction.

Patients presenting in respiratory distress with pneumonia and low baseline SpO_2 are managed conventionally with respect to antibiotic therapy, hydration, chest physical therapy, and nutrition. However, intubation may be necessary. Once the patient is intubated, minute ventilation is increased as needed to maintain $PaCO_2$ between 30 and 40 cmH_2O. As long as $PaCO_2$ is below 40 mmHg, the patient's SpO_2 remains below 95% despite aggressive MI-E, and the patient is intubated, supplemental oxygen can be provided to titrate the SpO_2 to approach 95%. Too often in the emergency department and hospital settings oxygen delivery is increased instead of using MAC and airway suctioning to eliminate airway mucus-associated $dSpO_2$s or using adequate assisted ventilation to eliminate hypercapnia. This approach only worsens atelectasis, airway encumberment, and hypoventilation.

MI-E is used via the tube to eliminate mucus whenever the SpO_2 decreases below 95% or baseline, whenever the patient requests it, or on a regular frequent schedule until SpO_2

baseline has returned to normal. Pressures ranging from +40 to –40 cmH$_2$O are typically used via tracheostomy tubes with diameters of 6 mm or greater. Higher pressures must be provided through smaller tubes to achieve rapid chest expansion and lung emptying with adequate exsufflation flows. For patients with profuse airway secretion, MAC may be needed (as provided by family members) every few minutes around the clock.

Unlike conventional management in which supplemental oxygen is delivered and ventilator weaning is attempted at the expense of hypercapnia, an approach that can ultimately "wean the patient to death," ventilator weaning must not be attempted at the expense of hypercapnia for patients with primarily ventilatory impairment. Before extubation of weanable patients, we use the assist-control mode with minimal pressure support (to compensate for airway resistance due to the presence of the airway tube) to maximize breath volumes while minimizing breathing rate.

The patient is extubated when the following criteria are satisfied: no supplemental oxygen requirement to maintain SpO$_2$ greater than 94%, chest radiograph abnormalities cleared or clearing, respiratory depressants discontinued, airway secretions less than on admission, and any nasal congestion cleared. The nasogastric tube is first removed to facilitate postextubation nasal IPPV. Patients who used air-stacking, bilevel PAP, or noninvasive IPPV before intubation are easily extubated directly to high-span bilevel PAP or to mouthpiece or nasal IPPV. Thus, once the patient is afebrile with a normal white blood cell count and the SpO$_2$ is normal on room air, whether able to breathe or not, the patient is extubated to up to full-time noninvasive support in ambient air. He or she weans from ventilator use, as possible, by taking fewer and fewer assisted breaths, usually via a mouthpiece, as he or she recovers ventilatory function. Thus, the need to fulfill "weaning criteria" is irrelevant since the patient self-weans, as possible, after extubation or decannulation.[1045,1046] MAC is then provided via the upper airway, and the oximetry feedback protocol is followed. MI-E is usually provided via an oral-nasal interface, but some patients with excellent bulbar muscle function use it via a simple mouthpiece.

After extubation, too, the patient's care providers provide MAC with oximetry feedback every few minutes, as necessary, to keep the SpO$_2$ baseline above 94% while the patient is awake. This approach facilitates successful extubation, and the care providers become expert at how to prevent respiratory decompensation and hospitalization in the future.

Extubation succeeds if postextubation CPF, assisted or unassisted, can reach 160 L/min.[656] In a study of 67 consecutive extubations, while VC and the ability to breathe were almost irrelevant because of the use of noninvasive IPPV after extubation, the inability to achieve unassisted or assisted CPF of 160 L/min invariably resulted in re-intubation within 48 hours. One patient with no measurable VC was successfully extubated to continuous noninvasive IPPV. His assisted CPFs were adequate. Yet another patient with a VC of 2000 ml, although breathing comfortably on his own with normal SpO$_2$ upon extubation, had maximum assisted CPF of 120 L/min and required re-intubation for secretion encumberment 24 hours later. It was discovered that he had tracheal stenosis.

Acutely ill patients may require supportive therapies. Once adequate hydration is established and extubated patients are comfortable using noninvasive IPPV, they may be encouraged to eat pureed food or drink fluids through a straw. Swallowing is facilitated by first delivering a few quick, deep, assisted breaths. Episodic desaturations during or for the first 1–2 hours after a meal are dealt with by MI-E with or without gingerly applied abdominal thrusts. Gastrostomy feedings may be suspended if abdominal thrusts are required to supplement MI-E and maintain SpO_2 greater than 94%.

We and others[1047] have extubated numerous patients with no significant breathing tolerance. Many had been using noninvasive IPPV continuously for years before requiring surgery and general anesthesia. Postoperatively they were extubated to their usual method of noninvasive IPPV. Others used only nocturnal noninvasive IPPV and/or daily air-stacking when an intercurrent chest infection or surgical anesthesia caused them to develop pneumonia and respiratory failure (see Case 6).[655,959] They, too, are easily extubated to full-time noninvasive ventilatory support.

Other patients who had never been taught air-stacking or noninvasive aids were referred to us already intubated and incapable of ventilator weaning. Untrained patients with no breathing tolerance are the most difficult to extubate to noninvasive IPPV or bilevel PAP. In such cases, body ventilators can be used to support lung ventilation during and immediately after extubation so that the patient can be trained in noninvasive IPPV without experiencing dyspnea. Once noninvasive IPPV is mastered, the body ventilators are discontinued.[917,918] For postextubation patients not experienced in noninvasive IPPV, nasal IPPV is usually easier to learn quickly than is mouthpiece IPPV. The greatest number of patients with a specific diagnosis whom we have extubated despite absence of breathing tolerance and inability to cooperate were infantile patients with spinal muscular atrophy (SMA; Chapter 12).[1048] As can be seen from reported data, extubation of ventilator-dependent patients following the principles cited above and in Chapter 12 is usually successful.[1048]

An instructive example is that of a patient with DMD who, despite symptomatic hypercapnia, refused to consistently use nocturnal noninvasive IPPV because of "fear that [he] would become addicted to it." The patient had an oximeter and Cough-Assist at home but did not use them when he developed an upper respiratory tract infection and was admitted to a local hospital in December 1996. Then, in March 1997, he was hospitalized locally again and intubated for a respiratory tract infection and respiratory failure. When he failed extubation, he was transferred to our service. When asked why he had not used MI-E, he said that he "forgot how to use it." We used our respiratory aid extubation protocol, but he failed extubation twice with postextubation assisted CPF below 160 L/min. Fortunately, the third extubation attempt (fifth overall) succeeded, and he has been using 20 or more hours per day of noninvasive IPPV for 6 years. Because of his episodes of respiratory failure and close brush with tracheotomy, he has become a strong advocate of the oximetry protocol and noninvasive IPPV.

Decannulation and Conversion to Noninvasive Respiratory Aids

With the trach removed
I much better can breathe
The only cuff that remains
I wear on my sleeve

   ∙☜∙ Richard L. Clingman, Sr., Webmaster for DoctorBach.com

Any patient with an indwelling tracheostomy tube who has understandable speech when the tube cuff is deflated or when a cuffless tube is used is evaluated for decannulation. Patients without severe speech and swallowing impairment are usually excellent candidates. Because noninvasive ventilatory support is successful even for patients with no ability to breathe, decannulation indications depend primarily on bulbar function and, in particular, on the ability to effect glottic closure and then to maintain airway patency sufficiently for CPF to exceed 160 L/min.

Cross-sectional anatomy of the airway can be assessed by computed tomography (CT) scan. Flow-volume loops can also provide information about airway patency but do not assess glottic closure and, therefore, do not correlate with the ability to cough (CPF). Airway patency can be quantitated for patients with tracheostomies by measuring upper airway airflow resistance. This technique utilizes either a body plethysmograph or an oral pneumotach to measure airflow, while pressure is measured in the stoma through a sealed tracheostomy tube. Resistance to flow in $cmH_2O/L/sec$ is equal to the change in pressure (cmH_2O) across the resistor per unit volume of air over time (L/sec). The patient breathes with the mouth wide open to eliminate nasal or oral resistance. The pressure gradient is determined from the trachea to the atmosphere. Airflow is measured, pressure-flow curves are generated, and resistance is calculated 50 times per second. Normal resistance is under 1 $cmH_2O/L/sec$.[1049] It is unclear what values correspond to ineffective cough flows.

As noted, the most important criterion for safe decannulation is the ability to achieve assisted CPF of about 160 L/min (see Case 4 in Chapter 15 of reference 103). Somewhat lower flows are acceptable with the tube in place because air-stacking is usually impossible; the tube obstructs the upper airway; and air leakage occurs around the tube and out of the tracheostomy site during measurements of CPF. The problem of tube obstruction can be alleviated by placing a fenestrated tube to increase airflow between the upper airway and the lungs (see Fig. 3 of Chapter 8). Any cuff must be deflated and the tube capped as the patient receives IPPV via mouthpiece or nasal interface and attempts to air-stack. If the tube fits snugly into the tracheostomy tract and is capped, air-stacking occasionally can be done to some degree, and the assisted CPF better reflects posttracheostomy site closure levels. If the fit is not snug, a manual cough assist must be done without providing a deep insufflation.

If CPFs are much lower than 160 L/min with the tube in place, it is removed, at least temporarily, and the site is covered by hand or with a tracheostomy (Olympic) button to clear the airway. This approach allows more accurate measurement of assisted CPF and facilitates the use of noninvasive IPPV as well as autonomous breathing. Upon button placement or ostomy site covering, patients with no breathing tolerance are immediately placed on noninvasive IPPV (Fig. 7). If despite air-stacking and coordinated abdominal thrusts, levels still fail to approach 160 L/min, vocal cord paralysis, hypopharyngeal collapse, tracheal stenosis, or other reasons for fixed airway obstruction are considered, and the patient is referred for fiberoptic evaluation of the upper airway. If the tracheostomy tube is replaced after the CPF measurement and the patient has a lot of airway secretions, a fenestrated cuffed tracheostomy tube may be warranted. Although cuffs should be deflated for IPPV for patients with any bulbar function, inflation increases the effectiveness of MI-E.

While the vocal cords of intubated patients are kept open by the tube and tend to remain open, patients who are accustomed to tracheostomy IPPV and have never used noninvasive IPPV lose the reflexive glottic opening that normally occurs at the initiation of inspiration. Thus, the patient may have to relearn how to open the vocal cords and

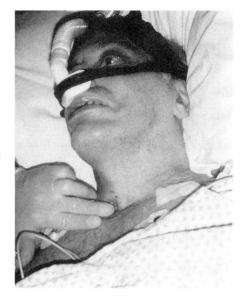

Figure 7. Tracheostomy tube is removed and the site occluded for assessment of maximum insufflation capacity, assisted cough peak flows, and training in noninvasive IPPV.

glottis to receive IPPV noninvasively. This process can take a few minutes or longer during trials of noninvasive IPPV. It may necessitate frequent, brief reconnecting to tracheostomy IPPV or body ventilator use until the patient "breathes" with the delivered air and prevents excessive insufflation leakage out of the mouth or nose. Occasionally, as soon as air enters from a mouthpiece or nasal interface, the patient reflexively opens the mouth to let the air leak. This scenario can occur whether the tube is left in the airway or the airway is clear and the site capped. Thus, it can take practice to be ventilated noninvasively, and nasal IPPV tends to be easier to learn under such circumstances (Fig. 8).

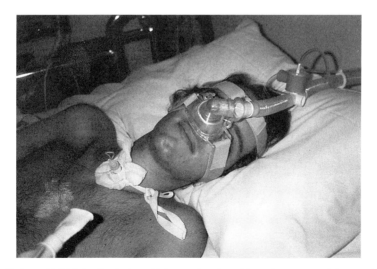

Figure 8. Patient with high-level spinal cord injury and no breathing tolerance practicing nasal IPPV and mouthpiece IPPV with tracheostomy tube capped before decannulation.

It must be realized that airway obstruction from an indwelling tracheostomy tube, even a cuffless one with a fenestration, can often make it difficult for patients to be adequately ventilated via the upper airway. High, uncomfortable oropharyngeal pressures can be generated during noninvasive IPPV in this manner. If these pressures are not excessive, it can be reassuring to let the patient use noninvasive IPPV for a day or 2 before removing the tube or button and letting the site close. Often when the tracheostomy tube has been removed for the more accurate measurement of CPF and noninvasive IPPV no longer induces high oropharyngeal pressures, the patient quickly becomes accustomed to it and the tracheostomy tube is simply left out. We no longer use body ventilators as a bridge to ventilate the lungs during training in noninvasive IPPV and tracheostomy site closure.[918,960] Because we have rarely had to replace a tracheostomy tube, we usually decannulate patients who meet the criterion of adequate assisted CPF, convert them directly to noninvasive IPPV, and let the tracheostomy sites close immediately upon decannulation. Thus, whereas the ability to achieve adequate CPF is critical, ability to autonomously sustain alveolar ventilation is unnecessary because ventilatory support can be provided noninvasively.[656] In addition to relying on noninvasive IPPV, IAPVs can be used (Chapter 10).

While the clinician is gaining confidence in using noninvasive IPPV for patients with little or no breathing tolerance, use of noninvasive ventilation with a tracheostomy button is advisable for a few days. In this way the tracheostomy tube can be replaced in the event that tracheal edema (or some other desire to recannulate) develops.

Soft silicon material in the form of a plugged donut of 2-inch diameter (Respironics, Inc., Murrysville, PA) (Fig. 9) or a cane tip (Fig. 10) cut short is placed over an occlusive tracheostomy site dressing (Fig. 11) (Tegaderm, 3M Company, St. Paul, MN). The latter decreases any tendency for silicon slippage and prevents airway secretions from wetting and loosening the overlying gauze and elastic dressing. Four-by-four-inch sterile gauze is placed over the silicon donut and can be covered and fixed in place by adhesive tape. Insufflation leakage through the site can then be further countered by placing an

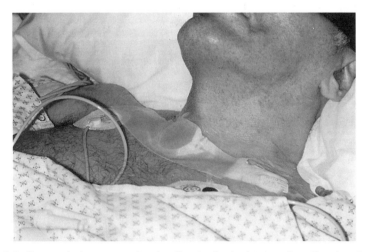

Figure 9. Soft silicon occlusive pressure dressing (Respironics, Inc.) to permit continued noninvasive IPPV after decannulation and before ostomy closure.

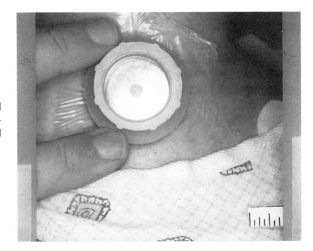

Figure 10. Cane tip cut short and placed over an occlusive tracheostomy site dressing (Tegaderm, 3M Company, St. Paul, MN).

elastic figure-of-8 strap. The strap crosses anteriorly across the neck; goes under the axillae, over the shoulders, and across the back; and inserts into an elastic band in front of the neck[546] (Fig. 12). This approach minimizes skin maceration from secretions leaking through the tracheostomy site and minimizes the amount of adhesive tape applied to the skin, thereby optimizing comfort and facilitating visualization of the ostomy as it closes. Although the tracheostomy site usually closes in 24–72 hours, it can be sutured if it has not closed after a few weeks. Once the tracheostomy site is closed, assisted CPF can be maximized and measured accurately, GPB can be taught, and MI-E use via the upper airway can be better assessed.

In 1990 we summarized the steps for the decannulation of patients admitted to an acute rehabilitation facility:

1. The patients were medically stabilized, supplemental oxygen therapy was discontinued, and MAC was used aggressively via the tube to clear secretions.

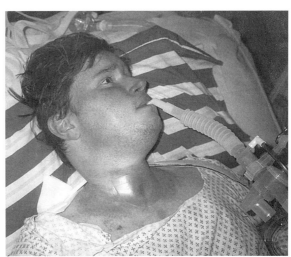

Figure 11. Occlusive tracheostomy site dressing (Tegaderm, 3M Company, St. Paul, MN) under cane tip or silicon plug.

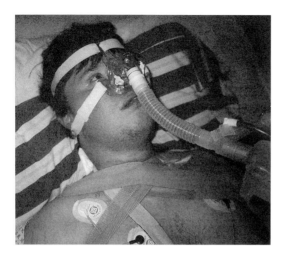

Figure 12. Post-decannulation pressure covering of occlusive ostomy dressing for patient with Duchenne muscular dystrophy and no autonomous breathing tolerance (see Fig. 8).

2. The patients were placed on portable volume-cycled ventilators. The cuffs were completely deflated hourly for increasing periods until cuff deflation could be tolerated throughout daytime hours. Partial-to-complete cuff deflation was then used overnight. To ensure adequate alveolar ventilation, the delivered insufflation volumes were increased to maintain the same airway pressures as with the cuff inflated. When necessary, the patient's tracheostomy tube diameter was changed to permit sufficient leakage for speech while maintaining adequate fit to permit effective assisted ventilation, with delivered ventilator volumes generally of 1–2 liters. The set volumes on assist/control mode, rate 10–12, were titrated to maintain pCO_2 levels between 35 and 40 mmHg. Tracheal integrity, tracheostomy tube width, and volitional glottic and vocal cord movements determined the amount of the delivered air to enter the lungs and the amount to "leak" upward through the vocal cords with each delivered volume. The insufflation leakage was used for crescendo/decrescendo inspiratory cycle speech.

A low speech volume indicated inadequate insufflation volume, a tracheostomy tube that was too wide, or subglottic obstruction, usually by granulation tissue. For such patients, optimal insufflation volumes for normal ventilation and more effective speech were obtained by cuff removal, by placing a narrower diameter tracheostomy tube, or by surgical ablation of the granulation tissue, when indicated. The expiratory valve was occasionally capped, permitting continuous speech without the expense of a Passy-Muir valve.

3. Patients were advanced to the use of 24-hour tracheostomy IPPV with a deflated cuff. The prolonged use of partial cuff deflation was discouraged because of the tendency of the nursing staff to gradually increase the amount of air in the cuff with time. Some patients were introduced to noninvasive ventilatory support by using an iron lung or chest shell ventilator with the tracheostomy tube open. Care was taken to maintain the tracheostomy tube above the iron lung collar.

4. The patients were trained in the use of mouthpiece IPPV for daytime ventilatory support with the tracheostomy tube capped. Each patient learned to close off the nasopharynx with the soft palate to prevent nasal leakage. Temporarily pinching the nostrils helped the patient to understand why this technique was necessary. Patients for whom

the cuffs had been inflated for long periods initially maintained their vocal cords fully adducted during attempts at mouthpiece IPPV. Each patient was unaware that he was obstructing flow. Each patient successfully re-learned the reflexive vocal cord abduction that permits effective mouthpiece IPPV. Nasal IPPV was also used successfully before decanulation. End-tidal carbon dioxide was evaluated by sampling end-tidal air under the interface and as close to the nostrils as possible (Fig. 13).

Once daytime mouthpiece IPPV was mastered, body ventilators were occasionally used for nocturnal support with the tracheostomy tube plugged. Body ventilator use facilitated tracheostomy site closure by relieving the stoma of the positive expulsive pressures that occur during IPPV and by providing ventilatory support. This approach prevented dyspnea and panic and facilitated the learning of noninvasive IPPV.

Mouthpiece IPPV normalized speech rhythm, provided normal daytime ventilation, and permitted air-stacking for volitional sighing, shouting, and assisted coughing when the tube fit tightly in the tracheostomy tract. The change to a fenestrated tracheostomy tube and its capping and cuff deflation often improved the efficacy of mouthpiece IPPV as well as the effectiveness of body ventilator use. It also improved speech volume during use of mouthpiece IPPV or autonomous breathing, whenever possible. The fenestration of the commercially available tubes, however, was at times malpositioned against the posterior tracheal wall, where invagination of the tracheal mucosa into the fenestration rendered it ineffective and caused bleeding, potentially exacerbating granulation formation. Proper positioning of the fenestration was accomplished by ordering a custom-made fenestrated tube or changing to a smaller tube.

5. Patients were advanced to the use of cuffless tracheostomy tubes. The great majority of patients did not require a change in tracheostomy diameter to maintain optimal ventilation and speech volume; however, ventilator volumes often needed to be as much as doubled to compensate for increased leakage. Then the tube was capped or at times replaced by a tracheostomy button for up to continuous practice with noninvasive IPPV for a few days before the tracheostomy site was allowed to close. Patients tried a variety

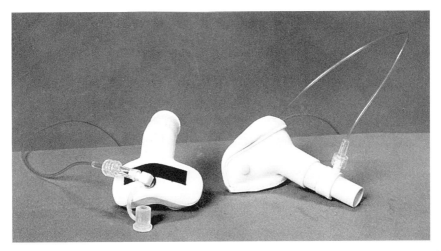

Figure 13. End-tidal sampler passed via nasal prongs interface for measurements of end-tidal carbon dioxide without discontinuing nasal ventilation.

of interfaces and chose accordingly. Once the patient was comfortable with noninvasive IPPV, the tracheostomy site was allowed to close.

Patients had trials of ventilatory support by the IAPV. Several trials were often necessary to determine the optimal belt size and position and the optimal buckle or Velcro strap pressures. Patients with measurable VC learned to coordinate breathing with the IAPV. With the site closed, ventilator weaning was facilitated by mouthpiece IPPV taken from a mouthpiece fixed adjacent to the patient's mouth and accessible to the patient by neck rotation. The patients took fewer and fewer assisted breaths as they weaned. This technique is free of the anxiety that ventilator users feel when they are disconnected and weaned from tracheostomy IPPV. Mouthpiece IPPV is used overnight with a lipseal.

Five centers have reported tracheostomy tube removal for conversion to noninvasive respiratory muscle aids.[101] We and others[1050] have reported the successful decannulation of over 40 patients with spinal cord injury (SCI) and no significant breathing tolerance to continuous noninvasive IPPV.[101] We have also decannulated 11 patients with non-DMD, 3 with nonbulbar ALS, 4 with post-poliomyelitis syndrome, 3 with DMD, 2 with multiple sclerosis, and 2 with SMA who had little or no breathing tolerance to continuous noninvasive IPPV. Only two of these patients, both with bulbar ALS, underwent tracheostomy a second time. We have also decannulated over 200 other part-time, mostly nocturnal, noninvasive ventilation users and others who were not using ventilators but had been told never to have their tubes removed.

> *With mask or with pillows*
> *I breathe through my nose*
> *And the hole in my throat*
> *Is ready to close*
>
> •☜• Richard L. Clingman, Sr., Webmaster for DoctorBach.com

Postsurgical Complications

With age, many patients with SCI, post-poliomyelitis syndrome, and NMD have respiratory difficulties after surgical interventions with general anesthesia. They may fail to wean from the ventilator in a timely manner, remain intubated, develop pneumonia, and be told that they need tracheostomy tubes. Even otherwise benign procedures such as colonoscopies performed under conscious sedation with oximetry monitoring and supplemental oxygen rather than carbon dioxide monitoring and assisted ventilation have typically resulted in tracheostomies or deaths from ventilatory failure. For example, patients with DMD and low plateau (lifetime maximum) VCs[610] invariably develop scoliosis that requires spinal stabilization. Postoperatively they may fail to wean from ventilatory assistance and undergo tracheotomy. However, tracheotomy is avoidable by training patients in the use of respiratory muscle aids before surgery so that, even with failure to wean from the ventilator postoperatively, they can be extubated to noninvasive IPPV and MAC with oximetry feedback. We often find it practical to maintain intubation for 2 or 3 days after spinal instrumentation to allow for opiod therapy for pain control before discontinuing or greatly curtailing opioid therapy and extubating ventilator-dependent patients to noninvasive aids.

Un artiste crèateur est comme un archer qui tire ses fleòhes dans le noir, sans jamais savoir si elles toucheront le but.

An artist is like an archer who shoots his arrows in the dark without ever knowing whether or not they will hit the target.

• Gustav Mahler

Noninvasive Respiratory Muscle Aid Outcomes and Clinical Considerations

From 1977 to 2002 the author managed 722 long-term users of noninvasive IPPV with the diagnoses listed in Table 1. The pulmonary function, extent of ventilator need, duration of use, and prolongation of survival for many of these ventilator users have been published.[655,742,750,1051] Although most used mouthpiece (daytime) and lipseal (nocturnal) IPPV, as early as 1990 we reported 43 noninvasive IPPV users of whom 33 used nocturnal nasal IPPV in a regimen of full-time noninvasive IPPV for over 20 months.[567]

Table 1. Diagnoses of Long-term Noninvasive IPPV Users at One Center	
Post-poliomyelitis	189
Duchenne muscular dystrophy	93
Diagnosis not confirmed	93
Spinal muscular atrophy	84
Amyotrophic lateral sclerosis	77
Non-Duchenne myopathies*	63
Spinal cord injury	60
Scoliosis	11
Chronic obstructive pulmonary disease	10
Obesity hypoventilation	9
Myasthenia gravis	7
Multiple sclerosis	5
Phrenic neuropathy	4
Polymyositis	3
Other respiratory disease[†]	3
Charcot-Marie-Tooth disease	3
Myelopathy other than traumatic	2
Miscellaneous[‡]	9
Total	725

* Including Emery-Dreifuss, limb-girdle, and myotonic muscular dystrophies and generalized myopathies, including acid maltase deficiency.
† Including pulmonary fibrosis, Milroy's disease, and tuberculosis.
‡ Including Friedreich's ataxia, neuropathy associated with cancer, osteogenesis imperfecta, Guillain-Barrè syndrome, central alveolar hypoventilation, brain stem astrocytoma, post-curarization paralysis, arthrogryposis, and Parkinson's disease.

Numerous other patients with many of the same diagnoses listed in Table 1 of Chapter 1, including 94 patients reported in a recent publication, avoided hospitalizations during chest infections with access to the oximetry respiratory aid protocol. That is, they became full-time ventilator-dependent without being hospitalized and experienced reversal of airway mucus plug-associated $dSpO_2$s by using MAC with oximetry feedback during chest colds. Sixteen of the patients avoided 1.02 ± 0.99 hospitalizations per patient per year over a period of 2.19 ± 1.84 years before requiring ongoing ventilator use. Forty-nine part-time ventilator users avoided 0.99 ± 1.12 hospitalizations per patient per year over 3.88 ± 3.45 years; and 18 full-time noninvasive ventilation users avoided 0.80 ± 0.85 hospitalizations per patient per year over 6.54 ± 5.00 years. All comparisons of preprotocol and protocol-access rates were statistically significant at $p < 0.004$.[655,959] After chest infections, patients generally weaned from full-time ventilator use to their pre-infection regimens.[655]

Although certain other groups have reported isolated cases of avoidance of respiratory complications and eventual use of up to 24-hour long-term noninvasive ventilatory support,[1052] thus far this scenario has resulted mostly from patient refusal of tracheostomy, continuance of nasal IPPV into daytime hours, and no occurrence of chest infections. The use of crucial noninvasive expiratory muscle aids has not been noted.[773] For example, Baydur et al. reported 46 years of experience using noninvasive ventilation for 79 patients with neuromusculoskeletal disorders.[757] They noted that hospital admissions increased 8-fold once patients began using NPBVs but decreased by 36% for those using noninvasive IPPV. Because of failure to use expiratory aids and noninvasive IPPV appropriately during daytime hours, 30 patients, including 10 of 15 with DMD, underwent tracheotomy. Most certainly none of these patients would have required tracheostomy if provided with the oximetry respiratory muscle aid protocol.[615]

Duchenne Muscular Dystrophy

Thirteen of 23 asymptomatic patients with DMD, ranging from 13 to 23 years of age, demonstrated sleep hypoxia, with SpO_2 decreasing below 90% during sleep. Twelve of the 13 had dips in SpO_2 associated with apneas. Sixty percent of the apneas were obstructive. With time hypoxemic periods became more frequent and associated with "pseudocentral" apneas[1053] or apneas due to inspiratory muscle weakness. However, treatment of sleep-disordered breathing before the development of symptoms is essentially treatment of the polysomnogram rather than the patient. Once symptoms develop, the patient is more appropriately managed by using a volume-cycled ventilator than by using CPAP or low-span bilevel PAP because in a few years the patient will require a volume-cycled ventilator for both nocturnal and daytime ventilatory assistance as well as for air-stacking.

Because patients with DMD breathe mostly with the diaphragm, their VCs are usually the same whether sitting or supine. As the VC decreases, as for other patients, maximum insufflation lung mobilizations are initiated 3 times/day, using a manual resuscitator. Soon afterward, unassisted CPFs decrease below 270 L/sec, and patients are taught MAC and the oximetry protocol to prevent acute respiratory failure during colds. Because respiratory tract infections are frequent in this young population, an oximeter and Cough-Assist are prescribed for home use. Many patients with DMD have airway secretion encumberment, often from chronic aspiration of upper airway secretions or from CHF, necessitating MAC multiple times every day.

Because such patients may also have scoliosis that decreases the efficacy of abdominal thrusts and because their bulbar musculature is dysfunctional (although never entirely impaired), MIC eventually decreases below 1000 ml, but assisted CPFs rarely decrease below 160 L/min.

The older the patient, the greater the risk of hypoventilation at higher VCs. As the VC decreases below 800 ml, patients with DMD often begin to rock back and forth in their wheelchairs to compress the abdomen during exhalation and thus increase tidal volumes. They also tend to develop sleep hypoxia and hypercapnia. They eventually use accessory breathing muscles. They usually remain grossly asymptomatic, however, until VC decreases below 450 ml and hypercapnia extends into daytime hours. Usually by this time nocturnal nasal IPPV with a portable volume-cycled ventilator is clearly indicated.

Patients usually require daytime mouthpiece IPPV with the ventilator on the back of the wheelchair and the mouthpiece adjacent to the mouth once the VC is less than 350 ml. About 15% of patients eventually lose the ability to use mouthpiece IPPV because of oromotor weakness. Such patients typically prefer to use nasal IPPV around the clock or an IAPV rather than undergo tracheotomy. Thus, the typical patient eventually requires a volume-cycled ventilator, a Cough-Assist, oximeter, and manual resuscitator and needs to use noninvasive IPPV on a full-time basis during intercurrent chest infections, for air-stacking, and eventually for continuous ventilatory support.

Some patients, even with VCs as high as 1500 ml, feel better and less fatigued with use of nocturnal nasal IPPV or even with low-span bilevel PAP in early stages of their disease. They may also have improvements in nocturnal SpO_2. Although mild evidence of sleep-disordered breathing often is seen in polysomnography studies long before the VC decreases to 700 ml, ongoing nocturnal nasal ventilation should not be recommended without symptomatic improvement. Such patients are likely to use noninvasive IPPV for 20 years or more. Burdening them in the absence of symptoms is unwarranted.

When patients are properly equipped and trained and when optimal personal care assistance is available in the home, respiratory complications of DMD can be completely avoided.[655] In our early study of patients referred after 1983, 86 patients (mean age: 26.0 ± 7.0 years) had become wheelchair-dependent at 9.7 ± 2.2 years of age. Their mean age at first visit was 19.2 ± 6.2 years. Fifty-one (59.3%) were still alive at 25.2 ± 5.9 years of age, and 35 (40.7%) died at 27.3 ± 8.2 years of age. The causes of death were respiratory (17), cardiac (12), other (2), and unknown (4). Although these early patients used up to full-time noninvasive IPPV, none of the patients with respiratory-related deaths had had access to oximetry or MAC. Of the 12 patients who died from CHF, the 9 who used mechanical ventilation died later than the nonventilator users at 26.8 ± 5.5 years of age. Of the 17 patients who died from respiratory complications, 14 died from acute respiratory tract illness and 3 died from ventilatory insufficiency when they were disconnected from the ventilator or slept without using it. These three patients had VCs of 411 ± 391 ml immediately before death and had been using IPPV for 16.3 ± 6.65 years when they died at 40 ± 10.15 years of age. Thus, in almost all cases, death occurred within days after onset of a chest infection or resulted from CHF in patients with extremely low cardiac ejection fractions. None of the 7 deaths for which autopsies were performed were due to pulmonary emboli or noncardiopulmonary causes.

Of the 34 patients with access to the oximetry protocol, 31 are still alive at 25.7 ± 4.5 years of age. They have been using the protocol for 5.3 ± 4.2 (range: 1–16) years and have been using noninvasive IPPV for 5.4 ± 4.0 years, including 1.6 ± 1.6 years of nocturnal-only noninvasive IPPV. None of these patients have died thus far from respiratory causes. The 3 who died had left ventricular ejection fractions below 15%. They were 25 ± 2 years of age at the time of death.

The longest periods for which our patients with DMD have been using 24-hour noninvasive IPPV are 26, 20, and 16 years to ages 43, 34, and 39 years, respectively. We also decannulated 3 full-time tracheostomy IPPV users and switched them to noninvasive IPPV. Five patients have required full-time noninvasive IPPV for 5 years or more without being hospitalized.[655] None of our DMD patients have undergone or needed to undergo tracheotomy since 1983.

Because patients with DMD retain adequate assisted CPF and can use MAC successfully at all ages, proper management of patients with intact cognitive function does not require tracheostomy tubes. A tube already in place need not be removed in all cases because such patients are usually not good candidates for effective GPB. However, 12 of our patients with mean VC of 265 ± 104 ml and no breathing tolerance using respiratory muscles were able to use GPB to volumes of 1273 ± 499 ml. This approach permitted them a mean of 5.3 ± 4.8 hours of breathing tolerance. Therefore, tubes should be removed if the patient desires it, if there have been complications of tracheostomy, or if tube removal can facilitate social functioning (e.g., de-institutionalization). Decannulation and transition to noninvasive IPPV from 24-hour tracheostomy IPPV result in discontinuance of daytime ventilator use for patients with over 200 ml of VC and facilitate returning home (see Case 8).

Since respiratory mortality can now be avoided, the limiting factor for survival in our center and in others in Japan has become cardiomyopathy. Death from cardiomyopathy can occur as early as 12 years of age but also can be delayed (Chapter 5). The Yakumo Byoin National Sanatorium in Hokkaido, Japan, under Dr. Yuka Ishikawa, and the Tokushima National Sanatorium Hospital in Tokushima, Japan, under Dr. Tatara have reported survival data for full-time mouthpiece/nasal IPPV users with DMD. Tatara's center recently reported a 5-year cumulative survival rate of 75% for 34 pediatric noninvasive IPPV users with NMD, including 25 with DMD. Tokushima is also the home of the rock group Dream Music Directory (see Dedication). At Ishikawa's center, 44 patients with DMD have used noninvasive IPPV since 20.3 ± 3.4 years of age. They have a 3-year survival rate of 97.7% and a 10-year survival rate of 93.3%. Before 1991 at the same center, tracheostomy IPPV was begun at age 20.0 ± 4.0 years for 26 patients with DMD and was the only method of ventilatory support. The 1-year survival rate 73.1%; the 3-year survival rate, 53.8%; the 5-year survival rate, 50%; and the 10-year survival rate, 42.3%. We are aware of no other centers with more than a few 24-hour noninvasive IPPV users with DMD.

Non-DMD Myopathies

Patients with non-DMD muscular dystrophies and other myopathies are managed similarly to patients with DMD except that their conditions are usually milder; therefore, they develop ventilatory insufficiency at older ages and at higher VCs. In addition, some of these patients, especially those with adult-onset muscular dystrophies and acid maltase deficiency, develop severe diaphragm weakness and lose breathing tolerance when supine but not when sitting. Often the VC in the supine position is less than half the VC in the sitting position. Such patients may require nocturnal ventilatory support for many years before needing daytime aid. Many can walk despite symptomatic daytime hypercapnia. As a result, they do not use assisted ventilation sufficiently during daytime hours to normalize diurnal carbon dioxide levels and thereby optimize nocturnal use (Chapter 10). Except for an occasional patient with facioscapulohumeral muscular dystrophy (FSH), bulbar muscles usually retain adequate function for effective speech, swallowing, GPB, and MAC. Therefore, few patients require tracheostomy tubes, and those with tracheostomy tubes are usually excellent candidates for decannulation and transition to noninvasive IPPV and GPB. They are introduced to air-stacking, assisted coughing, and GPB similarly to patients with DMD.

We reported that respiratory complications and hospitalizations were avoided for 25 ventilator users with non-Duchenne myopathies by using the oximetry protocol.[959] Because these patients have less bulbar muscle dysfunction and often less cardiomyopathy than patients with DMD, it is not surprising that 17 of our patients with non-DMD myopathy and a mean VC of 363 ml have now lived up to 30 years using full-time noninvasive ventilation.[752] There is also a recent report of prolongation of life by the use of the oximetry protocol for 2 patients with Fukuyama-type congenital muscular dystrophy in Japan.[1054]

Myotonic Dystrophy

Although myotonic dystrophy is essentially a non-DMD myopathy, it deserves special comment. The chemosensitivity of the respiratory centers as measured by $P_{0.1}$ is well preserved in patients with myotonic dystrophy, as it is for patients with other muscular dystrophies, but even in the absence of restricted lung volumes, output to breathing is modulated by impaired respiratory mechanics. This impairment causes chronic symptomatic alveolar hypoventilation despite VCs and MICs that are generally well preserved for many years.[1055] Even in the absence of significant central or obstructive sleep apneas[1056,1057] or chronic diurnal hypercapnia, however, such patients can exhibit sleep hypercapnia and hypersomnia (Chapter 1). More often, apneas and hypopneas, when present, are exacerbated by chronic alveolar hypoventilation due to weak and myotonic inspiratory muscles.

Despite severe hypercapnia and nocturnal ventilatory insufficiency, because these patients are usually able to walk, because of the general apathy and cognitive impairment that is often part of the primary pathology, and quite possibly because of the myotonic nature of the muscle impairment, patients often fail to use assisted ventilation sufficiently either during daytime hours or overnight. One study reported poor compliance with ventilator use by 62% of 38 patients compared with patients with other NMDs.[1058] Thus, many patients never cooperate sufficiently to benefit optimally from noninvasive IPPV. Most patients are hospitalized repeatedly before succumbing to cor pulmonale and CHF. With persistent hypercapnia and hypersomnolence, such patients are perhaps the most frustrating to treat by noninvasive ventilation. Nevertheless, those who do cooperate sufficiently to use at least nocturnal noninvasive IPPV have improved arterial blood gases and improved survival rates with greater alertness, less sleep disturbance, and fewer morning headaches, if not always less hypersomnolence.[1059]

When hypersomnolence persists despite apparently adequate alveolar ventilation, treatment with the central stimulant methylphenidate was reported to produce sustained benefit in 7 of 11 patients.[1060] Modafinil at 200–400 mg/day also benefited 9 other patients but should not be used for those with obstructive sleep apneas.[1061] Selegiline, an antioxidant used to treat the sleep attacks of narcolepsy, has not been shown to be effective.[1062]

Patients with myotonic dystrophy also have poor prognoses with tracheostomy tubes for the same reasons that they often fail to use noninvasive IPPV adequately. Although there are no long-term studies of the use of mechanical ventilation by patients with myotonic dystrophy, we have managed a handful with up to full-time dependence on tracheostomy IPPV and 8 others with noninvasive IPPV for a prolongation of survival of up to 8 years. In a recent study of 13 hypercapnic patients with some combination of hypersomnolence, dyspnea, morning headache, and sleep disturbance using nocturnal nasal or oronasal IPPV, diurnal $PaCO_2$ decreased from 64 to 53 mmHg, PaO_2 increased from 53 to 65 mmHg, mean nocturnal SpO_2 increased from 80.5 to 90.3%, and transcutaneous PCO_2 decreased from 59.3 to 41.4 mmHg. Three ventilator users died, but the other 10 had been using noninvasive IPPV for 27 months.[1059]

Amyotrophic Lateral Sclerosis/Motor Neuron Disease

When one patient was asked "What has it been like to be dependent upon a machine for your breathing?," without hesitation he responded via computer voice synthesizer, "It has been a friend. It has given me some extra years of life."[740]

Onset of generalized motor neuron disease is almost always after 19 years of age. As a result, patients are generally able to cooperate with the use of noninvasive respiratory muscle aids. There are essentially two types of presentation, bulbar and nonbulbar. Bulbar-onset patients can lose verbal communication and ability to swallow and may develop respiratory failure from aspiration of food or upper airway secretions while still able to walk and with a VC above 1500 ml. However, they often demonstrate stridor with severe airway collapsibility during inspiration, expiration, or both. Collapsibility during expiration has been shown to be associated with the obstructive apneas of sleep-disordered breathing.[1063] Five cm of negative pressure applied to the airway during expiration resulted in expiratory flow limitations and $dSpO_2$s in patients with sleep-disordered breathing but not in healthy controls.[1063] With ALS, collapsibility can be so severe as to render assisted CPF unmeasurable and MI-E useless. For patients with severe bulbar disease, glottic closure is lost, the MIC-VC difference becomes zero, assisted CPF becomes unmeasurable, and peak expiratory flows are inadequate for effective airway clearance.[910] Some patients with little or no volitional cough have reflex cough flows and can clear airway secretions to some degree. For such patients, although reflex coughing and MAC can at times be helpful,[849] eventually only repeated intubation or tracheotomy can maintain survival. As for others, tracheotomy is necessary when assisted CPFs are low and SpO_2 baseline decreases below 95% despite optimal access to respiratory muscle aids. Usually tracheotomy should be accompanied by laryngeal diversion (Chapter 4).

Patients with a strictly nonbulbar presentation, on the other hand, retain effective speech and swallowing despite the fact that VC can decrease to less than 100 ml and all breathing tolerance can be lost. MICs can remain greater than 3000 ml and assisted CPF much greater than 160 L/min for many years. These patients can often use GPB for breathing tolerance. Because they are not conventionally trained in noninvasive IPPV and MAC, tracheostomy tubes are often mistakenly placed during episodes of acute respiratory failure that arise from chest infections.

In one study, 57 ventilator users with ALS had been familiarized with the use of mouthpiece and nasal IPPV, IAPV, and MAC. Twenty-six of the 57 became dependent on 24-hour noninvasive IPPV with no breathing tolerance for 23.7 ± 20.3 months. This was 20.2 ± 23.4 months prior to tracheostomy for 13 patients, 24.1 ± 15.6 months for 7 patients who died without being intubated, and 32.2 ± 20.0 months for 6 patients still using noninvasive support.[545] Thus, noninvasive respiratory muscle aids can delay or eliminate the need for tracheostomy for patients with ALS who retain sufficient bulbar muscle function for assisted CPF to exceed 160 L/min.

We extubated or decannulated 6 patients with ALS who had been intubated or who had unnecessarily undergone tracheotomy for full-time ventilatory support. All 6 continued to require full-time aid but noninvasively, including two for 4 and 7 years, respectively. The former underwent repeat tracheotomy when it was necessitated by bulbar muscle dysfunction. The latter continues to use full-time noninvasive IPPV. One of the 6 patients was convinced by local physicians to undergo elective repeat tracheotomy within 2 months of decannulation despite not needing it. Another died 6 months after decannulation and full-time noninvasive IPPV when bulbar deterioration resulted in severe aspiration. He preferred death to tracheotomy a second time.

The other deceased patient was decannulated at her own request despite having no residual bulbar muscle function or measurable CPF. She subsequently developed respiratory failure again and was intubated at a local hospital. Because of full-time ventilator dependence, severe airway mucus encumberment, and refusal of repeat tracheotomy, she was transferred to our service for a trial of extubation to noninvasive IPPV. After aggressive MI-E via the tube had succeeded in clearing her airways and normalizing her SpO_2 in ambient air, she was extubated to full-time IPPV. However, her bulbar muscle dysfunction was too severe for effective nasal or lipseal IPPV; that is, she could not limit insufflation leakage during lipseal or nasal IPPV. Therefore, noninvasive IPPV had to be provided on a full-time basis via an oral-nasal interface. Unexpectedly, 1 month after hospital discharge she gradually weaned to nocturnal-only oral-nasal IPPV until she died suddenly 9 months later, probably of airway mucus-associated asphyxia. Thus, even in the absence of measurable assisted CPF, patients with bulbar ALS can be extubated to noninvasive IPPV. With such severe bulbar muscle dysfunction, however, long-term prognosis using noninvasive ventilation remains guarded.

Most patients with motor neuron disease develop some combination of bulbar and skeletal muscle weakness. As long as the MIC can exceed the VC and assisted CPFs remain greater than 160 L/min, they can benefit from air-stacking or maximal insufflations 3 times/day[545] and the oximetry protocol. At times such patients lose measurable CPF and require gastrostomy tubes, but if not aspirating upper airway secretions so much as to decrease SpO_2 baseline below 95%, they do not require invasive management. At least 5 other MDA clinics in the U.S.[615] as well as centers in other countries[1064] are using this noninvasive approach for patients with ALS.

For patients with no measurable CPF who drool or aspirate airway secretions, injections of botulinum toxin A into or irradiation of the salivary glands may be considered[1065] (Chapter 4). This approach may be particularly important when chronic aspiration causes a long-term decrease in SpO_2 baseline below 95%, indicating a very high risk of pneumonia and respiratory failure. Tracheotomy then becomes necessary if the SpO_2 cannot be normalized by assisted coughing, chest physical therapy, or chest percussion. If reduction in salivary production can decrease aspiration to the point of normalizing baseline SpO_2, the risk of pneumonia is greatly diminished and resort to tracheotomy is unnecessary; however, this point has not yet been demonstrated. Some investigators have tried to relieve trismus and the respiratory stridor associated with upper airway collapse and loss of measurable cough flows by the use of botulinum toxin.[1066]

Once intubated, patients with ALS and unmeasurable preintubation assisted CPF should be considered for tracheotomy rather than for extubation to noninvasive ventilation. Ventilator weaning attempts are almost always fruitless when patients are intubated under these conditions and should not be permitted to prolong hospitalization.

In general, patients with ALS and tracheostomy tubes are evaluated for decannulation by measuring assisted CPF, as for other patients with NMD. However, the rate of deterioration should also be ascertained by having monitored the VC, MIC, assisted CPF, and manual muscle testing every other month for at least 4–6 months. This approach, along with the patient's history, helps to determine whether bulbar muscle function is sufficiently stable to permit long-term benefit from decannulation. As for others with NMD, the MIC of many patients with ALS can increase with practice for months to years despite decreasing VC and rapidly progressive disease.[910] For patients with NMD and rapidly decreasing MIC or MIC that equals VC, decannulation should generally be avoided.

Spinal Muscular Atrophy Types 2–5

Although muscle strength is unchanged during adolescence, as for everybody else, physiologic deterioration begins at age 19 and weakness due to adult-onset SMA progresses at an increasingly greater rate in middle age. Nevertheless, these patients rarely lose the ability to speak, assisted CPF remains adequate, and ventilator use may be required initially only at night, with full-time ventilator use only during intercurrent chest infections, for many years after onset of muscle weakness. With advancing age, however, full-time noninvasive IPPV can be required, but tracheotomy is rarely if ever needed because of retention of adequate bulbar muscle function. The infantile SMAs are considered in Chapter 12.

Other Neurologic Conditions and Obesity-related Hypoventilation

Patients with multiple sclerosis, post-poliomyelitis syndrome, myasthenia gravis, myelopathies, SCI, and obesity-related hypoventilation can develop ventilatory failure and may require full-time noninvasive IPPV and the oximetry protocol over the long term as well as during acute episodes or exacerbations. Both acutely and over the long term, such patients can have inordinate diaphragm weakness that manifests itself by inability to breathe in the recumbent position. Patients benefit from ongoing nocturnal use of noninvasive IPPV so that they can sleep in the supine position. Depending on the extent of bulbar and expiratory muscle dysfunction, the protocol can be used to avert intubation. Indeed, the first patient ever to depend on full-time nasal IPPV with no breathing tolerance was a patient with multiple sclerosis.[674] Outcomes of noninvasive management of these conditions have been explored elsewhere.[101]

Difficulties in Initiating the Use of Noninvasive Aids

Patients and caregivers prefer noninvasive approaches.[699] These methods lower the cost of home mechanical ventilation;[1067] can eliminate the need for hospitalization, intubation, tracheostomy, and bronchoscopy;[14] and shorten hospitalizations.[14,655,742] They decrease the need for invasive ventilation[1068] and are associated with fewer complications[1069] and pneumonias[1070] than invasive ventilation in both the long-term and acute care settings. A recent study demonstrated that use of invasive mechanical ventilation, occurrence of pneumonia, need for surgery, and use of tracheostomy explain 60% of the variance in both length of stay and hospital costs for patients after cervical spine injury.[1071] Each of these variables, when considered independently, is a better predictor of hospital costs than level of injury. Thus, respiratory complications managed invasively rather than by exclusive use of noninvasive respiratory muscle aids, as can be done in many circumstances,[1072] can greatly increase hospital utilization and costs.

Despite these issues and their long-term safety and efficacy, noninvasive alternatives are not widely used. They are generally not part of health professional school curricula, and current invasive approaches are centered on the general tendency to resort to the highest available and most costly technology. Physician and hospital reimbursement is procedure-based and directed toward inpatient management rather than preventive care. One can be remunerated for hospitalizing patients for intubation, tracheotomy, and bronchoscopies, but outpatient management that prevents hospitalization by using noninvasive aids is poorly recognized and reimbursed by third-party payors, even though it costs only a small fraction of the alternative. The patients require equipment and training, which necessitate letters of justification and explanation. Furthermore, the initial use of noninvasive aids requires a significant time commitment for evaluating various IPPV interfaces to optimize comfort and effectiveness.

Even more important than using inspiratory muscle aids are the evaluation of CPFs and introduction of methods for increasing them. Although expiratory muscle aids must be used for noninvasive ventilation to be effective over the long term, in none of the studies in which the use of nocturnal nasal IPPV or bilevel PAP ultimately terminated in acute respiratory failure and tracheotomy or death was their use reported.[727,745,765,777,925]

Patients with neuromuscular disease are rarely taught to prevent acute respiratory failure before it occurs and leads to intubation. This is in part because only about 3% of the NMD clinics in the U.S. teach expiratory muscle aids, and even fewer use the oximetry protocol.[615] Certainly, our experience with patients with NMD has been consistent with the following statement by one of the many physicians knowledgeable of respiratory muscle aids 45 years ago:

As experience with exsufflation with negative pressure increased, bronchoscopy was performed less frequently for the removal of bronchial secretions. At times bronchoscopic aspiration did relieve acute obstructive anoxia; but it is clear from the case reports that bronchoscopy contributed little to the overall control of bronchial secretions.... Had not artificial coughing been available, death might well have followed bronchoscopy in (several cases). The only possible value of bronchoscopy is to relieve obstruction due to secretions in the trachea and main bronchi. This is usually only of transient benefit, and as the relief can be more easily achieved with exsufflation with negative pressure, bronchoscopic aspiration should rarely, if ever, be performed in patients undergoing artificial respiration.[1028]

Thus, the medical community has little knowledge of mouthpiece IPPV, IAPVs, and expiratory aids. However, even nasal ventilation, about which there are numerous publications, is used suboptimally or incorrectly. This problem is best typified by a recent publication in an otherwise reputable journal. In this article, entitled "Randomized trial of preventive nasal ventilation in Duchenne muscular dystrophy,"[745] 70 patients with DMD, 15–16 years of age, were randomized to nocturnal nasal IPPV or to a control group that did not use nasal IPPV. The patients were reported to have VCs of 20–50% of predicted normal but neither hypercapnia nor hypoxia (PaO_2 exceeded 60 mmHg). The 70 patients came from 17 centers. There was no standardization in ventilator use, nasal interface selection, caregiver or patient training, or follow-up. The authors stated that 15 of the 35 nasal IPPV users admitted that they did not use nasal ventilation for the minimal 6 hours per night. The authors concluded by history that only 20 were "effectively ventilated" and made no effort to substantiate ventilator use by employing ventilators that indicate hours of utilization. Indeed, historical claims tend to overestimate ventilator utilization, especially the claims by asymptomatic users. This finding is particularly true when patients are told to use ventilators by clinicians with little or no experience in noninvasive ventilation, who prescribe inappropriate ventilator settings, and who make little effort to try various styles of interfaces. We have found that no interface style, not even one that is custom-molded,[926] is tolerated by a majority of patients. In addition, in this study, ventilator adjustments were made during daytime hours, not during sleep when insufflation leakage occurs. Thus, delivered volumes of 15 ml/kg can be grossly inadequate for nocturnal nasal IPPV. The stated goal of lowering the $PaCO_2$ by 10% is arbitrary, and the goal of decreasing $PaCO_2$ by "at least 10% of recorded daytime value(s)" is inappropriate when one considers that daytime values were already normal. Furthermore, there is no reason to believe that the patients used nasal ventilation correctly because no effort was made to determine whether the interfaces were worn with sufficient snugness to provide effective IPPV during sleep. Rather than performing painful daytime arterial blood gas sampling for patients with normal pretreatment gases and other inappropriate pulmonary function testing, the authors might have documented efficacy by showing improvements in nocturnal oximetry or transcutaneous or end-tidal carbon dioxide.[567,1005]

The tragedy of publishing such a report lies in the perpetuation of misconceptions that dissuade clinicians from appropriate use of noninvasive IPPV.[745] The authors reported that the mortality rate of their "nasal IPPV users" may have actually been increased and even recommended earlier resort to tracheotomy! Although the predominant cause of death was mucus plugging during chest infections, the subjects were not offered mouthpiece IPPV, air-stacking, or any cough assistance during these episodes. During chest infections, nasal congestion can preclude effective use of nasal ventilation, and patients benefit by being switched to lipseal IPPV. So it is no surprise that the patients died, subjects and controls. For those with "left ventricular hypokinesis," cardiac ejection fractions under 20% would be predictive of early mortality,[383] but this, too, was not taken into account.

Thus, the "study" succeeded in perpetuating the following misconceptions:

1. Nasal ventilation is the only noninvasive method to be considered; IPPV via mouthpieces, lipseals, oral-nasal interfaces, and body ventilator use were ignored.

2. When nocturnal use of nasal ventilation is no longer adequate, one must resort to tracheotomy.

3. Simple prescription of nasal ventilation can be enough without the participation of a specifically trained respiratory therapist to evaluate IPPV trials with various interfaces and to train patients in assisted coughing and oximetry feedback.

4. The primary difficulty in preventing mortality in patients with DMD lies in assisting nocturnal ventilation rather than in assisted coughing and treating cardiomyopathy (Chapter 5).

Finally, it must be recognized that portable volume-cycled ventilators are useful not only for providing IPPV via tracheostomy tubes but also for mouthpiece and nasal IPPV and IAPV use. Likewise, bilevel PAP machines are useful not only for providing nasal ventilation but also for tracheostomy and mouthpiece ventilation. Paradigms are difficult to break.

Case Studies

Il n'y a qu'un seul moyen d'enseigner, c'est de donner l'exemple.
There is only one way to teach, that is to provide the example.

·☞· Gustav Mahler

The following are the most common errors in the evaluation and management of patients with respiratory muscle dysfunction (primarily ventilatory impairment):

1. Misinterpretation of symptoms
2. Failure to perform spirometry with the patient in various positions and circumstances and to evaluate maximum insufflation capacity
3. Failure to evaluate CPF
4. Use of arterial blood gas analyses rather than noninvasive monitoring of SpO_2 and carbon dioxide tensions
5. Unnecessary resort to bronchoscopy, endotracheal intubation, and tracheostomy
6. Failure to deflate or eliminate tracheostomy tube cuffs
7. Use of tracheal and airway suctioning, oxygen, and bronchodilators instead of MAC at optimal pressures
8. Use of body ventilators instead of noninvasive IPPV
9. Use of CPAP or suboptimal span bilevel PAP
10. Use of pressure- rather than volume-cycled ventilators for patients capable of air-stacking
11. Failure to vary IPPV interfaces for fit, comfort, and efficacy
12. Failure to use mouthpiece IPPV or to extend use of noninvasive IPPV into daytime hours
13. Unnecessary ventilator use or inappropriate weaning
14. Failure to train patients in glossopharyngeal breathing (GPB)
15. Failure to extubate patients with no breathing tolerance to MAC and high-span bilevel PAP or noninvasive IPPV in ambient air

Case 1: Failure to Perform Spirometry with the Patient Supine, Inappropriate Oxygen Therapy, and Failure to Offer Various IPPV Interfaces

A man born in 1951 with an undifferentiated myopathy had severe scoliosis and complained of increasing dyspnea, headaches, orthopnea and leg edema. He had reported decreased ability to concentrate since 1975, from which time he slept sitting and had no breathing tolerance in the supine position. By 1984 he had severe continuous headaches, sleep and arousal dysfunction, violent nightmares, obtundation, and massive pretibial edema, despite taking 120 mg of furosemide daily for 2 years. The man "felt like I was dreaming when I was awake, and I did things without being aware of what I was doing." Falling asleep at 5- to 15-minute intervals, he burned his arm twice on the stove while cooking.

He developed pneumonia in May 1984 and was intubated for 5 weeks. From August 19, 1984 to May 6, 1985, his $PaCO_2$ ranged from 40 to 51 mmHg and his SpO_2 from 85% to 92% during daytime hours. End-tidal carbon dioxide was between 60 and 80 mmHg, with a maximum of 90 mmHg during four sleep studies.

In December 1985 he had jugular vein distention at 45°, massive pretibial edema with severe chronic stasis dermatitis, anasarca, cardiomegaly, a tender and enlarged liver with elevated liver function enzymes, pulmonary congestion, and polycythemia (hematocrit: 52.6). His VC (sitting) was 1410 ml (31% of normal), and his FEV_1/FVC was 90%. SpO_2 was 87%; $PaCO_2$ was 57 mmHg and increased to 63 mmHg when he received 0.5 L/min of supplemental oxygen by nasal cannula. However, obtundation and cor pulmonale worsened, and he developed pneumonia, for which he was hospitalized, intubated, and mechanically ventilated on two further occasions through June 1986.

In June 1986 polysomnography and capnography were performed with the patient in the semisupine position (Grass Model 78 D Polysomnograph, Grass Instruments Co., Quincy, MA). He had 118 hypopneas per hour, a mean SpO_2 of 55.2%, and end-tidal carbon dioxide levels to 91 mmHg. He had neither REM nor slow-wave sleep.

In August 1986 he was rehospitalized for dyspnea, obtundation, and further elevations of plasma liver function enzymes. Furosemide was increased to 160 mg daily, and he was placed on nocturnal nasal IPPV, which he used in the supine position (Fig. 14). Two weeks later, polysomnography was repeated while he used nasal IPPV and breathed room air. The results revealed normal total sleep and sleep efficiency, normal sleep latency and sleep onset, and REM sleep. He had 13 apneas/hypopneas per hour. SpO_2 was 48–63% during the first hour (12–1 AM), then 70–96% for the rest of the night. He was

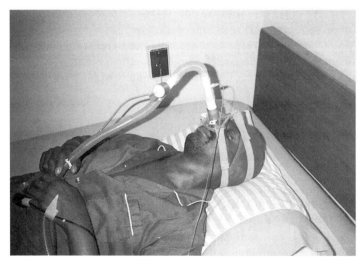

Figure 14. Nocturnal-only nasal IPPV corrected this patient's nocturnal SpO_2 from a mean of 55.2% to essentially normal.

discharged home using nasal IPPV and slept supine. His furosemide dosage was gradually lowered to 60 mg once per week. All hypoventilation symptoms resolved.

In January 1987, after 5 months of nocturnal nasal IPPV, he had only minimal residual dependent edema of the lower extremity. Liver size and enzymes were normal, and hematocrit was 40. VC was 1300 ml in the sitting position and 600 ml in the supine position. Breathing tolerance in the supine position continued to be negligible, but he did not require ventilator use when sitting. Although the baseline end-tidal carbon dioxide was 45–50 mmHg and SpO_2 was 88–92%, the $PaCO_2$ decreased to 33–38 mmHg, and the SpO_2 was greater than 95% within 2 minutes when he used nasal IPPV, sitting or supine, on assist/control mode with a delivered volume of 1150 ml (airway pressure: 30 cmH$_2$0).

Since he slept using nasal IPPV, insufflation leakage caused a decrease in air delivery pressure to a minimum of 26 cmH$_2$0. At this pressure the SpO_2 dropped to a low of 88%, and end-tidal carbon dioxide rose to the maximum of 49 mmHg. The airway pressure varied from 26 to 28 mmHg most of the night but was adequate to maintain a mean SpO_2 of 95%. His major complaint was that as soon as he discontinued nasal IPPV in the morning, he became dyspneic for the rest of the day. Nonetheless, he resisted using daytime mouthpiece IPPV.

He did well until he was hit by a truck and incurred fractures of the left tibia and fibula in January 1991. Even though he had been unable to walk for 8 years, his fractures were set under general anesthesia. However, because he was left supine and could not be weaned from the ventilator, he remained intubated, developed adult respiratory distress syndrome, self-extubated, and died while he was being re-intubated.

This patient demonstrates the following points:

1. Unessential surgery and general anesthesia should be avoided for people with minimal ventilatory reserve.
2. Because of failure to assess pulmonary function and ventilatory capacity with the patient recumbent and failure to use inspiratory muscle aids in a timely manner, he had ventilatory insufficiency for over 10 years, severe cor pulmonale, and ultimately fatal complications.
3. Exacerbation of hypoventilation by oxygen therapy can result in increased respiratory morbidity and hospitalizations.
4. A variety of IPPV interfaces, oral and nasal, should be tried, and the patient should be allowed to choose.

Case 2: Overreliance on Tracheostomy, Failure to Deflate Cuff, Failure to Evaluate for Home Care

A patient with DMD who had lost the ability to walk at age 10 years and had severe scoliosis developed symptomatic hypercapnia at age 26 with a VC of 46% of predicted normal. He was placed on nocturnal mouthpiece IPPV, which he used without lipseal retention. Three years later he required mouthpiece IPPV for increasing periods during daytime hours. He used it 24 hours per day from age 30 to 34, at which point his VC was 340 ml or 13% of predicted normal. Because he was never offered a lipseal retention system for nocturnal mouthpiece IPPV,[752] he had frequent sleep arousals and was convinced by his physicians to undergo elective tracheotomy during his first hospitalization at age 34. However, with the tracheostomy he developed pneumonia. His dysphagia worsened, malnutrition developed, and a gastrostomy tube and Hickman catheter were placed for alimentation and long-term antibiotic therapy.

Once the patient was stable, it was discovered that he could not be discharged home because his wife was a poliomyelitis survivor who could walk but had no upper extremity function and could not perform tracheal suctioning. Therefore, after a hospitalization of 6 months, the patient was forced to return to his parents' home. Because the tracheostomy tube cuff was never deflated, he could no longer verbalize. He received 24-hour oxygen therapy, and the Hickman catheter was not removed. At age 35, the family sent me a copy of his hospital records. The tracheostomy tube cuff was still inflated; he still received supplemental oxygen; he no longer had sufficient stamina to sit in a wheelchair and had not been placed into one since hospital discharge two and one-half years earlier; and he was extremely depressed because he could no longer live with his wife. I was told that the physicians had informed the family two and one-half years earlier that he was "being sent home to die and the oxygen will make him more comfortable." He died two months later, before he could be evaluated for decannulation, when he developed sepsis from the Hickman catheter.

This patient's depression and ultimate demise were the result of unnecessary tracheotomy, unnecessary long-term cuff inflation, an unnecessary central line, and failure to consider postdischarge tracheostomy management. It has been shown that with an optimal tracheostomy tube diameter and some residual vocal cord function, virtually no patient with primarily ventilation impairment requires cuff inflation unless pulmonary compliance is very poor.[754] Indeed, patients with DMD have sufficient bulbar musculature to speak and do not require tracheostomy tubes at any age.[655,1051]

Case 3: Inadequate Pressure Assist Ventilation, Inappropriate Use of Pressure- Rather Than Volume-cycled Ventilation, Failure to Extend Nocturnal Use of Noninvasive IPPV into Daytime Hours, Inappropriate Use of Oxygen, Unnecessary Emphasis on Tracheostomy

A cognitively intact patient with DMD underwent Harrington rod placement for scoliosis relief in 1989 at age 14 years. He remained stable until February 1995 when a chest infection caused fatigue and cyanosis. His $PaCO_2$ was found to be 88 mmHg. He was treated with low-span bilevel PAP (IPAP of 12 cmH_2O, EPAP of 6 cmH_2O) in a local emergency department with some improvement, then sent home using these settings nocturnally with supplemental oxygen. However, during the next month he had frequent nocturnal arousals with tachycardia, saying "breathe" to himself. He was, therefore, readmitted. Because the hospital had no policy regarding bilevel PAP, use of his ventilator was not permitted. On the first morning after admission he was found to be comatose with a $PaCO_2$ of 99 mmHg. The physicians advised his parents to "let him go," but they did not concur. He was placed back on low-span bilevel PAP and developed severe anoxic encephalopathy. I recommended discontinuing oxygen therapy and using the high spans of IPAP (18 cmH_2O) and EPAP (2 cmH_2O) to normalize SpO_2 without supplemental oxygen therapy. This recommendation, however, was not followed.

Because he remained precariously underventilated, his parents were urged to permit tracheotomy. At our urging against tracheostomy, his parents resisted and brought him to our clinic. However, because the hospital felt that it was hazardous to discharge or transfer him using a BiPAP machine (Respironics, Inc., Murrysville, PA) and the ambulance "did not have oxygen," his parents had to sign him out against medical advice and bring him themselves. We were advised to admit him for tracheotomy.

In our outpatient clinic we converted him to nasal IPPV, using the assist-control mode on a PLV-100 portable volume-cycled ventilator. He and his family were instructed in the MAC protocol that included discontinuing oxygen therapy. His SpO_2 became normal and remained so; he was sent home. Despite now requiring full-time noninvasive IPPV for 7 years, he has had no subsequent respiratory complications and has regained normal cognitive function.

This case demonstrates failure to use bilevel PAP at adequate spans, inappropriate use of pressure- rather than a volume-cycled ventilator for a patient who required more than nocturnal aid and was capable of air-stacking, unnecessarily protracted hospitalization, failure to use expiratory muscle aids to eliminate airway secretions, hazardous use of oxygen therapy, needless emphasis on tracheostomy, and the paradigm paralysis associating BiPAP machines with nasal-only low-span bilevel PAP and managing ventilatory failure like sleep-disordered breathing.

Case 4: Hazardous Oxygen Therapy, Overemphasis on Tracheostomy, Increased Respiratory Muscle Endurance by Rest with IPPV

A floppy neonate was clinically diagnosed with probable SMA at 2 years of age in 1958. Despite the inability to sit or walk and development of severe scoliosis, she achieved a Ph.D. and worked full-time as a leisure counselor from 1979 to 1991, when severe carbon dioxide retention caused symptoms that prevented continued employment. Her symptoms included hypersomnolence with sleep episodes every 5–10 minutes, confusion, "black-outs," depression, headaches, nightmares, frequent nocturnal arousals, and difficult morning arousals. She also had polycythemia (hematocrit: 55). She had been evaluated by physicians in three NMD clinics in Pennsylvania, had been prescribed continuous oxygen therapy that only exacerbated her hypercapnia and hypersomnolence, and was advised to undergo tracheotomy or she would die in a matter of weeks.

After reading an article about our approach, she came to our clinic. She was extremely depressed. Her VC was 120 ml, she weighed 37 lb, and she had greater than 120° of scoliosis. Her baseline SpO_2 while breathing room air was 70–78%; when she received 1 liter of oxygen, it was greater than 94%. End-tidal carbon dioxide, however, increased to over 80 mmHg. As she fell asleep breathing room air, her oximeter read 37–44%; with oxygen therapy it read 70%.

Oxygen therapy was discontinued, and she was instructed in the use of respiratory muscle aids and oximetry feedback. She was immediately able to maintain normal SpO_2 when using mouthpiece IPPV and breathing room air while awake. She also maintained normal SpO_2 when using nasal IPPV during sleep. All symptoms of hypercapnia cleared, and she returned to gainful employment in 1 month. Because her compensatory metabolic alkalosis cleared and her ventilatory drive normalized, she almost immediately became dependent on noninvasive IPPV with virtually no breathing tolerance. However, after 1–2 months, she developed up to 4 hours of breathing tolerance while maintaining normal SpO_2. Despite increased ventilatory ability, no change was observed in her VC. Over the past 11 years she has had no hospitalizations despite four chest infections that she managed at home with continuous noninvasive IPPV and MAC. She continues to work full-time.

This patient demonstrates the hazards of oxygen therapy and unnecessary insistence on tracheostomy. She also demonstrates that breathing tolerance (inspiratory muscle endurance) can initially be entirely lost while ventilatory drive resets but can subsequently increase with the inspiratory muscle rest provided by noninvasive IPPV.

Case 5: Overreliance on Tracheostomy, Benefits of Glossopharyngeal Breathing

A 43-year-old journalist with limb-girdle muscular dystrophy had been using IPPV via a tracheostomy with a VC of 200 ml and no breathing tolerance for 5.5 years. During this time, like other tracheostomy IPPV users, she could not be safely left alone to work and had experienced numerous febrile episodes that were treated with intravenous antibiotics. In July of 1992 her tracheostomy tube was removed and the site closed. She was converted to using daytime mouthpiece and nighttime nasal IPPV (see Fig. 2 of Chapter 1). She also mastered GPB sufficiently for up to 8 hours of breathing tolerance. GPB permitted her to work safely at home alone. With a maximum GPB single-breath capacity of 1200 ml, she was also able to better raise her voice and cough.

Case 6: Unnecessary Endotracheal Intubation, Extubation and Conversion to 24-hour Noninvasive IPPV, Postextubation Ventilator Weaning

In 1990 an 18-year-old boy with DMD developed acute respiratory failure during an otherwise benign chest infection and, without access to expiratory aids, was intubated in a local hospital. He was intubated even though he had been previously instructed in how to use mouthpiece and nasal IPPV and air-stacked daily. During intubation his VC decreased from an 800-ml baseline to 200 ml, and he had no breathing tolerance. I was called at this point. Because he knew how to receive IPPV noninvasively, he was extubated and switched directly to continuous noninvasive IPPV and the use of MAC. With aggressive MAC, his VC immediately increased to 400 ml, but he continued to have no breathing tolerance and airway secretions remained profuse for 5 days, at which point he weaned to nocturnal nasal IPPV and went home using MAC as needed. In 1996 he began to require daytime mouthpiece as well as nocturnal nasal IPPV. He has thus far had five chest infections that have been managed at home with the oximetry, MAC protocol, and no further hospitalizations. During one such episode, nasal congestion rendered nasal IPPV ineffective, and he developed respiratory distress with a $PaCO_2$ of 55 mmHg. When given the choice between switching to lipseal IPPV or using nasal decongestants, he chose the latter and had no further elevations of end-tidal carbon dioxide or significant $dSpO_2s$. Hospitalization was avoided despite temperature elevations to 104° and leucocytosis during at least three of the five infections. This patient also demonstrates postextubation ventilator weaning. He has required continuous noninvasive IPPV for 7 years.

Case 7: Noninvasive Nocturnal Blood Gas Monitoring, Need to Customize and Vary Interfaces, Oximetry Feedback, Improvement in Respiratory Muscle Endurance by Rest with IPPV

A patient with DMD had stopped walking at 30 months of age in 1972. His VC plateaued at 1050 ml before 9 years of age. Spinal surgery was refused, and his spinal curve was 114° to the left (Cobb technique) in 1994. From January 1985 to September 1987 he was hospitalized five times for dyspnea, difficulties with managing airway secretions, and chest infections. His mother said that he had frequent "mucus attacks," which she described as episodes of profuse salivation, airway congestion, and uncontrolled drooling.

In October of 1987, he presented with a temperature of 104°, complaints of chronic headaches, difficulty with swallowing, weight loss, VC of 280 ml, and profuse mucopurulent airway secretions. Manually assisted coughing was not effective because of severe scoliosis. He received antibiotics and required intravenous fluids because of dehydration. $PaCO_2$ on admission was 57 mmHg. His SpO_2 varied from 89 to 94% when awake with an end-tidal carbon dioxide of 50–54 mmHg.

Trials of mouthpiece IPPV failed because of inadequacy of oropharyngeal muscles to grab the mouthpiece. He was taught and used nasal IPPV during the daytime with end-tidal carbon dioxide and pulse oximetry feedback. In this manner end-tidal carbon dioxide was maintained below 43 mmHg and SpO_2 over 94%. He napped using nasally delivered assist/control volumes of 560 ml (mask pressure: 23–25 cmH_2O) at a rate of 16 per minute. His expiratory volumes were 500 ml while awake, with the mouth open or closed. During overnight sleep monitoring using nasal IPPV, end-tidal carbon dioxide varied from 40 to 47 mmHg, and SpO_2 averaged 95%, with a low of 85%, and few $dSpO_2$s. He was discharged home using nasal IPPV nocturnally.

The following week his mother stated that he felt stronger and was eating better. "Mucus attacks" were less frequent and less severe but were not completely relieved until he began cardiac medications (Chapter 5). He no longer required daytime ventilatory aid to maintain SpO_2 greater than 94%, except occasionally, when he was tired. Repeat nocturnal sleep studies were performed with ventilator-delivered volumes of 1200 ml. The mean SpO_2 was 96–97%, and the maximum recorded end-tidal carbon dioxide was 40 cmH_2O. The low pressure alarm, which was set at 14 cmH_2O, sounded often for a few seconds and about twice per night for longer periods. The alarms correlated with the SpO_2 dips that at no time were lower than 82%. He now had excellent control of his secretions, and his swallowing improved. His VC increased from 270 ml on October 27, 1987 to 330 ml on February 3, 1988. He gained weight and was able to sit in his wheelchair all day without fatigue.

This patient had four subsequent chest infections with fevers, elevated white blood cell counts, and profuse mucopurulent airway secretions during his first 15 months using nocturnal nasal IPPV. With each one he was managed at home using the oximetry MAC protocol and full-time noninvasive IPPV. On no occasion was supplemental oxygen administered. Sudden dips in SpO_2 that could not be corrected by taking large insufflation volumes were corrected by MAC. With only 1 L/sec of unassisted CPF, he required MAC about 4 times per hour during chest infections.

During a severe chest infection in August 1988 his SpO_2 ranged from 88 to 93%, PaO_2 from 62 to 70 mmHg, and end-tidal carbon dioxide remained normal as he used nasal IPPV and frequent MAC around the clock. The patient apparently had diffuse microscopic atelectasis that could not be identified on chest radiographs. Desaturations as low as 70% were immediately corrected to a baseline of 91–93% following MAC. With continued aggressive MAC his SpO_2 baseline returned to normal over a 4-day period, and he weaned back to nocturnal-only nasal IPPV.

Except during chest infections the patient used nasal IPPV only overnight and for short periods during the day until July 1989 when his total sitting time was down to less than 2 hours per day. He complained of extreme fatigue, frequent "mucus attacks," dysphagia, and weight loss. His VC was 250 ml. He then began to use nasal IPPV 24 hours per day. As a result, his symptoms once again cleared, and he returned to sitting in his wheelchair 16 hours per day and maintained an active lifestyle that included frequent interstate travel with his family. Because of the need for 24-hour aid, he alternated the use of four commercial CPAP and two custom-made nasal interfaces. For 3 years he used only IVALs (interfaces for ventilator-assisted living),[926] which he alternated over 12-hour periods around the clock (see Fig. 12 of Chapter 10). This approach sufficiently redistributed pressure around his nose to avert discomfort and skin irritation despite the requirement of increasingly higher pressures on the retention straps to avert insufflation leaks because mask pressures gradually increased to over 40 cmH_2O as a result of a chronic pneumothorax and severe scoliosis.

Nocturnal SpO_2 monitoring, which was repeated every 12 months since August 1988, demonstrated mean SpO_2 at 95% or greater with a mean of 1.7 4% dips in SpO_2 per hour and infrequent dips below 90%. His unassisted CPFs were less than 50 L/min. With air-stacking of the nasal insufflations he generated CPF of 110 L/min; although fully assisted CPFs were only 110 L/min, he used MI-E very effectively.[265]

On May 3, 1995 the ventilator-delivered volumes were generating interface pressures averaging 52 cmH_2O; nocturnal mean SpO_2 had decreased to 92% (on room air); airway secretion production had increased; and he had become febrile with a white blood cell count of 16,000. He decompensated from a massive pneumothorax with complete collapse of the right lung. After chest tube placement the mild dyspnea was relieved, and ventilator pressures normalized with the same delivered volumes. Seven hours later, however, he developed repeated episodes of ventricular tachyarrhythmias and died. This patient had a severe cardiomyopathy. Correction of his hemodynamic status led to acute cardiac decompensation. This was the only patient of the 725 noted in Table 1 who developed a clinically apparent pneumothorax.

This patient demonstrates the following points:

1. The utility of oximetry feedback and sleep monitoring
2. The need for switching between various nasal interfaces for IPPV
3. Nasal IPPV can be used effectively 24 hours per day over the long term when the lips are too weak for effective mouthpiece IPPV, when scoliosis is too severe for use of an IAPV, and even when patients have no breathing tolerance, pulmonary compliance is poor, and ventilator-delivered volumes generate interface pressures exceeding 40 cmH_2O,
4. Breathing tolerance can increase with the respiratory muscle rest provided by noninvasive IPPV.
5. Use of respiratory muscle aids can be critical for avoiding pulmonary complications and hospitalizations.
6. Volume-cycled ventilator gauge pressures should be monitored and, when they are increasing, chest radiographs should be performed.
7. MAC can be effective even when manually assisted CPF cannot exceed 180 L/min.
8. "Mucus attacks," which were most likely due in large part to heart failure, can be relieved by normalizing alveolar ventilation.

Case 8

A 49-year-old woman with a congenital myopathy had a long history of fatigue, difficulties with concentration, dyspnea, and hypersomnolence. She developed pneumonia, was hospitalized, and underwent tracheotomy in February 1990. She was weaned from IPPV and breathed through an open tracheostomy tube. Unfortunately, she was also placed on continuous supplemental oxygen therapy and developed increasing hypercapnia ($PaCO_2$: 55–93 mmHg) over a 3-week period. She could not tolerate plugging of the tube. Because of chronic fatigue she was placed again on tracheostomy IPPV and continued to receive continuous oxygen therapy. Further attempts at ventilator weaning involved alternating the use of diminishing rate and periods of SIMV with CPAP. Her arterial blood gases typically demonstrated normal pH, PaO_2 of 130–170 mmHg, $PaCO_2$ of 65 up to 74 mmHg, and elevated bicarbonate levels. The patient lived in a communal Ashram. Her caregivers were not relatives. Because no one could or would be permitted to take responsibility for tracheal suctioning, she could not be discharged.

After 5 months of unsuccessful ventilator weaning she was transferred to our service for decannulation on July 27, 1990. Supplemental oxygen therapy, bronchodilators, and theophylline were discontinued on admission with no untoward effects. Using oximetry feedback, she normalized SpO_2 and $PaCO_2$ by breathing more deeply through an open tracheostomy tube for short periods before tiring. Decannulation was performed on admission, and she was ventilated by a chest shell ventilator for 18 hours while the tracheostomy site closed (see Fig. 12 in Chapter 1). During overnight chest shell use her mean SpO_2 was 89%; she had a maximum end-tidal carbon dioxide of 55 mmHg; and she had been uncomfortable and had vomited twice. With discontinuance of the chest shell ventilator she could maintain normal SpO_2 by deep breathing supplemented by periods of mouthpiece IPPV. She was placed on nasal IPPV for nocturnal ventilatory aid. Using nocturnal nasal IPPV her mean SpO_2 was 97% with a low of 89%. The airway secretions that had been due to tracheostomy tube irritation were cleared by MAC for two days, at which point she no longer had sputum to clear. She was discharged to the Ashram on the fourth day after admission. Although at discharge her breathing tolerance was less than 2 hours, the maintenance of normal alveolar ventilation around the clock by noninvasive IPPV kept her symptom free. She returned to her active career as a professional writer and counselor and used noninvasive IPPV for 16–20 hours per day for 10 years without further respiratory difficulties.

Case 9

A 26-year-old man with DMD had become wheelchair-dependent at age 12 in 1983. He remained in good health until October 1996 when a cold developed into pneumonia and respiratory failure. He was hospitalized for 7 days without requiring intubation. In November another chest infection developed into pneumonia and respiratory failure, for which he was hospitalized for 4 more days, again without requiring intubation. Then, one morning in December 1996, he was found in hypercapnic coma. He was hospitalized for 32 days and intubated for 4 days and then underwent tracheotomy. He was discharged to a nursing home, where he remained for the next 7 months for tracheostomy care and continuous ventilator dependence that his parents felt they could not manage at home. However, since his parents wanted him to return home, they arranged for him to be transferred to our service in July 1997 for decannulation and transition to noninvasive aids.

On admission supplemental oxygen was discontinued. The patient's VC was 650 ml, SpO_2 averaged 92%, and end-tidal carbon dioxide was 38 mmHg. He had gross atelectasis on chest radiograph. His tracheostomy tube was changed to a fenestrated cuffed Shiley tube, and trials using mouthpiece and nasal IPPV were begun. He had no breathing tolerance and noted that he had had none since being intubated. At one point the patient's VC was 250 ml and SpO_2 was 87%. After MAC the VC immediately returned to 650 ml and the SpO_2 increased to the 92% baseline. MAC was used at intervals of at least 30 minute for 24 hours while he was awake to reverse $dSpO_2$s. Within 24 hours after admission his baseline SpO_2 had normalized to 97%. The fenestrated tracheostomy tube was then removed, and nasal IPPV was begun using the PLV-100 portable volume-cycled positive-pressure ventilator. After continuous nasal IPPV for 2 days, he was switched to daytime mouthpiece IPPV and required 2–3 mouthpiece IPPVs per minute. Over the next 4 days, he required assisted ventilation less and less frequently. His tracheostomy closed completely after 1 week, and SpO_2 continued to be normal. By the time of discharge home on day 8, VC was 840 ml, assisted CPFs were 200 L/m, and he required only nocturnal ventilatory assistance using a PLV-100, an oximeter, and a Cough-Assist for home use. He has subsequently had one chest infection that was managed at home with continuous noninvasive IPPV, expiratory aids, and oximetry feedback. Six years after discharge home he remains without a tracheostomy tube and has had no further hospitalizations.

This patient had never had any speech or swallowing difficulties and was also a good candidate for decannulation because his assisted CPFs were over 160 L/min. In addition, the patient and his care providers were cooperative in learning the respiratory aid/oximetry protocol. This case demonstrates that, despite 7 months of continuous ventilator dependence with no breathing tolerance, decannulation and transition to noninvasive IPPV can result in weaning to nocturnal-only aid for the reasons noted in Chapter 10. Even patients with DMD who are generally not good candidates for GPB should, under certain circumstances, be decannulated and switched to noninvasive alternatives. Decannulation and access to a variety of noninvasive inspiratory muscle aids and IPPV interfaces can facilitate discharge to the community.

Believe in noninvasive ventilation. Indeed, "When ye encounter the nonbelievers, strike off their heads 'til ye have made a great slaughter among them, and of the rest, make fast the fetters."

"And by troops shall the unbelievers be driven towards hell until when they reach it its gates shall be open....and it shall be said to them enter ye the gates of hell, therein, to dwell forever, and wretched the abode of the arrogant."

ꞏ☞ꞏ Sura 47, "Mohammed", page 382, and Sura 39, "The Troops," page 260. In The Qur'an, translation by J. M. Rodwell in 1909, London, J. M. Dent & Sons, Ltd., 1978.

Chapter 12

Pediatric Respiratory Management

Is it worth the investment?
Is it worthy of your time?
What is the value of this one life?

　　　　　　　　•☞• Richard Clingman, Web Master for DoctorBach.com

Incidence of Ventilator Use

There are 500,000 people in the United States, or 0.15% of the population, with pediatric neuromuscular diseases (NMDs)[1073] and many more with thoracic wall restrictive lung disease. Neonatal ventilatory failure requiring ventilatory support is most common in NMDs such as spinal muscular atrophy (SMA) type 1. It also occurs with certain congenital malformations such as Pierre Robin syndrome, congenital central hypoventilation, and bronchopulmonary dysplasia. It can result from subglottic stenosis due to damage from intubation or tracheostomy. Ventilatory/respiratory failure also occurs in older children and adolescents; the diagnoses are listed in Table 1 of Chapter 1 (see Chapters 9 through 11). Surveys of the United States, Western Europe, and Japan indicate that the use of home mechanical ventilation is increasing rapidly for children.[1074] In young patients with NMD, most episodes of acute respiratory failure result from inability to eliminate effectively airway secretions and mucus during otherwise benign intercurrent chest infections;[14] for patients with Duchenne muscular dystrophy (DMD) the rate is as high as 90%.

Conventional Invasive Mechanical Ventilation

Although the use of bilevel PAP and noninvasive IPPV as alternatives to intubation for acute respiratory failure has now been extensively described for adults,[1044] there have been no comparable pediatric studies. Indeed, small children with weak expiratory muscles and inability to cooperate with MAC are much less likely to avoid intubation during intercurrent chest infections than older cooperative patients.[742] Intubated children who have difficulty weaning from ventilatory support or who are thought to be unable to expectorate airway secretions effectively through conventional methods undergo tracheotomy. When the tubes are not removed after the acute episode, the users remain full-time ventilator-dependent for the same reasons that adults with tubes and minimal vital capacity (VC) become or remain continuously ventilator-dependent (see Chapter 9). In addition, ventilator-dependent infants with tubes do not develop the ability to speak. Although the complications of intubation and tracheotomy described for adults (Chapter 8) also occur in children, incidences are less well known. The trachea, however, is much more easily damaged by tracheostomy and cuff inflation in young children than it is in adults. The most common complication is subglottic stenosis.[1075] Because of the growth and greater plasticity of pediatric tissues, orthodontic deformities and facial flattening are more likely in children. The incidence of tracheostomy tube dislodgment in a 59-bed pediatric subacute facility was recently reported. A total of 561 dislodgments resulted in six emergency calls over a period of 4.5 years. There were 5.4 dislodgments per 1000 days (total of 35,096 patient-days) for patients with tracheostomy tubes who were not using ventilators and 18.8 dislodgments per 1000 days (total of 19,564 patient days) for patients using IPPV. Thus, life-threatening dislodgments are more common with ventilator use.[1076] There has also been one case report of a premature infant who developed cerebellar necrosis as a result of using ventilation via an oronasal interface.[1077] On the other hand, small children are less susceptible to skin pressure discomfort and ulcers.

Only uncuffed tracheostomy tubes should be used for children with primarily ventilatory impairment unless aspiration of upper airway secretions causes a continuous decrease in baseline SpO_2 below 95%. As for adults, excessive insufflation leakage can usually be managed by some combination of increasing the diameter of the tube, increasing air delivery volumes, or, if necessary, placing a tracheostomy tube with a cuff but leaving the cuff deflated.

After 10 years of age the shape of the larynx changes from conical to cylindrical, and the narrowest part of the airway and the trachea becomes more resilient to contact with the tube and cuff.[1075] Silver tubes are then often used because of their greater internal-to-external diameter ratio for patients with very narrow airways. The position and size of the tubes relative to the patient should be checked by radiograph at least every 6–12 months to optimize air delivery and minimize tracheal damage.

Goals of Intervention

As for older patients, the goals of intervention are to maintain lung compliance and normal alveolar ventilation at all times and to maximize cough flows. In addition, because of difficulties with cooperation in very young children, acute episodes of respiratory failure must be managed in the manner described in this chapter so that the child can reach the age when cooperation is no longer a problem and morbidity and mortality can be avoided without hospitalization.[1048]

Lung Mobilization

The lungs and chest walls of infants with NMD do not grow normally because of inability to take deep breaths. The results include severely restricted pulmonary volumes, decreased pulmonary compliance, and undergrowth of the thoracic cage (Chapter 9). In addition to maintaining compliance, range-of-motion therapy in pediatric patients promotes more normal lung growth and prevents chest deformity. Because small infants cannot air-stack or cooperate to receive maximal insufflations, all infants with SMA or other NMDs who have paradoxical chest wall motion require nocturnal high-span bilevel PAP to rest inspiratory muscles, prevent pectus excavatum, and promote lung growth. Even without the use of maximal insufflation therapy, the use of high-span bilevel PAP during sleep completely prevents pectus excavatum for children with SMA type 1[742] and quite possibly for other infants with paradoxical breathing.

Inspiration-timed deep insufflations can be provided via an oral-nasal interface for children over 9 months of age, along with concomitant abdominal compression to prevent abdominal expansion while directing the air into the upper thorax. Children can become cooperative with deep insufflation therapy by 11–30 months of age. This therapy is usually performed two or three times daily with the delivery of 10–15 maximal insufflations via a manual resuscitator or a Cough-Assist (J. H. Emerson Co., Cambridge, MA) at a pressure of 40 cmH$_2$O timed to inspiration. Although no data support this approach, periodic maximal insufflations may complement nocturnal bilevel PAP in preventing pectus excavatum and promoting lung growth. Barois has treated over 100 infants with SMA, 9 months and older, with regular deep insufflation therapy and later provided them with mouthpieces or nasal interfaces for nocturnal aid. She reported that this treatment ameliorated the restrictive pulmonary syndrome.[1078,1079] She also used an abdominal binder so that the insufflated air entered the upper thorax rather than ventilated only the lower lobes. We recommend the use of this maximal insufflation technique by children over 9 months of age, but we also recommend using the palm of the hand to restrict abdominal expansion rather than an abdominal binder. By becoming accustomed to the positive-pressure insufflations, some infants have become able to use MI-E effectively via oronasal interfaces for airway clearance during chest infections by as early as 11 months of age. Nocturnal high-span bilevel PAP and perhaps daytime maximal insufflations are usually the only respiratory interventions that such children need between chest infections.

Maintenance of Alveolar Ventilation

Intermittent Abdominal Pressure Ventilator

The Exsufflation Belt (Respironics) is made in three sizes for adults. IAPVs can also be improvised for children from blood pressure cuffs. Adult and pediatric sizes are also custom-made in France (Hôpital Gui de Chauliac, Montpelier).[1080,1081]

Negative-pressure Body Ventilators

Although negative-pressure body ventilators (NPBVs; Fig. 1) were the first methods of long-term ventilatory support for children as well as adults, there is little interest in them today because of the efficacy of noninvasive positive-pressure ventilation and the fact that NPBVs often cause obstructive sleep apneas. Nevertheless, occasional reports continue to suggest their utility for infants and other children.[1082]

Noninvasive Positive-pressure Interfaces

Whereas adults play the major role in choosing the appropriate interface, for infants the success of noninvasive ventilation depends on the clinician's choice of appropriate interfaces and ventilator. The choice is especially important because children have greater difficulties with synchronization to and triggering of the ventilator. There are also greater limitations in commercially available pediatric interfaces. The interface often has to be tailored to fit the child. One can often improvise its construction from supplies commonly available in the pediatric intensive care unit.

The simple Respironics (Murrysville, PA) 15-mm and 22-mm angled mouthpieces that are so commonly used for adults (see Fig. 21 of Chapter 10) can also be used by

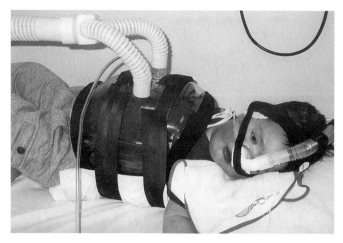

Figure 1. Child, now 8.5 years old, with SMA type 1 who has required high-span nasal bilevel PAP continuously since 5 months of age. He used an Adam circuit with small nasal pillows around the clock. CPAP prongs of an infant CPAP circuit (Hudson, Inc., Temecula, CA; 15.0-French CPAP Nasal Prongs) were cut off and taped into the pillows. Chest shell ventilator use was tried, but delivery of comparable volumes of air was not possible and application of the shell was considered by the parents to be inconvenient and by the patient to be less comfortable. He now uses a Nasal-Aire interface that does not impair vision.

children who have good oromotor control after age 4 years. The air flow resistance or back pressure created by the 15-mm angled mouthpiece prevents the low-pressure alarm of the volume ventilator from sounding when the alarm is set at its minimum level (2 cmH$_2$O). Thus, the alarms will not sound between mouthpiece-assisted insufflations when the patient is eating or speaking. The standard pulmonary function study mouthpieces can also be used. They are, however, straight and too wide for young children and may not prevent the low-pressure alarms from sounding.

For nocturnal use, mouthpiece IPPV is best delivered via a mouthpiece with Lipseal phalange and cloth retention straps with Velcro closures (see Fig. 6 of Chapter 10) or via Oracle. Unfortunately, the Lipseal comes only in sizes for adolescents and adults. The youngest child who has used this device was 12 years of age.

There are now many manufactures of adult-size disposable noninvasive interfaces and headgear of various sizes. Some can also be used by children (see Table 1 of Chapter 10). The Adam circuit consists of a nasal shell (standard or narrow sizes) into which nasal pillows are inserted (small, medium, or large) and connected to a swivel adapter and headgear. An angle adapter is also available for more angled noses. Only the model with small pillows and narrow shell is useful for children (Fig. 1). The Adam circuit is nondisposable and can be sterilized for reuse. One advantage of this system is the lack of contact with the bridge of the nose. The system also has an easier and more comfortable seal when pressure requirements are high. Some patients experience nasal irritation or congestion when using this interface. For very small infants, another option is to cut off the CPAP prongs of infant CPAP circuits (Hudson 15.0-French CPAP Nasal Prongs) and tape them into the prongs of the small adult Adam circuit (see Fig. 1). The larger prongs of the Adam circuit seal the child's nostrils, and the circuit's suspension system retains the interface.

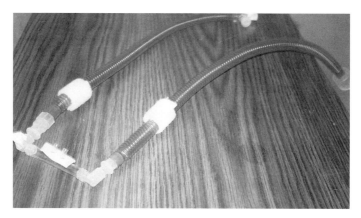

Figure 2. Hudson nasal prongs sealed at one end and connected to the ventilation circuit using intervening tubing adapters.

Another option for infants below 6 months age is to seal one end of the Hudson nasal prongs circuit and connect the other end to the ventilation circuit using intervening tubing adapters (Fig. 2). The prongs themselves are passed through foamy material such as the nasal bridge cushions of a Respironics CPAP mask (Fig. 3) or the center of a Duoderm patch (Bristol Myers Squibb Co., New York) that adheres to the nostril linings and seals the nasal orifices. These prongs are designed for infants weighing between 1500 and 2000 grams. Custom headgear is prepared to secure the interface. We have had success with these prongs in infants up to 2 years of age, at which time we often switch to the Respironics pediatric petite nasal interface (Fig. 4). The latter is generally effective for children from 6 months to 4 years of age and is the most widely used interface for small children.

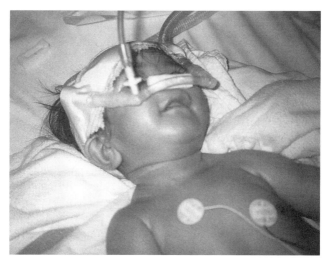

Figure 3. Infant with SMA type 1 using CPAP prongs passed through the nasal bridge cushions of a Respironics CPAP mask that adheres to the nostril linings and seals the nasal orifices.

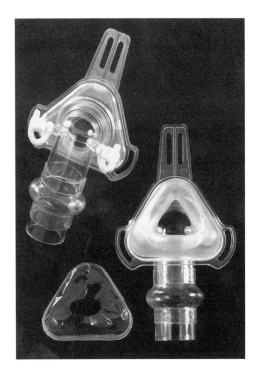

Figure 4. Respironics small-child mask/comfort flap, front and back views.

Respironics, Inc. makes nondisposable pediatric oral-nasal interfaces for children from 6 months to 4 years of age and 2–8 years of age as well as a petite mask for older children. These inexpensive interfaces are adequate for the majority of children. During use, the bridge of the nose is the most likely site of discomfort. Respironics, Inc. also makes pediatric "bubble" nasal and oral-nasal interfaces. These interfaces include inner flaps that act like valves as ventilator-delivered air pushes them against the face. They are available in various sizes and shapes. Occasionally, adult-sized nasal interfaces can be used as oral-nasal interfaces for small children. Because of their wider surface area, however, it is much more difficult to eliminate air leaks when oral-nasal designs are used.

Nasal ventilation is the most practical means of noninvasive support for small children for several reasons: lipseals are not made for small children, small children have no teeth, their lips are too weak to grab a mouthpiece, they may not be able to cooperate with a mouthpiece, pediatric exsufflation (IAPV) belts are difficult to procure, and infants are obligate nasal breathers. All patients are offered trials of various styles of interfaces and the ones that are most comfortable and associated with the least leakage are used. Occasionally, interfaces of different styles are alternated nightly and during the day as well when ventilatory assistance is needed around the clock. A design that can be used for daytime as well as nocturnal aid without hindering a child's vision is molded to cover the nostrils (Fig. 5). The retention system also serves as the conduit for the air delivery (see Figs. 2 and 13 of Chapter 10). The Nasal-Aire interface (Fisher-Paykel, Inc.) similarly ventilates without hindering vision.

No attempt is made to eliminate all insufflation leakage by tightening the interface straps. Ventilator volumes and pressures are adjusted to compensate for small air leakages.

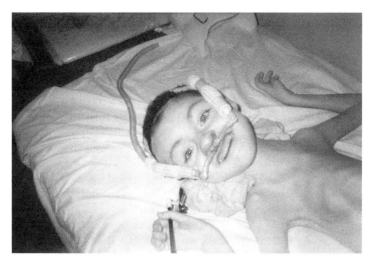

Figure 5. Patient using nasal interface molded to seal the nostrils and attached to the Hudson prongs circuit.

Lipseal IPPV is recommended for older children with signs of discomfort, skin irritation, or nasal congestion, as during upper respiratory tract infections.

Ventilator Choice and Settings

Ventilator choice depends on age; VC; lung and chest wall compliance; extent of gas exchange impairment; size and mobility of the patient; and ability to cooperate. As for adults, pressure- and volume-cycled portable ventilators are available for noninvasive ventilation. In general, pressure-cycled ventilators have the advantage that they are triggered by flow sensing. In intubated patients, flow-sensing ventilators significantly decrease the work of breathing by comparison with pressure-sensing ventilators. Flow sensing also results in a shortened response time for ventilators and, therefore, can be effective even with the high respiratory rates of small children. This approach tends to prevent ventilator-patient dyssynchrony and increases patient tolerance. Use of pressure-cycled ventilators may involve a lesser risk of barotrauma, but effectiveness is limited in patients with poor pulmonary compliance who may not receive adequate tidal volumes.

Patient-triggering is not always possible for very small and weak patients for whom rate adjustment becomes highly important. This is typically the case for infants extubated to nasal bilevel PAP. To facilitate patient-ventilator synchrony for patients unable to trigger the machine, the spontaneous timed mode of pressure-cycled machines is used with a back-up rate set slightly higher than that of the spontaneous breathing rate of the infant. In general, back-up rates of 25–30 breaths per minute are required for infants, 15–20 breaths per minute for small children, and 10–12 breaths per minute for adolescents.

After the patient tolerates nocturnal bilevel PAP, only high IPAP-EPAP spans are used, typically 15–18 cmH$_2$O for IPAP and 2–3 cmH$_2$O for EPAP. However, when high rates are required, as for infants immediately after extubation, lower IPAPs may be needed so that the machine can deliver the air during the very brief inspiratory time. Because the augmented assisted tidal volumes result in a decrease in the infant's spontaneous rate, the machine's back-up rate is decreased and IPAP increased. This effect facilitates a slower breathing rate with more normal tidal volumes and minute ventilation.

Ventilator settings are adjusted to achieve good excursion of the chest wall and resolution of tachypnea and any hypercapnia. The initial goal is to have the infant become accustomed to high-span nasal bilevel PAP. Noninvasive ventilation during sleep is adequate with a mean nocturnal SpO_2 of at least 94%, chest expansion during insufflation, resolution of pectus excavatum, and relief of sleep disturbances and diaphoresis. Inspiratory times of 0.5–1 second and inspiratory-to-expiratory ratios of 1:1 to 1:2 are usually used. If the spontaneous rate is greater than the pressure-cycled ventilator's highest set rate, a volume ventilator with highly sensitive triggering can be tried, such as the LTV-900 or VIP (Innovative Product Technologies, Inc., Gainesville, FL). Once spontaneous rates decrease, the infant can continue to use the machines or be switched to simpler, much less expensive pressure-cycled units.

In general, low-span nasal bilevel PAP is used by children of all ages with obstructive apneas or primarily respiratory insufficiency and adequate pulmonary compliance, whereas high-span nasal bilevel PAP is used by children under 5 years of age with primarily ventilatory impairment. Ventilator settings are tailored to the underlying disease. The EPAP can replace the normal PEEP generated by the larynx, especially during coughing, talking, and crying. Typically, EPAP levels of 2–3 cmH_2O are adequate to diminish carbon dioxide rebreathing from the interface. EPAP levels may be increased in the rare patient with NMD and severe hypoxemic insufficiency or air trapping to increase mean airway pressures and counter auto-PEEP if it can be shown to improve oxygenation (SpO_2). EPAP levels as high as 10 cmH_2O have been used safely in children (Padman et al).[1083] EPAP is rarely needed for children with primarily ventilatory impairment and normal lung compliance; however, it is often beneficial for older children with SMA type 1.

Nasal bilevel PAP is typically introduced in the home while small children sleep. IPAP levels are initially set low (6–8 cmH_2O) to facilitate patient acceptance. They are quickly increased to high spans as tolerated. Soon children tolerate it even when awake. Because the lesser respiratory rates of older children decrease the need for flow-sensing pressure-cycled ventilators and older children need to air-stack, we usually switch children from pressure- to volume-cycled ventilators after age 5.

Portable volume-cycled ventilators also vary. The PLV-100 is quiet, extremely reliable, relatively inexpensive, and ideal for the self-directed patient to learn to operate. For small children or ambulatory patients who require the smallest and lightest machines, however, the LTV-900 or Newport HT-50 ventilators may be more appropriate (Chapter 8).

Humidification

The need for humidification is individualized. Heated-water humidifiers are usually needed during ventilation via tracheostomy tube and also in children under 3 years of age who autonomously breathe through a tracheostomy. After discontinuation of Puritan-Bennett's Cascade humidifier because of unsubstantiated allegations that it caused a fire during use by a hospitalized patient in New York, Fisher and Paykel introduced the MR410 humidifier, which has now been adopted by virtually all ventilator manufactures. It is small, lacks the many delicate assembly parts of the Cascade, and is easy to clean and fill with sterile water. However, inappropriate temperature settings can result in "rain out" in the circuit. For units without temperature gauges, trial and error are required to determine proper temperature settings.

Older children breathing autonomously via tubes may use a regenerative humidifier or heat and moisture exchanger (HME). The original HME was a metal coil placed in the ventilator circuit, often directly to the tracheostomy tube itself. Exhaled water vapor is picked up by the coil and humidifies the next inhalation. Although they are not nearly as effective as standard humidifiers, they do not cause rain out; they eliminate the danger of introducing hot air into the patient's breathing mechanism; they are simple to use; and they create sufficient back pressure (about 2 cmH$_2$O) to block minimally set low-pressure alarms to permit use of mouthpiece IPPV. They eliminate the need to clean and refill standard humidifiers. Perhaps the most effective HME currently on the market is manufactured by Ballard, Inc. (Draper, UT). It can be so effective that some patients on nocturnal Lipseal IPPV have been able to use it rather than standard humidifiers. Standard humidifiers, however, become necessary during respiratory tract infections.

Nasal interface users do not generally require supplemental humidification. If, however, the patient has nasal congestion, sinusitis, or expresses discomfort, an HME can be tried. It is usually inadequate because most patients exhale from the mouth. When used, the regenerative humidifier is connected to the tubing as close to the patient as possible. When it is inadequate, heated humidification is used. In a series of 15 patients, ranging from 4 to 21 years of age, who used noninvasive nighttime support for up to 21 months, Padman et al. used no humidification.[1083] Heated humidification is almost always required when oral interfaces are used for nocturnal, but not for daytime, noninvasive IPPV.

Optimized Clearance of Airway Secretions

As for adults with NMD, inability to clear the airway of debris is the most common cause of pneumonia, acute respiratory failure, and death in pediatric NMD. Airway encumberment can result from retained airway mucus during intercurrent chest colds or aspiration of food or saliva. The bulbar dysfunction of adult patients with ALS may not permit effective use of expiratory aids; their baseline SpO$_2$s decrease below 95% and necessitate tracheotomy to avoid respiratory failure. For infants and small children, however, the situation is quite different. Even infants with severe bulbar dysfunction who cannot articulate or swallow are protected from aspirating food and saliva for anatomic reasons until 8 months of age (Chapter 4). Airway mucus during colds, uncommon at this age, and aspiration secondary to gastric reflux are the principal causes of airway encumberment in such infants, and aspiration due to reflux can be prevented surgically (Chapter 4). Interestingly, even after 8 months of age our 8- to 9-year-old patients with SMA type 1 who have insufficient bulbar function for verbal communication and swallowing still maintain normal baseline SpO$_2$ and appear to be spared from overwhelming aspiration of saliva and, therefore, have not required tracheotomy. Thus, in general, care provider efforts need principally address clearing airway mucus during intercurrent respiratory tract infections.

In pediatric patients who are unable to cough adequately to eliminate secretions, chest physical therapy and assisted coughing are used as for adults (Chapter 11). Chest percussion with postural drainage can help mobilize peripheral airway secretions, but it causes dSpO$_2$ and imposes respiratory work that can also fatigue respiratory muscles. As for adults, mechanical chest percussors can also be very useful. Small, inexpensive percussors are of optimal size for small children (see Figure 38 of Chapter 10).

Whereas in adult airways 160 L/min, measured at the mouth, appears to be the critical level for effective coughing,[656] no one has determined the critically effective level for children. However, perhaps lower total flows are effective in the airways of small children because cough effectiveness is more a function of the velocity of air rather than its flow (Chapter 9).[834]

Expectoration can be facilitated and fatigue eased by providing deep insufflations and nasal IPPV or high-span bilevel PAP for infants. Infants under 1 year of age learn how to close the glottis to hold the IPAP and subsequently open the glottis quickly to expel secretions. They can be heard to "grunt" during these forced expiratory maneuvers.

Caregivers provide the positive pressure of MI-E timed to diaphragm movement (abdominal protrusion) via oral-nasal interfaces to 9- to 30-month-old infants on a daily basis to allow maximal lung expansion and to accustom them to the technique so that they will use MI-E effectively during chest infections. The use of MI-E via the upper airway can be effective for children as young as 11 months of age. Even at this age patients can permit its effective use by not crying or closing the glottis. Between 2.5 and 5 years of age most children become able to cooperate and cough on cue with MI-E.

When airway secretions need to be cleared in small children not yet cooperative with MI-E, MI-E with an exsufflation-timed abdominal thrust (MAC) is used via an oral-nasal interface on manual mode to coincide insufflation and exsufflation with an infant's inspiration and expiration. Manually assisted coughing is avoided for the first 1.5 hours after a meal so that if assisted coughing is needed, only MI-E is done or MAC is done without aggressive manual thrusting. Although timing MI-E to an infant's breathing and crying may be helpful, when the patient does not cooperate, MI-E can be optimally effective only when used via a translaryngeal or tracheostomy tube with the cuff inflated. Relative contraindications for the insufflation phases of MI-E are the same as for adults (see Table 3 of Chapter 10).

When used through oronasal interfaces, settings of +20 to −20 cmH$_2$O are used initially and advanced quickly, as tolerated, to the more effective setttings of +40 to −40 cmH$_2$O via oronasal interfaces. When used via pediatric translaryngeal or tracheostomy tubes, a severe drop-off in flows and pressures often necessitates 4 or more seconds each for full-lung insufflation and subsequent emptying. Machine pressures much greater than 40 cmH$_2$O are usually required to achieve the clinical goal of observing full chest expansion and subsequently complete lung emptying in 2–4 seconds. Even the maximum capabilities of the Cough-Assist can be suboptimal for effective cough flows across infants' tubes. We routinely use MI-E via the translaryngeal tubes of infants as young as 3 months old.

Although no large series related to the use of MI-E in small children are available, we recently reported the use of MI-E with no untoward effects in series of pediatric patients.[655,1084] Our recommendations for pressures of 35–40 cmH$_2$O across oronasal interfaces are based on observed clinical efficacy. They are also the pressures that patients almost invariably want to use. It has also been found that they are the optimal pressures for maximizing deflation volumes and flows in Rhesus monkeys.[1009] They also happen to be the standard pressure pop-off for the manual resuscitators used for cardiopulmonary resuscitation.

Conventional Management Outcomes

Just for this evening when I run my finger through your hair as you pray, I will simply be grateful that God has given me the greatest gift ever given. I will think about the mothers and fathers who are searching for their missing children, the mothers and fathers who are visiting their children's graves instead of their bedrooms, and mothers and fathers who are in hospital rooms watching their children suffer senselessly, and screaming inside that they can't handle it anymore. And when I kiss you good night I will hold you a little tighter, a little longer. It is then, that I will thank God for you, and ask Him for nothing, except one more day....

Mother of a child with SMA

SMA type 1 is the most widely studied NMD presenting in infants because it is the most common. The principles of evaluation and management of other infant NMDs are or should be the same.

Members of pediatric sections of national medical societies, including 75 intensivists, 61 physiatrists, and 51 neurologists, responded to a survey asking about their recommendations for treatment of an infant with SMA type 1 in respiratory distress. Noninvasive ventilation (most likely CPAP or low-span bilevel PAP) would be offered by 70% of the respondents but recommended by only 23% and neither offered nor recommended by 7%. Intubation would be offered and recommended by 38%, offered but not recommended by 48%, and neither offered nor recommended by 14%. Tracheotomy would be offered and recommended by 29%, offered but not recommended by 47%, and neither offered nor recommended by 24%.[1085] In another survey of 33 Japanese pediatricians, 80% thought that quality of life was inadequate to justify survival, but about 50% said that they would begin ventilatory assistance for infants with SMA. They noted that strong familial endorsement, general pro-life beliefs, and secure medical funding could affect decisions in favor of providing life-sustaining treatments.[1086] Over 80% of infants with SMA type 1 who do not benefit from respiratory interventions die by 1 year of age.[63] Thus, it is not surprising that physicians almost invariably tell parents that children with SMA cannot survive infancy.

A few studies have reported long-term outcomes of tracheostomy and NPBV use for a variety of conditions, but the information is not particularly useful for extrapolating potential use by children with NMDs.[1074] In one study 17 of 54 children with tracheostomy tubes died over a 20-year period. Nine deaths were related to complications from the tube or electrical supply. The outcomes were very poor by comparison with those of children with primarily ventilatory impairment who were managed noninvasively.

Other than from our center, there have been no reports of 2-year survival of children with SMA type 1 who do not undergo tracheotomy. Considering infants with NMD who do undergo tracheotomy, one study reported a 57% mortality rate within an average of 23 months for 7 children supported by invasive ventilation following an intubation before age 2.[1087] Two children had SMA; two had nemaline myopathy; and one each had congenital myotonic dystrophy, congenital muscular dystrophy, and fiber-type disproportion myopathy. Three of the children died from pneumonia and the other from aspiration after ventilator use was discontinued. Total duration of mechanical ventilation was an average of 23 months, of which 19 were spent in hospitals. Two of the 4 children who were discharged home, all with professional nursing support, died. All 7 patients had recurrent atelectasis and pneumonia. Three of the 4 who died had evidence of cor pulmonale at autopsy.

Despite the above study, long-term survival of tracheostomy IPPV users is very possible. Our center is managing 17 tracheostomy IPPV users with SMA type 1. Although 16 of the 17 have no breathing tolerance, they have a mean age of 73 ± 57 months. All of these 16 children lost any ability to breathe autonomously immediately after tracheotomy for the reasons stated in Chapter 10 as well as because of severe inspiratory muscle weakness and hypoplastic lungs and chest walls. Once tracheostomy tubes were placed, hospitalization rates were 0.58 per year from birth to the third birthday and 0.21 per year from 3 to 19 years of age. One child died within 3 months of tracheotomy because of lung collapse. However, respiratory infections, hemorrhage, other tube-related complications, and cardiac arrhythmias were also related to tracheostomy. Only 1 of the 17 children developed the ability to speak. In addition, a 20-year-old man and a 14-year-old boy with SMA type 1, both of whom use continuous tracheostomy IPPV, are living in Japan, a 10-year-old patient lives in Hong Kong, and a 19-year-old man who has used tracheostomy IPPV on a full-time basis since 2 months of age is living in Pennsylvania. All four of our ventilator users with SMA type 1 who are older than 10 years and the three elsewhere are averbal but communicate by a Morse code system of grunting or by computer-driven voice synthesizers. One child used a highly sophisticated combination of guttural sounds in a Morse code-like system developed with his mother to communicate needs and even to spell out letters of the alphabet from as early as 3 years of age. All seven patients are straight A students in school, including the two patients in college. The 19-year-old man from Pennsylvania graduated third in his high school class. Even at these ages they retain muscle function sufficient to operate computers. A recent study demonstrated that older children and adolescents with SMA have significantly higher intelligence quotients than unaffected children (113.8 vs. 104.6). It suggested that by adolescence environmentally mediated aspects of intelligence are higher in children with SMA and that the development of cognitive skills and knowledge is a creative way to compensate for their physical disabilities.[1088]

Improvements in prognosis have not been demonstrated by using nocturnal-only low-span nasal bilevel PAP with or without supplemental oxygen. In one such study of infants with SMA type 1, all four patients died from inadequate ventilatory assistance or failure to intubate or use expiratory aids during chest infections, once the parents were told that there was no alternative to tracheotomy or letting their children die.[1089]

Infant Evaluation

Infants are evaluated for airway secretions (auscultation), cry VC,[1090] VC when over 2 years of age, the presence and extent of paradoxical breathing and pectus excavatum or carinatum, SpO_2, and end-tidal carbon dioxide. Although especially helpful in older children and adults, end-tidal carbon dioxide is less accurate than transcutaneous carbon dioxide monitoring in infants and toddlers.[1091] SpO_2 tends to decrease when infants cry and during periods of diaphoresis and arousals associated with inspiratory muscle weakness. Patients are also surveyed for history of frequent arousals, nocturnal flushing, and diaphoresis. Limb and trunk muscle strength is assessed. Older children are evaluated like adults (Chapter 11).

Management of Spinal Muscular Atrophy Type 1 or Other Congenital NMDs

Patient Classification

Children with SMA type 1 can be categorized most simply and perhaps best according to three levels of severity: most severe, typical and intermediate, and mild. About 10% of children with SMA type 1 are most severely affected. They develop chronic respiratory muscle failure and require ongoing continuous ventilatory support, whether invasive or noninvasive, before 6 months of age—regardless of whether the need was triggered by a respiratory infection. Such children conventionally either undergo tracheotomy for full-time IPPV or are left to die. They do not develop the ability to speak even when continuous noninvasive ventilation is used over the long term.

Most children with SMA type 1 (typical and intermediate level) have less severe involvement. They all develop paradoxical breathing and respiratory failure before age 2 during intercurrent chest infections, primarily because of inability to cough effectively. They usually require intubation, but conventionally they either are not intubated and die or undergo tracheotomy because of inability to wean from ventilator use or because the clinician is uneasy about extubation because of anticipated difficulties with clearing airway secretions. If intubated during acute respiratory infections, patients can be extubated according to a new protocol (Table 1)[1048] and weaned back to nocturnal-only nasal bilevel PAP as much as 3 weeks after extubation. They develop the ability to speak. However, about 20% of typical patients with SMA type 1 (intermediate level) develop only moderately dysarthric speech and require varying periods of daytime as well as nocturnal noninvasive ventilatory assistance by 5 years of age.

Another 10% of patients have mild SMA type 1 or type 1+. They can never sit independently but can roll. They may not develop respiratory failure or require gastrostomy feedings before 2 years of age. In this text such patients are not categorized as having SMA type 1. Infants with myopathic diseases who can never sit can also be considered in severe, intermediate, typical, and mild functional categories for the purposes of management.

All children with SMA type 1 demonstrate paradoxical thoracic retraction during inspiration.[1048] If untreated this condition results in a severe pectus deformity, lung and chest wall undergrowth, and pulmonary restriction. Usually, after a period of sleeping comfortably without noticeable arousals, the child begins to awaken every hour or two and has frequent periods of diaphoresis. Episodes of diaphoresis can be associated with bradycardias.

The Three Management Approaches

The parents can decide to "let nature take its course." Often parents decide to have the child undergo gastrostomy for parenteral nutrition but later decide against intubation once the child is in respiratory failure. Most often, perhaps about 96% of the time, children are intubated during respiratory tract infections, but once conventionally managed extubations fail, the parents are convinced by clinicians that repeat intubation would be futile and the child dies.[1089] The second approach is for the child to undergo tracheotomy once intubation is required for an episode of acute respiratory failure.

The third approach is to place the child on high-span bilevel PAP during sleep and use the extubation protocol described in this chapter during episodes of acute respiratory failure. Nocturnal high-span bilevel PAP alleviates diaphoresis, permits more restful

Table 1.   **Conventional vs. Protocol Management of Intubated Patients with SMA type 1 or Other Congenital NMDs**

Conventional

1. Oxygen is administered arbitrarily in concentrations that maintain SpO_2 well above 95%.
2. Frequent airway suctioning via the tube.
3. Supplemental oxygen is increased when desaturations occur.
4. Ventilator weaning is attempted at the expense of hypercapnia.
5. Extubation is not attempted unless the patient appears to be ventilator-weaned.
6. Extubation to CPAP or low-span bilevel PAP with continued oxygen therapy.
7. After extubation, deep airway suctioning is done by catheterizing the upper airway, along with postural drainage and chest physical therapy.
8. With increasing carbon dioxide retention or hypoxia, supplemental oxygen is increased and ultimately the patient is reintubated or dies.
9. After repeat intubation tracheostomy is thought to be the only long-term option *or*
   After successful extubation bronchodilators and ongoing routine chest physical therapy are used.
10. Eventually the patient is discharged home with a tracheostomy, often after an extended rehabilitation stay for family acceptance and training.

Protocol

1. Oxygen administration is limited only to approach 95% SpO_2.
2. Mechanical insufflation-exsufflation is used via the tube up to every few minutes, as needed to fully expand and quickly empty the lungs to reverse oxyhemoglobin desaturations due to airway mucus accumulation, and when auscultatory evidence suggests secretion accumulation. Abdominal thrusts are applied during exsufflation. Tube and upper airway are suctioned after use of expiratory aids as needed.
3. Ventilator weaning is attempted without permitting hypercapnia.
4. Extubation is attempted whether or not the patient is ventilator-weaned when the following criteria are met:
   - Afebrile with normal white blood cell count
   - No supplemental oxygen requirement to maintain SpO_2 > 94% for greater than 24 hours
   - Chest radiograph abnormalities cleared or clearing
   - All respiratory depressants discontinued with no residual effects
   - Airway secretions normal and suctioning required less than 1–2 times/8 hr
   - Coryza diminished sufficiently to permit use of nasal ventilation
5. Extubation to continuous high-span, high-rate bilevel PAP with no supplemental oxygen.
6. Oximetry feedback is used to guide the use of MAC, postural drainage, and chest physical therapy to reverse any desaturations due to airway mucus accumulation.
7. With carbon dioxide retention or ventilator synchronization difficulties, nasal interface leaks are eliminated; pressure support and ventilator rate are increased; or the patient is switched from bilevel PAP to a sensitively triggered volume-cycled ventilator. During use of bilevel PAP, spans may need to be decreased to permit adequate cycling time. Persistent oxyhemoglobin desaturation despite eucapnia and aggressive MAC can indicate oxygen therapy, impending respiratory distress, and need to re-intubate.
8. After repeat intubation the protocol is used for a second trial of extubation to high-span nasal bilevel PAP *or*
   After successful extubation, bronchodilators and chest physical therapy are discontinued, and the patient is weaned to nocturnal-only high-span nasal bilevel PAP, often after discharge home.
9. Discharge home after the SpO_2 remains within normal limits for at least 24 hours.

sleep, prevents or reverses pectus deformity, and promotes lung growth (Fig. 6; also see Figure 5 of Chapter 10 of reference 103). It is indicated for all infants with NMD from the time of diagnosis and observation of paradoxical breathing. High-span bilevel PAP also normalizes nocturnal SpO2 and end-tidal carbon dioxide when they are abnormal. IPAPs of 15–20 cmH$_2$O are used with minimal (about 2 cmH$_2$O) EPAP.

Outpatient Protocol and Hospitalization

At times auscultatory evidence of airway mucus is confused with the wheezing of reversible bronchospasm. Family physicians often prescribe ongoing oxygen supplementation, bronchodilators, nebulizer treatments, and chest physical therapy even when the children are well. Without a history of asthma or bronchospasm, these treatments are usually unnecessary and waste care provider time. Oxygen therapy can also be harmful (Chapter 9). Bronchodilators, however, may be helpful during acute respiratory tract infections.

When such children develop respiratory failure, it is most often the result of a respiratory syncytial virus (RSV) or other acute viral infection. Because of the difficulty in preventing respiratory failure during upper respiratory tract infections and the high risk of RSV in early childhood, RSV-specific human immune globulin (palivizumab, Synagis Intramuscular, MedImmune, Inc.), an intramuscularly delivered synthetic monoclonal antibody to RSV, should be provided monthly to high-risk children during the high RSV infection months.

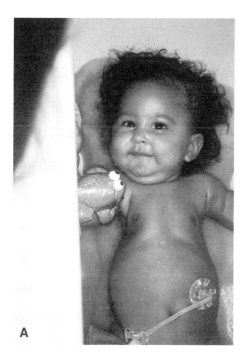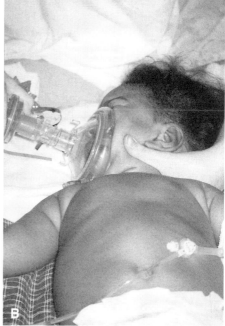

Figure 6. *A* and *B*, Child with SMA type 1 at 7 months of age demonstrates severely hypoplastic chest and early pectus excavatum just before beginning nocturnal high-span bilevel PAP. Nineteen months later with bilevel PAP therapy the child has excellent chest development and expansion and no residual pectus excavatum.

Small children often require hospitalization for dehydration, high fever, or a steady decrease in SpO$_2$ baseline below 95%. Supplemental oxygen is avoided unless SpO$_2$ baseline is less than 94%, in which case patients need to be carefully monitored for sudden respiratory arrest due to airway mucus plugging and fatigue. Once the SpO$_2$ baseline decreases below 95%, patients often require intubation to manage respiratory failure.

Because parents have refused tracheotomy when we and others have recommended it, we were forced to modify and apply the noninvasive approaches that we use successfully for older children and adults. As a result, we found that children can survive and actually do better without tracheostomy tubes. Most if not all children with SMA type 1 avoid chronic aspiration of upper airway secretions to the extent of causing a decrease in baseline SpO$_2$ below 95% and recurrent aspiration pneumonias. Even our severe, averbal, continuously ventilator-dependent patients with SMA type 1 do not demonstrate this problem.

From the time of diagnosis an oximeter is prescribed, along with a manual resuscitator and nocturnal high-span nasal bilevel PAP. The family is told to use the oximeter continuously during colds, to guide in the use of manually assisted coughing and MAC in chest physical therapy, including possible use of chest vibrators (see Fig. 39 of Chapter 10), and in postural drainage to maintain or return SpO$_2$ levels to normal (oximetry protocol; see Chapter 11). MAC is ideally timed to the infant's own coughing attempts. In addition to using carefully timed manually assisted coughing, coughs can be facilitated by holding the child against the shoulder and gently squeezing his or her belly against the shoulder as he or she coughs. In addition to assisting the cough, this position is also less likely to result in reflux and aspiration of stomach contents.

If infants with NMD use manual resuscitators or the positive pressure of MI-E for regular daily maximal insufflations, if they use nasal bilevel PAP nightly, and especially if they have had frequent episodes of respiratory failure and intubation and have experienced MI-E via invasive tubes, they may cooperate with MI-E via oral-nasal interfaces before 1 year of age. They simply relax, keep the airways open, and let MI-E bring up airway secretions. Full cooperation with the oximetry protocol is vital to avoid pneumonia and hospitalizations. More typically, children need to be old enough (usually 2.5–4.5 years of age) to cooperate fully with the protocol, at which point most chest infections that would otherwise necessitate hospitalization and intubation can be avoided.

Long hospitalization associated with intubation and tracheotomy (a mean of 72 days for adults and often longer for infants)[14] and family acceptance and training in tracheostomy management can result in weakening due to poor nutritional support. Nutrition is often poorly maintained during intercurrent chest infections or after surgery (Chapter 3). Such children may not recover their strength.

Intubation and Extubation

Intubated infants receive antibiotics and hydration as is usual for patients with pneumonia, gross atelectasis, or lung collapse. Chapter 3 summarizes nutritional management. They also receive MI-E via the tube at up to the maximum capacity of the Cough-Assist until essentially full chest expansion and lung emptying are observed. Abdominal thrusts concomitant with exsufflation are applied during the exsufflation cycle (MAC), just as they are when MI-E is used via the upper airway. When this technique is used to full lung inflation and emptying, whether via a tube or upper airway, children neither show

discomfort nor develop evidence of barotrauma. If aggressive airway secretion management and MI-E via the tube fail to maintain normal SpO_2, oxygen supplementation is
provided to increase SpO_2 to approach 95% only. This limit is set because of the tendency of hospital personnel to treat $dSpO_2$s by increasing oxygen administration rather
than by clearing airway debris, the principal cause of pneumonia and lung collapse.

Once the SpO_2 is normal on room air, one should attempt to wean the patient from
ventilatory support without supplemental oxygen. Hypercapnia is avoided. Once the
criteria noted in Table 1 are satisfied, the child is extubated, whether weaned from ventilator use or not.

Criteria for extubation are similar to but more restrictive than those for older children
and adults (Chapter 11). Even continuously ventilator-dependent children can be safely
extubated and effectively ventilated after extubation by immediately placing them on
high-span nasal bilevel PAP at rates slightly greater than their autonomous breathing
rates (Fig. 7). For small children who cannot trigger the bilevel PAP delivery and who

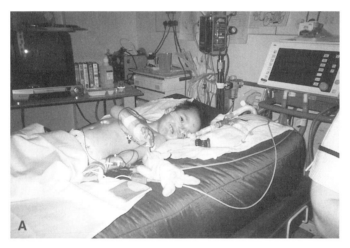

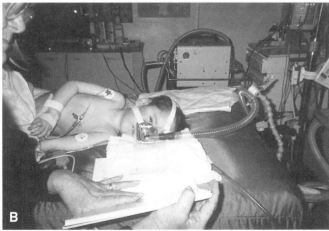

Figure 7. *A* and *B*, Third successful extubation to high-span bilevel PAP for a small child with SMA type 1.

require a very rapid rate that does not permit an adequate bilevel PAP span, sensitively triggered volume-cycle ventilators can be tried (see "Ventilator Choice and Settings" above). Because these children with SMA type 1 or comparable NMD should have been using nasal bilevel PAP nightly before the hospitalization, transition from tube to nasal ventilation is usually smooth. We have never had to keep children with SMA type 1 intubated for more than 10 days. However, they must not be extubated prematurely.

Bronchomalacia is a common complication of infants born prematurely and especially of infants who require frequent or prolonged intubations. Airway and lung collapse occurs peripherally to an underdeveloped central bronchial wall. In prematurely born infants, the cartilaginous-connective tissue structure of the central bronchial walls is underdeveloped. The children outgrow the problem, usually by 2 years of age. Recently, we have observed bronchomalacia in at least two infants with SMA type 1. In one case it resulted in repeated intubations and tracheotomy and sudden death 3 months later. In at least one other case it involved a more peripheral right upper lobe bronchus. These cases required repeat intubations but, like unaffected children, these patients seem to be outgrowing the problem. Bronchomalacia should be suspected in any child who fails extubation with recurrent lobar collapse despite benefiting from the intensive care protocol and despite having minimal airway secretions and no sign of acute respiratory tract infection. It is diagnosed by lobar collapse and bronchoscopic evidence of cyclical airway collapse despite absence of offending airway mucus. Such children require EPAP of 5 cmH$_2$O or perhaps greater.

Since it is difficult if not impossible to expect intensive care nurses and respiratory therapists to use manually assisted coughing and MI-E every few minutes or so, essentially around the clock while the patient is awake, we rely heavily on the child's parents. Family members apply MI-E via translaryngeal tubes or oral-nasal interfaces.

After extubation airway secretions continue to be removed by some combination of chest physical therapy, postural drainage, and MAC for a few days until they "dry up" and the airways are clear on auscultation. The family continues to provide most of the airway secretion management and is trained in respiratory resuscitation, including manual resuscitation with oxygen supplementation. The family needs this knowledge and skill to avoid future hospitalizations and to resuscitate children susceptible to bradycardias or sudden respiratory arrests associated with mucus plugging or fatigue. Transmitted sounds from throat and pharyngeal secretions are not a reason to continue chest physical therapy. Thus, chest physical therapy and postural drainage usually can be discontinued, the premorbid routine of nocturnal nasal bilevel PAP and daytime insufflations is continued, and the patient is discharged home whether or not able to breathe autonomously. Most children wean from full-time to nocturnal-only ventilator use 1 or 2 weeks after hospital discharge.[1048] Many infants "grunt" out pharyngeal secretions using IPAP, as noted above. If these children had undergone tracheotomy, lifetime 24-hour ventilator dependence would have resulted. Most of these children can be managed by predominantly nocturnal noninvasive IPPV at least to 10 years of age.[1048]

For children with NMD who undergo tracheotomy, the use of MI-E via the tube is a more comfortable and effective alternative to deep tracheal suctioning. In addition, as for other patients, oxygen supplementation must be avoided in favor of adequate ventilatory support and aggressive airway secretion management to maintain SpO$_2$ greater than 94%. It may be largely because of MAC that our patients with tracheostomies have much better prognoses than those described in the literature.[14]

In a recent study we compared extubation outcomes using our extubation protocol vs. conventional management (see Table 1). Fifty-six infants with SMA type 1 were intubated a total of 145 times for respiratory failure. Thirty-two of 37 protocol extubations were successful. Fourteen of 24 other extubations to high-span PIP-PEEP were also successful, although most of the 14 children had been using nocturnal bilevel PAP before intubation. Only 3 of 52 conventional extubations without postextubation bilevel PAP were successful (p < 0.001). The other extubations were done following tracheotomy.[742,1048] Thus, although intercurrent chest infections will necessitate periods of hospitalization and intubation until the children are old enough to cooperate with the oximetry protocol, extubation can be successful and tracheotomy avoided for most of them.

A chief concern in caring for chronic respirator-dependent children in hospitals has been the enormous financial and psychosocial burden.[1092,1093] Kettrick reported a mean ICU stay of over 200 days for children with NMD receiving invasive mechanical ventilation.[1094] Because patients with SMA type 1 who undergo tracheotomy usually remain ventilator-dependent and hospitalized for extensive periods and avoidance of tracheostomy usually results in avoidance of continuous ventilator dependence, the cost and quality of life benefits are obvious. We have two brothers with SMA type 1 who have been continuously dependent on high-span bilevel PAP for 8 years and 4 years, respectively, since early infancy (see Figure 17 of Chapter 1). The first was hospitalized briefly at the initiation of bilevel PAP, and the second has never been hospitalized. It is much easier to avoid invasive ventilation in the first place than it is to decannulate children. This is true because of the tendency of children to be fearful and to develop airway damage and deformity from having a tube.

Outcomes of Noninvasive/Protocol Management

Of our 57 patients with typical and severe SMA type 1 who used nocturnal high-span nasal bilevel PAP, 3 died suddenly at 6, 13, and 16 months of age. The other 54 are now 52.8 ± 26.0 months old, and one child is 10.5 years old. Twenty-one children are over age 4 years; 13 are over age 5; and 5 are over age 7. Although the hospitalization rate was 1.52 per year until the third birthday, it has been 0.20 from 3–9 years of age, with only one hospitalization after the fifth birthday in 37 patient-years. Fifty-one of the 57 noninvasively managed children have developed the ability to speak, and only four require continuous high-span nasal bilevel PAP. Thus, the great majority of children with SMA type 1 can require nocturnal-only bilevel PAP and develop the ability to speak. Even children with severe type 1 disease who become continuously ventilator-supported during the first 6 months of life can often be managed noninvasively. Another recent study of extubation of 28 pediatric patients to noninvasive IPPV also supports this approach.[1095]

Spinal Muscular Atrophy Types 2-5 and Other Conditions

SMA type 2 also has a wide range of severity. Affected children may initially recover from chest infections without hospitalization. Depending on severity, they usually first develop pneumonia and respiratory failure at some time between 2 and 12 years of age.

They are managed like children with SMA type 1 with hospitalization and intubation, when needed, until they are old enough to cooperate with the oximetry protocol, at which point they are equipped at home to prevent further respiratory difficulties. Because of a frequent incidence of upper respiratory tract infections, they, too, require oximeters and Cough-Assists from the time of diagnosis.

Nocturnal nasal ventilation is used for the 30–50% of children with SMA type 2 and comparable NMDs who have paradoxical thoracic movement with decreased upper thoracic volumes during inspiration[793] or who have symptoms of hypoventilation. They, too, may come to awaken frequently from sleep with diaphoresis and flushing. Nocturnal oximetry, end-tidal carbon dioxide monitoring, and even polysomnography or plethysmography may be helpful in deciding whether or not to introduce nocturnal nasal ventilation. Some children with SMA type 2 do not benefit from ongoing nocturnal nasal IPPV until adulthood. Many patients with SMA type 2 also require gastrostomy tubes after age 2 years. However, they should rarely if ever require tracheostomy tubes. Often their VCs continue to increase into early adulthood and plateau at more than 50% of predicted normal. As they become older, they can use respiratory muscle aids quite effectively to avert hospitalizations and tracheostomy.[64]

Patients with SMA types 3–5 can walk for a certain period. They should not require tracheostomy tubes and usually require noninvasive IPPV and expiratory aids only during severe chest infections. Concomitant scoliosis, obesity, or other factors that hamper lung or respiratory muscle functioning, when combined with underlying respiratory muscle weakness, the effect of aging on muscles, and senescent loss of anterior horn cells, result in the need for nighttime and even full-time noninvasive IPPV in middle age or later.

In a study in which 12 ventilator users with infantile and adult-type SMA had thus far survived 9.7 ± 8.3 years with ventilatory support, five had received only IPPV via oral and/or nasal interfaces for 5.5 ± 6.1 years, and seven had used tracheostomy IPPV (including one patient who had used both methods). The tracheostomy IPPV users had significantly more pulmonary complications than the noninvasive IPPV users. The noninvasive IPPV users had access to MI-E to clear airway secretions. All patients could communicate verbally and take nutrition by mouth. Five of the seven tracheostomy IPPV users but none of the noninvasive IPPV users remained institutionalized. Except for the ventilator users with SMA type 1, all remained socially active and four were gainfully employed. Thus, noninvasive IPPV methods are effective and practical alternatives to tracheostomy for patients of all ages with SMA.[742]

Patients with congenital NMDs other than SMA, such as those listed in Table 2 of Chapter 1, often have the four patterns of severity described for children with SMA types 1–4. Children who do not attain the ability to sit usually have paradoxical breathing and require nocturnal high-span bilevel PAP. They often develop respiratory failure during intercurrent chest infections before age 2 years, as is the case in SMA type 1. Those who attain the ability to sit but not walk follow the pattern for SMA type 2 and develop respiratory failure later in childhood. Those who walk develop more like patients with SMA type 3 and rarely develop respiratory failure before adolescence. Thus, prognosis and requirement for respiratory interventions and protocols parallel those for SMA. From the perspective of patient management, this pattern is fortunate because the inability to cooperate with air-stacking and CPF testing and the relative anatomic protection that small children have from aspiration of upper airway secretions (see above) make the use of CPF analysis irrelevant for indicating tracheotomy or tracheostomy tube decannulation. In general, tracheotomy does not need to be considered until bulbar muscle function and anatomic protective mechanisms are lost and aspiration of upper airway secretions causes a sustained decrease in SpO_2 baseline below 95%. Children with mild NMDs who typically live into adulthood using noninvasive IPPV are considered in Chapters 9–11.

All over the place nothing was to be heard except the barking of dogs, which deafened the ears of Don Quixote and troubled the heart of Sancho. "The fact that the dogs are barking, Sancho, means that we are moving forward."

•֍• Don Quixote de la Mancha

Chapter 13

Quality of Life and Ethical Issues

N'oublie jamais que chaque être est un monde en soi, que l'on connait en grande partie, mais seulement dans la mesure où nous possédons cette même partie en nous-mêmes. Le reste, pourtant, demeurera toujours secret pour nous. Si l'on veut établir des lois nouvelles, elles ne sont valables que pour cette partie des autres que nous connaissons, parce qu'elle existe en nous.

Don't ever forget that each person is a world unto himself and that we can only understand that part of the character of each individual that is in ourselves. The rest will always remain incomprehensible for us. If you want to establish new laws, they can only be valid for that part of others that we understand in ourselves.

•❦• Gustav Mahler to Justi Mahler, Briefe, 1891[1]

It is now clear that life can be greatly prolonged by ventilator use for many people with respiratory muscle weakness or paralysis and that such people can be happy, productive members of society. However, few health care professionals seem to appreciate this fact.[615] Indeed, there is little written in medical literature about the productivity, social reintegration, and life satisfaction of ventilator users with NMDs. This chapter will review these issues along with ventilator style preferences, complications of ventilator use, and the related ethical issues.

Survey of 700 Ventilator Users

Comment donc parvient-on à connaitre les hommes, qui sont bien plus profonds et plus complexes que leurs oeuvres? Il faut les observer avec attention et tendresse.

How can we understand men, who are much more profound and complex than their works? One must observe them with attention and affection.

•❦• Gustav Mahler

From a mailing to about 1000 community-based users of equipment provided by a single portable ventilator manufacturer (Respironics, Inc.), 695 users responded to a survey. Four hundred ninety-four of the respondents were supported by noninvasive means and 92 by tracheostomy IPPV; 35 did not indicate the means by which they were ventilated or did not fill out the Likert satisfaction scales; and 74 had used both tracheostomy and noninvasive methods of ventilatory support and responded only to questions concerning ventilator-style preferences. Excluding the 74 who did not respond to the satisfaction items, the remaining 621 respondents were wheelchair users, of whom 585 were completely unable to walk and were dependent on attendant care for virtually all activities of daily living (ADL). The seven ventilator users with intrinsic lung disease could walk short distances using a rolling walker with a ventilator tray. The diagnoses, mean ages, residual function, hours per day and years of ventilator use, and life satisfaction indices are listed in Table 1. Respondents included 313 males with a mean age of 46.5 years, 306 females with a mean age of 52.2 years, and two whose gender was not indicated. The 621 ventilator users had been dependent on ventilatory support for a mean of 21.1 years and, at the time of the survey, used aid for a mean of 15.7 hours per day. An additional 46 autonomously breathing patients with spinal cord injury (SCI), who were randomly identified from the medical records of a rehabilitation facility, were also included in the survey.

Table 1	**Duration of Ventilator Use and Life Satisfaction Index**					
Diagnosis	No. of Patients	Age (yrs)[a]	Residual Function	Years of Ventilator Use	Hours[b] per day	Life Satisfaction[c]
Individuals using noninvasive aids (n = 494)						
Poliomyelitis	336	54.5 ± 8.9	1.2 ± 0.9	27.8 ± 12.6	15.4 ± 9.7	5.2 ± 1.6
Duchenne dystrophy	47	27.3 ± 7.2	0.6 ± 0.5	7.6 ± 5.0	18.0 ± 6.8	5.1 ± 1.5
Unknown[d]	29	54.3 ± 16.2	1.6 ± 1.3	14.2 ± 12.7	13.9 ± 6.7	4.8 ± 1.3
Traumatic SCI	23	33.7 ± 11.0	0.3 ± 0.7	8.8 ± 6.4	17.5 ± 8.1	4.0 ± 1.3
Non-Duchenne myopathy	23	40.2 ± 17.1	1.5 ± 1.2	8.7 ± 10.4	15.9 ± 6.7	4.6 ± 1.9
ALS	8	48.3 ± 12.5	0.4 ± 0.5	7.0 ± 7.8	19.3 ± 8.1	4.1 ± 1.7
Intrinsic[e]	7	57.1 ± 10.2	2.3 ± 1.2	6.3 ± 7.7	11.6 ± 6.8	4.6 ± 1.4
Myasthenia gravis	5	57.6 ± 11.0	2.0 ± 1.0	18.4 ± 12.1	9.4 ± 2.5	4.6 ± 2.3
Kyphoscoliosis	4	60.3 ± 13.7	2.8 ± 0.5	9.5 ± 3.0	8.5 ± 1.3	4.7 ± 1.9
Polymyositis	3	46.3 ± 11.0	1.7 ± 1.2	11.3 ± 7.8	18.0 ± 5.6	5.0 ± 0.9
Obesity/hypoventilation syndrome	3	39.3 ± 11.5	1.3 ± 0.6	7.0 ± 5.6	7.7 ± 2.5	4.0 ± 2.6
Myelopathy	3	54.7 ± 13.7	0.0 ± 0.0	10.9 ± 10.1	18.2 ± 10.1	5.5 ± 1.5
Multiple sclerosis	2	59.0 ± 24.0	0.5 ± 0.7	20.5 ± 12.0	5.8 ± 6.0	4.7 ± 1.1
Arthrogryposis	1	26.0	2.5	11.0	8.0	5.5
Tracheostomy IPPV users (n = 92						
Poliomyeltitis	44	53.1 ± 10.0	1.4 ± 0.9	24.1 ± 11.8	16.0 ± 6.6	4.6 ± 1.8
Duchenne dystrophy	13	30.8 ± 4.8	0.6 ± 0.5	5.0 ± 3.0	20.8 ± 5.5	4.8 ± 1.3
Non-Duchenne myopathy	12	34.2 ± 13.6	1.3 ± 1.0	9.4 ± 6.5	19.9 ± 6.7	4.9 ± 1.6
ALS	5	51.8 ± 21.7	0.6 ± 0.9	11.4 ± 10.5	20.2 ± 6.1	2.5 ± 1.5
Unknown[d]	5	50.8 ± 20.5	2.4 ± 0.5	8.2 ± 1.5	11.8 ± 7.1	5.5 ± 2.6
Traumatic SCI	4	31.3 ± 9.1	0.0 ± 0.0	30.8 ± 18.2	20.0 ± 8.0	5.4 ± 1.7
Polymyositis	2	41.0 ± 9.9	1.0 ± 1.4	4.0 ± 1.4	23.0 ± 0.0	3.0 ± 2.8
Charcot-Marie-Tooth disease	2	53.5 ± 0.8	1.5 ± 0.7	6.5 ± 4.9	24.0 ± 0.0	4.5 ± 3.5
Kyphoscoliosis	1	47.0	3.0	11.0	8.0	5.5
Myelopathy	1	40.0	1.0	27.0	8.0	5.5
Multiple sclerosis	1	62.0	0.0	6.0	24.0	3.0
Spinal muscular atrophy	1	40.0	1.0	26.0	16.0	7.0
Polyneuropathy	1	17.0	0.0	7.0	24.0	5.5

[a] Age at the time of the survey.
[b] Hours per day of ventilator use.
[c] Patient satisfaction with life in general, where 1 is very dissatisfied and 7 is very satisfied.
[d] Not reported in the survey.
[e] Intrinsic lung disease, including pulmonary fibrosis and chronic obstructive pulmonary disease.

Marriage/Divorce

Those who deem me unworthy at a glance and pass me on by, have my blessing to keep walking, for they have a long way to go. They have not reached the point in their journey where they are able to see and appreciate me for who I am.

❧ Terri McPherson, Words from a Simple Heart, terri@wisehearts.com

Two hundred seventy-seven of the 621 respondents (45%), 157 men and 120 women, had not married. One hundred eighty-six, 97 men and 89 women, were married before requiring ventilatory support and remained married and living with their spouses. This figure includes four respondents who were widowed before requiring ventilatory support and later remarried while using support and two men who were divorced before requiring support and remarried while using support. These 186 people had been using ventilatory support for a mean of 22.7 years and required 13.7 hours of support per day. Twenty other respondents were married before requiring ventilatory aid and subsequently widowed. Thirty-six respondents, 10 men and 26 women, were married before requiring ventilatory support and have been divorced and remained so while using ventilatory aids. An additional 60 respondents (20%), 32 men and 28 women, who were single before requiring ventilator support were married as ventilator users and live with their spouses. Forty-two people did not respond to this question. Therefore, only 16.2% of the ventilator users who were married before onset of ventilator dependence were divorced subsequently and have not remarried over a mean period of 22.7 years (individual ages: 28–51 years) of ventilator use. This group became ventilator users at the mean age of 28 years. The general nondisabled population has a divorce rate of 30% for people married at the mean age of 28 years.[1096]

In one report, 12 women with SMA with onset from 8 months to 29 years delivered a total of 17 infants. Complications included premature labor, prolonged labor, and delayed postpartum recovery; cesarean section was performed for 3 cases. There were no deleterious effects on fetal outcome. Exacerbation of muscle weakness was noted by 8 women during the second trimester. Three had recovery in strength in the puerperium.[1097] As noted in Chapter 1, a 27-year-old woman with SMA type 1 also had a successful pregnancy.[66]

Employment

We must all—people with disabilities in particular—be allowed the opportunity to satisfy the need we all have to prove ourselves, to contribute to our chosen field, and to our quality of life. Anything to the contrary sends the message that we no longer have any contribution to make, that—for example in my case—unless I am physically capable of transporting myself to the seat of justice, I am incapable of rendering it.[602]

❧ Justice Sam Filer

Two hundred thirty-four ventilator users (134 men, 99 women, and 1 respondent whose gender was not indicated) were gainfully employed (Table 2). Seventeen other ventilator users reported being active on a daily basis as volunteers for various philanthropic causes, and 24 were students. In addition, 32 married women ventilator users

Table 2. Occupations of Ventilator Users with Neuromuscular Conditions	
Accounting/banking	28
Social work/counseling	27
Business owners	21
Teachers	18
Engineers/scientists	13
Business/corporation executives/administration	12
Journalism/freelance writers	10
Computer work (programming, systems analysis)	10
Lawyers	10
College professors	8
Artists (including mouthstick)	8
Insurance sales	6
Investment brokers and analysts	4
Real estate brokers	4
Physicians	2
Architects	2
College administrators	2
Mail order sales	2
Dispatchers (police, trucking)	2
Speech-language pathologist	1
Clergy	1
Receptionist	1
Librarian	1
Travel agent	1
Not specified	42

reported being homemakers. In another report of employment profiles in NMDs, 40% of 154 people with progressive NMDs, including SMA and FSH, Becker, limb-girdle, and myotonic muscular dystrophies, were employed in the competitive market at the time of the study; 50% had been employed in the past; and only 10% had never been employed. The major barrier to employment was education. Intellectual capacity, psychosocial adjustment, and the belief by most people that their physical disability was the only or major barrier to obtaining a job were also identified. Physical impairment and disability were not associated with level of employment. The myotonic and limb-girdle muscular dystrophy diagnostic groups had significantly lower employment rates, lower educational levels, and fewer employed professional, management, and technical workers.[1098] However, a recent study of 1000 Dutch patients with myotonic dystrophy, hereditary motor and sensory neuropathy, SMA, and myasthenia gravis noted that the majority were employed. Employment levels decreased after age 34, but the availability of work adaptations made it possible to prolong employment. Limiting factors were loss of effective communication, limited cognitive function, and the effect of weakness on facial expression.[1099] It is likely that, with the influence of the Internet, employment rates for ventilator users will increase.

Life Satisfaction

Six hundred fifteen of the 621 ventilator users who responded to a 1–7 Likert scale for overall life satisfaction had a mean response of 5.1. The 586 respondents whose methods of ventilatory support were known had a mean age of 49.4 ± 14 years (range = 16–84 years) and reported a mean life satisfaction index of 4.98 ± 1.68. In addition, 242 nondisabled health care professionals with an average age of 33.0 ± 8 years (range = 21–59 years) reported scores of 5.33 ± 1.2 for satisfaction with their own lives, with no one reporting a score of 1. This score was significantly higher than the mean 4.98 score of the ventilator users ($p < 0.005$). When asked how ADL-dependent ventilator users would respond to this question, the mean estimate of health care professionals was 2.42 ± 1.37. This score was significantly worse than the ventilator users' actual responses ($p < 0.0001$).

Differences arose between respondents using noninvasive ventilatory aids and respondents using tracheostomy IPPV. Both groups were compared for level of upper extremity function in the following manner: 0, for no upper extremity function; 1, for sufficient finger movement to operate a motorized wheelchair; 2, for adequate function to feed oneself; and 3, for normal or near-normal function. The ages, levels of function, years of ventilator use, hours per day of use, and life satisfaction index for the tracheostomy and the noninvasive groups are listed in Table 3. The noninvasive group was older than the tracheostomy group (50 vs. 45.8 years; $p < 0.001$), had significantly less upper extremity function (1.13 vs. 1.21; $p < 0.05$), and had used ventilatory support for fewer hours per day (15.5 vs. 17.7; $p < 0.05$) but for more years (22 vs. 17; $p < 0.005$). However, the tracheostomy IPPV group had a mean satisfaction index of 4.68 as opposed to 5.04 for the noninvasive group ($p < 0.05$). These figures are compared for various diagnostic subgroups in Table 1.

Table 3. **Characteristics of Ventilator Users**	
Variable	Mean ± Standard Deviation
Using tracheostomy IPPV (n = 92)	
Age	45.8 ± 15.33
Function	1.21 ± 0.97
Ventilator use (yr)	17.05 ± 14.74
Ventilator use (hr/day)	17.65 ± 6.81
Satisfaction index	4.64 ± 1.85
Using noninvasive methods of ventilatory support (n = 494)	
Age	50.03 ± 13.69
Function	1.13 ± 0.97
Ventilator use (yr)	22.01 ± 14.29
Ventilator use (hr/day)	15.47 ± 8.95
Satisfaction index	5.03 ± 1.64

None of the variables studied were significantly different at the 95% confidence level for any of the diagnostic groups except for the post-poliomyelitis ventilator users. For this subgroup, age, years of ventilator use, hours per day of use, and level of function were not significantly different for the tracheostomy and noninvasive groups. However, the life satisfaction index for the noninvasive group was significantly greater than that of the tracheostomy group (5.20 vs. 4.55, p < 0.02).

Quality of Life and Satisfaction Domains

Dios, que es proveedor de todas las cosas, no nos faltara. No les falta a los mosquitos del aire, ni a los gusanillos de la tierra, ni a los renacuajos del agua. Es tan piadoso que hace salir su sol sobre los buenos y los malos, y llueve sobre los injustos y justos.

ᶜᵒ᷈ᵃ Don Quijote de La Mancha

The mean score of the overall life satisfaction in Campbell's survey of 2134 random subjects responding to a 1–7 Likert scale was 5.54 compared with 5.36 for our 273 health care professionals. Although the 5.1 mean score of the ventilator users was significantly less than the scores of the physically able population, it was still very positive (> 4.0) and significantly greater than the 2.42 anticipated by the health care professionals. In addition to the overall life satisfaction item, 380 ventilator users with post-poliomyelitis syndrome,[1100] 60 ventilator users with DMD,[1101] and 273 health care professionals (controls) were asked to respond to various Life Domain Satisfaction Measures and to 1–7 Semantic Differential Scales of General Affect, with 7 being the most positive response.[1102] The controls were also asked how they thought ventilator users with little or no extremity function would respond. A summary of the responses is presented in Tables 4 and 5.

Ninety-three percent of Campbell's 2134 subjects, 91% of our 273 health care professional controls, 85% of ventilator users with post-polio syndrome, and 87.5% of ventilator users with DMD reported being satisfied with their lives (response of 4 or greater). The ventilator users with post-polio syndrome, DMD, and spinal cord injury were significantly less satisfied with their transportation, education, health, social lives, sexual lives, and life in general than were the controls. They were significantly more satisfied with their housing. There were no significant differences in satisfaction with family life and employment. Except for health (post-polio ventilator users) and sexual activity (DMD ventilator users), the ventilator users were generally satisfied in each domain and reported means greater than 4.0.

The controls felt that their lives were significantly easier, more worthwhile, fuller, more hopeful, freer, and more rewarding than the ventilator users. However, the controls significantly misjudged that the ventilator users would give negative responses for each semantic differential (see Table 5). In fact, the ventilator users' mean responses were greater than 4 for each differential, except "hard—easy" (poliomyelitis and DMD ventilator users), and "tied down—free" (DMD ventilator users). The post-polio ventilator users even judged their lives to be more interesting and friendly than did the controls, although the differences did not reach statistical significance. There was no significant difference in the "miserable—enjoyable" differential between the two groups.

Table 4. **Life Domain Satisfaction Measures***

Ventilator Users	Post-polio		DMD		SCI	
	n	Mean ± SD	n	Mean + SD	n	Mean ± SD
Housing	386	5.7 ± 1.7	78	5.6 ± 1.4	42	5.6 ± 2.1
Transportation	351	5.3 ± 2.1	77	4.7 ± 2.0	41	4.5 ± 2.3
Education	388	5.2 ± 1.9	82	5.2 ± 1.5	42	4.6 ± 2.1
Job	216	5.2 ± 1.9	29	4.6 ± 1.7	15	5.2 ± 2.2
Health	384	3.9 ± 1.9	82	3.8 ± 2.0	42	4.1 ± 2.1
Family life	364	5.6 ± 1.8	77	5.6 ± 1.7	41	5.7 ± 1.7
Social life	360	5.8 ± 1.8	75	4.4 ± 1.9	41	4.5 ± 2.0
Sexual life	324	4.1 ± 2.2	51	3.6 ± 2.3	36	3.1 ± 2.2
Life in general	380	5.1 ± 1.7	80	4.9 ± 1.3	42	4.4 ± 1.8
Life in general[†]	273	2.5 ± 1.7				

	Controls		SCI Controls	
	n	Mean ± SD	n	Mean ± SD
Housing	263	5.2 ± 1.5	47	5.0 ± 1.5
Transportation	268	5.7 ± 1.6	47	4.6 ± 2.0
Education	266	5.5 ± 0.1	46	4.8 ± 1.8
Job	269	5.2 ± 1.4	33	3.5 ± 2.0
Health	269	5.7 ± 1.2	47	3.9 ± 1.7
Family life	268	5.6 ± 1.4	47	4.9 ± 1.8
Social life	268	5.4 ± 1.4	47	4.4 ± 1.9
Sexual life	227	5.5 ± 1.5	46	3.2 ± 2.0
Life in general	259	5.4 ± 1.2	47	4.1 ± 1.7

DMD = Duchenne muscular dystrophy, SCI = spinal cord injury, SD = standard deviation.

* The ventilator users were asked to rate their satisfaction with the dimension under question from 1 to 7, where 1 indicates extreme dissatisfaction and 7 indicates extreme satisfaction. The controls were autonomously breathing.

† Controls' responses assessing the ventilator users' satisfaction with life.

Social Integration

> *Compter...*
> *Apprendre à compter sur soi-même*
> *A compter pour ceux qui vous aiment*
> *Pour faire aussi partie du nombre*
> *Pouvoir enfin sortir de l'ombre*
>
> ・◉・ *Apprendre* by Yves Duteil

Home mechanical ventilation has proved to be safe and to optimize quality of life. A total of 307 ventilator users, or about one-half of the 621 in our study, maintained active and productive lives in their communities, as seen by their social and occupational

Table 5. **Semantic Differential Scale of General Affect***			
Ventilator Users	Post-Polio	DMD	SCI
Number of respondents	368	256	41
Responses to each item	> 360	> 249	> 39
	Mean ± SD	Mean ± SD	Mean ± SD
Boring–Interesting	5.6 ± 1.6	4.5 ± 1.6	4.7 ± 2.0
Miserable–Enjoyable	5.6 ± 1.5	4.9 ± 1.5	4.9 ± 1.9
Hard–Easy	3.8 ± 1.8	2.9 ± 1.7	3.2 ± 1.8
Useless–Worthwhile	5.9 ± 1.7	5.0 ± 1.9	5.0 ± 2.1
Lonely–Friendly	5.9 ± 1.7	5.3 ± 1.7	5.1 ± 2.3
Empty–Full	5.5 ± 1.6	5.0 ± 1.5	4.8 ± 1.8
Discouraging–Hopeful	5.4 ± 1.8	4.9 ± 1.5	4.9 ± 2.1
Tied down–Free	4.0 ± 2.0	3.5 ± 2.1	3.2 ± 2.1
Disappointing–Rewarding	5.3 ± 1.8	4.5 ± 1.4	4.1 ± 2.3
	Controls[†]	SCI	Controls[‡]
Number of respondents	256	46	239
Responses to each item	> 249	> 43	> 232
	Mean ± SD	Mean ± SD	Mean ± SD
Boring–Interesting	5.4 ± 1.5	4.7 ± 2.2	2.4 ± 1.5
Miserable–Enjoyable	5.7 ± 1.2	4.5 ± 1.6	2.4 ± 1.4
Hard–Easy	4.1 ± 1.5	3.4 ± 1.7	1.8 ± 1.1
Useless–Worthwhile	6.2 ± 1.1	5.0 ± 2.0	2.8 ± 1.7
Lonely–Friendly	5.8 ± 1.4	4.9 ± 1.9	3.0 ± 1.9
Empty–Full	5.8 ± 1.2	4.6 ± 1.8	2.7 ± 1.4
Discouraging–Hopeful	5.9 ± 1.2	4.8 ± 1.8	2.8 ± 1.7
Tied down–Free	5.0 ± 1.6	3.8 ± 2.0	1.8 ± 1.2
Disappointing–Rewarding	5.8 ± 1.1	4.5 ± 1.8	2.4 ± 1.5

DMD = Duchenne muscular dystrophy, SCI = spinal cord injury, SD = standard deviation.

* The subjects were asked to indicate the extent that each heuristic dimension describes them by indicating a number from 1 to 7, where 1 and 7 reflect the extremes of the polar adjective pairs in a seven-point Likert-type scale.

† The controls were 256 health care professionals, who provided at least 250 responses to each item, and 46 autonomously breathing patients after spinal cord injury, who provided at least 44 responses to each item.

‡ Controls' estimates of the ventilator users' responses.

activities. The male/female ratio was equal. Since other activities such as visits with friends, going to restaurants, sporting events, or other spectacles were not surveyed, it is clear that over one-half of this population maintains a considerable degree of mobility despite severe disability and ventilatory dependence. Technologic advances in environmental control systems, personal computers, and robot aids[752] as well as in ventilators and home health care delivery have also greatly facilitated a more active and higher-quality lifestyle.

Il ne suffit pas de lire que les sables des plages sont doux; je veux que mes pieds nus le sentent.

It does not suffice to read that the sands of the beaches are smooth, I want to feel them with my bare feet.

                •◉• André Gide, *Les Nourritures Terrestres*, 1897, ed. Gallimard.

Assessment Issues

Campbell et al. recognized the difficulty in dealing with subjective perceptions of well-being in that reports of "excellent," "good," or "poor" overall quality of life may have different meanings for different people. He concluded, nonetheless, that these subjective parameters yielded consistent results when compared between different populations and that they are essential for assessing individual personal values and for self-assessment of quality of life.[1103] He found that the single-item measure of overall life satisfaction closely fit the measures of satisfaction with the specific domains of life, and as such, it was one of the most important measures. Kammann et al. also demonstrated that the items with the highest validities were those which had a global frame of reference, such as feeling that life is going well in general.[1104] Not one subject who expressed satisfaction with life in general was dissatisfied with his or her family life. The strongest association for all ventilator user groups was between general life satisfaction and satisfaction with social life.

Campbell noted that different life domains have different importance to different people. The downgrading of importance of any particular life domain can be explained by denial or adaptation to situations.[1102] Likewise, it appears that family life and housing issues—domains less affected by physical disability—take on the greatest significance for ventilator users. Campbell found that satisfaction with family life was one of the most effective predictors of general life satisfaction in his study population and correlated even more significantly with general life satisfaction for ventilator users in his study.

More recently it has become evident that there are more relevant ways of assessing the impact of disability, including disability associated with ventilator use, on the quality of a person's life. The impact of disability on the activities or domains most important to individual patients can be determined by asking patients to list favorite activities in order of importance to them and then to consider the impact of the disability on each one.[1105,1106]

Physicians' Consideration of Quality of Life

Physicians' perceptions of the patients' quality of life are extremely variable.[1107] Surveys have demonstrated the extent to which health care professionals underestimate the satisfaction with life of severely disabled, ventilator-assisted people. This point is important because physicians' assessment of patients' quality of life and the relative desirability of certain types of existence determine the likelihood that patients will receive therapeutic interventions.[1108,1109] Physicians consider patients' quality of life more often to support decisions to withhold therapy than to support decisions to use mechanical ventilation ($p < 0.01$).[1107] This situation is further revealed by the fact that despite the widespread use of nocturnal bilevel PAP for patients with ALS, less than 10% of patients with ALS ever use ventilatory support, and virtually none are offered the respiratory muscle aids that could spare them morbidity and mortality.[100] Some neurologists openly profess their "therapeutic nihilism."[644]

Why Life Satisfaction in Ventilator Users?

Happiness = reality ÷ expectations

At first it is surprising that people with such severe disability might be satisfied with their lives. However, habituation tends to produce a decline in the subjective pleasurableness or unpleasantness of any input.[1104] Campbell stated that "where an [unpleasant] situation is fixed for a person over a long term, there may be a tendency toward accommodation to it, reflected in gradual increases in satisfaction."[1102] Perhaps for ventilator users with ever-greater disability and decreasing expectations, habituation occurs along with maturity and acceptance, thereby decreasing the unpleasantness of the circumstances. Constricted horizons may also lead to satisfaction with the status quo.[1102] In addition, the ventilator serves as a daily reminder of the tenuousness of human existence. Unless the person uses nontracheostomy aids and is capable of GPB,[917] the ventilator is all that stands between the user and death. In a concrete way these people appear to appreciate that their quality of life is closely tied to their family lives and personal relationships, and their use of a ventilator takes on a positive aspect in permitting continued appreciation of human ties. Campbell described other populations of people with limited horizons who, although severely oppressed by society, remained satisfied until their status in society improved. With less limited horizons, they became aware that more could be obtained, and with new frustration came discontent. Thus, such severe disability may lead to a general scaling down of expectations and shifts in the importance of life domains. In addition, ventilator users may come to experience life satisfaction as a consequence of cognitive dissonance. They overcame the greatest of obstacles and challenges simply to be alive; therefore, life must be meaningful and satisfying.

Whiteneck studied the psychosocial outcomes of people with spinal cord injury at least 20 years after the injury occurred.[1110] Three-fourths of the subjects rated their current quality of life as good or excellent on a 5-point scale. There were no significant differences by level of injury, but satisfaction correlated inversely with age. Whiteneck et al. also demonstrated that ventilator users with spinal cord injury rated their quality of life higher than autonomously breathing traumatic tetraplegics. They reported that fewer of the former than of the latter considered suicide at least once and six times or more and that more of the former were happy to be alive and had greater self-esteem.[1111] Our survey also demonstrated that, while ventilator users with spinal cord injury were dissatisfied only with sexual function, autonomously breathing traumatic tetraplegics were dissatisfied (mean responses below 4.0) with the domains of job satisfaction, health, and sexual functioning.[1112] The ventilator users with spinal cord injury reported a significantly greater satisfaction with housing, job, and family life and a greater satisfaction with social life, health, and life overall in comparison with the autonomously breathing traumatic tetraplegics. They also felt that life was somewhat friendlier, more interesting, more enjoyable, fuller, and more hopeful than the latter group. This level of psychosocial adjustment and well-being is remarkable, considering that, in addition to ventilator use, people with spinal cord injury also had less upper extremity function than autonomously breathing tetraplegics. Thus, ventilator use had to be the difference in their more positive perceptions of life. The level of disability may not be as important a factor as aging in determining overall long-term life satisfaction in ventilator users.[1113]

The more positive well-being scores of patients with polio and DMD compared with the scores of ventilator users with ALS may also be explained by the fact that the former were initially managed by noninvasive methods of long-term ventilatory assistance and their ventilator use requirement usually increased gradually. Thus, the patients with polio and DMD generally had more time to adjust to both physical disability and ventilator use than did ventilator users with ALS and other motor neuron diseases (MNDs).

Other studies have confirmed the positive view of life held by the great majority of ventilator users with NMD.[1114] One study reported that 92% of ventilator users with DMD "had positive feelings of life" more than half of the time.[1115] In one study of 19 patients with ALS/MND, over two-thirds were satisfied with their lives; 84% felt that they had made the right choice; and 18 felt that ventilator-assisted breathing had been a worthwhile option and would choose it again. In another study of 92 long-term tracheostomy IPPV users with ALS, 20 lived 8 to 17 years using IPPV and 9 became locked in. Although most wanted to live as long as possible, 14 eventually requested that mechanical ventilation be withdrawn.[1116] In the study by Ganzini et al. of 100 patients with ALS, 84% said they would not consider physician-assisted suicide and looked "forward to the future with hope and enthusiasm."[1117] Although still positive, the views of patients with ALS/MND in these studies were less positive toward assisted ventilation and life satisfaction than were those of patients with DMD.

In a recent study of sexuality in 200 patients who used noninvasive IPPV for a mean of 41 ± 27 months, 34.5% reported that they were sexually active. For 46% "nothing changed" after beginning noninvasive IPPV; 36% were less active; and 13% were more active. The sexually active noninvasive IPPV users reported having intercourse 5.4 ± 4.8 times per month.[1118] The rocking bed ventilator has been used by some to facilitate sexual intercourse (and to conserve energy during intercourse) as well as for ventilatory assistance. The rocking bed also has beneficial effects on alleviating constipation.

Ventilator Style Preference:
Tracheostomy vs. Noninvasive Approaches

A survey of a subset of the 695 ventilator users—the 170 with greater than 1 month experience in the use of both tracheostomy and noninvasive methods—was undertaken to compare ventilator use preferences.[699] Participants had the following diagnoses: postpoliomyelitis, 129; non-Duchenne myopathies, 14; spinal cord injury, 13; severe kyphoscoliosis, 3; chronic obstructive pulmonary disease, 3; DMD, 2; Guillain-Barrè syndrome, 2; and myasthenia gravis, multiple sclerosis, ALS/MND, and polymyositis, 1 each. This group had a mean age of 54.7 ± 11.4 years, was using ventilatory support for 17.1 ± 6.5 hours per day, and had been ventilator users for 22.7 ± 13.1 consecutive years. Of the 170, 155 required both nocturnal and at least some daytime ventilatory aid. Over 155 had required 24-hour support for some period. The group was divided into two subgroups: the 111 noninvasive ventilation users who were switched to tracheostomy IPPV (group 1) and the 59 ventilator users who were switched from tracheostomy IPPV to noninvasive aids (group 2). There were no significant differences between the groups in age ($p = 0.22$), hours per day of ventilator use ($p = 0.11$), or years of ventilator use ($p = 0.10$). Group 1 respondents used noninvasive aids for 13.7 ± 11.5 years before being switched to tracheostomy IPPV, which they used for another 10.5 ± 10.3 years. Group 2 respondents used tracheostomy IPPV for 1.6 ± 4.8 years before switching to noninvasive ventilatory aids for another 18.8 ± 14.8 years.

Of the 170 patients who used noninvasive ventilation, 84 used a body ventilator for a mean of 14.3 ± 14.1 years overnight and 10.7 ± 14.1 years during waking hours; 24 used noninvasive IPPV for a mean of 9 ± 8.2 years for nocturnal support and 4.5 ± 7.5 years during waking hours; and 62 used both body ventilators and noninvasive IPPV methods for a mean of 21.7 ± 10.0 years overnight and 21.7 ± 12.9 years during waking hours. Figures 1–3 present the respondents' preferences for the quality-of-life issues included in the survey. Table 6 demonstrates concordance of the principal caregivers' preferences with those of the ventilator users. Other reasons cited for preferring tracheostomy or noninvasive aids are listed in Table 7.

In addition, the ventilator users reported that during use of indwelling tracheostomy tubes they required tracheal suctioning a mean of 7.6 ± 8.3 times per day; 27 patients (16%) reporting 10 or more times per day. Thirteen of the latter group cited numerous respiratory complications before switching to as much as 24-hour use of noninvasive aids. Thirty-five percent of group 1 ventilator IPPV users expressed the desire to return to noninvasive aids, whereas none of the group 2 ventilator users wished to switch back to

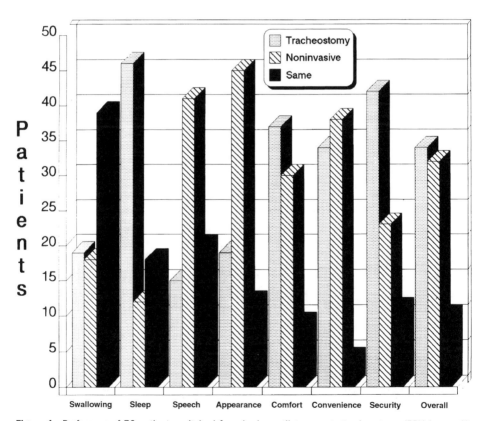

Figure 1. Preference of 76 patients switched from body ventilator use to tracheostomy IPPV (group 1). (From Bach JR: A comparison of long-term ventilatory support alternatives from the perspective of the patient and care giver. Chest 1993;104:1702–06; with permission.)

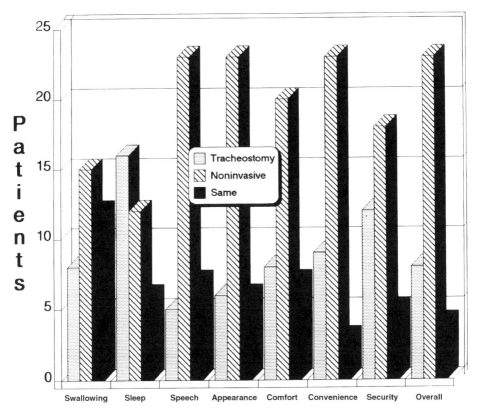

Figure 2. Preferences of 35 patients switched from a regimen of body ventilators and/or noninvasive IPPV to tracheostomy (group 1). (From Bach JR: A comparison of long-term ventilatory support alternatives from the perspective of the patient and care giver. Chest 1993;104:1702–06; with permission.)

tracheostomy IPPV. Two of the ventilator users in group 1 (2%) and 8 in group 2 (14%) had regular access to MI-E during respiratory infections. Twenty-eight of the ventilator users in group 1 (25%) and 22 in group 2 (37%) had mastered GPB sufficiently to achieve or increase ventilator-free breathing tolerance while they were using noninvasive ventilation.

In miscellaneous survey questions, every ventilator user without exception indicated that ventilatory assistance should be offered to every person who could benefit from it; that finances should not be a consideration; and, if having to do it over, each ventilator user would have made the same choice.

Respiratory Complications

The 621 ventilator users were surveyed for the number of times that they were hospitalized for respiratory distress after an initial respiratory hospitalization under the following circumstances: (1) before use of ventilators on an ongoing daily basis, (2) during use of ongoing oxygen therapy, (3) during use of noninvasive aids predominantly overnight, (4) during use of noninvasive aids greater than 16 hours per day, and (5)

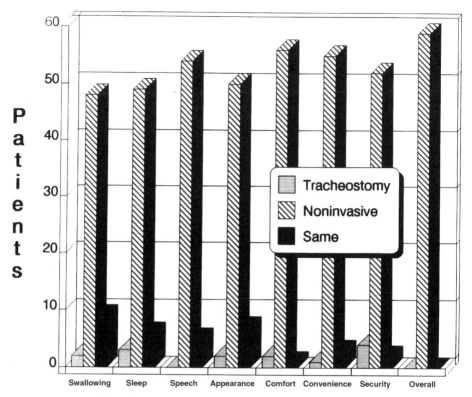

Figure 3. Preferences of 59 patients switched from tracheostomy to noninvasive aids (group 2), including 8 who switched to body ventilators, 18 to noninvasive IPPV methods, and 33 to a combination of body ventilators and noninvasive IPPV methods. (From Bach JR: A comparison of long-term ventilatory support alternatives from the perspective of the patient and care giver. Chest 1993;104:1702–06; with permission.)

during use of indwelling tracheostomy tubes and daily IPPV. The groups were controlled for level of extremity function. All comparisons were statistically significant. The highest incidence of hospitalizations for respiratory complications was in patients receiving oxygen therapy, followed by those using tracheostomy IPPV and those using noninvasive aids predominantly overnight. The lowest incidence was for the full-time

Table 6.	**Patient and Principal Caregiver Ventilator Method Preferences**		
	Noninvasive	Tracheostomy	No Preference
Group 1			
Patients	55	42	14
Caregivers	50	38	23
Group 2			
Patients	59	0	0
Caregivers	48	1	8

Table 7.	**Other Reasons Cited for Preferring Tracheostomy or Noninvasive Aids**

For preferring tracheostomy
Facility in clearing airway secretions during respiratory tract infections: 57 (31%)
Greater mobility by comparison with body ventilator use: 8 (9%)
Better speech than by using mouth IPPV: 1 (1%)

For preferring noninvasive aids
Greater independence and control of breathing: 24 (14%)
Facilitation of management in the community: 17 (10%)
Suctioning no longer needed/absence of secretions: 17 (10%)
Greater portability (less equipment, supply needs, and upkeep): 14 (8%)
Greater mobility: 11 (7%)
Fewer infections: 11 (7%)
More natural: 9 (5%)
Compatibility with glossopharyngeal breathing/air-stacking: 3 (2%)

noninvasive aid users.[14] The fact that the lowest incidence was in the noninvasive aid users with the greatest need for ventilatory support can be explained by the following factors: noninvasive aid users avoid the complications associated with indwelling tracheostomy tubes; nighttime-only ventilator users are often underventilated during daytime hours and, when not using a ventilator, may not increase insufflation volumes for optimal elimination of airway secretions, as needed; and nighttime-only ventilator users are less likely to have been introduced to MI-E.

In addition to the fact that noninvasive IPPV is associated with fewer respiratory complications and pneumonias for long-term ventilator users, a prospective epidemiologic survey from a single ICU recently demonstrated that noninvasive IPPV is also associated with a significantly lower incidence of ventilator-associated pneumonias compared with tracheal intubation in the acute setting.[1070] The groupings taken into account in this study were patients going from noninvasive IPPV to IPPV via tracheal intubation, patients going from tracheal intubation to noninvasive IPPV, users of IPPV via tracheal intubation only, and users of noninvasive IPPV only.

Tracheostomy IPPV vs. Noninvasive Physical Medicine Alternatives

Whether switched to or from noninvasive ventilatory support regimens that include noninvasive IPPV, the great majority of ventilatory users considered noninvasive methods to be superior to tracheostomy IPPV for every item on the survey, including safety, convenience, swallowing, speech, appearance, comfort, and overall satisfaction.[14] Both ventilator users and their principal caregivers unanimously preferred the noninvasive methods overall to tracheostomy IPPV. Except for sleep, those switched from a noninvasive aid regimen, including noninvasive IPPV, to tracheostomy also preferred the noninvasive regimen for every item evaluated.

There are many reasons that patients prefer noninvasive aid and that noninvasive aid users express greater life satisfaction than tracheostomy IPPV users. Tracheostomy IPPV users with little breathing tolerance are fearful of sudden apnea resulting from tracheostomy disconnection or ventilator failure. Unlike noninvasive ventilation, IPPV via tracheostomy tends to cause continuous ventilator dependence (Chapter 8). Tracheostomy IPPV users also require ongoing tracheostomy care, including tracheal suctioning and regular uncomfortable tube changes. Sudden detachment of mucus plugs from the tube or cuff can cause acute respiratory distress. It is more difficult to obtain attendant care in the home for tracheostomized patients. In addition, tracheostomy IPPV users cannot use the sense of smell to taste their food and require supplemental humidification because air does not pass through the nasal passages and upper airway. They often complain of unpleasant taste sensations, which appear to be associated with chronic pathogenic bacterial colonization of the tracheostomy site and upper airways.

Patients using noninvasive aids, on the other hand, maintain more normal speech, do not require deep airway suctioning, and usually require assisted elimination of airway secretions only during respiratory tract infections. The fear of tracheostomy disconnection and sudden ventilator failure is eliminated by decannulation, use of noninvasive IPPV, and mastery of GPB (Chapter 10). Physiologic use of the upper airway permits the noninvasive ventilator user to maintain normal airway humidification and olfactory and taste sensations. All of these factors facilitate self-confidence and more active community living and may have contributed to the noninvasive aid users' greater life satisfaction.

Patients who were switched from body ventilator use-only to tracheostomy IPPV preferred the former for appearance, convenience, and speech and the latter for comfort, security, swallowing, sleep, and overall satisfaction. Most of these ventilator users were never introduced to noninvasive IPPV methods. Nocturnal mouthpiece IPPV with a lipseal was used almost exclusively in one center,[752] and nasal IPPV was not comprehensively described until 1987, long after most of these ventilator users had been switched to tracheostomy.[674] Their general preference for tracheostomy IPPV was understandable because body ventilators are less effective and more restrictive than IPPV; airway secretion clearance can be impossible without use of noninvasive IPPV and MI-E; and, except for the chest shell ventilator and IAPV, body ventilators must be used while the patient is reclining.[935] Of the ventilator users who "preferred" tracheostomy, none had mastered GPB and none had had access to MI-E. It is not surprising, therefore, that 31% of the ventilator users who preferred tracheostomy IPPV indicated that they did so because of the use of tracheal suctioning to clear airway secretions during respiratory tract infections. When more than nocturnal ventilatory support was required, resort to tracheostomy IPPV appeared to be desirable because noninvasive IPPV and MAC were unavailable.

The preferences for noninvasive ventilation are contrary to the views of physicians who think that IPPV via tracheostomy can facilitate voice production or swallowing or that it is safer than noninvasive methods because it provides better control of ventilator-delivered volumes and a convenient portal for airway suctioning. On the contrary, as noted in Chapters 4 and 8, tracheostomy tubes tie down the strap muscles in the neck and impede swallowing.[228,286,1119] Even when a cuffless tracheostomy tube or a deflated cuff is used, speech is of poorer quality than when noninvasive aids are used. Rhythm and voice tone are less natural than when the patient uses an IAPV with GPB or noninvasive IPPV. The use of GPB for deep breaths to increase voice volume, improve cough efficacy, and ensure safety in the event of ventilator failure is not possible during tracheostomy IPPV.[792] Indeed, a lower percentage of effective glossopharyngeal breathers would be expected and was found in the group that was ultimately switched to tracheostomy IPPV. All of these factors have considerable bearing on quality of life.

Ethics

Beware of bringing the hospital into the home.

Beware of astronomical costs involved with ventilation or society will choose the more economical alternative: no ventilators.

Beware of underestimating the limitless potential of individuals with disability.

Independence for a ventilator user means that one can say, "So I use a ventilator, I am in charge of it. I direct my own life and take my own risks. I am the one who decides about my quality of life."[1120]

⋅☞⋅ Gini Laurie's Ventilator User Caveats

Purtilo[1121] observed that most discussion of ventilator use has focused on the critically ill patient maintained by tracheostomy IPPV in ICUs. She pointed out that this focus has "fostered misconceptions and stereotypes" about other appropriate uses of ventilators. There is, likewise, great potential for "misunderstanding of the ethical issues involved in treating patients whose chronic maintenance depends on either positive or negative long-term ventilator support."

Quality of life is difficult, if not impossible, to measure by objective criteria that can be applied to all people. Most efforts at measurement, however, appear to have been based on factors relevant for physically able people.[1122] Jonsen et al. noted that the important point is the subjective satisfaction experienced by a person in physical, mental, and social situations, even though these experiences may be deficient in some manner.[1123] Thus, potential satisfaction with life and with the various aspects of existence should be considered in questioning the appropriateness of vital therapeutic options. Informed decisions about ethically and financially complex matters such as long-term ventilator use should be made by examining the life satisfaction of competent people who have already chosen these options. The great majority of severely disabled ventilator users with NMD are satisfied with their lives despite the inability to achieve many of the "usual" goals associated with quality of life in the physically able population. Their principal life satisfaction derives from their social relationships, reorganization of goals, and immediate environment.

In a study of 98 ventilator users, most of whom had neuromuscular weakness or chest wall disease, the impact of using a mechanical ventilator was found to be overwhelmingly positive (87%) in regard to sustaining life, facilitating mobility, improving physical symptoms, and overall satisfaction. Tracheostomy IPPV users volunteered significantly fewer positive statements than users of noninvasive ventilation. Whereas 53% of users indicated that they had initially experienced difficulties in coping with the ventilator, only 11% identified difficulties at the time of the survey.[1124] Although the willingness of and hardship imposed on care providers and community resources need to be taken into consideration, it is unethical not to consider the life satisfaction of people who have already chosen to use mechanical ventilation and who are living with the consequences of their decisions when decisions about about long-term ventilator use are made for others.[1108,1125] Eighty to 97% of tracheostomy continuous IPPV users with ALS are glad to have chosen mechanical ventilation, are satisfied with their lives, and would use mechanical ventilation again if they had to do so.[97,100,1126–1128] The longer that totally ADL-dependent patients with ALS/MND use continuous ventilatory support (from 1 to 15 years with only the ability to blink), the more life satisfaction they report.[1128] Only about 8% ever seriously consider discontinuing ventilatory support.[1126] Yet many physicians inappropriately judge the "lack of quality" of their patients' lives to justify withholding mechanical ventilation, even during episodes of acute respiratory failure. Indeed, less than 3% of patients with ALS undergo tracheotomy in the U.S.,[746] less than 10% are offered the option, and death from respiratory complications is almost ubiquitous.[100]

The right of the disabled person to live freely is often jeopardized by health care and societal issues. Zola described the "dehumanizing indignity in safety"[1129]: "Life entails risk and to try to create an environment without risk ultimately devalues the person with the disability by suggesting that he/she is not capable of coping except in the most restrictive and supportive environment."[1130] What is often appropriate and necessary in the protective environment of the acute care setting is not appropriate in the rehabilitation setting and has led many patients to express "intense frustration at the double messages given by rehabilitation professionals: you must learn to be independent as a disabled person, but we will make all your decisions for you."[1130]

A common reason for constraining the actions of institutionalized patients is to avoid risk to them and liability to the institution. However, this controlling focus does not always change once the person returns home because the daily care of "patients" is often directed by licensed nurses contracted by professional nursing agencies. Thus, the activities of the severely disabled person continue to be circumscribed by the rules of institutional health care organizations that hamper the client's self-determination and individuality. The solution for this problem lies in the formation of client-maintained personal assistance services (PAS) and the provision of adequate PAS for the severely disabled, self-directed people who require them. In the words of Gill:

> Our people are still being warehoused without hope of ever having a home or family or lifestyle of their own. When you think about it, in contrast to the vast numbers of us demanding our rights to first-class citizenship, only a handful of disabled people have publicly sought death. Yet...laws are being passed at record speed to ease the way to our demise. Prominent "experts" [argue] for our right to die...as defenders of our freedom, dignity, humane treatment, and even "independence"...[yet it] has taken almost 20 years of exhausting struggle to get a basic civil rights law for disabled people.[1131]

Although the Americans with Disabilities Act (ADA) is seen as an important step to prevent discrimination against disabled people, it does little or nothing for the self-directed disabled person who, like most patients with neuromuscular disorders, is not informed by physicians about potentially vital therapeutic options,[1108] nor does it help those who are warehoused in institutions because of lack of a national PAS policy. The false beliefs that prohibitively expensive continuous nursing care is required and that disabled ventilator users are unable to take responsibility for and manage their own care are the greatest obstacles to returning them to the community. This position is ironic since the provision of PAS for the home care of ventilator users can greatly reduce cost[1067] as well as enhance quality of life.

One large group of ventilator users with respiratory failure was institutionalized for 24–31 years before obtaining release to enter the community in 1979. The ventilator users were authorized to develop a client-maintained organization, Concepts of Independence, Inc., that permits self-directed clients, themselves and others, to hire, train, direct, and dismiss their own personal care attendants.[1132] Virtually all of the current 1156 clients of Concepts of Independence, Inc. require continuous attendant care. This population includes 25 noninvasive and 11 tracheostomy IPPV users. The program has now successfully expanded throughout New York State, and there have been no significant accidents or litigation in its 23-year history. Indeed, the home health care industry has had virtually no history of tort litigation.[1132,1133] The efforts of these courageous and tenacious ventilator users succeeded in establishing a precedent for humanizing the care of severely disabled, self-directed people in private domiciles and, in doing so, greatly increased the quality of their lives with 70% cost savings to the taxpayers of New York.[1067] As Kafka observed, "Without effective community options we lose our humanity. More and more people are choosing to die rather than exist in institutions...warehoused for 'cost' and 'efficiency.'"[1134]

The institutional control of chronic care, whether in an institution or in the community with PAS managed by nursing organizations, can impersonalize and dehumanize care in the name of safety. It reduces the client's sense of personal control and self-efficacy and suggests inadequacy in coping. Physicians who train their patients in how to manage and take responsibility for their care need to play a more active role in advocating for the procurement of the services needed to permit them to return to or remain in the community.

Typical counterproductive regulations include the prohibition of tracheal suctioning by unlicensed personal care attendants. In 46 states young children who are relatives of the user may perform tracheal suctioning, but third-party payors and home nursing care agencies will not sanction this activity by trained PAS. Such regulations too often serve to protect private interests under the pretext of avoiding liability and ensuring the patient's safety. These restrictions continue despite the fact that the American College of Chest Physicians[1135] and others[1136] support the use of properly trained PAS for self-directed ventilator users. So far, regulations have been modified to permit this practice in at least Colorado, Massachusetts, and New York.[1137]

We routinely close tracheostomy sites and convert ventilator users to noninvasive respiratory aids. Because this service is performed by very few institutions,[932] most ventilator users are never made aware of it, and many, without adequate family support, must remain tracheostomized and institutionalized. It is the ethical responsibility of the health care community to inform ventilator users about noninvasive alternatives to tracheostomy before considering advanced medical directives. Patients should be offered training in their use and decannulation to noninvasive supports, especially when these methods can facilitate community living with or without PAS. This approach benefits both the patient and the taxpayer. In the face of calls to limit entitlement spending, it should be noted that a society willing to provide free room, board, health care, legal and educational services, vocational training, and cable television for murderers, rapists, drug dealers, and other felons at a cost of billions of dollars, including $30,000 per year per inmate just for internment, has the ethical responsibility to provide PAS to those in need, some of whom are crime victims themselves.[1067] Further information about the need for and status of PAS is available in various sources.[1137–1139]

Despite the consternation about growing medical costs, little is being done to limit costs and optimize care for users of mechanical ventilation. Instead of preventing the otherwise inevitable episodes of respiratory failure for patients with NMD by using the methods discussed in this book, patients are left to develop respiratory failure and undergo tracheotomy. However, the average length of hospital stay for patients with NMD when they undergo tracheotomy is 72.1 days, most of which are spent in intensive care; for 16.2 of these days the patient is intubated.[655] The prolonged hospitalization is due to failed weaning and extubation attempts; in addition, the family is often ill prepared to care for a tracheostomy IPPV-dependent member and requires considerable time for acceptance, training, and home preparation. Most of these costly hospitalizations can be avoided with proper patient follow-up, education, training, and equipment.

In another example of waste of financial resources, the initial costs of placement and training in phrenic nerve pacing exceed $300,000, and the technique has a realistic long-term success rate of only 33%.[882] Furthermore, patients using electrophrenic respiration (EPR) most often retain tracheostomy tubes, which create additional expenses for disposable suction catheters, tracheostomy tube changes, related stomal care, and possibly home nursing services. In contrast, removal of the tracheostomy tube, teaching of GPB to free the patient from vital ventilator dependence, and use of noninvasive ventilatory support alternatives are significantly less expensive. Mouthpieces cost $3–27 each; nasal interfaces, $30–200 each; and Exsufflation Belts, $350 each. The $300,000 initial cost of EPR often comes out of a limited insurance policy. This money often can be used with much better effect to provide ADL-enhancing equipment and personal care. Unfortunately, the profits from pacemaker placement and use and the intensive marketing of this approach obscure the more reasonable but less immediately profitable alternative of using respiratory muscle aids. One still earns more money by placing tracheostomy tubes and pacemakers than by removing them.

With the growing emphasis on cost containment and reform of the health care delivery system in the United States, quality-of-life issues are being evoked to justify withholding life-sustaining medical interventions, including mechanical ventilation.[1107,1108] Although it would appear that an intelligent, self-directed person should be fully informed about therapeutic options and prognosis, in the frenzy of seeking a less expensive health care delivery system, some physicians have suggested eliminating the patient from the decision-making process. As recently as 1989 it was recommended that the physician's assessment of patients' quality of life should be "independent of the patient's feelings" in determining whether or not to institute mechanical ventilation.[1125]

Besides the fact that most physicians underestimate the life satisfaction of ventilator users with NMD, the great majority of physicians caring for such people are ignorant of noninvasive methods that offer prolonged survival. It should not be surprising, therefore, that many, if not most, physicians are biased against the long-term use of ventilatory assistance, which they wrongly associate with the need for an indwelling tracheostomy tube. This misconception was documented in a survey of NMD clinic directors.[1108] Forty-one percent of 273 MDA clinic directors openly discouraged ventilator use, whereas only 30% ever recommended it. Fifty-five percent of the directors cited "poor quality of life" to justify their position. Only two physicians who discouraged ventilator use were familiar with noninvasive IPPV. Not surprisingly, the directors who most underestimated the ventilator users' life satisfaction were also the least likely to encourage ventilator use and to be familiar with noninvasive respiratory aids.[1108] More recent surveys of MDA clinic directors in the United States[615] and Canada[1140] unfortunately demonstrated similar results. In the Canadian study, most physicians had a negative bias against assisted ventilation; 53% cited poor quality of life as the reason not to offer assisted ventilation; and 25% of them never even broached the subject of mechanical ventilation. A manuscript demonstrating a 2-year prolongation of survival by the use of strictly noninvasive methods for people with ALS/MND and no breathing tolerance was recently rejected by the *Journal of Neurology* when the reviewer stated that, in his opinion, "these patients did not need to use ventilators." Did his opinion reflect disbelief in the efficacy of the methods, the view that the patients were simply better off dead, or both? Other clinicians have frankly stated that "the use of chronic assisted ventilation should be avoided."[1141] Still others consider the long-term use of assisted ventilation for people with DMD to be "most controversial" and to raise "enormous ethical difficulties."[1142]

Indeed, some physicians appear to impose hardly any limits on their self-determined right to make life-and-death decisions for their patients. Ventilator use is a situation "in which the support system does not replace the diseased organ. The ventilator assists an organ system that is not primarily diseased. The model of renal dialysis does not apply, since the diseased organ is replaced by the function of the machine."[740] This rationale has been used despite the fact that the cost of ventilator use is about 30% of the cost of renal dialysis and far less disruptive of the patient's day-to-day life.

In the words of Goldblatt, "Patients should be encouraged as much as possible to direct their own lives, but, if they are incapable of reaching an unequivocal and seemingly rational decision, they should be able to trust their doctor to act in their best interest...the physician will consult the family and will look as objectively as possible at the quality of the patient's life."[1143] Negative physician attitudes make it imperative for patients to have sources other than their health care professionals to learn about therapeutic options. For many the Internet has provided the needed patient-networking capabilities. Health care providers must ethically avoid a paternalistic stance when working with the disabled. Self-directed people, once properly informed, should be treated as competent to make decisions about their own welfare. Paternalism undermines the goals of rehabilitation.

The Futility of Advanced Directives: When Does No Really Mean No?

Advanced directives are valid only if the patient is fully informed about treatment options and, in particular, the likely clinical course if they are not used. Patients with NMD are rarely properly informed because few clinicians are knowledgeable about noninvasive options. In part as a result of this problem, some clinicians argue that "the patient, his or her family, the physician, and other care providers may not be able to adhere to a planned decision to withhold [invasive] ventilatory support in the presence of impending respiratory failure, when the instinctive urge to preserve life supplants the rational conclusion that, in this particular instance, death is preferable to life under such profoundly altered conditions."[1143]

When asked early in the course of their disease, many patients with ALS/MND indicate that they would rather die than use respiratory support. In a recent study, 38% of 640 physicians also stated that they would prefer to end their lives rather than use ventilators for ALS.[1144] Many people change their minds during episodes of acute respiratory failure, however, particularly when dyspnea can be relieved by the simple use of noninvasive respiratory muscle aids. The patient's attitude toward the use of ventilatory aids more closely reflects the physician's attitude and the nature of the treatment options than an informed rational decision.[1108] There were no differences in scores of depression, hopelessness, overall quality of life, or psychological well-being in patients with ALS/MND who required ventilatory support for 1–120 months and patients with ALS/MND who had less disability and did not require ventilator use.[1127] It should be recognized that a decision for ventilatory support is probably the best predictor of an acceptable quality of life using a ventilator.[1127]

Few if any clinicians would consider the use of respiratory muscle aids to be "heroic" interventions. Yet, to the health care professional offering advance directives, heroic measures to be avoided include "mechanical ventilation," which to most clinicians means intubation and tracheostomy. The belief is that intubation will result in failure to wean from the ventilator, tracheotomy, and long-term dependence on tracheostomy IPPV. In reality, this belief is true only for patients with severe bulbar ALS/MND and a persistent decrease in baseline SpO_2 due to chronic aspiration.

Although most patients say that they would refuse tracheotomy, as VCs and CPF decrease, few if any refuse the occasional use of noninvasive respiratory muscle aids to relieve dyspnea or to facilitate airway secretion elimination. Some patients initially use mouthpiece IPPV only to increase voice volume. With time and further decreases in VC, the patient eventually uses noninvasive IPPV continuously. Once accustomed to it, the patient may be more likely to accept tracheotomy when it is warranted by decreasing SpO_2.

Because of avoidance of noninvasive aids, patients are unfamiliar with ventilator use when respiratory failure unexpectedly occurs. At that time, desperate, intubated, suboptimally managed, and poorly informed patients are given a tracheostomy ultimatum that they accept with fear and anger. Patients and families feel overwhelmed and inadequately counseled;[740] they rarely understand the wide-reaching financial, social, and physical consequences of acquiescing to tracheotomy. To avoid this scenario, which is often incorrectly thought to be inevitable, some physicians prescribe euthanasia with supplemental oxygen and morphine.[648,1145]

Should the patient's desire to live be ignored because "death is preferable to life under these conditions," or should morbidity be avoided by using noninvasive aids? Noninvasive aids can postpone or entirely obviate the "crisis" of deciding whether or not to "go on a ventilator" (to undergo tracheotomy). Furthermore, the use of noninvasive methods eliminates the ethical considerations related to suicide by withdrawal of ventilatory support because users of noninvasive methods are not passively attached to a respirator but actively control their alveolar ventilation. The personal sense of controlling one's own life is also better maintained. Physicians have the ethical responsibility to inform patients about noninvasive respiratory aids.

Children and Quality of Life

"Terminal illness" is a self-fulfilling prophecy.

Children's physicians often intentionally withhold information about the potentially life-saving use of respiratory muscle aids, feeling that the quality of life of severely disabled children is too poor to warrant letting them survive and that their parents cannot make the "appropriate" decision to "let nature take its course." In one study, over 70 health care professionals were asked to judge the quality of life of children with SMA type 1 using a Likert scale of 0–10, on which 10 is maximum and 0 is minimum. Their replies averaged less than 2, and most said that they would advise against any ventilator use. Not surprisingly, parents are often told that there is no point in keeping their children alive because their quality of life is too poor and too much effort is required to raise them. Yet, in a study of 104 responding care providers, mostly parents, of 66 children with SMA type 1 (Chapters 1 and 12), the responses were significantly more positive (Table 8) than the estimates of the health care professionals. Except for effort required to raise the child, the responses were not significantly different from the responses of parents of unaffected children. The parents and other care providers of children with SMA type 1 noted that the children were happy and that their lives were worthwhile despite the relatively high effort that it took to raise them. The ongoing use of noninvasive ventilation was clearly not considered an intolerable burden for these children or their care providers.[1146]

On the other hand, the emotional status of the children with SMA needs to be assessed. It has been noted that 5 patients with SMA type 2 and 3 had intense and recurrent anguish about death and the image of "a narcissistically injured self."[1147] However, the title of the paper, which cites onset of "a terminal disease," can in part explain the anguish. Patients and their families are told that they are terminally ill because their physicians are unaware of how to help them avoid morbidity and mortality. Nevertheless,

Table 8. Responses of 104 Care Providers of 66 Children with SMA Type 1	
Likert scale 0 (minimum) to 10 (maximum) except where noted	
Quality of the child's life	7.8
Quality of the provider's life	8.0
Effort in raising the child (compared with 5 for average child)	8.3
Burden in raising the child (compared with 5 for average child)	5.8
Child's happiness	8.5
Child's life worthwhile	9.6
Likert scale 0 (minimum) to 7 (maximum)	
Child's satisfaction with life	6.0
Semantic differential 1 to 7	
Life with your child is:	
Boring–Interesting	6.7
Hard–Easy	3.8
Lonely–Friendly	6.1
Miserable–Enjoyable	6.3
Useless–Worthwhile	6.7
Empty–Full	6.6
Disappointing–Rewarding	5.9
Tied down–Free	4.0

now that even patients with SMA type 1 can live into adulthood, more work is required to evaluate their emotional needs.

Interestingly, children with SMA, including those with type 1, do very well in school. They have been found to have IQs significantly higher than normal (Chapter 12). Even before age 2 they can often cooperate with VC measurements and Cough-Assist use. People with all severities of SMA have gone to college and achieved meaningful social relationships. Those with types 2–5 have achieved professional employment. We are following 5 children with SMA type 1 over the age of 10 years who are continuously dependent on ventilatory support via tracheostomy tubes. All are doing very well in school. One 19-year-old man graduated third in his high school class and now attends college, despite being unable to speak or eat and having only minimal residual finger and eye movement. In another study of ventilatory support via tracheostomy for patients with SMA, three of the 10 patients over 18 years of age had college degrees, 2 were college students, 3 graduated from high school, and 2 completed eleventh grade. One patient is the mother of a healthy child. Two patients are employed, and 2 others do volunteer work.[741]

Purtilo summarized an article about ethical issues related to the management of ventilator users by saying that misconceptions about the undesirability of "'going on a respirator' have far-reaching negative effects for persons now happily being supported on a respirator, and mitigate the positive effects it could have for some types of chronically impaired persons whose quality of life also could be enhanced by the use of a ventilator."[1121] Freed stressed the importance of professionals not imposing their own concepts, values and judgments onto the disabled person.[1148] Clinicians should be cognizant of their inability to gauge disabled patients' life satisfaction and potential for social and vocational productivity and thus refrain from letting inaccurate and unwarranted judgment of subjective factors associated with quality of life in the general population affect patient management decisions.

> *Surprendre...*
> *Cueillir ses mots comme des fleurs*
> *Semer des graines au long des coeurs*
> *Confier son âme et sa mèmoire*
> *A celui qui viendra plus tard*
>
>   Apprendre by Yves Duteil

References

1. de La Grange H-L. Gustav Mahler, vol. 1. Fayard, Paris, 1979.
2. Kraft GH. Multiple sclerosis: future directions in the care and the cure. J Neurol Rehabil 1989;3:61–4.
3. LaPlante MP, Hendershot GE, Moss AJ. Assistive technology devices and home accessibility features: prevalence, payment, need, and trends. Adv Data 1992;217:1–11.
4. Lapena JF Jr, Berkowitz RG. Neuromuscular disorders presenting as congenital bilateral vocal cord paralysis. Ann Otol Rhinol Laryngol 2001;110:952–5.
5. Emery AEH. Duchenne muscular dystrophy: genetic aspects, carrier detection and antenatal diagnosis. Br Med Bull 1980;36:117–22.
6. Meryon E. On granular or fatty degeneration of the voluntary muscles. Medico-Chirurgical Trans 1852;35: 73–84.
7. Bach JR. The Duchenne de Boulogne - Meryon controversy and pseudohypertrophic muscular dystrophy. J Hist Med Appl Sci 2000;55:158–178.
8. Hattori N, Kaido M, Nishigaki T, Inui K, Fujimura H, Nishimura T, Naka T, Hazama T. Undetectable dystrophin can still result in a relatively benign phenotype of dystrophinopathy. Neuromuscul Disord 1999;9:220–6.
9. McDonald CM, Abresch RT, Carter GT, et al. Profiles of neuromuscular diseases: Duchenne muscular dystrophy. Am J Phys Med Rehabil 1995;74:S70–92.
10. Cohen L, Morgan J, Babbs R Jr, Karrison TG, Giacomoni M. Fast walking velocity in health and Duchenne muscular dystrophy: a statistical analysis. Arch Phys Med Rehabil 1984;65:573–8.
11. Johnson EW. Pathokinesiology of Duchenne muscular dystrophy: implications for management. Arch Phys Med Rehabil 1977;58:4–7.
12. Bach JR, McKeon J. Orthopedic surgery and rehabilitation for the prolongation of brace-free ambulation of patients with Duchenne muscular dystrophy. Am J Phys Med Rehabil 1991;70:323–331.
13. Billard C, Gillet P, Barthez M, Hommet C, Bertrand P. Reading ability and processing in Duchenne muscular dystrophy and spinal muscular atrophy. Dev Med Child Neurol 1998;40:12–20.
14. Bach JR, Rajaraman R, Ballanger F, Tzeng AC, Ishikawa Y, Kulessa R, Bansal T. Neuromuscular ventilatory insufficiency: the effect of home mechanical ventilator use vs. oxygen therapy on pneumonia and hospitalization rates. Am J Phys Med Rehabil 1998;77:8–19.
15. Rideau Y, Gatin G, Bach J, Gines G. Prolongation of life in Duchenne muscular dystrophy. Acta Neurol 1983;5:118–24.
16. Phillips MF, Quinlivan RC, Edwards RH, Calverley PM. Changes in spirometry over time as a prognostic marker in patients with Duchenne muscular dystrophy. Am J Respir Crit Care Med 2001;164: 2191–4.
17. Thomas NST, Williams H, Elsas LJ, Hopkins LC, Sarfarazi M, Harper PS. Localisation of the gene for Emery-Dreifuss muscular dystrophy to the distal long arm of the X chromosome. J Med Genet 1986;23:596–98.
18. Miller RG, Layzer RB, Mellenthin MA, Golabi M, Francoz RA, Mall JC. Emery-Dreifuss muscular dystrophy with autosomal dominant transmission. Neurology 1985;35:1230–33.
19. Cartegni L, di Barletta MR, Barresi R, et al. Heart-specific localization of emerin: new insights into Emery-Dreifuss muscular dystrophy. Hum Mol Genet 1997;6:2257–64.
20. Mascarenhas DA, Spodick DH, Chad DA, et al. Cardiomyopathy of limb-girdle muscular dystrophy. J Am Coll Cardiol 1994;24:1328–33.
21. McDonald CM, Johnson ER, Abresch RT, Carter GT, Fowler WM Jr, Kilmer DD. Profiles of neuromuscular diseases: limb-girdle syndromes. Am J Phys Med Rehabil 1995;74:S117–S130.
22. Walton JN, Gardner-Medwin D. The muscular dystrophies. In: Walton J (ed). Disorders of Voluntary Muscle, ed. 5. Churchill Livingstone, London: 1988:519–568.
23. Jung D, Leturcq F, Sunada Y, et al. Absence of gamma-sarcoglycan in autosomal recessive muscular dystrophy linked to chromosome 13q12. FEBS Lett 1996;381:15–20.
24. McMenamin JB, Becker LE, Murphy EG. Congenital muscular dystrophy: a clinicopathologic report of 24 cases. J Pediatr 1982;100:692–97.

25. O'Brien MD. An infantile muscular dystrophy: report of a case with autopsy findings. Guy's Hosp Rep 1962;111:98–106.
26. Wharton BA. An unusual variety of muscular dystrophy. Lancet 1965;1:603–604.
27. Zellweger H, Afifi A, McCormick WF, Mergner W. Severe congenital muscular dystrophy. Am J Dis Child 1967;114:591–602.
28. Bailey RO, Marzulo DC, Hans MB. Infantile fascioscapulohumeral muscular dystrophy: new observations. Acta Neurol Scand 1986;74:51–58.
29. Bushby KM, Pollitt C, Johnson MA, Rogers MT, Chinnery PF. Muscle pain as a prominent feature of facioscapulohumeral muscular dystrophy: four illustrative case reports. Neuromuscul Disord 1998;8:574–9.
30. Kilmer DD, Abresch MA, McCrory MA, Carter GT, Fowler WM Jr, Johnson ER, McDonald CM. Facioscapulohumeral muscular dystrophy. Am J Phys Med Rehabil 1995;74:S131–139.
31. Brooke MH. A Clinician's View of Neuromuscular Diseases, ed. 2. Williams & Wilkins, Baltimore: 1986:194–212.
32. Aslanidis C, Jansen G, Amemiya C, et al. Cloning of the essential myotonic dystrophy region and mapping of the putative defect. Nature 1992;355:548–551.
33. Rutherford MA, Heckmatt JZ, Dubowitz V. Congenital myotonic dystrophy: respiratory function at birth determines survival. Arch Dis Child 1989;64:191–195.
34. Abercrombie JF, Rogers J, Swash M. Faecal incontinence in myotonic dystrophy. J Neurol Neurosurg Psychiatry 1998;64:128–301.
35. Salomonson J, Kawamoto H, Wilson L. Velopharyngeal incompetence as the presenting symptom of myotonic dystrophy. Cleft Palate J 1988;25:296–300.
36. Misra D, DeSilva S, Fellerman H, Dufour DR, Streeten DH, Nylen ES. Hyperkalemia and selective hypoaldosteronism in myotonic dystrophy. Clin Endocrinol 2002;56:271–5.
37. Johnson ER, Abresch RT, Carter GT, et al. Profiles of neuromuscular disease: myotonic dystrophy. Am J Phys Med Rehabil 1995;74:S104–S116.
38. Hayashi T, Ichiyama T, Tanaka H, Koga M, Okino A. Successful treatment of incontinence of feces in myotonic muscular dystrophy by mexiletine. No To Hattatsu 1991;23:310–2.
39. Finlay M. A comparative study of disopyramide and procainamide in the treatment of myotonia in myotonic dystrophy. J Neurol Neurosurg Psychiatry 1982;45:461–3.
40. Kashiwagi K, Nagafuchi S, Sekiguchi N, et al. Troglitazone not only reduced insulin resistance but also improved myotonia in a patient with myotonic dystrophy. Eur Neurol 1999;41:171–2.
41. Sechi GP, Traccis S, Durelli L, Monaco F, Mutani R. Carbamazepine versus diphenylhydantoin in the treatment of myotonia. Eur Neurol 1983;22:113–8.
42. Milner-Brown HS, Miller RG. Myotonic dystrophy: quantification of muscle weakness and myotonia and the effect of amitriptyline and exercise. Arch Phys Med Rehabil 1990;71:983–87.
43. Sugino M, Ohsawa N, Ito T, et al. A pilot study of dehydroepiandrosterone sulfate in myotonic dystrophy. Neurology 1998;51:586–9.
44. Merlini L, Granata C, Bonfiglioli S, et al. Scoliosis in spinal muscular atrophy: natural history and management. Dev Med Child Neurol 1989;31:501–8.
45. Achiron A, Barak Y, Magal N, Shohat M, Cohen M, Barar R, Gadoth N. Abnormal liver test results in myotonic dystrophy. J Clin Gastroenterol 1998;26:292–5.
46. Rimmer KP, Whitelaw WA. The respiratory muscles in multicore myopathy. Am Rev Respir Dis 1993;148:227–231.
47. Brownell AKW, Gilbert JJ, Shaw DT, Garcia B, Wenkebach GF, Lam AKS. Adult onset nemaline myopathy. Neurology 1978;28:1306–1309.
48. Jerusalem F, Ludin H, Bischoff A, Hartmann G. Cytoplasmic body neuromyopathy presenting as respiratory failure and weight loss. J Neurol Sci 1979;41:1–9.
49. Carpenter S, Karpati G, Holland P. New observations in reducing body myopathy. Neurology 1985;35:818–827.
50. Stanley CA, DeLeeuw S, Coates PM, et al. Chronic cardiomyopathy and weakness or acute coma in children with a defect in carnitine uptake. Ann Neurol 1991;30:709–716.
51. Selby R, Starzl TE, Yunis E, et al. Liver transplantation for type IV glycogen storage disease. N Engl J Med 1991;324:39–42.
52. Griggs RC, Mendell JR, Miller RG. Evaluation and treatment of myopathies. FA Davis Company, Philadelphia: 1995:294–313.
53. Fruch BR, Su CS. Medial tarsal suspension: a method of elevating the medial lower eyelid. Ophthal Plast Reconstr Surg 2002;18:133–7.

54. Wong VA, Beckingsale PS, Oley CA, Sullivan TJ. Management of myogenic ptosis. Ophthalmology 2002;109:1023–31.
55. Thompson CE. Infantile myositis. Dev Med Child Neurol 1982;24:307–313.
56. Simpson JA. Myasthenia gravis and myasthenic syndromes. In: Walton JN (ed). Disorders of Voluntary Muscle, ed. 5. Churchill Livingstone, London: 1988:628–665.
57. Tsujimoto Y. Role of anti-apoptotic Bcl-2 protein in spinal muscular atrophy. J Neural Transm Suppl 2000;58:41–52.
58. Kerr DA, Nery JP, Traystman RUJ, Chau BN, Hardwick JM. Survival motor neuron protein modulates neuron-specific apoptosis. Proc Natl Acad Sci USA 2000;24f:13312–7.
59. Iannaccone ST. Spinal muscular atrophy. Semin Neurol 1998;18:19–26.
60. Grohmann K, Weinker TF, Saar K, et al. Diaphragmatic spinal muscular atrophy with respiratory distress is heterogeneous, and one form is linked to chromosome 11q13-q21. Am J Hum Genet 1999;65:1459–62.
61. Yamamoto K, Sakai H, Hadano S, Gondo Y, Ikeda JE. Identification of two distinct transcripts for the neuronal apoptosis inhibitory protein gene. Biochem Biophys Res Commun 1999;264:998–1006.
62. Rubio-Gozalbo ME, Smeitink JA, Ruitenbeek W, et al. Spinal muscular atrophy-like picture, cardiomyopathy, and cytochrome c oxidase deficiency. Neurology 1999;52:383–6.
63. Dubowitz V. Very severe spinal muscular atrophy (SMA type 0): an expanding clinical phenotype. Europ J Paediatr Neurol 1999;3:49–51.
64. Wang TG, Bach JR, Avilez C, Alba AS, Yang GF. Survival of individuals with spinal muscular atrophy on ventilatory support. Am J Phys Med Rehabil 1994;73:207–11.
65. Fok ML. Living with SMA in Hong Kong. International Ventilator Users Network 2002;16:1–2.
66. Yim R, Kirschner K, Murphy E, Parson J, Winslow C. A successful pregnancy in a patient with spinal muscular atrophy type 1 and severe kyphoscoliosis. Am J Phys Med Rehabil 2003;82:222–5.
67. Russman BS, Buncher CR, White M, Samaha FJ, Iannaccone ST. Function changes in spinal muscular atrophy II and III: the DCN/SMA Group. Neurology 1996;47:973–6.
68. Koch BM, Simenson RL. Upper extremity strength and function in children with spinal muscular atrophy type 2. Arch Phys Med Rehabil 1992;73:241–5.
69. Iannaccone ST, Russman BS, Browne RH, et al. Prospective analysis of strength in spinal muscular atrophy. J Child Neurol 2000;15:97–101.
70. Zerres K, Rudnik-Schoneborn S, Forrest E, Lusakowska A, Borkowska J, Hausmanowa-Petrusewicz I. A collaborative study on the natural history of childhood and juvenile onset proximal spinal muscular atrophy: 569 patients. J Neurol Sci 1997;27:67–72.
71. Rudnik-Schoneborn S, Hausmanowa-Petrusewicz I, Borkowska J, Zerres K. The predictive value of achieved motor milestones assessed in 441 patients with infantile spinal muscular atrophy types II and III. Eur Neurol 2001;45:174–81.
72. Bach JR, Wang TG. Noninvasive long-term ventilatory support for individuals with spinal muscular atrophy and functional bulbar musculature. Arch Phys Med Rehabil 1995;76:213–217.
73. Houston K, Buschang PH, Iannaccone ST, Seale NS. Craniofacial morphology of spinal muscular atrophy. Pediatr Res 1994;36:265–9.
74. Popnick JM, Jacobs I, Supiuski G, DiMarco A. Effect of upper respiratory track infection in patients with neuromuscular disease. Am J Respir Crit Care Med 1997;156:659–664.
75. Mier-Jedrzejowicz A, Brophy C, Green M. Respiratory muscle weakness during upper respiratory tract infections. Am Rev Respir Dis 1988;138:5–7.
76. Hattori N, Nishigaki T, Inui K, Kaido M, Nishimura T, Hazama T, Nakata T. A case of spinal muscular atrophy with marked calf hypertrophy and adolescent onset. Rinsho Shinkeigaku 2000;40:170–3.
77. Bach JR. Perspectives, indications, and the ethics of prolonging "meaningful life" for individuals with progressive neuromuscular disease. J Neuro Rehab 1992;6:61–66.
78. Ostermeyer-Shoaib B, Patten BM. IgG subclass deficiency in amyotrophic lateral sclerosis. Acta Neurol Scand 1993;87:192–4.
79. Moulignier A, Moulonguet A, Pialoux G, Rozenbaum W. Reversible ALS-like disorder in HIV infection. Neurology 2001;57:995–1001.
80. Rijnders B, Decramer M. Reversibility of paraneoplastic bilateral diaphragmatic paralysis after nephrectomy for renal cell carcinoma. Ann Oncol 2000;11:221–5.
81. Veldink JH, van den Berg LH, Cobben JM, et al. Homozygous deletion of the survival motor neuron 2 gene is a prognostic factor in sparadic ALS. Neurology 2001;56:749–52.

82. Forsyth PA, Dalmau J, Graus F, Cwik V, Rosenblum MK, Posner JB. Motor neuron syndromes in cancer patients. Ann Neurol 1997;41:722–30.

83. Nobile-Orazio E, Carpo M, Meucci N. Are there immunologically treatable motor neuron diseases? Amyotroph Lateral Scler Other Motor Neuron Disord 2001;2:S23–30.

84. Orrell RW, Habgood JJ, de Belleroche JS, Lane RJ. The relationship of spinal muscular atrophy to motor neuron disease: investigation of SMN and NAIP gene deletions in sporadic and familial ALS. J Neurol Sci 1997;145:55–61.

85. Bentes C, deCarvalho M, Evangelista T, Sales-Luis ML. Multifocal motor neuropathy mimicking motor neuron disease: nine cases. J Neurol Sci 1999;169:76–9.

86. Van den Berg-Vos RM, Franssen H, Wokke JH, Van Es HW, Van den Berg LH. Multifocal motor neuropathy: diagnostic criteria that predict the response to immunoglobulin treatment. Ann Neurol 2000;48:919–26.

87. Hazouard E, Bergemer-Fouquet AM, Hommet C, et al. Amyotrophic lateral sclerosis manifesting as cognitive disorders: value of brain perfusion scintigraphic tomography in intensive care. Press Med 2000;29:299–302.

88. Portet F, Cadilhac C, Touchon J, Camu W. Cognitive impairment in motor neuron disease with bulbar onset. Amyotroph Lateral Scler Other Motor Neuron Disord 2001;2:23–9.

89. Newsom-Davis IC, Lyall RA, Leigh PN, Moxham J, Goldstein LH. The effect of non-invasive positive pressure ventilation on cognitive function in amyotrophic lateral sclerosis: a prospective study. J Neurol Neurosurg Psychiatry 2001;71:482–7.

90. Norris F, Shepherd R, Denys E, Kwei U, Mukai E, Elias L, Holden D, Norris H. Onset, natural history and outcome in idiopathic adult motor neuron disease. J Neurol Sci 1993;118:48–55.

91. Bradley MD, Orrell RW, Williams AJ, et al. Motor neurone disease presenting with acute respiratory failure. ALS and Other Motor Neuron Disorders 2000;1:21–22.

92. Strong MJ, Ferguson KA, Ahmad D. The pulmonary function testing as a predictor of survival in amyotrophic lateral sclerosis (abstract). Chest 1992;102:180S.

93. Jablecki CK, Berry C, Leach J. Survival prediction in amyotrophic lateral sclerosis. Muscle Nerve 1989;12:833–41.

94. Norris F, Shepherd R, Denys E, et al. Natural history and outcome in idiopathic adult motor neuron disease. J Neurol Sci 1993;118:48–55.

95. Cazzoli PA. The use of noninvasive and tracheostomy positive pressure ventilation in amyotrophic lateral sclerosis survival, long-term outcomes, factors for success and failure, and quality of life. 8th Journées Internationales de Ventilation a Domicile, abstract 120, March 7, 2001, Hôpital de la Croix-Rousse, Lyon, France.

96. Tucker T, Layzer RB, Miller RG, Chad D. Subacute, reversible motor neuron disease. Neurology 1991;41:1541–44.

97. Bach JR. Amyotrophic lateral sclerosis: communication status and survival with ventilatory support. Am J Phys Med Rehabil 1993;72:343–349.

98. Lechtzin N, Wiener CM, Clawson L, Chaudhry V, Diette GB. Hospitalization in amyotrophic lateral sclerosis: causes, costs, and outcomes. Neurology 2001;56:753–7.

99. Oppenheimer EA. Respiratory management and home mechanical ventilation in amyotrophic lateral sclerosis. In: Mitsumoto H, Norris FH (eds). Amyotrophic Lateral Sclerosis: A Comprehensive Guide to Management. New York, Demos, 1994.

100. Moss AH, Casey P, Stocking CB, Roos RP, Brooks BR, Siegler M. Home ventilation for amyotrophic lateral sclerosis patients: outcomes, costs, and patient, family and physician attitudes. Neurol 1993;43:438–443.

101. Bach JR. Respiratory muscle aids: diagnosis-related outcomes. In: Bach JR: Noninvasive Mechanical Ventilation. Philadelphia: Hanley & Belfus 2002:189–202.

102. Bach JR, Alba AS, Bohatiuk G, Saporito L, Lee M. Mouth intermittent positive pressure ventilation in the management of post-polio respiratory insufficiency. Chest 1987;91:859–864.

103. Bach JR (ed). Noninvasive Mechanical Ventilation. Philadelphia, Hanley and Belfus 2002.

104. Halstead L, Grimby G (eds). Post-Polio Syndrome. Philadelphia, Hanley & Belfus 1995:89–111.

105. Carter GT, Abresch RT, Fowler WM JR, Johnson ER, Kilmer DD, McDonald CM. Profiles of neuromuscular diseases: hereditary motor and sensory neuropathy, types 1 and 2. Am J Phys Med Rehabil 1995;74:S140–S149.

106. Rowland LP, Bach JR, Borg K, et al. Post-Polio Syndrome: Identifying Best Practices in Diagnosis and Care. White Plains, N.Y.: March of Dimes Birth Defects Foundation, 2001.

107. Kirshblum S, Campagnolo DI, DeLisa JA. Spinal cord medicine. Philadelphia: Lippincott/Williams & Wilkins, 2002:1–655.
108. Burks JS, Johnson KP. Multiple Sclerosis: Diagnosis, medical management and rehabilitation. New York: Demos, 2000:1–598.
109. Bach JR (ed). Pulmonary Rehabilitation: The Obstructive and Paralytic Conditions. Hanley & Belfus, Philadelphia: 1996.
110. Bach JR. Disease profiles of noninvasive ventilation users. In: Bach JR (ed). Noninvasive Mechanical Ventilation. Hanley & Belfus, Philadelphia: 2002:1–24.
111. Persky AM, Brazeau GA. Clinical pharmacology of the dietary supplement creatine monohydrate. Pharmacological Reviews 2001;53:161–76.
112. Walter MC, Lochmuller H, Reilich P, Klopstock T, Huber R, Hartard M, Hennig M, Pongratz D, Muller-Felber W. Creatine monohydrate in muscular dystrophies: a double-blind, placebo-controlled clinical study. Neurology 2000;54:1848–50.
113. Ikeda K, Iwasaki Y, Kinoshita M. Oral administration of creatine monohydrate retards progression of motor neuron disease in the wobbler mouse. Amyotroph Lateral Scler Other Motor Neuron Disord 2000;1:207–12.
114. Felber S, Skladal D, Wyss M, Kremser C, Koller A, Sperl W. Oral creatine supplementation in Duchenne muscular dystrophy: a clinical and 31P magnetic resonance spectroscopy study. Neurol Res 2000;22:145–50.
115. Mazzini L, Balzarini C, Colombo R, Mora G, Pastore I, DeAmbrogio R, Caligari M. Effects of creatine supplementation on exercise performance and muscular strength in amyotrophic lateral sclerosis: preliminary results. J Neurol Sci 2001;191:139–44.
116. Beal MF. Coenzyme Q10 as a possible treatment for neurodegenerative diseases. Free Radic Res 2002;36:455–60.
117. Ende N, Chen F, Weinstein L, Bagtas-Ricafort, Ende M. Human umbilical cord blood and effect on SOD mice (abstract). Modern Pathology 2000;13:1137.
118. Chen R, Ende N. The potential for the use of mononuclear cells from human umbilical cord blood in the treatment of amyotrophic lateral sclerosis in SOD1 mice. J Med 2000;31:21–30.
119. Torrente Y, Tremblay JP, Pisati F, et al. Intraarterial injection of muscle-derived CD34(+)Sca-1(+) stem cells restores dystrophin in mdx mice. J Cell Biol 2001;152:335–48.
120. Law PK, Goodwin TG, Fang Q, et al. Cell transplantation as an experimental treatment for Duchenne muscular dystrophy. Cell Transplant 1993;2:485–505.
121. Drachman DB, Toyka RV, Myer E. Prednisone in Duchenne muscular dystrophy Lancet 1974;2:1409–12.
122. Backman E, Henriksson KG. Low dose prednisolone treatment in Duchenne and Becker muscular dystrophy. Neuromusc Disord 1995;5:233–41.
123. Mendell JR, Moxley RC, Griggs RC, et al. Randomized, double-blind six-month trial of prednisone in Duchenne's muscular dystrophy. N Engl J Med 1989;320:1592–97.
124. Hirano K, Sakamoto Y. Urinary excretion of acid-soluble peptides in children with Duchenne muscular dystrophy. Acta Paediatr Jpn 1994;36:627–31.
125. Rifai Z, Welle S, Moxley RT 3rd, Lorenson M, Griggs RC. Effect of prednisone on protein metabolism in Duchenne dystrophy. Am J Physiol 1995;268:E67–74.
126. Rahman MM, Hannan MA, Mondol BA, Bhoumick NB, Haque A. Prednisolone in Duchenne muscular dystrophy. Bangladesh Med Res Counc Bull 2001;27:38–42.
127. DeSilva S, Drachman DB, Mellits D, Kunel RW. Prednisone treatment in Duchenne muscular dystrophy: long-term benefit. Arch Neurol 1987;44:818–22.
128. Johnsen SD. Prednisone therapy in Becker's muscular dystrophy. J Child Neurol 2001;16:870–1.
129. Urbanek K, Chudackova J, Veliskova J. ACTH and steroids in Kugelberg-Welander disease. Acta Univ Palacki Olomuc Fac Med 1990;126:147–50.
130. Tawil R, McDermott MP, Pandya S, King W, Kissel J, Mendell JR, Griggs RC. A pilot trial of prednisone in facioscapulohumeral muscular dystrophy. FSH-DY Group. Neurology 1997;48:46–9.
131. Talim B, Malaguti C, Gnudi S, Politano L, Merlini L. Vertebral compression in Duchenne muscular dystrophy following deflazacort. Neuromuscul Disord 2002;12:294–5.
132. Bonifati MD, Ruzza G, Bonometto P, et al. A multicenter, double-blind, randomized trial of deflazacort versus prednisone in Duchenne muscular dystrophy. Muscle Nerve 2000;23:1344–7.
133. Biggar WD, Gingras M, Fehlings DL, Harris VA, Steele CA. Deflazacort treatment of Duchenne muscular dystrophy. J Pediatr 2001;138:45–50.

134. Dubrovsky AL, Mesa L, Marco P, et al. Deflazacort treatment in Duchenne muscular dystrophy. Neurology 1991;41(Suppl 1):136–41.
135. Pourmand R (ed). Neuromuscular Diseases: Expert Clinicians' Views. Boston: Butterworth Heinemann, 2001.
136. Perkins KJ, Burton EA, Davies KE. The role of basal and myogenic factors in the transcriptional activation of utrophin promoter A: implications for therapeutic up-regulation in Duchenne muscular dystrophy. Nucleic Acids Res 2001;29:4843–50.
137. Zdanowicz MM, Slonim AE, Bilaniuk I, O'Connor MM, Moyse J, Teichberg S. High protein diet has beneficial effects in murine muscular dystrophy. J Nutr 1995;125:1150–8.
138. Kenichel GM, Griggs RC, Kissel J, et al. A randomized efficacy and safety trial of oxandrolone in the treatment of Duchenne dystrophy. Neurology 2001;56:1075–9.
139. Hankard RG, Hammond D, Haymond MW, Darmaun D. Oral glutamine slows down whole body protein breakdown in Duchenne muscular dystrophy. Pediatr Res 1998;43:222–6.
140. Chen SS, Wang DC, Chen TJ, Yang SL. Administration of Chinese herbal medicines facilitates the locomotor activity in dystrophin-deficient mice. Am J Chin Med 2001;29:281–92.
141. Buetler TM, Renard M, Offord EA, Schneider H, Ruegg UT. Green tea extract decreases muscle necrosis in mdx mice and protects against reactive oxygen species. Am J Clin Nutr 2002;75:749–53.
142. Kissel JT, McDermott MP, Mendell JR, et al. Randomized, double-blind, placebo-controlled trial of albuterol in facioscapulohumeral dystrophy. Neurology 2001;57:1434–40.
143. Tellez-Zenteno JF, Remes-Troche JM, Garcia-Ramos G, Estanol B, Garduno-Espinoza J. Prognostic factors of thymectomy in patients with myasthenia gravis: a cohort of 132 patients. Eur Neurol 2001;46:171–7.
144. Gourie-Devi M, Naline A, Subbakrishna DK. Temporary amelioration of symptoms with intravenous cyclophosphamide in amyotrophic lateral sclerosis. J Neurol Sci 1997;150:167–72.
145. Savery F, Hang LM. Immunodeficiency associated with motor neuron disease treated with intravenous immunoglobulin. Clin Ther 1986;8:700–2.
146. Quality Standards Subcommittee of the American Academy of Neurology. Practice advisory on the treatment of Amyotrophic Lateral Sclerosis with riluzole. Neurology 1997;49:657–59.
147. Lacomblez L, Bensimon G, Leigh PM, et al. Long-term safety of riluzole in amyotrophic lateral sclerosis. Amyotroph Lateral Scler Other Motor Neuron Disord 2002;3:23–9.
148. Desnuelle C, Dib M, Garrel C, Favier A. A double-blind, placebo-controlled randomized clinical trial of alpha-tocopherol in the treatment of amyotrophic lateral sclerosis. Amyotroph Lateral Scler Other Motor Neuron Disord 2001;2:9–18.
149. Eisen A, Stewart H, Schulzer M, Cameron D. Anti-glutamate therapy in amyotrophic lateral sclerosis: a trial using lamotrigine. Can J Neurol Sci 1993;20:297–301.
150. Apostolski S, Marinkovic Z, Nikolic A, Blagojevic D, Spasic MB, Michelson AM. Glutathione peroxidase in amyotrophic lateral sclerosis: the effects of selenium supplementation. J Environ Pathol Toxicol Oncol 1998;17:325–9.
151. Miller RG, Smith SA, Murphy JR, et al. A clinical trial of verapamil in amyotrophic lateral sclerosis. Muscle Nerve 1996;19:511–5.
152. Miller RG, Shepherd R, Dao H, Khramstov A, Mendoza M, Graves J, Smith S. Controlled trial of nimodipine in amyotrophic lateral sclerosis. Neuromuscul Disord 1996;6:101–4.
153. Testa D, Caraceni T, Fetoni V, Girotti F. Chronic treatment with L-threonine in amyotrophic lateral sclerosis: a pilot study. Clin Neurol Neurosurg 1992;94:7–9.
154. Vyth A, Timmer JG, Bossuyt PM, Louwerse ES, deJong JM. Survival in patients with amyotrophic lateral sclerosis, treated with an array of antioxidants. J Neurol Sci 1996;139:99–103.
155. Szczudlik A, Tomik B, Slowik A, Kasprzyk K. Assessment of the efficacy of treatment with pimozide in patients with amyotrophic lateral sclerosis. Introductory notes. Neurol Neurochir Pol 1998;32:821–9.
156. Ochs G, Penn RD, York M. A phase I/II trial of recombinant methionyl human brain derived neurotrophic factor administered by intrathecal infusion to patients with amyotrophic lateral sclerosis. Amyotroph Lateral Scler Other Motor Neuron Disord 2000;1:201–6.
157. Kriz J, Nguyen M, Julien J. Minocycline slows disease progression in a mouse model of amyotrophic lateral sclerosis. Neurobiol Dis 2002;10:268.
158. Carter GT, Rosen BS. Marijuana in the management of amyotrophic lateral sclerosis. Am J Hosp Palliat Care 2001;18:264–70.
159. Ohno T, Shimizu T, Kato S, Hayashi H, Hirai S. Effect of tamsulosin hydrochloride on sympathetic hyperactivity in amyotrophic lateral sclerosis. Auton Neurosci 2001;88:94–8.

160. Miller RG, Moore DH, Dronsky V, et al. A placebo-controlled trial of gabapentin in spinal muscular atrophy. J Neurol Sci 2001;191:127–31.
161. Angelini C, Micaglio GR, Trevisan C. Guanidine hydrochloride in infantile and juvenile spinal muscular atrophy: a double blind controlled study. Acta Neurol (Napoli) 1980;2:460–5.
162. Frey JR, Kaeser HE, Krause R. Therapeutic trials with an anabolic steroid and hexahydrocoenzyme Q4 in a case of spinal muscular atrophy. Eur Neurol 1970;3:308–318.
163. Tzeng AC, Cheng JF, Fryczynski H, Niranjan V, Stitik T, Sial A, Takeuchi Y, Foye P, DePrince M, Bach JR. Randomized double-blind prospective study of thyrotropin-releasing hormone for the treatment of spinal muscular atrophy: a preliminary report. Am J Phys Med Rehabil 2000;79:435–440.
164. Chang JG, Hsieh-Li HM, Jong YJ, Wang NM, Tsai CH, Li H. Treatment of spinal muscular atrophy by sodium butyrate. Proc Natl Acad Sci USA 2001;98:9808–13.
165. Andreassi C, Jarecki J, Zhou J, et al. Aclarubicin treatment restores SMN levels to cells derived from type I spinal muscular atrophy patients. Hum Mol Genet 2001;10:2841–9.
166. Baron-Delage S, Abadie A, Echaniz-Laguna A, Melki J, Beretta L. Interferons and IRF-1 induce expression of the survival motor neuron (SMN) genes. Mol Med 2000;11:957–68.
167. Kinali M, Mercuri E, Main M. Pilot trial of albuterol in spinal muscular atrophy. Neurology 2002;59:609–10.
168. Recommended Dietary Allowances, 10th ed. National Academy Press, Washington, D.C., 1989.
169. The Manual of Clinical Dietetics, 5th ed. American Dietetic Association, Chicago, Ill, 1996.
170. Blackburn GL, Bistrian BR, Maini BS, Schlamm HT, Smith MF. Nutritional and metabolic assessment of the hospitalized patient. JPEN 1977;1:11.
171. Gacad G, Dickie K, Marraro D. Protein synthesis in the lung: influence of starvation on amino acid incorporation in protein. J Appl Physiol 1972;33:381–85.
172. Weiss HS, Jurus E. Effects of starvation on compliance and surfactant of the rat lung. Respir Physiol 1971;12:123–29.
173. Sahebjami H, MacGee J. Changes in connective tissue composition of the lung in starvation and refeeding. Am Rev Respir Dis 1983;128:644–47.
174. Sahebjami H, MacGee J. Effects of starvation and refeeding on lung biochemistry in rats. Am Rev Respir Dis 1982;126:483–87.
175. Goldberg AL, Odessy R. Oxidation of amino acids by diaphragms from fed and fasted rats. Am J Physiol 1972;233:1384–96.
176. McMurray DN, Loomis SA, Casazza LJ, Rey H, Miranda R. Development of impaired cell mediated immunity in mild and moderate malnutrition. Am J Clin Nutr 1981;34:68–77.
177. Good RA. Nutrition and immunity. J Clin Immunol 1981;1:3–11.
178. Moriguchi S, Sonc S, Kishino Y. Changes of alveolar macrophages in protein deficient rats. J Nutr 1983;113:40–46.
179. Martin TR, Altman LC, Alvares OF. The effects of severe protein-calorie malnutrition on antibacterial defense mechanisms in the rat lung. Am Rev Respir Dis 1983;128:1013–19.
180. Niederman MS, Merrill WW, Ferranti RD, et al. Nutritional status and bacterial binding in the lower respiratory tract in patients with chronic tracheostomies. Ann Intern Med 1984;100:795–800.
181. Aubier M, Murciano D, Lecocguie Y, et al. Effect of hypophosphatemia on diaphragmatic contractility in patients with acute respiratory failure. N Engl J Med 1985;313:420–24.
182. Baier H, Somani P. Ventilatory drive in normal man during semi-starvation. Chest 1984;85:222–25.
183. Doekel RC Jr, Zwillich CW, Scoggin CH, Kryger M, Weil JV. Clinical semistarvation: depression of hypoxic ventilatory response. N Engl J Med 1976;295:358–61.
184. Askanazi J, Rosembaum SH, Hyman AI, et al. Effects of parenteral nutrition on ventilatory drive (Abstract). Anesthesiology 1980;53(Suppl):185.
185. Tilton AH, Miller MD, Khoshoo V. Nutrition and swallowing in pediatric neuromuscular patients. Seminars in Pediatric Neurology 1998;5:106–15.
186. Hankard R, Gottrand F, Turek D, et al. Resting energy expenditure and energy substrate utilization in children with Duchenne's muscular dystrophy. Pediatr Res 1996;40:29–33.
187. Balkom R, Dekhuijzen PN, Folgering H, et al. Effects of long-term low-dose methylprednisolone on rat diaphragm function and structure. Muscle Nerve 1997;20:983.
188. Wagner MB, Vignos PJ, Carlozzi C, Hull AL. Assessment of hand function in Duchenne muscular dystrophy. Arch Phys Med Rehabil 1993;74:801–4.
189. Bach JR, Zeelenberg A, Winter C. Wheelchair mounted robot manipulators: long term use by patients with Duchenne muscular dystrophy. Am J Phys Med Rehabil 1990;69:59–69.

190. Kelley R. Nutrition: a new understanding of muscle metabolism in spinal muscular atrophy and other muscle disorders. Direction Fall/1993;7:7.
191. Morrison G, Hark L. Medical Nutrition and Disease. Blackwell Science Inc., Cambridge Ma, 1996: 48–59.
192. McDonald B, Rosenthal SA. Hypokalemia complicating Duchenne muscular dystrophy. Yale J Biol Med 1987;60:405–08.
193. Fried M, Pencharz P. Energy and nutrient intakes of children with spastic quadriplegia. J Pediatr 1991;119:947–51.
194. Aparicio LF, Jurkovic M, DeLullo J. Decreased bone density in ambulatory patients with Duchenne muscular dystrophy. J Pediatr Orthop 2002;22:179–81.
195. Gray B, Hsu JD, Furumasu J. Fractures caused by falling from a wheelchair in patients with neuro-muscular disease. Dev Med Child Neurol 1992;34:589–92.
196. Bennett MJ, Spotswood SD, Ross KF, et al. Fatal hepatic short-chain L-3-hydroxyacl-coenzyme A de-hydrogenase deficiency: clinical, biochemical, and pathological studies on three subjects with this re-cently identified disorder of mitochondrial beta-oxidation. Pediatr Dev Pathol 1999;2:337–45.
197. Tein I, Sloane AE, Donner EJ, et al. Fatty acid oxidation abnormalities in childhood-onset spinal mus-cular atrophy: primary or secondary defects? Pediatr Neurol 1995;12:21–30.
198. Crawford TO, Sladky JT, Hurko O, Besner-Johnston A, Kelley RI. Abnormal fatty acid metabolism in childhood spinal muscular atrophy. Ann Neurol 1999;45:337–43.
199. Iannaccone ST, Browne RH, Samaha FJ, Buncher CR. Prospective study of spinal muscular atrophy before age 6 years. Pediatr Neurol 1993;9:187–93.
200. Haber II, Bach JR, Gaydos J. Nutrition. In: Bach JR (ed) Noninvasive mechanical ventilation. Philadelphia, Hanley and Belfus 2002:285–302.
201. Frisancho AR. Anthropometric Standards for the Assessment of Growth and Nutritional Status. Ann Arbor, MI, University of Michigan Press, 1993.
202. Spender QW, Cronk CE, Charney EB, Stallings VA. Assessment of linear growth of children with cere-bral palsy: use of alternative measures to height or length. Dev Med Child Neurol 1989;31:206–14.
203. Jin L, Lalone C, Demling R. Lung dysfunction after thermal injury in relation to prostanoid and oxygen radical release. J Appl Physiol 1986;61:103–12.
204. National Academy of Sciences Recommended Dietary Allowances, 10th ed. Washington DC, National Academy Press, 1989.
205. Gong QY, Phoenix J, Kemp GJ, Garcia-Finana M, Frostick SP, Brodie DA, Edwards RH, Whitehouse GH, Roberts N. Estimation of body composition in muscular dystrophy by MRI and stereology. J Magn Reson Imaging 2000;12:467–75.
206. Willig TN, Gilardeau C, Kazandjian MS, Bach JR, Varille V, Navarro J, Dikeman KJ. Dysphagia and nutrition in neuromuscular disorders. In: Bach JR (ed). Pulmonary Rehabilitation: The Obstructive and Paralytic Conditions. Philadelphia, Hanley & Belfus 1996:353–369.
207. Slaughter MH, Lohman TG, Boileau RA, et al. Skinfold equations for estimation of body fatness in children and youth. Hum Biol 1988;60:709–23.
208. Brook CGD. Determination of body composition of children from skinfold measurement. Arch Dis Child 1971;46:182–84.
209. Tanner JH, Whitehouse RH, Takaishi M. Standards from birth to maturity for height, weight, height velocity, and weight velocity: British Children, Part II, 1965. Arch Dis Child 1966;41:613–35.
210. Willig TN, Carlier L, Legrand M, Riviere H, Navarro J. Nutritional assessment in Duchenne muscular dystrophy. Dev Med Child Neurol 1993;35:1074–82.
211. Pessolano FA, Suarez A, Dubrovsky A, Mesa L, Monteiro S, Roncoroni AJ, DeVito EL. Assessment of the nutritional status in patients with neuromuscular disease. Am J Phys Med Rehabil 2002;81:506–11.
212. Axen KV. Nutrition in chronic obstructive pulmonary disease. In: Haas F, Axen K (eds): Pulmonary Therapy and Rehabilitation Principles and Practice, ed. 2. Williams & Wilkins, Baltimore, 1991: 95–105.
213. Kagan RJ. Restoring nitrogen balance after burn injury. Compr Ther 1991;17:60–67.
214. Harpey JP, Charpentier C, Paturneau-Jonas M, et al. Secondary metabolic defects in spinal muscular atrophy type II. Lancet 1990;336:629–30.
215. Kelley RI. Octenylsuccinic aciduria in children fed protein-hydrolysate formulas containing modified cornstarch. Pediatr Res 1991;30:564–569.
216. Bruce AK, Jacobsen E, Dossing H, Kondrup J. Hypoglycaemia in spinal muscular atrophy. Lancet 1995;346:609–10.

217. Okada K, Sachinobu M, Sadaichi S, Masaharu O, Yoshiaki N. Protein and energy metabolism in patients with progressive muscular dystrophy. J Nutr Sci Vitaminol 1992;38:147–54.
218. McCrory MA, Wright NC, Kilmer DD. Nutritional aspects of neuromuscular diseases. Phys Med Rehabil Clin N Am 1998;9:127–43.
219. Lin CH, Hudson AJ, Strickland KP. Palmitic acid-1-^{14}C oxidation by skeletal muscle mitochondria of dystrophic mice. Can J Biochem 1969;48:566–72.
220. Hudecki MS, Pollina CM, Heffner RR. Parenteral branched-chain amino acid treatment and avian dystrophy. Muscle Nerve 1982;5:447–57.
221. Edwards RHT, Round JM, Jackson MJ, Griffiths RD, Lilburn MF. Weight reduction in boys with muscular dystrophy. Dev Med Child Neurol 1984;26:384–90.
222. Appel V, Calvin S, Smith G, Woehr D. Meals for easy swallowing. Muscular Dystrophy Association, Tucson, 1986.
223. Willig TN. Tous á table: cuisine adaptée aux difficultés d'alimentation. Association Contre les Myopathies et l'Association des Paralysés de France, Paris, 1993.
224. Miller RG, Rosenberg JA, Gelinas DF, et al. The care of the patient with amyotrophic lateral sclerosis: report of the Quality Standards Subcommittee of the American Academy of Neurology ALS Practice Parameters Task Force. Neurology 1999;52:1311–23.
225. Shimizu T, Hayashi H, Tanabe H. Energy metabolism of ALS patients under mechanical ventilation and tube feeding. Clin Neurol 1991;31:255–59.
226. Edmonds CJ, Smith T, Griffiths RD, et al. Total body potassium and water, and exchangeable sodium in muscular dystrophy. Clin Sci 1985;68:379–85.
227. Lespargot A. Les fausses routes trachéales chez l'enfant I M C ou poly-handicapé. Motricité Cérébrale 1989;10:141–60.
228. Logeman JA. Evaluation and Treatment of Swallowing Disorders. San Diego: College-Hill Press Inc., 1983:119.
229. Shaker R, Li Q, Ren J, et al. Coordination of deglutition and phases of respiration: effect of aging, tachypnea, bolus volume and chronic obstructive pulmonary disease. Am J Physiol 1992;263:750–55.
230. Nishino T, Yonezawa T, Honda Y. Effects of swallowing on the pattern of continuous respiration in human adults. Am Rev Respir Dis 1985;132:1219–22.
231. Martin BJW, Robbins J. Physiology of swallowing: protection of the airway. Semin Respir Crit Care Med 1995;16:448–58.
232. Nutman J, Nitizan M, Grunebaum M. Swallowing disturbances in Werdnig-Hoffmann disease. Harefuah 1990;101:301–03.
233. Granger NW, Buschang PH, Throckmorton GS, Iannaccone ST. Masticatory muscle function in patients with spinal muscular atrophy. Am J Orthod Dentofacial Orthop 1999;115:697–702.
234. Ashby DW. Bone dystrophy in association with muscular dystrophy. British Medical Journal 1951;1:1486–88.
235. Jaffe KM, Craig M, McDonald IE, Hass J. Symptoms of upper gastrointestinal dysfunction in Duchenne muscular dystrophy: case-control study. Arch Phys Med Rehabil 1990;71:742–44.
236. Goldberg MH. Correction of facial skeletal deformities in two patients with facio-scapulo-humeral dystrophy. J Oral Maxillo Fac Surg 1989;47:996–99.
237. Leonard RJ, Kendall KA, Johnson R, McKenzie S. Swallowing in myotonic muscular dystrophy: a videofluoroscopic study. Arch Phys Med Rehabil 2001;82:979–85.
238. Cox MS, Petty J. A videofluoroscopy chair for the evaluation of dysphagia in patients with severe neuromotor disease. Arch Phys Med Rehabil 1991;72:157–59.
239. Pruzanski W, Profis A. Dysfunction of the alimentary tract in myotonic dystrophy. Isr J Med Sci 1966;2:59–64.
240. Pruzanski W. Respiratory tract infections and silent aspiration in myotonic dystrophy. Dis Chest 1962;42:608–10.
241. Grob D. Myasthenia gravis. Arch Intern Med 1961;108:615–38.
242. Sonies BC, Dalakas MC. Dysphagia in patients with the post-polio syndrome. N Engl J Med 1991;324:1162–67.
243. Coelho CA, Ferrante R. Dysphagia in postpolio sequelae: report of three cases. Arch Phys Med Rehabil 1988;69:634–36.
244. Buchholz D. Dysphagia in post-polio patients. Birth Defects 1987;23:55–62.
245. Mayberry JF, Atkinson M. Swallowing problems in patients with motor neuron disease. J Clin Gastroenterol 1986;8:233–34.

246. Hillel AD, Miller R. Bulbar amyotrophic lateral sclerosis: patterns of progression and clinical management. Head Neck 1989;11:651–59.
247. Logeman JA. Management of tracheostomy tubes, intubation, ventilators during swallowing assessment and treatment. Presented at Special Consultations in Dysphagia, Northern Speech Services, Chicago, IL, 1993.
248. Dworkin JP. Tongue strength measurement in patients with amyotrophic lateral sclerosis: qualitative vs. quantitative procedures. Arch Phys Med Rehabil 1980;61:422–4.
249. Teba L, Omert LA. Postoperative respiratory insufficiency. Am Fam Phys 1995;51:1473–80.
250. Zenner PM, Losinski DS, Mills RH. Using cervical auscultation in the clinical dysphagia examination in long-term care. Dysphagia 1995;10:27–31.
251. Vice FL, Heinz JM, Giuriati G, Hood M, Bosma JF. Cervical auscultation of suckle feeding in newborn infants. Dev Med Child Neurol 1990;32;760–68.
252. Dikeman KJ, Kazandjian MS. Communication and Swallowing Management of Tracheostomized and Ventilator Dependent Adults. San Diego, Singular Publishing Group, Inc., 1995.
253. Wilson DJ. The reliability and validity of the methylene blue test to detect aspiration in patients with a tracheostomy tube. (Abstract) Am Rev Respir Dis 1993;147:A409.
254. Dean S, Bach JR. The use of noninvasive respiratory muscle aids in the management of patients with progressive neuromuscular diseases. Respir Care Clin N Am 1996;2,2:223–40.
255. Potts RG, Zaroukian MD, Guerrero PA, Baker CD. Comparison of blue dye visualization and glucose oxidase test strip methods for detecting pulmonary aspiration of enteral feedings in intubated adults. Chest 1993;103:117–21.
256. Langmore SE, Schatz K, Olsen N. Fiberoptic endoscopic evaluation of swallowing safety: a new procedure. Dysphagia 1988;2:216–19.
257. Murray J, Langmore SE, Ginsberg S, Dostie A. The significance of accumulated oropharyngeal secretions and swallowing frequency in predicting aspiration. Dysphagia 1996;11:99–103.
258. Aviv JE, Martin JH, Keen MS, Debell M, Blitzer A. Air pulse quantification of supraglottic and pharyngeal sensation: a new technique. Ann Otol Rhinol Laryngol 1993;102:777–80.
259. Aviv SE, Sacco RL, Diamond K, et al. FEEST: A new bedside endoscopic test of the motor and sensory components of swallowing. Ann Otol Rhino Laryngol 1998;107:378–87.
260. Johnson ER, McKenzie SW. Kinematic pharyngeal transit times in myopathy: evaluation for dysphagia. Dysphagia 1993;8:35–40.
261. Zaidi NH, Smith HA, King SC, et al. Oxygen desaturation on swallowing as a potential marker of aspiration in acute stroke. Age and Aging 1995;24:267–70.
262. Rogers B, Msall M, Shucard D. Hypoxemia during oral feedings in adults with dysphagia and severe neurologic disabilities. Dysphagia 1993;8:43–48.
263. Bach JR. Update and perspectives on noninvasive respiratory muscle aids: part 2—the expiratory muscle aids. Chest 1994;105:1538–44.
264. Iskowitz M. Evaluation of the efficacy of pulse oximetry in the detection of dysphagia. Advance for Speech and Language Pathologists and Audiologists 1997;7:13–14.
265. Bach JR. Mechanical insufflation-exsufflation: comparison of peak expiratory flows with manually assisted and unassisted coughing techniques. Chest 1993;104:1553–62.
266. Buchfinder D, Currivan R. Evaluation of mobilization regimens for jaw hypomobility. Abstract, 73rd Annual Meeting of the American Academy of Oral and Maxillofacial Surgery, Chicago, 1991.
267. Leinbach TE. Prosthetic treatment of malocclusion in patients with muscular dystrophy. J Prosthet Dent 1987;58:604–6.
268. Appel V, Calvin S, Smith G, Woehe D. Meals for Easy Swallowing. Tucson, AZ, Muscular Dystrophy Association.
269. DeLisa JA, Mikulic MA, Miller RM, Melnick RR. Amyotrophic lateral sclerosis: comprehensive management. Am Fam Pract 1989;19:137–42.
270. Bach JR, Tippett DC, McCrary MM. Bulbar dysfunction and associated cardiopulmonary considerations in polio and neuromuscular disease. J Neuro Rehab 1992;6:121–28.
271. Rocco G, Deschamps C, Martel E, et al. Results of reoperation on the upper esophageal sphincter. J Thorac Cardiovasc Surg 1999;117:28–30.
272. Short SO, Hillel AD. Palliative surgery in patients with bulbar amyotrophic lateral sclerosis. Head Neck 1989;11:364–9.
273. Ibanez J, Penafiel A, Raurich JM, et al. Gastroesophageal reflux in intubated patients receiving enteral nutrition: effect of supine and semirecumbent positions. J Parenter Enteral Nutr 1992;16: 419–22.

274. Dotson RG, Robinson RG, Pingleton SK. Gastroesophageal reflux with nasogastric tubes: effect of nasogastric tube size. Am J Respir Crit Care Med 1994;149:1659–62.
275. Horowitz M, Maddox A, Maddern GJ, Wishart J, Collins PJ, Shearman DJ. Gastric and esophageal emptying in dystrophia myotonica: effect of metoclopramide. Gastroenterology 1987;92:570–7.
276. Veen A, Molenbuur B, Richardson FJ. Epidural anaesthesia in a child with possible spinal muscular atrophy. Paediatr Anaesth 2002;12:556–8.
277. Mathieu J, Allard P, Gobeil G, Girard M, DeBraekeleer M, Begin P. Anesthetic and surgical complications in 219 cases of myotonic dystrophy. Neurology 1997;49:1646–50.
278. Shime N, Hosokawa T, Hori Y, Hashimoto T, Miyazaki M. Anesthetic management of a patient with progressive spinal muscular atrophy. Masui 1990;39:918–20.
279. Capozzoli G, Auricchio F, Accinelli G. Total intravenous anaesthesia without muscle relaxants in a child with diagnosed Duchenne muscular dystrophy. Minerva Anestesiol 2000;66:839–40.
280. Wappler F, Scholz J, von Richthofen V, et al. Incidence of disposition for malignant hyperthermia in patients with neuromuscular diseases. Anasthesiol Intensivmed Notfallmed Schmerzther 1998;33:373–80.
281. Breucking E, Mortier W. Anesthesia in neuromuscular diseases. Acta Anaesthesiologica Belgica 1990;41:127–32.
282. Stamm M. Gastrostomy by a new method. Medical News 1894;65:324–26.
283. Pope JF, Birnkrant DJ, Martin JE, Repucci AH. Noninvasive ventilation during percutaneous gastrostomy placement in Duchenne muscular dystrophy. Pediatr Pulmonol 1997;23:468–71.
284. Zickler RW, Barbagiovanni JT, Swan KG. A simplified open gastrostomy under local anesthesia. American Surgeon 2001;67:806–08.
285. Bach JR. Update and perspectives on noninvasive respiratory muscle aids: part 1—the inspiratory muscle aids. Chest 1994;105:1230–40.
286. Bonanno P. Swallowing dysfunction after tracheostomy. Ann Surg 1971;174:29–33.
287. Feldman SA, Deal CW, Urqhart W. Disturbance of swallowing after tracheotomy. Lancet 1966;1:954–55.
288. Martin F. Dysphagia due to tracheotomy (in German). Med Klin 1999;94:43–44.
289. Tolep K, Getch CL, Criner GJ. Swallowing dysfunction in patients receiving prolonged mechanical ventilation. Chest 1996;109:167–72.
290. DeVita MA, Spierer Rundback L. Swallowing disorders in patients with prolonged orotracheal intubation or tracheostomy tubes. Crit Care Med 1990;18:1328–30.
291. Stauffer JL, Olson DE, Petty TL. Complications and consequences of endotracheal intubation and tracheostomy. Am J Med 1981;70:65–75.
292. Tippett D, Siebens A. Speaking and swallowing on a ventilator. Dysphagia 1991;6:94–99.
293. Buchwalter JA, Sasaki CT. Effect of tracheotomy on laryngeal function. Otolaryngol Clin N Am 1984;17:41–48.
294. McConnel FMS, Cerenko D, Mendelsohn MS. Manofluorographic analysis of swallowing. Otolaryngol Clin N Am 1988;21:625–37.
295. Stackler RJ, Hamlet SL, Choi J, Fleming S. Scintigraphic quantification of aspiration reduction with the Passy Muir Valve. Laryngoscope 1996;106:231–34.
296. Leder SB, Tarro JR, Burrell MI. Effect of occlusion of a tracheotomy tube on aspiration. Dysphagia 1996;11:254–58.
297. Ikari T, Sasaki CT. Glottic closure reflex: control mechanisms. Ann Otol Rhinol Laryngol 1980;89:220–24.
298. Sasaki CT, Buchwalter J. Laryngeal function. Am J Otolaryngol 1984;5:281–91.
299. Charlieflue RJ, Fernandez LB, Peres CJ, Gonzalez E, Marzi A. Functional studies of the parotid and pancreas glands in amyotrophic lateral sclerosis. J Neurol Neurosurg Psych 1974;37:863–67.
300. Blasco PA, Stansbury JCK. Glycopyrrolate treatment of chronic drooling. Arch Pediatr Adolesc Med 1996;150:932–35.
301. Stern LM. Preliminary study of glycopyrrolate in the management of drooling. J Paediatr Child Health 1997;33:52–54.
302. Goode RL, Smith RA. The surgical management of sialorrhea. Laryngoscope 1970;80:1078–89.
303. Camp-Bruno JA, Winsberg BG, Green-Parsons AR, Abrams JP. Efficacy of benztropine therapy for drooling. Dev Med Child Neurol 1989;31:309–19.
304. Reddihough D, Johnson H, Staples M, Hudson I, Exarchos H. Use of benzhexol hydrochloride to control drooling of children with cerebral palsy. Dev Med Child Neurol 1990;32:985–89.

305. Talmi YP, Finkelstein Y, Zohar Y, Laurian N. Reduction of salivary flow with scopoderm TTS. Ann Otol Rhinol Laryngol 1988;97:128–30.
306. Brodtkorb E, Wyzocka-Bakowska MM, Lillevold PE, et al. Transdermal scopolamine in drooling. J Mental Deficiency Res 1988;32:233–37.
307. Lewis DW, Fontana C, Mehallick LK, Everett Y. Transdermal scopolamine for reductions in drooling in developmentally delayed children. Dev Med Child Neurol 1994;36:484–86.
308. Dworkin JP, Nadal JC. Nonsurgical treatment of drooling in a patient with closed head injury and severe dysarthria. Dysphagia 1991;6:40–49.
309. Newall AR, Orser R, Hunt M. The control of oral secretions in bulbar ALS/MND. J Neurol Sci 1996;139:43–4.
310. Adderley RJ, Goddard K, Hay J. Low dose parotid irradiation for amelioration of drooling in paediatric patients with progressive neuropathies. 8th Journées Internationales de Ventilation à Domicile, abstract 57, March 7, 2001, Hôpital de la Croix-Rousse, Lyon, France.
311. Harriman M, Morrison M, Hay J, Revonta M, Eisen A, Lentle B. Use of radiotherapy for control of sialorrhea in patients with amyotrophic lateral sclerosis. J Otolaryngol 2001;30:242–5.
312. Newell AR, Orser R, Hunt M. The control of oral secretions in bulbar ALS/MND. J Neurological Sci 1996;139 (suppl):43–44.
313. Giess R, Naumann M, Werner E, et al. Injections of botulinum toxin A into the salivary glands improve sialorrhoea in amyotrophic lateral sclerosis. J Neurol Neurosurg Psychiatry 2000;69:121–23.
314. Tan EK, Lo YL, Seah A, Auchus AP. Recurrent jaw dislocation after botulinum toxin treatment for sialorrhoea in amyotrophic lateral sclerosis. J neurol Sci 2001;190:95–7.
315. Moulding MB, Koroluk LD. An intraoral prosthesis to control drooling in a patient with amyotrophic lateral sclerosis. Spec Care Dentist 1991;11:200–2.
316. Krespi YP, Quatela VC, Sisson GA, Som ML. Modified tracheoesophageal diversion for chronic aspiration. Laryngoscope 1984;94:1298–1301.
317. Takano Y, Suga M, Sakamoto O, et al. Satisfaction of patients treated surgically for intractable aspiration. Chest 1999;116:1251–56.
318. Nakasaki H, Sugihara T, Tajima T, Mitomi T, Osamura Y, Onoda N, Fujii K. Tracheoesophageal anastomosis for intractable aspiration pneumonia. Ann Thorac Surg 1991;51:23–9.
319. Lacau Saint Guilly J, Pri S, Willig TN, et al. Swallowing disorders in muscular diseases: functional assessment and indications of cricopharyngeal myotomy. ENTJ 1994;73:34–40.
320. MacDougall G, Wilson JA, Pryde A, Grant R. Analysis of the pharyngoesophageal pressure profile in amyotrophic lateral sclerosis. Otolaryngol Head Neck Surg 1995;112:258–61.
321. Norris FH, Denys EH, Lebo CP. Surgery in patients with amyotrophic lateral sclerosis: experience with cricopharyngeal myotomy in 100 cases (abstract). Excerpta Medica International Congress Series No. 427, 1977:45.
322. Leighton SE, burton MJ, Lund WS, Cochrane GM. Swallowing in motor neurone disease. J R Soc Med 1994;87:801–5.
323. Brouillette D, Martel E, Chen LQ, Duranceau A. Pitfalls and complications of cricopharyngeal myotomy. Chest Surg Clin N Am 1997;7:457–75.
324. Muller H, Punt-Van Manen JA. Maxillo-facial deformities in patients with dystrophia myotonica and the anaesthetic implications. J Maxillofac Surg 1982;10:224–28.
325. Ronsick SO, Pingleton SK, Kerby GR, et al. Effects of lower diaphragmatic contraction on lower esophageal sphincter pressure. Chest 1994;106S:75S.
326. Sonies BC, Baum BJ. Scintigraphy and manometry. Otolaryngol Clin N Am 1988;21:637–48.
327. Boonyaprapa S, Alderson PO, Garfinkel DJ, Chipps BE, Wagner HN Jr. Detection of pulmonary aspiration in infants and children with respiratory disease: concise communication. J Nucl Med 1980;21:314–18.
328. Latini G, Del Vecchio A, De Mitri B, et al. Scintigraphic evaluation of gastroesophageal reflux in newborns. Pediatr Med Chir 1999;21:115–17.
329. Evans SRT, Jackson PG, Czerniach DR, Kalan MMH, Iglesias AR. A stepwise approach to laparoscopic Nissen fundoplication. Arch Surg 2000;135:723–28.
330. Hui TT, Fass SM, Giurgiu DI, et al. Gastroesophageal disease and nausea: does fundoplication help or hurt? Arch Surg 2000;135:545–49.
331. Jamieson GG. An emerging trend in anti-reflux surgery? Aust N Z J Surg 2000;70:473–74.
332. Subramaniam R, Dickson AP. Long-term outcome of Boix-Ochoa and Nissen fundoplication in normal and neurologically impaired children. J Pediatr Surg 2000;35:1214–16.
333. Chung BC, Park HJ, Yoon SB, Lee HW, Kim KW, Lee SI, Park IS. Yonsei Med J 1998;39:175–9.

334. Torretta A, Mascagni D, Zeri KP, et al. The megacolon in myotonic dystrophy: case report and review of the literature. Ann Ital Chir 2000;71:729–32.
335. Kusunoki M, Hatada T, Ikeuchi H, Okamoto T, Sakanoue Y, Utsunomiya J. Gastric volvulus complicating myotonic dystrophy. Hepatogastroenterology 1992;39:586–8.
336. Robin GC, Falewski de Leon GH. Acute gastric dilatation in progressive muscular dystrophy. Lancet 1963;2:171–72.
337. Love R, Choe E, Lippton H, et al. Positive end-expiratory pressure decreases mesenteric blood flow despite normalization of cardiac output. J Trauma 1995;39:195–199.
338. Aneman A, Ponten J, Fandriks L, et al. Hemodynamic sympathetic and angiotensis II responses to PEEP ventilation before and during administration of isoflurane. Acta Anaesthesiol Scand 1997;41: 41–48.
339. Physicians Desk Reference, 56th edition. Medical Economics Company, Inc., Montvale, N.J. 2002:2935–8.
340. Li T, Oi N, Shioya K, Kawano T, Nakahara S, Matsukura S. A case of progressive spinal muscular atrophy with disorder of intestinal motility improved by administration of erythromycin. Nippon Naika Gakkai Zasshi 1992;81:1261–2.
341. Weber KT, Janicki JS, Shroff S, Likoff MJ. The cardiopulmonary unit: the body's gas transport system. Clin Chest Med 1983;4:101–10
342. Sharp J, Griffith G, Bunnell I, Greene DG. Ventilatory mechanics in pulmonary edema in man. J Clin Invest 1958;37:111–17.
343. Faggiano P. Abnormalities of pulmonary function in congestive heart failure. Int J Cardiol 1994;44:1–8.
344. Lee TH, Hamilton MA, Stevenson LW, et al. Impact of left ventricular cavity size on survival in advanced heart failure. Am J Cardiol 1993;72:672–76.
345. Conte G, Goija L. Scrofola del sistema muscolare. Ann Clin Osp Incur 1836;2:66–79.
346. Ross J. On a case of pseudo-hypertrophic paralysis. Br Med J 1883;1:200–03.
347. Borgeat A, Goy JJ, Sigwart U. Acute pulmonary edema as the inaugural symptom of Becker's muscular dystrophy in a 19-year old patient. Clin Cardiol 1987;10:127–29.
348. Seay AR, Ziter F, Thompson JA. Cardiac arrest during anesthesia in Duchenne muscular dystrophy. J Pediatr 1978;93:88–90.
349. Brooke MH, Fenichel GM, Griggs RC, et al. Duchenne muscular dystrophy: patterns of clinical progression and effects of supportive therapy. Neurol 1989;39:475–80.
350. Mingo PU, Romero JT, Barbero JLT, Jalon EI. Miocardiopatia dilatada en una mujer portadora de la enfermedad de Duchenne de Boulogne. Rev Clin Esp 1987;181:468.
351. Wiegand V, Rahlf G, Meinck M, Kreuzer H. Kardiomyopathie bei Tragerinnen des Duchenne-Gens. Z Kardiol 1984;73:188–91.
352. Mirabella M, Servidei S, Manfredi G, et al. Cardiomyopathy may be the only clinical manifestation in female carriers of Duchenne muscular dystrophy. Neurology 1993;43:2342–45.
353. Hagiwara Y, Nishio H, Kitoh Y, et al. A novel point mutation (G-1 to T) in a 5' splice donor site of intron 13 of the dystrophin gene results in exon skipping and is responsible for Becker muscular dystrophy. Am J Hum Genet 1994;54:53–61.
354. Steare SE, Dubowitz V, Benatar A. Subclinical cardiomyopathy in Becker muscular dystrophy. Br Heart J 1992;68:304–08.
355. Yoshioka M, Saida K, Itagaki Y, Kamiya T. Follow up study of cardiac involvement in Emery-Dreifuss muscular dystrophy. Arch Dis Childh 1989;64:713–15.
356. Church SC. The heart in myotonia atrophica. Arch Intern Med 1967;119:176–81.
357. Lazzeroni E, Favaro L, Botti G. Dilated cardiomyopathy with regional myocardial hypoperfusion in Becker's muscular dystrophy. Int J Cardiol 1989;22:126–29.
358. Hoogerwaard EM, Bakker E, Ippel PF, et al. Signs and symptoms of Duchenne muscular dystrophy and Becker muscular dystrophy among carriers in the Netherlands: a cohort study. Lancet 1999;353: 2116–19.
359. Towbin JA, Hejtmancik F, Brink P, et al. X-linked dilated cardiomyopathy: molecular genetic evidence of linkage to the Duchenne muscular dystrophy (dystrophin) gene at the Xp21 locus. Circulation 1993;87:1854–65.
360. Berko BA, Swift M. X-linked dilated cardiomyopathy. N Engl J Med 1987;316:1186–91.
361. Muntoni F, Cau M, Ganau A, et al. Brief report: deletion of the dystrophin muscle-promoter region associated with X-linked dilated cardiomyopathy. N Eng J Med 1993;329:921–25.

362. Towbin JA, Bowles NE. Genetic abnormalities responsible for dilated cardiomyopathy. Curr Cardiol Rep 2000;2:475–80.

363. Oldfors A, Eriksson BO, Kyllerman M, Martinsson T, Wahlstrom J. Dilated cardiomyopathy and the dystrophin gene: an illustrated review. Br Heart J 1994;72:344–48.

364. Fatkin D, MacRae C, Sasaki T, et al. Missense mutations in the rod domain of the lamin A/C gene as causes of dilated cardiomyopathy and conduction system disease. N Engl J Med 1999;341: 1715–24.

366. Roberds SL, Ervasti JM, Anderson RD, et al. Disruption of dystrophin-glycoprotein complex in the cardiomyopathic hamster. J Biol Chem 1993;268:11496–99.

367. Kasper EK, Agema WRP, Hutchins GM, et al. The causes of dilated cardiomyopathy : a clinicopathologic review of 673 consecutive patients. J AM Coll Cardiol 1994;23:586–90.

368. Nagasawa H, Nakajima T, Arakaki Y, et al. Normalization of left ventricular dimension in normal children by two-dimensional echocardiogram. The Journal of The Japan Pediatric Society (Jpn) 1994;98: 1857–61.

369. Raynolds MV, Bristow MR, Bush EW, et al. Angiotensin-converting enzyme DD genotype in patients with ischaemic or idiopathic dilated cardiomyopathy. Lancet 1993;342:1073–75.

371. Yotsukura M, Miyagawa M, Tsuya T, Ishihara T, Ishikawa K. Pulmonary hypertension in progressive muscular dystrophy of the Duchenne type. Japan Circulation J 1988;52:321–26.

372. Yotsukura M, Fujii K, Katayama A, et al. Nine year follow-up study of heart rate variability in patients with Duchenne-type progressive muscular dystrophy. Am Heart J 1998;136:289–96.

373. Gaffney JF, Kingston WJ, Metlay LA, Gramiak R. Left ventricular thrombus and systemic emboli complicating the cardiomyopathy of Duchenne's muscular dystrophy. Arch Neurol 1989;46:1249–51.

374. Riggs T. Cardiomyopathy and pulmonary emboli in terminal Duchenne's muscular dystrophy. Am Heart J 1990;119:690–93.

375. Cobos E, Phy M, Keung YK. Thrombotic risk of muscular dystrophy: protein C deficiency, factor V Leiden, and myotonic dystrophy. Clin Appl Thrombosis/Hemostasis 1999;5:185–86.

376. Porreca E, Guglielmi MD, Uncini A, et al. Haemostatic abnormalities, cardiac involvement and serum tumor necrosis factor levels in X-linked dystrophic patients. Thromb Haemost 1999;81:543–46.

377. Forst J, Forst R, Leithe H, Maurin N. Platelet function deficiency in Duchenne muscular dystrophy. Neuromuscular Disorders 1998;8:46–49.

378. Noordeen MH, Haddad FS, Muntoni F, et al. Blood loss in Duchenne muscular dystrophy: vascular smooth muscle dystrophin? J Pediatr Orthop B 1999;8:212–15.

379. Bies RD, Friedman D, Roberts R, Perryman MB, Caskey CT. Expression and localization of dystrophin in human cardiac purkinje fibers. Circulation 1992;86:147–53.

380. Kunkel LM. Analysis of deletions in DNA from patients with Becker and Duchenne muscular dystrophy. Nature 1986;322:73–77.

381. Tanaka H, Nishi S, Katanasako H. Natural course of cardiomyopathy in Duchenne muscular dystrophy. Jpn Circulation J 1979;43:974–84.

382. Nigro G, Comi LI, Limongelli FM, et al. Prospective study of X-linked progressive muscular dystrophy in Campania. Muscle Nerve 1983;6:253–62.

383. Stewart CA, Gilgoff I, Baydur A, Prentice W, Applebaum D. Gated radionuclide ventriculography in the evaluation of cardiac function in Duchenne's muscular dystrophy. Chest 1988;94:1245–48.

384. Backman E, Nylander E. The heart in Duchenne muscular dystrophy: a non-invasive longitudinal study. Europ Heart J 1992;13:1239–44.

385. Sarma RJ, Stewart C, Gilgoff IS, Bach JR. Cardiovascular considerations in the management of Duchenne muscular dystrophy. J Neuro Rehab 1992;6:113–19.

386. Farah MG, Evans EB, Vignos PJ. Echocardiographic evaluation of left ventricular function in Duchenne's muscular dystrophy. Am J Med 1980;69;248–54.

387. Tamura T, Shibuya N, Hashiba K, et al. Evaluation of myocardial damage in Duchenne's muscular dystrophy with thallium-201 myocardial SPECT. Jpn Heart J 1993;34:51–61.

388. Goldberg SJ, Feldman L, Reinecke C, et al. Echocardiographic determination of contraction and relaxation measurements of the left ventricular wall in normal subjects and patients with muscular dystrophy. Circulation 1980;62:1061–69.

389. Reeves WC, Griggs R, Nanda NC, et al. Echocardiographic evaluation of cardiac abnormalities in Duchenne's dystrophy and myotonic muscular dystrophy. Arch Neurol 1980;37:273–77.

390. Sanyal SK, Leung RKF, Tierney RC, et al. Mitral valve prolapse syndrome in children with Duchenne's progressive muscular dystrophy. Pediatrics 1979;63:116–22.

391. Lane RJM, Gardner-Medwin D, Roses AD. Electrocardiographic abnormalities in carriers of Duchenne muscular dystrophy. Neurology 1980;30:497–507.
392. Gilroy J, Cahalan JL, Berman R, et al. Cardiac and pulmonary complications in Duchenne's progressive muscular dystrophy. Circulation 1963;27:484–93.
393. Ishikawa K, Yanagisawa A, Ishihara T, et al. Sequential changes of orthogonal electrocardiograms in progressive muscular dystrophy of the Duchenne type. Am Heart J 1979;98:73–82.
394. Yotsukura M, Ishizuka T, Shimada T, Ishikawa K. Late potentials in progressive muscular dystrophy of the Duchenne type. Am Heart J 1991;121:1137–42.
395. Hilton T, Orr RD, Perkin RM, Ashwal S. End of life care in Duchenne muscular dystrophy. Pediatr Neurol 1993;9:165–77.
396. Waters DD, Nutter DO, Hopkins LC, Dorney ER. Cardiac features of an unusual X-linked humeroperoneal neuromuscular disease. N Eng J Med 1975;293:1017–22.
397. Fowler WM, Nayak NN. Slowly progressive proximal weakness: limb-girdle syndromes. Arch Phys Med Rehabil 1983;64:527–38.
398. Merlini L, Granata C, Domenici P, Bonfiglioli S. Emery-Dreifuss muscular dystrophy. Muscle Nerve 1986;9:481–85.
399. Walker S, Levy T, Rex S, Paul VE. Biventricular implantable cardioverter defibrillator use in patients with heart failure and ventricular tachycardia secondary to Emery-Dreifuss syndrome. Europace 1999;1:206–9.
400. Motta J, Guilleminault C, Billingham M, Barry W, Mason J. Cardiac abnormalities in myotonic dystrophy: electrophysiologic and histopathologic studies. Am J Med 1979;67:467–73.
401. Phillips MF, Harper, PS. Cardiac disease in myotonic dystrophy. Cardiovascular Research 1997;33: 13–22.
402. Child JS, Perloff JK. Myocardial myotonia in myotonic muscular dystrophy. Am Heart J 1995;129: 982–990.
403. Merino JL, Carmona JR, Fernandez-Lozano I, Peinado R, Basterra N, Sobrino JA. Mechanisms of sustained ventricular tachycardia in myotonic dystrophy: implications for catheter ablation. Circulation 1998;98:541–46.
404. Olofsson B, Forsberg H, et al. Electrocardiographic findings in myotonic dystrophy. Br Heart J 1988;59:47–52.
405. Hawley R, Milner M, Gottdiener JS, Cohen A. Myotonic heart disease: a clinical follow-up. Neurology 1991;41:259–62.
406. Fragola PV, Luzi M, Calo L, et al. Cardiac involvement in myotonic dystrophy. Am J Cardiol 1994;74:1070–72.
407. Perloff J, Stevenson W, Roberts N, et al. Cardiac involvement in myotonic muscular dystrophy (Steinert's disease): a prospective study of 25 patients. Am J Cardiol 1984;54:1074–81.
408. Fox R. The heart in myotonic dystrophy. Lancet 1992;339:528–29.
409. Holt JM, Lambert EHN. Heart disease as the presenting feature in myotonia atrophica. Br Heart J 1964;26:433–36.
410. Hartwig GB, Rao KR, Radoff FM, et al. Radionuclide angiocardiographic analysis of myocardial function in myotonic muscular dystrophy. Neurology 1983;33:657–60.
411. Segawa I, Kikuchi M, Tashiro A, Hiramori K, Sato M, Satodate R. Association of myotonic dystrophy and sick sinus syndrome, with special reference to electrophysiological and histological examinations. Intern Med 1996;35:185–8.
412. Reardon W, Newcombe R, Fenton I, et al. The natural history of congenital myotonic dystrophy: mortality and long term clinical aspects. Arch Dis Child 1993;68:177–81.
413. Berman EJ, DiBenedetto RJ, Causey DE, et al. Right ventricular hypertrophy detected by echocardiography in patients with newly diagnosed obstructive sleep apnea. Chest 1991;100:347–50.
414. Lavie P, Yoffe N, Berger I, Peled R. The relationship between the severity of sleep apnea syndrome and 24-h blood pressure values in patients with obstructive sleep apnea. Chest 1993;103:717–21.
415. Tilkian AG, Motta J, Guilleminault C. Cardiac arrhythmias in sleep apnea. In Guilleminault C, Dement WC (eds): Sleep Apnea Syndromes. Alan R Liss, New York, 1978:177–96.
416. Zwillich C, Devlin T, White D, et al. Bradycardia during sleep apnea. J Clin Invest 1982;69:1286–92.
417. Huang JJ, Jong YJ, Huang MY, Chiang CH, Huang TY. Electrocardiographic findings in children with spinal muscular atrophy. Jpn Heart J 1996;37:239–42.
418. Elkohen M, Vaksmann G, Elkohen MR, Francard C, Foucher C, Rey C. Cardiac involvement in Kugelberg-Welander disease. A prospective study of 8 cases. Arch Mal Coeur Vaiss 1996;89:611–7.

419. Mulleners WM, van Ravenswaay CM, Gabreels FJ, Hamel BC, van Oort A, Sengers RC. Spinal muscular atrophy combined with congenital heart disease: a report of two cases. Neuropediatrics 1996;27:333–4.

420. Swash M, Schwartz MS. Cardiac involvement in neuromuscular disease. In: Russell JML (ed), Handbook of Muscle Disease, Marcel Dekker, New York, 1996:655–62.

421. Ishikawa Y, Bach JR, Sarma RJ, et al. Cardiovascular considerations in the management of neuromuscular disease. Seminars in Neurology 1995;15:93–108.

422. Perloff JK, De Leon AC, O'Doherty D. The cardiomyopathy of progressive muscular dystrophy. Circulation 1966;33:625–48.

423. D'Orsogna L, O'Shea JP, Miller G. Cardiomyopathy of Duchenne muscular dystrophy. Pediatr Cardiol 1988;9:205–13.

424. Weisenfeld A, Messinger WJ. Cardiac involvement in progressive muscular dystrophy. Am Heart J 1952;43:170–87.

425. Perloff JK. Cardiac rhythm and conduction in Duchenne's muscular dystrophy: a prospective study of 20 patients. J Am Coll Cardiol 1984;3:1263–68.

426. Sudoh T, Kangawa K, Minamino N, et al. A new natriuretic peptide in porcine brain. Nature 1988;332:78–81.

427. Mukoyama M, Nakao K, Hosoda K, et al. Brain natriuretic peptide as a novel cardiac hormone in humans. J Clin Invest 1991;87:1402–12.

428. Cohn JN, Levine B, Olivari MT, et al. Plasma norepinephrine as a guide to prognosis in patients with chronic congestive heart failure. N Engl J Med 1984;311:819–23.

429. Francis GS, Cohn JN, Johnson G, et al. Plasma norepinephrine, plasma renin activity, and congestive heart failure: relations to survival and the effects of therapy in V-HeFT. Circulation 1993;87: 40–48.

430. Floras JS. Clinical aspects of sympathetic activation and parasympathetic withdrawal in heart failure. J Am Coll Cardiol 1993;22:72A–84A.

431. Cowie RM, Struthers AD, Wood DA, et al. Value of natriuretic peptides in assessment of patients with possible new heart failure in primary care. Lancet 1997;350:1347–51.

432. Kashiwagi S, Akaike M, Kawai H, et al. Estimation of cardiac function by plasma concentration of brain natriuretic peptide in patients with Duchenne muscular dystrophy. Clin Neurol (Tokyo) 1996; 36:7–11.

433. McDonagh TA, Robb SD, Murdoch DR, et al. Biochemical detection of left-ventricular systolic dysfunction. Lancet 1998;351:9–13.

434. Yoshimura M, Yasue H, Okumura K, et al. Different secretion patterns of atrial natriuretic peptide and brain natriuretic peptide in patients with congestive heart failure. Circulation 1993;87:464–69.

435. Yamada Y, Goto J, Yokota M. Brain natriuretic peptide is a sensitive indicator of impaired left-ventricular function in elderly patients with cardiovascular disease. Cardiol 1997;88:401–07.

436. Burnett JC, Kao PC, Hu DC, et al. Atrial natriuretic peptide elevation in congestive heart failure in humans. Science 1968;231:1145–47.

437. Gottlieb SS, Kukin ML, Ahern D, Packer M. Prognostic importance of atrial natriuretic peptide in patients with chronic heart failure. J Am Col Cardiol 1989;13:1534–39.

438. Yanagisawa A, Yokata N, Miyagawa M, et al. Plasma levels of atrial natriuretic peptide in patients with Duchenne's muscular dystrophy. Am Heart J 1990;120:1154–58.

439. Kawai H, Adachi K, Kimura C, et al. Secretion and clinical significance of atrial natriuretic peptide in patients with muscular dystrophy. Arch Neurol 1990;47:900–04.

440. Kameda K. Clinical significance of the relationship between cardiac insufficiency and atrial natriuretic peptide and dystrophin in patients with Duchenne muscular dystrophy. Sapporo Medical Journal 1991;60:535–43.

441. Davis M, Espiner E, Richards G, et al. Plasma brain natriuretic peptide in assessment of acute dyspnoea. Lancet 1994;343:440–44.

442. Ishikawa Y, Bach JR, Minami R. Cardioprotection for Duchenne's muscular dystrophy. Am Heart J 1999;137:895–902.

443. Davidson NC, Naas AA, Hanson JK, et al. Comparison of atrial natriuretic peptide, B-type natriuretic peptide, and N-terminal proatrial natriuretic peptide as indicators of left ventricular systolic dysfunction. Am J Cardiol 1996;77:828–31.

444. Sanyal SK, Johnson WW, Dische MR, et al. Dystrophic degeneration of papillary muscle and ventricular myocardium. Circulation 1980;62:430–37.

445. Slucka C. The electrocardiogram in Duchenne progressive muscular dystrophy. Circulation 1968;38: 933–40.
446. Schott J, Jacobi M, Wald MA. Electrocardiographic patterns in the differential diagnosis of progressive muscular dystrophy. Am J Med Sci 1955;229:517–24.
447. Perloff JK, Roberts WC, DeLeon AC, et al. The distinctive electrocardiogram of Duchenne's progressive muscular dystrophy: an electrocardiographic-pathologic correlative study. Am J Med 1967;42: 179–88.
448. Emery AEH. Abnormalities of the electrocardiogram in hereditary myopathies. J Med Genet 1972;9:8–12.
449. Emery AEH. Abnormalities of the electrocardiogram in female carriers of Duchenne muscular dystrophy. Br Med J 1969;2:418–20.
450. Nigro G, Comi LI, Politano L, Bain RJI. The incidence and evolution of cardiomyopathy in Duchenne muscular dystrophy. Int J Cardiol 1990;26:271–77.
451. Fitch CW, Ainger LW. The Frank vectorcardiogram and the electrocardiogram in Duchenne progressive muscular dystrophy. Circulation 1967;35:1124–40.
452. Frankel KA, Rosser RJ. The pathology of the heart in progressive muscular dystrophy: epimyocardial fibrosis. Human Pathology 1976;7:375–86.
453. Ahmad M, Sanderson JE, Dubowitz V, et al. Echocardiographic assessment of left ventricular function in Duchenne's muscular dystrophy. Br Heart J 1978;40:734–40.
454. Biddison JH, Dembo DH, Spalt H, et al. Familial occurrence of mitral valve prolapse in X-linked muscular dystrophy. Circulation 1979;59:1299–304.
455. Danilowicz D, Rutlowski M, Myung D, et al. Echocardiography in Duchenne muscular dystrophy. Muscle Nerve 1980;3:298–303.
456. de Kermadec JM, Becane HM, Chenard A, Tertain F, Weiss Y. Prevalence of left ventricular systolic dysfunction in Duchenne muscular dystrophy: an echocardiographic study. Am Heart J 1994;127: 618–23.
457. Heymsfield SB, McNish T, Perkins JV, et al. Sequence of cardiac changes in Duchenne muscular dystrophy. Am Heart J 1978;95:283–94.
458. Goldberg SJ, Stern LZ, Feldman L, et al. Serial two dimensional echocardiography in Duchenne muscular dystrophy. Neurology 1982;32:1101–05.
459. Goldberg SJ, Stern LZ, Feldman L, et al. Serial left ventricular wall measurements in Duchenne's muscular dystrophy. J Am Coll Cardiol 1983;2:136–45.
460. Mor-Avi V, Vignon P, Koch R, et al. Segmental analysis of color kinesis images: a new method for quantification of the magnitude and timing of endocardial motion during left ventricular systole and diastole. Circulation 1997;95:2082–97.
461. Lang RM, Vignon P, Weinert L, et al. Echocardiographic quantification of regional left ventricular wall motion with color kinesis. Circulation 1996;93:1877–85.
462. Devaux J-Y, Duboc D, Caldera R, et al. Dipyridamole and thallium myocardial tomography in muscular dystrophy. Eur J Nucl Med 1989;15:471.
463. Stewart CA, Hung G-L, Gilgoff I, Baydur A, Sarma R. Response to vasodilator therapy in Duchenne's muscular dystrophy: evaluation by radionuclide ventriculography. Clin Nucl Med 1991;16:719.
464. Perloff JK, Henze E, Schelbert H. Alterations in regional myocardial metabolism, perfusion, and wall motion in Duchenne muscular dystrophy studied by radionuclide imaging. Circulation 1984;69: 33–42.
465. Conference on Respiratory Problems in Poliomyelitis, March 12-14, 1952, Ann Arbor, National Foundation for Infantile Paralysis - March of Dimes, White Plains, N.Y.
467. Ishikawa Y, Ishikawa Y, and Minami R. Beneficial and adverse effects of angiotensin-converting enzyme inhibitor in patients with severe congestive heart failure associated with Duchenne muscular dystrophy. Iryo 1993;47:720–24.
468. Tamura T, Shibuya N, Iida M, et al. Clinical evaluation of captopril in chronic cardiac dysfunction in patients with Duchenne muscular dystrophy. Rinsho Iyaku (Japan) 1996;12:3635–46.
469. Bristow MR. Beta-adrenergic receptor blockade in chronic heart failure. Circulation 2000;101:558–69.
470. Shaddy RE, Tani LY, Gidding SS, Pahl E, Orsmond GS, Gilbert EM, Lemes V. Beta-blocker treatment of dilated cardiomyopathy with congestive heart failure in children: a multi-institutional experience. J Heart Lung Transplant 1999;18:269–74.
471. CONSENSUS (Cooperative north scandinavian enalapril survival study) Trial Study Group. Effects of enalapril on mortality in severe congestive heart failure. N Engl J Med 1987;316:1429–35.

472. The SOLVD investigators. Effect of enalapril on survival in patients with reduced left ventricular ejection fractions and congestive heart failure. N Engl J Med 1991;325:293–302.
473. Konstam MA, Kronenberg MW, Rousseau MF, et al. For SOLVD Investigators. Effects of the angiotensin converting enzyme inhibitor enalapril on the long-term progression of left ventricular dilatation in patients with asymptomatic systolic dysfunction. Circulation 1993;88:2277–83.
474. Coirault C, Hagege A, Chemla D. Angiotensin-converting enzyme inhibitor therapy improves respiratory muscle strength in patients with heart failure. Chest 2001;119:1755–60.
475. Sabbah HN, Shimoyama H, Kono T, et al. Effects of long-term monotherapy with enalapril, metoprolol, and digoxin on the progression of left ventricular dysfunction and dilation in dogs with reduced ejection fraction. Circulation 1994;89:2852–59.
476. Rubler S, Perloff JK, Roberts WD. Duchenne's muscular dystrophy. Am Heart Journal 1977;94:776–84.
477. Heidenreich PA, Lee TT, Massie BM. Effect of Beta-blockade on mortality in patients with heart failure: a meta-analysis of randomized clinical trials. J Am Coll Cardiol 1997;30:27–34.
478. Yoshikawa T, Handa S, Anzai T, et al. Early reduction of neurohumoral factors plays a key role in mediating the efficacy of beta-blocker therapy for congestive heart failure. Am Heart J 1996;131:329–36.
479. Waagstein F, Bristow MR, Swedberg K, et al. for the Metoprolol in Dilated Cardiomyopathy (MDC) Trial Study Group: Beneficial effects of metoprolol in idiopathic dilated cardiomyopathy. Lancet 1993;342:1441–46.
480. The cardiac insufficiency bisoprolol study (CIBIS) Investigators and Committees. A randomized trial of alpha blockade in heart failure: The Cardiac Insufficiency Bisoprolol Study. Circulation 1994;90: 1765–73.
481. Regitz-Zagrosek V, Leuchs B, Krulls-Munch J, et al. Angiotensin-converting enzyme inhibitors and beta blockers in long-term treatment of dilated cardiomyopathy.Am Heart J 1995;129:754–61.
482. Steinfath M, Lavicky J, Schmitz W, et al. Changes in cardiac B-adrenoceptors in human heart diseases: relationship to the degree of heart failure and further evidence for ethiology-related regulation of B 1 and B 2 subtypes. Journal of Cardiothoracic and Vascular Anesthesia 1993;7:668–73.
483. Heilbrunn SM, Shah P, Bristow MR, et al. Increased B-receptor density and improved hemodynamic response to catecholamine stimulation during long-term metoprolol therapy in heart failure from dilated cardiomyopathy. Circulation 1989;79:483–90.
484. Ducceschi V, Nigro G, Sarubbi B, et al. Autonomic nervous system imbalance and left ventricular systolic dysfunction as potential candidates for arrhythmogenesis in Becker muscular dystrophy. Int J Cardiol 1997;59:275–79.
485. Xi H, Shin WS, Suzuki J, et al. Dystrophin disruption might be related to myocardial cell apoptosis caused by isoproterenol. J Cardiol Pharmacol 2000;36(suppl2):S25–29.
486. Kim MH, Devlin WH, Das SK. Effects of beta-adrenergic blocking therapy on left ventricular diastolic relaxation properties in patients with dilated cardiomyopathy. Circulation 1999;100:729–35.
487. Bach JR, Kang SW. Disorders of ventilation: weakness, stiffness, and mobilization. Chest 2000; 117:301–03.
488. Panchal AR, Stanley WC, Kerner J, Sabbah HN. Beta-receptor blockade decreases carnitine palmitoyl transferase activity in dogs with heart failure. J Cardiac Failure 1998;4:121–26.
489. Stanley WC, Lopaschuk GD, Hall JL, McCormack JG. Regulation of myocardial carbohydrate metabolism under normal and ischaemic conditions: potential for pharmacological interventions. Cardiovasc Res 1997:33:243–57.
490. Katz AM. Mechanisms and abnormalities of contractility and relaxation in the failing heart. Cardiologia 1993;38:39–43.
491. Eichhorn EJ, Heesch CM, Barnett JH, et al. Effect of metoprolol on myocardial function and energetics in patients with non-ischemic dilated cardiomyopathy: a randomized, double-blind, placebo controlled study. J Am Coll Cardiol 1994;24:1310–20.
492. Rupp H, Schulze W, Vetter R. Dietary medium-chain triglyceride can prevent changes in myosin and sarcoplasmic reticulum due to carnitine palmitoyl transferase inhibition by etomoxir. Am J Physiol 1995;269:630–40.
493. Turcani M, Rupp H. Etomoxir improves left ventricular performance of pressure-overloaded rat heart. Circulation 1997;96:3681–86.
494. Haber HL, Simek CL, Gimple LW, et al. Why do patients with congestive heart failure tolerate the initiation of beta-blocker therapy? Circulation 1993;88:1610–19.
495. Matsumura T, Saito T, Miyai I, Mozaki S, Kang J. Effective milrinone therapy to a Duchenne muscular dystrophy patient with advanced congestive heart failure. Rinsho Shinkeigaku 1999;39:643–8.

496. Cleland JGF, Dargie HJ, Mcalpine H, et al. Severe hypotension after first dose of enalapril in heart failure. Br Med J 1985;291:1309–12.
497. Herrlin B, Nyquist O, Sylven C. Induction of a reduction in haemoglobin concentration by enalapril in stable, moderate heart failure:a double blind study. Br Heart J 1991;66:199–205.
498. Todd PA, Goa KL. Enalapril an update of its pharmacological properties and therapeutic use in congestive heart failure. Drugs 1989;37:141–61.
499. Swedberg K. Effects of ACE-inhibition on renal function in severe congestive heart failure. Z Kardiol 1991;80:50–54.
500. Flapan AD, Davies E, Williams BC, et al. The relationship between diuretic dose, and the haemodynamic response to captopril in patients with cardiac failure. Eur Heart J 1992;13:971–75.
501. Di Lenarda A, Secoli G, Perkan A, et al. Changing mortality in dilated cardiomyopathy. Br Heart J 1994;72:S46–51.
502. Doing AH, Renlund DG, Smith RA. Becker muscular dystrophy related cardiomyopathy: a favorable response to medical therapy. J Heart Lung Transplant 2002;21:496–98.
503. Ishikawa Y, Bach JR, Ishikawa Y, et al. A management trial for Duchenne cardiomyopathy. Am J Phys Med Rehabil 1995;74:345–50.
504. Mattioli L, Melhorn M. Duchenne's muscular dystrophy. Journal of Kansas Medical Society 1982; March:115–21.
505. Young JB. Do digitalis glycosides still have a role in congestive heart failure? Cardiol Clin 1994;12:51–61.
506. Adam KF Jr, Gheorrghiade M, Uretsky BF, et al. Clinical predictors of worsening heart failure during withdrawal from digoxin therapy. Am Heart J 1998;135:389–97.
507. Acosta B, DiBenedetto R, Rahimi A, et al. Hemodynamic effects of noninvasive bilevel positive airway pressure on patients with chronic congestive heart failure with systolic dysfunction. Chest 2000;118: 1004–09.
508. Barr CS, Lang CC, Hanson J, Arnott M, Kennedy N, Struthers AD. Effects of adding spironolactone to an angiotensin-converting enzyme inhibitor in chronic congestive heart failure secondary to coronary artery disease. Am J Cardiol 1995;76:1259–65.
509. Struthers AD. Aldosterone escape during angiotensin-converting enzyme inhibitor therapy in chronic heart failure. J Card Fail 1996;2:47–54.
510. Weber KT, Brilla CG. Pathological hypertrophy and cardiac interstitium: fibrosis and renin-angotensin-aldosterone system. Circulation 1991;83:1849–65.
511. Wang W. Chronic administration of aldosterone depresses baroreceptor reflex function in the dog. Hypertension 1994;24:571–5.
512. Rocha R, Chander PN, Khanna K, Zuckerman A, Stier CT Jr. Mineralocorticoid blockade reduces vascular injury in stroke-prone hypertensive rats. Hypertension 1998;31:451–8.
513. Duprez DA, De Buyzere ML, Rietzschel ER, et al. Inverse relationship between aldosterone and large artery compliance in chronically treated heart failure patients. Eur Heart J 1998;19:1371–6.
514. Pitt B. "Escape" of aldosterone production in patients with left ventricular dysfunction treated with an angiotensin converting enzyme inhibitor: implications for therapy. Cardiovasc Drugs Ther 1995;9: 145–9.
515. The RALES Investigators. Effectiveness of spironolactone added to an angiotensin-converting enzyme inhibitor and a loop diuretic for severe chronic congestive heart failure (the Randomized Aldactone Evaluation Study [RALES]). Am J Cardiol 1996;78:902–7.
516. Pitt B, Zannad F, Remme WJ, Cody R, Castaigne A, Perez A, Palensky J, Wittes J, for the randomized aldactone evaluation study investigators. The effect of spironolactone on morbidity and mortality in patients with severe heart failure. N Eng J Med 1999;341:709–17.
517. Brilla CG, Matsubara LS, Weber KT. Anti-aldosterone treatment and the prevention of myocardial fibrosis in primary and secondary hyperaldosteronism. J Mol Cell Cardiol 1993;25:563–75.
518. Vasotec: enalapril maleate. In: Physicians' desk reference. 52nd ed. Montvale, N. J.: Medical economics, 1998:1771–4.
519. Yanagisawa A, Miyagawa M, Yotsukura M, et al. The prevalence and prognostic significance of arrhythmias in Duchenne type muscular dystrophy. Am Heart J 1992;124:1244–50.
520. Munoz J, Sanjuan R, Morell JS, et al. Ventricular tachycardia in Duchenne's muscular dystrophy. Int J of Cardiology 1996;54:259–62.
521. Matsumura T, Saito T, Miyai I, Nozaki S, Kang J. Electrolyte abnormalities and metabolic acidosis in two Duchenne muscular dystrophy patients with advanced congestive heart failure. Rinsho Shinkeigaku 2000;40:439–45.

522. Rusterholtz T, Kempf J, Berton C, et al. Noninvasive pressure support ventilation with face mask in patients with acute cardiogenic pulmonary edema. Intensive Care Med 1999;25:21–28.
523. Newberry DL III, Noblett KE, Kolhouse L. Noninvasive bilevel positive pressure ventilation in severe acute pulmonary edema. Am J Emerg Med 1995;13:479–82.
524. Massip J, Betbese' AJ, Paez J, et al. Non-invasive pressure support ventilation versus conventional oxygen therapy in acute cardiogenic pulmonary oedema: a randomised trial. Lancet 2000;356: 2126–32.
525. Hoffmann B, Welte T. Noninvasive pressure support ventilation as therapy for severe respiratory insufficiency due to pulmonary edema. Pneumologie 1999;53:316–21.
526. LoCoco A, Vitale G, Marchese S, et al. Treatment of acute respiratory failure secondary to pulmonary oedema with bi-level positive airway pressure by nasal mask. Monaldi Arch Chest Dis 1997;52: 444–46.
527. Sacchetti AD, Harris RH, Paston C, Hernandez Z. Bi-level positive airway pressure support system use in acute congestive heart failure: preliminary case series. Acad Emerg Med 1995;2:714–18.
528. Mehta S, Jay GD, Woolard RH, et al. Randomized prospective trial of bilevel versus continuous positive airway pressure in acute cardiogenic edema. Crit Care Med 1997;25:620–28.
529. Park M, Lorenzi-Filho G, Feltrim MI, et al. Oxygen therapy, continuous airway pressure, or noninvasive bilevel positive pressure ventilation in the treatment of acute cardiogenic pulmonary edema. Arq Bras Cardiol 2001;76:226–30.
530. Conraads VM, Beckers PJ, Vorlat A, Vrints CJ. Importance of physical rehabilitation before and after cardiac transplantation in a patient with myotonic dystrophy: a case report. Arch Phys Med Rehabil 2002;83:724–6.
531. Rees W, Schuler S, Hummel M, Hetzer R. Heart transplantation in patients with muscular dystrophy associated with end-stage cardiomyopathy. J Heart Lung Transplant 1993;12:804–7.
532. Riggs T, Oak R. Cardiomyopathy and pulmonary emboli in terminal Duchenne's muscular dystrophy. Am Heart J 1990;119:690–93.
533. Greenberg S, Frishman WH. Co-enzyme Q10: a new drug for cardiovascular disease. J Clin Pharmacol 1990;30:596–608.
534. Folkers K, Wolaniuk J, Simonsen R, et al. Biochemical rationale and the cardiac response of patients with muscle disease to therapy with coenzyme Q10. Proc Natl Acad Sci 1985;82:4513–16.
535. Folkers K, Simonsen R. Two successful double-blind trials with coenzyme Q10 on muscular dystrophies and neurogenic atrophies. Biochim Biophys Acta 1995;1271:281–6.
536. Hochleitner M, Hortnagl H, Hg CK, et al. Usefulness of physiological dual-chamber pacing in drug-resistant idiopathic dilated cardiomyopathy. Am J Cardiol 1990;66:198–202.
537. Hochleitner M, Hortnagl H, Hortnagl H, Fridich L, Gschnitzer F. Long-term efficacy of physiological dual-chamber pacing in the treatment of end-stage idiopathic dilated cardiomyopathy. Am J Cardiol 1992;70:1320–25.
538. Kubler W, Haas M. Cardioprotection: definition, classification, and fundamental principles. Heart 1996;75:330–33.
539. Shimizu T, Hayashi H, Kato S, et al. Circulatory collapse and sudden death in respiratory-dependent amyotrophic lateral sclerosis. J Neurol Sci 1994;124:45–55.
540. Rousseau M, Konstam MA, Benedict CR, et al. Progression of left ventricular dysfunction secondary to coronary artery disease, sustained neurohormonal activation and effects of ibopamine therapy during long-term therapy with angiotensin-converting enzyme inhibitor. Am J Cardiol 1994;73:488–93.
541. Andersson B, Blomstrom-Lundqvist C, Hedner T, Waagstein F. Exercise hemodynamics and myocardial metabolism during long-term beta-adrenergic blockade in severe heart failure. J Am Col Cardiol 1991;1059–66.
542. Armstrong PW, Moe GW. Medical advances in the treatment of congestive heart failure. Circulation 1994;88:2941–52.
543. Miyai I, Kang Jin, Nozaki S, Matsumura T. Alteration of atrial natriuretic peptide in progressive muscular dystrophy with congestive heart failure. Clin Neurol 1992;32:588–92.
544. Bach JR. Pulmonary rehabilitation considerations for Duchenne muscular dystrophy: the prolongation of life by respiratory muscle aids. Crit Rev Phys Rehabil Med 1992;3:239–69.
545. Bach JR. Amyotrophic lateral sclerosis: predictors for prolongation of life by noninvasive respiratory aids. Arch Phys Med Rehabil 1995;76:828–32.
546. Bach JR, Saporito LS. Indications and criteria for decannulation and transition from invasive to noninvasive long-term ventilatory support. Respir Care 1994;39:515–31.

547. Bach JR. Pulmonary rehabilitation in neuromuscular disorders. Seminars in respiratory medicine 1993;14:515–29.
548. Thomas MA, Fast A, Bach JR. Diseases of the motor unit. In: DeLisa JD (ed). Rehabilitation Medicine: Principles and Practice, ed. 3. Philadelphia, Lippincott-Raven, 1998:1545–1573.
549. deLateur BJ, Giaconi RM. Effect on maximal strength of submaximal exercise in Duchenne muscular dystrophy. Am J Phys Med 1979;58:26–36.
550. Vignos PJ, Watkins MP. The effect of exercise in muscular dystrophy. J Am Med Assoc 1966;197:843–8.
551. Milner-Brown HS, Miller RG. Muscle strengthening through high-resistance weight training in patients with neuromuscular diseases. Arch Phys Med Rehabil 1988;69:14–19.
552. Kelm J, Ahlhelm F, Regitz T, Pape D, Schmitt E. Controlled dynamic weight training in patients with neuromuscular disorders. Fortschr Neurol Psychiatr 2001;69:359–66.
553. McCartney N, Moroz D, Garner SH, McComas AJ. The effects of strength training in patients with selected neuromuscular disorders. Med Sci Sports Exerc 1988;20:362–8.
554. Lindeman E, Leffers P, Spaans F, Drukker J, Reulen J, Kerckhoffs M, Koke A. Strength training in patients with myotonic dystrophy and hereditary motor and sensory neuropathy: a randomized clinical trial. Arch Phys Med Rehabil 1995;76:612–20.
555. Tollback A, Eriksson S, Wredenberg A, et al. Effects of high resistance training in patients with myotonic dystrophy. Scand J Rehabil Med 1999;31:9–16.
556. Drory VE, Goltsman E, Reznik JG, Mosek A, Korczyn AD. The value of muscle exercise in patients with amyotrophic lateral sclerosis. J Neurol Sci 2001;191:133–7.
557. Bach JR. Pulmonary rehabilitation. In: DeLisa JD (ed), Rehabilitation Medicine: Principles and Practice, ed 2. Philadelphia, J. B. Lippincott Company, 1993:952–972.
558. Sockolov R, Irwin B, Dressendorfer RH, Bernauer EM. Exercise performance in 6-to-11 year old boys with Duchenne muscular dystrophy. Arch Phys Med Rehabil 1977;58:195–201.
559. Pinto AC, Alves M, Nogueira A, et al. Can amyotrophic lateral sclerosis patients with respiratory insufficiency exercise? J Neurol Sci 1999;169:69–75.
560. Highcock MP, Smith IE, Shneerson JM. The effect of noninvasive intermittent positive pressure ventilation during exercise in severe scoliosis. Chest 2002;121:1555–60.
561. Wanke T, Toifl K, Merkle M, Formanek D, Lahrmann H, Zwick H. Inspiratory muscle training in patients with Duchenne muscular dystrophy. Chest 1994;105:475–82.
562. Winkler G, Zifko U, Nader A, Frank W, Zwick H, Toifl K, Wanke T. Dose-dependent effects of inspiratory muscle training in neuromuscular disorders. Muscle Nerve 2000;23:1257–60.
563. Koessler W, Wanke T, Winkler G, Nader A, Toifl K, Kurz H, Zwick H. Two years' experience with inspiratory muscle training in patients with neuromuscular disorders. Chest 2001;120:765–9.
564. Klefbeck B, Lagerstrand L, Mattsson E. Inspiratory muscle training in patients with prior polio who use part-time assisted ventilation. Arch Phys Med Rehabil 2000;81:1065–71.
565. Gozal D, Thiriet P. Respiratory muscle training in neuromuscular disease: long-term effects on strength and load perception. Med Sci Sports Exerc 1999;31:1522–7.
566. Smeltzer SC, Lavietes MH, Cook SD. Expiratory training in multiple sclerosis. Arch Phys Med Rehabil 1996;77:909–12.
567. Bach JR, Alba AS. Management of chronic alveolar hypoventilation by nasal ventilation. Chest 1990;97:52–57.
568. Willig TN, Bach JR, Rouffet MJ, Krivickas LS, Maquet C. Correlation of flexion-contractures with upper extremity function for spinal muscular atrophy and congenital myopathy patients. Am J Phys Med Rehabil 1995;74:33–38.
569. Abresch RT, Carter GT, Jensen MP, Kilmer DD. Assessment of pain and health-related quality of life in slowly progressive neuromuscular disease. Am J Hosp Palliat Care 2002;19:39–48.
570. Forst J, Forst R. Lower limb surgery in Duchenne muscular dystrophy. Neuromuscular Disorders 1999;9:176–81.
571. Paul WD. Medical management of contractures in muscular dystrophy. In: Proceedings Third Medical Conference of Muscular Dystrophy Associations of America, New York, 1954.
572. Hyde SA, Filytrup I, Glent S, Kroksmark AK, Salling B, Steffensen BF, Werlauff U, Erlandsen M. A randomized comparative study of two methods for controlling tendo Achilles contracture in Duchenne muscular dystrophy. Neuromuscul Disord 2000;10:257–63.
573. Rideau Y, Bach J. Efficacite' therapeutique dans la dystrophie musculaire de Duchenne. J Readapt Med 1982;2:96–100.

574. Archibald DC, Vignos PJ Jr. A study of contractures in muscular dystrophy. Arch Phys Med Rehabil 1959;40:150–7.

575. Bach JR, Lieberman JS. Rehabilitation of the patient with disease affecting the motor unit. In: DeLisa JD (ed), Rehabilitation Medicine: Principles and Practice, ed. 2. Philadelphia, J. B. Lippincott Company, 1993:1099–1110.

576. Bakker JP, deGroot IT, Beckerman H, deJong BA, Lankhorst GJ. The effects of knee-ankle-foot orthoses in the treatment of Duchenne muscular dystrophy: review of the literature. Clin Rehabil 2000;14:343–59.

577. Bach JR. Standards of care in Muscular Dystrophy Association clinics. J Neuro Rehab 1992;6: 67–73.

578. Miller GM, Hsu JD, Hoffer MM, Rentfro R. Posterior tibial tendon transfer: a review of the literature and analysis of 74 procedures. J Pediatr Orthop 1982;2:363–70.

579. Scher DM, Mubarak SJ. Surgical prevention of foot deformity in patients with Duchenne muscular dystrophy. J Pediatr Orthop 2002;22:384–91.

580. Taktak DM, Bowker P. Lightweight, modular knee-ankle-foot orthosis for Duchenne muscular dystrophy: design, development, and evaluation. Arch Phys Med Rehabil 1995;76:1156–62.

581. Valenza J, Guzzardo SL, Bach JR. Functional interventions for individuals with neuromuscular disease. In: Bach JR (ed). Pulmonary Rehabilitation: The Obstructive and Paralytic Conditions. Philadelphia, Hanley & Belfus 1996:371–394.

582. Rideau Y, Duport G, Delaubier A, Guillou C, Renardel-Irani A, Bach JR. Early treatment to preserve quality of locomotion for children with Duchenne muscular dystrophy. Semin Neurol 1995; 15:9–17.

583. Goertzen M, Baltzer A, Voit T. Clinical results of early orthopaedic management in Duchenne muscular dystrophy. Neuropediatrics 1995;26:257–9.

584. Hsu JD, Jackson R. Treatment of symptomatic foot and ankle deformities in the nonambulatory neuromuscular patient. Foot Ankle 1985;5:238–44.

585. Wong CK, Wade CK. Reducing iliotibial band contractures in patients with muscular dystrophy using custom dry floatation cushions. Arch Phys Med Rehabil 1995;76:695–700.

586. Granata C, Magni E, Merlini L, Cervellati S. Hip dislocation in spinal muscular atrophy. Chir Organi Mov 1990;75:177–84.

587. Thompson CE, Larsen LJ. Recurrent hip dislocation in intermediate spinal atrophy. J Pediatr Orthop 1990;10:638–41.

588. Chan KG, Galasko CS, Delaney C. Hip subluxation and dislocation in Duchenne muscular dystrophy. J Pediatr Orthop B 2001;10:219–25.

589. Frischhut B, Krismer M, Stoeckl B, Landauer F, Auckenthaler T. Pelvic tilt in neuromuscular disorders. J Pediatr Orthop B 2000;9:221–8.

590. Copeland SA, Levy O, Warner GC, Dodenhoff RM. The shoulder in patients with muscular dystrophy. Clin Orthop 1999;368:80–91.

591. Jakab E, Gledhill RB. Simplified technique for scapulocostal fusion in facioscapulohumeral dystrophy. J Pediatr Orthop 1993;13:749–51.

592. Bunch WH, Siegel IM. Scapulothoracic arthrodesis in facioscapulohumeral muscular dystrophy. Review of seventeen procedures with three to twenty-one-year follow-up. J Bone Joint Surg Am 1993; 75:372–6.

593. Heller KD, Prescher A, Forst J, Stadtmuller A, Forst R. Anatomo-experimental study for lace fixation of winged scapula in muscular dystrophy. Surg Radiol Anat 1996;18:75–9.

594. Barnett ND, Mander M, Peacock JC, Bushby K, Gardner-Medwin D, Johnson GR. Winging of the scapula: the underlying biomechanics and an orthotic solution. Proc Inst Mech Eng 1995;209:215–23.

595. Roper BA, Tibrewal SB. Soft tissue surgery in Charcot-Marie-Tooth disease. J Bone Joint Surg Br 1989;71:17–20.

596. Medhat MA, Krantz H. Neuropathic ankle joint in Charcot-Marie-Tooth disease after triple arthrodesis. Orthop Rev 1988;17:873–80.

597. Wetmore RS, Drennan JC. Long-term results of triple arthrodesis in Charcot-Marie-Tooth disease. J Bone Joint Surg Am 1989;71:417–22.

598. Wukich DK, Bowen JR. A long-term study of triple arthrodesis for correction of pes cavovarus in Charcot-Marie-Tooth disease. J Pediatr Orthop 1989;9:433–7.

599. Sinaki M, Mulder DW. Rehabilitation techniques for patients with amyotrophic lateral sclerosis. Mayo Clin Proc 1978;53:173–8.

600. Rahman T, Sample W, Seliktar R, Alexander M, Scavina M. A body-powered functional upper limb orthosis. J Rehabil Res Dev 2000;37:675–80.

601. Sinaki M, Wood MB, Mulder DW. Rehabilitative operation for motor neuron disease: tendon transfer for segmental muscular atrophy of the upper extremities. Mayo Clin Proc 1984;59:338–42.

602. Filer S. Quality of life...whose the judge? Abilities Fall/1995:20–22.

603. Johnson EW, Yarnell SK. Hand dominance and scoliosis in Duchenne muscular dystrophy. Arch Phys Med Rehabil 1976;57:462–4.

604. Oda T, Shimizu N, Yonenobu K, Ono K, Nabeshima T, Kyoh S. Longitudinal study of spinal deformity in Duchenne muscular dystrophy. J Pediatr Orthop 1993;13:478–88.

605. Cambridge W, Drennan JL. Scoliosis associated with Duchenne muscular dystrophy. J Pediatr Orthop 1987;7:436–40.

606. Rodillo E, Marini ML, Heckmatt JZ, Dubowitz V. Scoliosis in spinal muscular atrophy: review of 63 cases. J Child Neurol 1989;4:118–23.

607. Brown JC, Zeller JL, Swank SM, Furumasu J, Warath SL. Surgical and functional results of spine fusion in spinal muscular atrophy. Spine 1989;14:763–70.

608. Phillips DP, Roye DP, Farcy JC, Leet A, Shelton YA. Surgical treatment of scoliosis in a spinal muscular atrophy population. Spine 1990;15:942–5.

609. Colbert AP, Craig C. Scoliosis management in Duchenne muscular dystrophy: prospective study of modified Jewett hyperextension brace. Arch Phys Med Rehabil 1987;68:302–4.

610. Rideau Y, Glorion B, Delaubier A, Tarle O, Bach J. Treatment of scoliosis in Duchenne muscular dystrophy. Muscle Nerve 1984;7:281–286.

611. Yamashita T, Kanaya K, Kawaguchi S, Murakami T, Yokogushi K. Prediction of progression of spinal deformity in Duchenne muscular dystrophy: a preliminary report. Spine 2001;26:E223–6.

612. Jenkins JG, Bohn D, Edmonds JF, Levison H, Barker GA. Evaluation of pulmonary function in muscular dystrophy patients requiring spinal surgery. Crit Care Med 1982;10:645–9.

613. Kumano K, Tsuyama N. Pulmonary function before and surgical correction of scoliosis. J Bone Joint Surg 1982;64A:242–8.

614. Smith AD, Koreska J, Moseley CF. Progression of scoliosis in Duchenne muscular dystrophy. J Bone Joint Surg 1989;71A:1066–74.

615. Chaudhry SS, Bach JR. Management approaches in muscular dystrophy association clinics. Am J Phys Med Rehabil 2000;79:193–96.

616. Ramirez N, Richards BS, Warren PD, Williams GR. Complications after posterior spinal fusion in Duchenne's muscular dystrophy. J Pediatr Orthop 1997;17:109–14.

617. Piasecki JO, Mahinpour S, Levine DB. Long-term follow-up of spinal fusion in spinal muscular atrophy. Clin Orthop 1986;207:44–54.

618. Robinson D, Galasko CS, Delaney C, Williamson JB, Barrie JL. Scoliosis and lung function in spinal muscular atrophy. Eur Spine J 1995;4:268–73.

619. Gayet LE. Surgical treatment of scoliosis due to Duchenne muscular dystrophy. Chirurgie 1999;124:423–31.

620. Bell DF, Moseley CF, Koreska J. Unit rod segmental spinal instrumentation in the management of patients with progressive neuromuscular spinal deformity. Spine 1989;14:1301–7.

621. Duport G, Gayet E, Pries P, Thirault C, Renardel-Irani A, Fons N, Bach JR, Rideau Y. Spinal deformities and wheelchair seating in Duchenne muscular dystrophy: twenty years of research and clinical experience. Semin Neurol 1995;15:29–37.

622. Marchesi D, Arlet V, Stricker U, Aebi M. Modification of the original Luque technique in the treatment of Duchenne's neuromuscular scoliosis. J Pediatr Orthop 1997;17:743–9.

623. Miladi LT, Ghanem IB, Draoui MM, Zeller RD, Dubousset JF. Iliosacral screw fixation for pelvic obliquity in neuromuscular scoliosis: a long-term follow-up study. Spine 1997;22:1722–9.

624. Mubarak SJ, Morin WD, Leach J. Spinal fusion in Duchenne muscular dystrophy-fixation and fusion to the sacropelvis? J Pediatr Orthop 1993;13:752–7.

625. Alman BA, Kim HK. Pelvic obliquity after fusion of the spine in Duchenne muscular dystrophy. J Bone Joint Surg Br 1999;81:821–4.

626. Bridwell KH, Baldus C, Iffrig TM, Lenke LG, Blanke K. Process measures and patient/parent evaluation of surgical management of spinal deformities in patients with progressive flaccid neuromuscular scoliosis. Spine 1999;24:1300–9.

627. Kennedy JD, Staples AJ, Brook PD, Parsons DW, Sutherland AD, Martin AJ, Stern LM, Foster BK. Effect of spinal surgery on lung function in Duchenne muscular dystrophy. Thorax 1995;50:1173–8.

628. Matsumura T, Kang J, Nozaki S, Takahashi MP. The Effects of spinal fusion on respiratory function and quality of life in Duchenne muscular dystrophy. Rinsho Shinkeigaku 1997;37:87–92.

629. Yasuda YL, Bowman K, Hsu JD. Mobile arm supports: criteria for successful use in muscle disease patients. Arch Phys Med Rehabil 1986;67:253–6.

630. Takai VL. Case report: the development of a feeding harness for an ALS patient. Am J Occup Ther 1986;40:359–61.

631. Trail M, Nelson N, Van JN, Appel SH, Lai EC. Wheelchair use by patients with amyotrophic lateral sclerosis: a survey of user characteristics and selection preferences. Arch Phys Med Rehabil 2001;82: 98–102.

632. Cherry DB. Transfer techniques for children with muscular dystrophy. Phys Ther 1973;53:970–1.

633. Amir A, Wolf Y, Ezra Y, Shohat M, Sher C, Hauben DJ. Pharyngeal flap for velopharyngeal incompetence in patients with myotonic dystrophy. Ann Plast Surg 1999;42:549–52.

634. McGuirt WF, Blalock D. The otolaryngologist's role in the diagnosis and treatment of amyotrophic lateral sclerosis. Laryngoscope 1980;90:1496–501.

635. Gonzalez JB, Aronson AE. Palatal lift prosthesis for treatment of anatomic and neurologic palatopharyngeal insufficiency. Cleft Palate J 1970;7:91–104.

636. Esposito SJ, Mitsumoto H, Shanks M. Use of palatal lift and palatal augmentation prostheses to improve dysarthria in patients with amyotrophic lateral sclerosis: a case series. J Prosthet Dent 2000;83:90–8.

637. Kubota M, Sakakihara Y, Uchiyama Y, et al. New ocular movement detector system as a communication tool in ventilator-assisted Werdnig-Hoffmann disease. Dev Med Child Neurol 2000;42:61–4.

638. Kubler A, Kotchoubey B, Hinterberger T, et al. The thought translation device: a neurophysiological approach to communication in total motor paralysis. Exp Brain Res 1999;124:223–32.

639. Bach JR, Alba AS. Tracheostomy ventilation: a study of efficacy with deflated cuffs and cuffless tubes. Chest 1990;97:679–83.

640. Reynolds J. Noninvasive ventilation for acute respiratory failure. Journal of Emergency Nursing 1998;23:608–10.

641. Bach JR, Bach GA. Paradigm paralysis. In: Interventions, Respironics Inc., Murrysville, PA, 1993;93: 3,13.

642. Barker JL. Discovering the future (video), Infinity Limited Inc and Film Media Inc., St. Paul-Minneapolis.

643. Krause JS. Employment after spinal cord injury. Arch Phys Med Rehabil 1992;73:163–169.

644. Dubowitz V. Management of muscular dystrophy in 1977. Isr J Med Sci 1977;235–38.

645. Yoshida Y, Kato B, Mizushima Y, Arai N, Matsui S, Maruyama M, Kobayashi M. Syndrome of inappropriate secretion of antidiuretic hormone associated with amyotrophic lateral sclerosis in respiratory failure. Respirology 1999;4:185–7.

646. Cinel D, Markwell K, Lee R, Szidon P. Variability of the respiratory gas exchange ratio during arterial puncture. Am Rev Respir Dis 1991;143:217–18.

647. Polkey MI, Lyall RA, Davidson AC, Leigh PN, Moxham J. Ethical and clinical issues in the use of home non-invasive mechanical ventilation for the palliation of breathlessness in motor neurone disease. Thorax 1999;54:367–71.

648. Sykes NP. People with MND/ALS using noninvasive positive pressure ventilation: how do they die? Amyotrophic Lateral Sclerosis and Other Motor Neuron Disorders, 11th International Symposium, World Federation of Neurology, ALS Foundation, London, 2000:40.

649. Neudert C, Oliver D, Wasner M, Borasio GD. The course of the terminal phase in patients with amyotrophic lateral sclerosis. J Neurol 2001;248:612–6.

650. Poponick JM, Jacobs I, Supiski G, DiMarco AF. Effect of upper respiratory tract infection in patients with neuromuscular disease. Am J Respir Crit Care Med 1997;156:659–64.

651. Bach JR. Home mechanical ventilation for neuromuscular ventilatory failure: conventional approaches and their outcomes. In: Bach JR (ed). Noninvasive mechanical ventilation. Philadelphia, Hanley & Belfus 2002:103–128.

652. Ogata K, Nakayama T, Kawai M. Treatment of nocturnal periodic hypoxemia with safrazine hydrochloride in patients with Duchenne muscular dystrophy under nasal intermittent positive pressure ventilation [Japanese]. Rinsho Shinkeigaku 1998;38:776–8.

653. Goldstein RS. Supplemental oxygen in chronic respiratory disease. In: Bach JR (ed). Pulmonary Rehabilitation: The Obstructive and Paralytic Conditions. Philadelphia: Hanley & Belfus. 1996: 55–84.

654. Stark P. Atelectasis: types and pathogenesis. Up to Date in Pulmonary and Critical Care Medicine, CD ROM. New York, American Thoracic Society, 1997.

655. Bach JR, Ishikawa Y, Kim H. Prevention of pulmonary morbidity for patients with Duchenne muscular dystrophy. Chest 1997;112:1024–28.

656. Bach JR, Saporito LR. Criteria for extubation and tracheostomy tube removal for patients with ventilatory failure: a different approach to weaning. Chest 1996;110:1566–71.

657. Gatin G. Intêret de la ventilation assistée dans les dystrophies musculaires. Ann Readapt Med Phys 1983;26:111–28.

658. Brimacombe J, Keller C, Hormann C. Pressure support ventilation versus continuous positive airway pressure with the laryngeal mask airway: a randomized crossover study of anesthetized adult patients. Anesthesiology 2000;92:1621–23.

659. Aslanian P, El Atrous S, Isabey D, et al. Effects of flow triggering on breathing effort during partial ventilatory support. Am J Respir Crit Care Med 1998;57:135–43.

660. Calderini E, Confalonieri M, Puccio PG, et al. Patient-ventilator asynchrony during noninvasive ventilation: the role of expiratory trigger. Intensive Care Med 1999;25:662–67.

661. Pinto AC, Evangelista T, Carvalho M, Alves MA, Sales Luis ML. Respiratory assistance with a non-invasive ventilator in MND/ALS patients: survival rates in a controlled trial. J Neurol Sci 1995;129(Suppl): 19–26.

662. Kleopa KA, Sherman M, Neal B, Romano GJ, Heiman-Patterson T. Bipap improves survival and rate of pulmonary function decline in patients with ALS. J Neurol Sci 1999;164:82–88.

663. Montner PK, Greene ER, Murata GH, et al. Hemodynamic effects of nasal and face mask continuous positive airway pressure. 1994;149:1614–18.

664. Ferguson KA, Strong MJ, Ahmad D, George CFP. Sleep-disordered breathing in amyotrophic lateral sclerosis. Chest 1996;110:664–69.

665. Robert D, Willig TN, Paulus J, Leger P. Long-term nasal ventilation in neuromuscular disorders: report of a consensus conference. Eur Respir J 1993;6;599–606.

666. Clinical indications for noninvasive positive pressure ventilation in chronic respiratory failure due to restrictive lung disease, COPD, and nocturnal hypoventilation—a consensus conference report. Chest 1999;116:521–34.

667. Gelinas D. Nocturnal oximetry as an early indicator of respiratory involvement in ALS - correlation with FVC plus symptoms and response to NIPPV therapy. ALS and Other Motor Neuron Disorders 2000;1:38–39.

668. Jackson CE, Rosenfeld J, Moore DH, et al. A preliminary evaluation of a prospective study of pulmonary function studies and symptoms of hypoventilation in ALS/MND patients. J Neurol Sci 2001;191:75–8.

669. Elman LB, Siderowff AD, MacCluskey LF. Nocturnal oximetry: utility in the respiratory management of ALS. Am J Phys Med Rehabil (in press).

670. Gries RE, Brooks LJ. Normal oxyhemoglobin saturation during sleep. Chest 1996;110:1489–92.

671. Estournet-Mathiaud B. La ventilation non invasive à domicile dans les maladies neuromusculaires. Arch Pediatr 2000;7 (Suppl2):210–12.

672. Wood KE, Flaten AL, Backes WJ. Inspissated secretions: a life-threatening complication of prolonged noninvasive ventilation. Respir Care 2000;45:491–93.

673. Claman DM, Piper A, Sanders MH, Stiller RA, Votteri BA. Nocturnal noninvasive positive pressure ventilatory assistance. Chest 1996;110:1581–88.

674. Bach JR, Alba AS, Mosher R, Delaubier A. Intermittent positive pressure ventilation via nasal access in the management of respiratory insufficiency. Chest 1987;92:168–70.

675. Ellis ER, Bye PTP, Bruderer JW, Sullivan CE. Treatment of respiratory failure during sleep in patients with neuromuscular disease, positive-pressure ventilation through a nose mask. Am Rev Respir Dis 1987;135:148–52.

676. Kerby GR, Mayer LS, Pingleton SK. Nocturnal positive pressure ventilation via nasal mask. Am Rev Respir Dis 1987;135:738–40.

677. Kirshblum SC, Bach JR. Walker modification for ventilator assisted individuals. Am J Phys Med Rehabil 1992;71:304–06.

678. Mehta S, Hill NS. Noninvasive ventilation. Am J Respir Crit Care Med 2001;163:540–77.

679. Kreit JW, Capper MW, Eschenbacher WL. Patient work of breathing during pressure support and volume-cycled mechanical ventilation. Am J Respir Crit Care Med 1994;149:1085–91.

680. Ferguson GT, Gilmartin M. CO_2 rebreathing during BiPAP^{TM} ventilatory assistance. Am J Respir Crit Care Med 1995;151:1126–35.

681. Smina M, Salam A, Khamiees M, Gada P, Amoateng-Adjepong Y, Manthous CA. Cough peak flows and extubation outcomes. Chest (in press).

682. Le Bourdelles G, Viires N, Boczkowski J, et al. Effects of mechanical ventilation on diaphragmatic contractile properties in rats. Am J Respir Crit Care Med 1994;149:1539–44.

683. Vasilyev S, Schaap RN, Mortensen JD. Hospital survival rates of patients with acute respiratory failure in modern respiratory intensive care units: an international, multicenter, prospective survey. Chest 1995;107:1083–88.

684. Bellamy R, Pitts FW, Stauffer S. Respiratory complications in traumatic quadriplegia. J Neurosurg 1973;39:596–600.

685. Craven DE, Kunches LM, Kilinsky V, et al. Risk factors for pneumonia and fatality in patients receiving continuous mechanical ventilation. Am Rev Respir Dis 1986;133:792–96.

686. Johanson WG, Pierce AK, Sanford JP, Thomas GD. Nosocomial respiratory infections with gram-negative bacilli: the significance of colonization of the respiratory tract. Ann Int Med 1972;77: 701–06.

687. Johanson WG, Seidenfeld JJ, Gomez P, De Los Santos R, Coalson JJ. Bacteriologic diagnosis of nosocomial pneumonia following prolonged mechanical ventilation. Am Rev Respir Dis 1988;137: 259–64.

688. Niederman MS, Ferranti RD, Ziegler A, Merrill W, Reynolds HY. Respiratory infection complicating long-term tracheostomy: the implication of persistent gram-negative tracheobronchial colonization. Chest 1984;85:39–44.

689. Deutschman CS, Wilton P, Sinow J, et al. Paranasal sinusitis associated with nasotracheal intubation: a frequently unrecognized and treatable source of sepsis. Crit Care Med 1986;14:111–14.

690. Moar JJ, Lello GE, Miller SD. Stomal sepsis and fatal haemorrhage following tracheostomy. Int J Oral Maxillofac Surg 1986;15:339–41.

691. Dee PM, Suratt PM, Bray ST, Rose CE. Mucous plugging simulating pulmonary embolism in patients with quadriplegia. Chest 1984;85:363–66.

692. Cohn JR, Steiner RM, Posuniak E, Northrup BE. Obstructive emphysema due to mucus plugging in quadriplegia. Arch Phys Med Rehabil 1987;68:315–17.

693. de Groot REB, Dik H, Groot HGW, Bakker W. A nearly fatal tracheal obstruction resulting from a transtracheal oxygen catheter. Chest 1993;104:1634–35.

694. Berk JL, Levy MN. Profound reflex bradycardia produced by transient hypoxia or hypercapnia in man. Eur Surg Res 1977;9:75–84.

695. Mathias CJ. Bradycardia and cardiac arrest during tracheal suction - mechanisms in tetraplegic patients. Europ J Intens Care Med 1976;2:147–56.

696. Welply NC, Mathias CJ, Frankel HL. Circulatory reflexes in tetraplegics during artificial ventilation and general anesthesia. Paraplegia 1975;13:172–82.

697. Splaingard ML, Frates RC, Harrison GM, Carter RE, Jefferson LS. Home positive-pressure ventilation: twenty years' experience. Chest 1984;4:376–82.

698. Carter RE, Donovan WH, Halstead L, Wilkerson MA. Comparative study of electrophrenic nerve stimulation and mechanical ventilatory support in traumatic spinal cord injury. Paraplegia 1987; 25:86–91.

699. Bach JR. A comparison of long-term ventilatory support alternatives from the perspective of the patient and care giver. Chest 1993;104:1702–06.

700. Pingleton SK. Complications of acute respiratory failure. Am Rev Respir Dis 1988;37:1463–93.

701. Korber W, Laier-Groeneveld G, Criee CP. Endotracheal complications after long-term ventilation: noninvasive ventilation in chronic thoracic diseases as an alternative to tracheostomy. Med Klin 1999;94:45–50.

702. Hedden M, Ersoz C, Safar P. Tracheoesophageal fistulas following prolonged artificial ventilation via cuffed tracheostomy tubes. Anesthesiology 1969;31:281–89.

703. Malingue S, Prunier F, Egreteau JP. Four cases of tracheoesophageal fistula associated with prolonged ventilation (in French). Ann Anesthesiol Fr 1978;l19:539–44.

704. Elpern EH, Scott MG, Petro L, Ries M. Pulmonary aspiration in mechanically ventilated adults with tracheostomies. Am Rev Respir Dis (Abstract) 1993;147:A409.

705. Colice GL. Resolution of laryngeal injury following translaryngeal intubation. Am Rev Respir Dis 1992;145:361–64.

706. Heffner JE. Timing of tracheotomy in mechanically ventilated patients. Am Rev Respir Dis 1993;147: 768–71.

707. Castella X, Gilbert J, Torner F. (letter) Chest 1990;98:776–77.

708. Richard I, Giraud M, Perrouin-Verbe B, et al. Laryngotracheal stenosis after intubation or tracheostomy in patients with neurological disease. Arch Phys Med Rehabil 1996;77:493–96.

709. Konrad F, Schreiber T, Brecht-Kraus D, Georgieff M. Mucociliary transport in ICU patients. Chest 1994;105:237–41.

710. Sanada Y, Kohima Y, Fonkalsrud EW. Injury of cilia induced by tracheal tube cuffs. Surg Gynecol Obstet 1982;154:648–52.

711. Rumbak MJ, Walsh FW, Anderson WM, Rolfe MW, Solomon DA. Significant tracheal obstruction causing failure to wean in patients requiring prolonged mechanical ventilation: a forgotten complication of long-term mechanical ventilation. Chest 1999;115:1092–5.

712. Newth CJL, Lipton JJ, Gould RG, Stretton M. Varying tracheal cross-sectional area during respiration in infants and children with suspected upper airway obstruction by computed cineotomagraphy scanning. Pediatr Pulmonol 1990;9:224–32.

713. Haber II, Bach JR. Normalization of blood carbon dioxide levels by transition from conventional ventilatory support to noninvasive inspiratory aids. Arch Phys Med Rehabil 1994;75:1145–50.

714. Todd DA, John E, Osborn RA. Epithelial damage beyond the tip of the endotracheal tube. Early Hum Dev 1990;24:187–200.

715. Czarnik RE, Stone KS, Everhart CC Jr, Preusser BA. Differential effects of continuous versus intermittent suction on tracheal tissue. Heart Lung 1991;20:144–51.

716. Clini E. Patient ventilator interfaces: practical aspects in the chronic situation. Monaldi Arch Chest Dis 1997;52:76–79.

717. Kleiber C, Krutzfield N, Rose EF. Acute histologic changes in the tracheobronchial tree associated with different suction catheter insertion techniques. Heart Lung 1988;17:10–14.

718. Brodsky L, Reidy M, Stanievich JF. The effects of suctioning techniques on the distal tracheal mucosa in intubated low birth weight infants. Int J Pediatr Otorhinolaryngol 1987;14:1–14.

719. Bailey C, Kattwinkel J, Teja K, Buckley T. Shallow versus deep endotracheal suctioning in young rabbits: pathologic effects on the tracheobronchial wall. Pediatrics 1988;82:746–51.

720. Thompson CL, Wiggins W, Sheppard L, Sims K. Criteria for tracheal suction of ventilated intensive care adults. Am Rev Respir Dis (Abstract) 1993;147:A410.

721. Fishburn MJ, Marino RJ, Ditunno JF. Atelectasis and pneumonia in acute spinal cord injury. Arch Phys Med Rehabil 1990;71:197–200.

722. Bach JR, Sortor S, Sipski M. Sleep blood gas monitoring of high cervical quadriplegic patients with respiratory insufficiency by non-invasive techniques [abstract]. Abstracts Digest, 14th Annual Scientific Meeting of the American Spinal Cord Injury Association, available from L. H. Johnson, 2020 Peachtree Road, NW, Atlanta, GA, 1988:102.

723. Bach JR, Haber II, Wang TG, Alba AS. Alveolar ventilation as a function of ventilatory support method. Eur J Phys Med Rehabil 1995;5:80–84.

724. Watt JWH, Oo T, Salva P. Biochemical profile and long-term hyperventilation in high tetraplegia. 8th Journées Internationales de Ventilation à Domicile, abstract 128, March 7, 2001, Hôpital de la Croix-Rousse, Lyon, France.

725. Popova LM, Moiseev AN. Mechanics of breathing during prolonged artificial ventilation. Resuscitation 1980;8:29–41.

726. Sakakihara Y, Yoneyama A, Kamoshita S. Chronic ventilator-assisted children in university hospitals in Japan. Acta Paediatr Jpn 1993;35:332–5.

727. Baydur A, Gilgoff I, Prentice W, Carlson M, Fischer DA. Decline in respiratory function and experience with long-term assisted ventilation in advanced Duchenne's muscular dystrophy. Chest 1990;97:884–89.

728. Soudon P. Tracheal versus noninvasive mechanical ventilation in neuromuscular patients: experience and evaluation. Monaldi Arch Chest Dis 1995;50:228–31.

729. Eagle M, Chandler C, Giddings D, Bullock R, Bushby K. Survival and cause of death in Duchenne muscular dystrophy. 8th Journées Internationales de Ventilation à Domicile, abstract 121, March 7, 2001, Hôpital de la Croix-Rousse, Lyon, France.

730. Bach JR, O'Brien J, Krotenberg R, Alba A. Management of end stage respiratory failure in Duchenne muscular dystrophy. Muscle Nerve 1987;10:177–82.

731. Vianello A, Bevilacqua M, Arcaro G, Gallan F, Serra E. Non-invasive ventilatory approach to treatment of acute respiratory failure in neuromuscular disorders. A comparison with endotracheal intubation. Int Care Med 2000;26:384–90.

732. Nomori H, Ishihara T. Pressure controlled ventilation via a mini-tracheostomy tube for neuromuscular disease patients. Neurology 2002;55:698–702.

733. Ishihara T. Respiratory management in muscle disease. In: Itoyama Y, Kobayashi S, Sobue G (eds). Medical Topics in CNS and Neuromuscular Disease. Medical Topics Series 14. Tokyo, Sentan-Iryogijyutsu-Kenkyusho (Japanese) 2001:259–63.

734. Kang J. Widespread application of NPPV in respiratory failure associated with neuromuscular diseases (in Japanese). Kokyo To Jyunkan (Respiration and Circulation). 2000;48:11–16.

735. Salamand J, Robert D, Leger P, Langevin B, Barraud J. Definitive mechanical ventilation via tracheostomy in end stage amyotrophic lateral sclerosis, in Proceedings of the International Conference on Pulmonary Rehabilitation and Home Ventilation. Denver, National Jewish Center, 1991:51.

736. Gabinski CL, Barthe A, Castaing Y, Favarel-Garrigues JC. Sclérose latérale amyotrophique et réanimation. Concours Medical 1983;105:249–52.

737. Goulon M, Goulon-Goeau C. Sclérose latérale amyotrophique et assistance respiratoire. Rev Neurol (Paris) 1989;145:293–98.

738. Oppenheimer EA, Baldwin-Myers A, Tanquary P. Ventilator use by patients with amyotrophic lateral sclerosis. In Proceedings of the International Conference on Pulmonary Rehabilitation and Home Ventilation. Denver, National Jewish Center, 1991, p 49.

739. Iwata M. Clinico-pathological studies of long survival ALS cases maintained by active life support. Adv Exper Med Biol 1987;209:223–25.

740. Sivak ED, Gipson WT, Hanson MR. Long-term management of respiratory failure in amyotrophic lateral sclerosis. Ann Neurol 1982;12:18–23.

741. Gilgoff IS, Kahlstrom E, MacLaughlin E, Keens TG. Long-term ventilatory support in spinal muscular atrophy. J Pediatr 1989;115:904–09.

742. Bach JR, Baird JS, Plosky D, Nevado J, Weaver B. Spinal muscular atrophy type 1: management and outcomes. Pediatr Pulmonol 2002:34:16–22.

743. Smith PEM, Calverley PMA, Edwards RHT. Hypoxemia during sleep in Duchenne muscular dystrophy. Am Rev Respir Dis 1988;137:884–88.

744. Simonds AK, Muntoni F, Heather S, Fielding S. Impact of nasal ventilation on survival in hypercapnic Duchenne muscular dystrophy. Thorax 1998;53:949–52.

745. Raphael J-C, Chevret S, Chastang C, Bouvet F. Randomised trial of preventive nasal ventilation in Duchenne muscular dystrophy. Lancet 1994;343:1600–04.

746. Melo J, Homma A, Iturriaga E,et al. Pulmonary evaluation and prevalence of noninvasive ventilation in patients with amyotrophic lateral sclerosis: a multicenter survey and proposal of a pulmonary protocol. J Neurol Sci 1999;169:114–17.

747. Aboussouan LS, Khan SU, Mecker DP, Stelmach K, Mitsumoto H. Effect of noninvasive positive-pressure ventilation on survival in amyotrophic lateral sclerosis. Ann Intern Med 1997;127:450-53

748. Sherman MS, Paz HL. Review of respiratory care of the patient with amyotrophic lateral sclerosis. Respiration 1994;61:61–67.

749. Lyall RA, Donaldson N, Fleming T, et al. A prospective study of quality of life in ALS patients treated with non-invasive ventilation. Neurology 2001;57:153–6.

750. Bach JR. Amyotrophic lateral sclerosis: prolongation of life by noninvasive respiratory aids. Chest 2002;122:92–8.

751. Bach JR, Robert D, Leger P, Langevin B. Sleep fragmentation in kyphoscoliotic individuals with alveolar hypoventilation treated by nasal IPPV. Chest 1995;107:1552–58.

752. Bach JR, Alba AS, Saporito LR. Intermittent positive pressure ventilation via the mouth as an alternative to tracheostomy for 257 ventilator users. Chest 1993;103:174–82.

753. Masa JF, Celli BR, Riesco JA, et al. The obesity hypoventilation syndrome can be treated with noninvasive mechanical ventilation. Chest 2001;119:1102–07.

754. Mohn CH, Hill NS. Long-term follow-up of nocturnal ventilatory assistance in patients with respiratory failure due to Duchenne-type muscular dystrophy. Chest 1990;97:91–96.

755. Leger P, Langevin B, Guez A, et al. What to do when nasal ventilation fails for neuromuscular patients. Eur Respir R 1993;3:279–83.

756. Neri M, Donner CF, Grandi M, Robert D. Timing of tracheostomy in neuromuscular patients with chronic respiratory failure. Monaldi Arch Chest Dis 1995;50:220–22.

757. Baydur A, Layne E, Aral H, et al. Long term non-invasive ventilation in the community for patients with musculoskeletal disorders: 46 year experience and review. Thorax 2000;55:4–11.

758. Lofaso F, Brochard L, Touchard D, et al. Evaluation of carbon dioxide rebreathing during pressure support ventilation with airway management system devices. Chest 1995;108:772–78.

759. DiMarco AF, Connors AF, Altose MD. Management of chronic alveolar hypoventilation with nasal positive pressure breathing. Chest 1987;92:952–54.

760. Ellis ER, Grunstein RR, Chan RR, et al. Noninvasive ventilatory support during sleep improves respiratory failure in kyphoscoliosis. Chest 1988;94:811–15.

761. Carroll N, Branthwaite MA. Control of nocturnal hypoventilation by nasal intermittent positive pressure ventilation. Thorax 1988;43:349–53.
762. Guilleminault C, Stoohs R, Schneider H, et al. Central alveolar hypoventilation and sleep: treatment by intermittent positive pressure ventilation through nasal mask in an adult. Chest 1989;96:1210–12.
763. Heckmatt JZ, Loh L, Dubowitz V. Night-time nasal ventilation in neuromuscular disease. Lancet 1990;335:579–82.
764. Goldstein RS, DeRosie JA, Avendano MA, Dolmage TE. Influence of noninvasive positive pressure ventilation on inspiratory muscles. Chest 1991;99:408–15.
765. Gay PC, Patel AM, Viggiano RW, Hubmayr RD. Nocturnal nasal ventilation for treatment of patients with hypercapnic respiratory failure. Mayo Clin Proc 1991;66:695–703.
766. Laier-Groeneveld G, Huttemann V, Criee C-P. Nasal ventilation can reverse chronic ventilatory failure in both chest wall diseases and COPD. International Conference on Pulmonary Rehabilitation and Home Ventilation. National Jewish Center for Immunology and Respiratory Medicine, Denver, CO, Proceedings 1991, p. 104.
767. Thommi G, Nugent K, Bell GM, Liu J. Termination of central sleep apnea episodes by upper airway stimulation using intermittent positive pressure ventilation. Chest 1991;99:1527–29.
768. Hill NS, Eveloff SE, Carlisle CC, Goff SG. Efficacy of nocturnal nasal ventilation in patients with restrictive thoracic disease. Am Rev Respir Dis 1992;145:365–71.
769. Waldhorn RE. Nocturnal nasal intermittent positive pressure ventilation with bi-level positive airway pressure in respiratory failure. Chest 1992;101:516–21.
770. Paulus J, Willig T-N. Nasal ventilation in neuromuscular disorders: respiratory management and patients' experience. Eur Respir Rev 1993;3:245–49.
771. Delguste P, Rodenstein. Implementation and monitoring of mechanical ventilation via nasal access. Eur Respir Rev 1993;3:266–69.
772. Barois A, Estournet-Mathiaud B. Nasal ventilation in congenital myopathies and spinal muscular atrophies. Eur Respir R 1993;3:275–78.
773. Chetty KG, McDonald RL, Berry RB, Mahutte CK. Chronic respiratory failure due to bilateral vocal cord paralysis managed with nocturnal nasal positive pressure ventilation. Chest 1993;103:1270–71.
774. Sekino H, Ohi M, Chin K, et al. Long term artificial ventilation by nasal intermittent positive pressure ventilation; 6 cases of domiciliary assisted ventilation. Nihon Kyobu Shikkan Gakkai Zasshi 1993;31:1377–84.
775. van Kesteren RG, Kampelmacher MJ, Dullemond-Westland AC, et al. Favorable results of nocturnal nasal positive-pressure ventilation in 64 patients with neuromuscular disorders: 5-year experience (in Dutch). Ned Tijdschr Geneeskd 1994;138:1864–68.
776. Vianello A, Bevilacqua M, Salvador V, Cardaioli C, Vincenti E. Long-term nasal intermittent positive pressure ventilation in advanced Duchenne's muscular dystrophy. Chest 1994;105:445–48.
777. Leger P, Bedicam JM, Cornette A, et al. Nasal intermittent positive pressure ventilation: long-term follow-up in patients with severe chronic respiratory insufficiency. Chest 1994;105:100–05.
778. Piper AM, Sullivan CE. Effects of short-term NIPPV in the treatment of patients with severe obstructive sleep apnea and hypercapnia. Chest 1994;105:434–40.
779. Robertson PL, Roloff DW. Chronic respiratory failure in limb-girdle muscular dystrophy: successful long-term therapy with nasal bilevel positive airway pressure. Pediatr Neurol 1994;10:328–31.
780. Yasuma F, Sakai M, Matsuoka Y. Effects of noninvasive ventilation on survival in patients with Duchenne's muscular dystrophy (letter). Chest 1996;109:590.
781. Escarrabill J, Estopa R, Farrero E, Monasterio C, Manresa F. Long-term mechanical ventilation in amyotrophic lateral sclerosis. Respir Med 1998;92:438-41.
782. Schlamp V, Karg O, Abel A, et al. Noninvasive intermittent self-ventilation as a palliative measure in amyotrophic lateral sclerosis. Nervenarzt 1998;69:1074–82.
783. Guilleminault C, Philip P, Robinson A. Sleep and neuromuscular disease: bilevel positive airway pressure by nasal mask as a treatment for sleep disordered breathing in patients with neuromuscular disease. J Neurol Neurosurg Psychiatry 1998;65:225–32.
784. Jardine E, O'Toole M, Paton JY, Wallis C. Current status of long term ventilation of children in the United Kingdom: questionnaire survey. BMJ 1999;318:295–98.
785. Annane D, Quera-Salva MA, Lofaso F, et al. Mechanisms underlying effects of nocturnal ventilation on daytime blood gases in neuromuscular diseases. Eur Respir J 1999;13:157–62.

786. Raffenberg M, Geerdes-Fenge H, Muller-Pawlowski H, et al. Invasive and noninvasive home ventilation-changes between 1982 and 1996 (in German). Med Klin 1999;94:18–21.
787. Pahnke J, Bullemer F, Heindl S, Kroworsch B, Karg O. Long-term breathing via traceostoma (in German). Med Klin 1999;94:40–42.
788. Hukins CA, Hillman DR. Daytime predictors of sleep hypoventilation in Duchenne muscular dystrophy. Am J Respir Crit Care Med 2000;161:166–70.
789. Ohi M, Kuno K. Effectiveness of domiciliary noninvasive positive pressure ventilation in improving blood gas levels and the performance of daily activities. NIPPV Study Group.Nihon Kokyuki Gakkai Zasshi 2000 38:166–73.
790. Round Table Conference on Poliomyelitis Equipment, Roosevelt Hotel, New York City, Sponsored by the National Foundation for Infantile Paralysis, Inc., May 28–29, 1953.
791. Hudgel DW, Martin RJ, Johnson B, Hill P. Mechanics of the respiratory system and breathing pattern during sleep in normal humans. J Appl Physiol 1984;56:133–37.
792. Bach JR, Alba AS, Bodofsky E, Curran FJ, Schultheiss M. Glossopharyngeal breathing and non-invasive aids in the management of post-polio respiratory insufficiency. Birth Defects 1987;23:99–113.
793. Lissoni A, Aliverti A, Molteni F, Bach JR. Spinal muscular atrophy: kinematic breathing analysis. Am J Phys Med Rehabil 1996;75:332–39.
794. Lechtzin N, Wiener CM, Shade DM, Clawson L, Diette GB. Spirometry in the supine position improves the detection of diaphragmatic weakness in patients with amyotrophic lateral sclerosis. Chest 2002;121:436–42.
795. West JB. Respiratory Physiology: The Essentials: Dystrophy. Acta Paediatr Jpn 1994;36:627–31.
796. Slonim NB, Hamilton LH (eds): Respiratory Physiology, ed. 5. C.V. Mosby Co, St. Louis; 1987: 123–130,281.
797. Inkley SR, Oldenburg FC, Vignos PJ Jr. Pulmonary function in Duchenne muscular dystrophy related to stage of disease. Am J Med 1974;56:297–306.
798. Slonim NB, Hamilton LH (eds): Respiratory Physiology ed. 5. C.V. Mosby Co, St. Louis; 1987: 143–49.
799. Bucher U, Reid L. Development of the mucus-secreting elements in human lung. Thorax 1961;16: 219–225.
800. Willson HG. Post natal development of lung. Am J Anat 1928;41:97–105.
801. Reid L. Autopsy studies of the lungs in kyphoscoliosis. In: Zorab PA, ed., Proceedings of a Symposium on Scoliosis: Action for the Crippled Child. Monograph, London: Academic Press, 1965:71–7.
802. Bach JR. Pulmonary assessment and management of the aging and older patient. In: Felsenthal G, Garrison SJ, Steinberg FU (eds): Rehabilitation of the Aging and Elderly Patient, Baltimore, Williams & Wilkins 1993:263–73.
803. Levison H, Cherniack RM. Ventilatory cost of exercise in chronic obstructive pulmonary disease. J Appl Physiol 1968;25;21–27.
804. Edwards RHT. Human muscle function and fatigue. In: Human Muscle Fatigue: Physiological Mechanisms. Pitman Medical, London (Ciba Foundation Symposium 82) 1981:1–18.
805. Braun NMT, Arora MS, Rochester DF. Respiratory muscle and pulmonary function in polymyositis and other proximal myopathies. Thorax 1983;38:616–23.
806. Begin P, Grassino A. Inspiratory muscle dysfunction and chronic hypercapnia in chronic obstructive pulmonary disease. Am Rev Respir Dis 1983;143:905–12.
807. Barton AD, Lourenço RV. Bronchial secretions and mucociliary clearance. Biochemical characteristics. Arch Intern Med 1973;131:140–44.
808. Jeffery PK. The origins of secretions in the lower respiratory tract. Eur J Respir Dis 1987;71(suppl 153):34–42.
809. Kaliner M, Marom Z, Patow C, Shelhamer J. Human respiratory mucus. J Allergy Clin Immunol 1984;73:318–23.
810. Lopez-Vidriero MT, Das I. Airway secretion: Source, biochemical and rheological properties. In: Brain JD, Proctor DF, Reid LM (eds): Respiratory Defense Mechanisms, Marcel Dekker, New York, 1977:288–301.
811. Lopez-Vidriero MT. Airway mucus production and composition. Chest 1981;80:799–804.
812. Richardson PS. The physical and chemical properties of airway mucus and their relation to airway function. Eur J Respir Dis 1980;61(suppl 111):13–15.
813. Toremalm NG. The daily amount of tracheobronchial secretions in man. Acta Oto-Laryng 1960; (suppl 185):43–53.

814. Asmundsson T, Kilburn KH. Mucociliary clearance rates at various levels in dogs' lungs. Am Rev Respir Dis 1970;102:388–97.
815. Lee PS, Gerrity TR, Hass FJ, Lourenço RV. A model for tracheobronchial clearance of inhaled particles in man and comparison with data. IEEE Transactions on Biomedical Engineering 1979;26: 624–30.
816. Kilburn KH. A hypothesis for pulmonary clearance and its implications. Am Rev Respir Dis 1968; 98:449–63.
817. Van As A. Pulmonary airway clearance mechanisms: a reappraisal. Am Rev Respir Dis 1977;115: 721–26.
818. Phipps RJ, Richardson PS. The effects of irritation at various levels of the airway upon tracheal mucus secretion in the cat. J Physiol 1976;261:561–81.
819. Richardson PS, Peatfield AC. The control of airway secretion. Eur J Respir Dis 1987;71(suppl 153): 43–51.
820. Pavia D, Agnew JE, Clarke SW. Physiological, pathological and drug-related alterations in tracheo-bronchial mucociliary clearance. In: Isles AF, von Wichert P (eds). Sustained-release theophylline and noctural asthma. Exerpta Medica, Amsterdam, 2000:44.
821. van As A. Pulmonary airway defense mechanisms: an appreciation of integrated mucociliary activity. Eur J Respir Dis 1980;61(suppl 111):21–24.
822. Newhouse M, Sanchis J, Bienenstock J. Lung defense mechanisms. N Eng J Med 1976;195:990–98.
823. Sleigh MA. The nature and action of respiratory tract cilia. In Brain JD, Proctor DF, Reid LM (eds): Respiratory Defense Mechanisms. Marcel Dekker, New York, 1977:247.
824. Wanner A. Clinical aspects of mucociliary transport. Am Rev Respir Dis 1977;115:73–125.
825. Jeffery PK, Reid L. New observations of rat airway epithelium: a quantitative and electron microscopic study. J Anat 1975;120:295–320.
826. Hoffman LA. Ineffective airway clearance related to neuromuscular dysfunction. Nursing Clin N Am 1987;22:151–166.
827. Williams R, Rankin N, Smith T, et al. Relationship between the humidity and temperature of inspired gas and the function of the airway mucosa. Crit Care Med 1996;24:1920–29.
828. Slonim NB, Hamilton LH (eds): Respiratory Physiology, ed. 5. C.V. Mosby Co, St. Louis; 1987:42–47.
829. Mullen JBM, Wright JL, Wiggs BR, Pare PD, Hogg JC. Structure of central airways in current smok-ers and ex-smokers with and without mucus hypersecretion: relation to lung function. Thorax 1987;42:843–48.
830. Leith DE. Lung biology in health and desease: respiratory defense mechainisms, part 2. In Brain JD, Proctor D, Reid L (eds): Cough. Marcel Dekker, New York, 1977:545–92.
831. von Leden H, Isshiki N. An analysis of cough at the level of the larynx. Arch Otol 1965;81:616–25.
832. Macchione M, Guimaraes ET, Saldiva PHN, Lorenzi-Filho G. Methods for studying respiratory mucus and mucus clearance. Braz J Med Biol Res 1995;28:1347–55.
833. Regnis JA, Robinson M, Bailey DL, et al. Mucociliary clearance in patients with cystic fibrosis and in normal subjects. Am J Respir Crit Care Med 1994;150:66–71.
834. Evans JN, Jaeger MJ. Mechanical aspects of coughing. Pneumonologie 1975;152:253–57.
835. Griggs RG, Donohoe KM, Utell MJ, Goldblatt D, Moxley TR. Evaluation of pulmonary function in neuromuscular disease. Arch Neurol 1981;38:9–12.
836. Profiles of neuromuscular diseases. Am J Phys Med Rehabil 1995;74:1–165.
837. Leiner GC, Abramowitz S, Small MJ, Stenby VB, Lewis WA. Expiratory peak flow rate. Standard values for normal subjects. Use as a clinical test of ventilatory function. Am Rev Respir Dis 1963;88:644.
838. Polgar G, Promadhat V. Pulmonary function testing in children: techniques and standards. W.B. Saunders, Philadelphia; 1971
839. Suarez AA, Pessolano F, Monteiro SG, et al. Peak flow and peak cough flow in the evaluation of expira-tory muscle weakness and bulbar impairment of neuromuscular patients. Am J Phys Med Rehabil 2002;81:506–11.
840. Rayl JE. Tracheobronchial collapse during cough. Radiology 1965;85:87–92.
841. Pedersen OF, Nielsen TM. The critical transmural pressure of the airway. Acta Physiol Scand 1976;97:426–46.
842. Scherer PW. Mucus transport by cough. Chest 1981;80:830–33.
843. Mead J, Turner JM, Macklem PT, Little JB. Significance of the relationship between lung recoil and maximum expiratory flow. J Appl Physiol 1967;22:95–108.
844. Agarwal M, King M, Rubin BK, Shukla JB. Mucus transport in a miniaturized simulated cough ma-chine: effect of constriction and serous layer simulant. Biorheology 1989;26:977–88.

845. van der Schans CP, Ramirez OE, Postma DS, Koëter GH, Rubin BK. Effect of airway constriction on the cough transportability of mucus. Am J Respir Crit Care Med 1994;149:A1023.

846. King M, Brock G, Lundell C. Clearance of mucus by simulated cough. J Appl Physiol 1985;58: 1776–85.

847. Cook NR, Evans DA, Scherr PA, et al. Peak expiratory flow rate and 5-year mortality in an elderly population. Am J Epidemiol 1991;133:784–94.

848. Wang TG, Bach JR. Pulmonary dysfunction in residents of chronic care facilities. Taiwan Journal of Rehabilitation 1993;21:67–73.

849. Hanayama K, Ishikawa Y, Bach JR. Amyotrophic lateral sclerosis: successful treatment of mucus plugging by mechanical insufflation-exsufflation. Am J Phys Med Rehabil 1997;76:338–39.

850. Jubran A, Tobin MJ. Use of flow-volume curves in detecting secretions in ventilator-dependent patients. Am J Respir Crit Care Med 1994;150:766–69.

851. Lambertsen CJ. Chemical control of respiration at rest. In: Mountcastle VB (ed): Medical Physiology, ed. 14. CV Mosby, St. Louis; 1980:1771–1827.

852. Bach JR. Physiology and pathophysiology of hypoventilation: ventilatory vs. oxygenation impairment. In: Bach JR (ed). Noninvasive Mechanical Ventilation. Philadelphia, Hanley and Belfus 2002: 25–45.

853. Milic-Emili J, Grassino AE, Whitelaw WA. Measurement and testing of respiratory drive. In: Hornbein TF (ed): Regulation of Breathing, Vol. 17, Lung Biology in Health and Disease, Marcel Dekker, New York; 1981:675–743.

854. Hugelin A, Cohen MI. The reticular activating system and respiratory regulation in the cat. Ann N Y Acad Sci 1963;109:586–603.

855. Lydic R, Orem J. Respiratory neurons of the pneumotaxic center during sleep and wakefulness. Neurosci Lett 1979;15:187–92.

856. Orem J, Montplaiser J, Dement WC. Changes in the activity of respiratory neurons during sleep. Brain Res 1974;82:309–15.

857. Becker HF. Pathophysiology and clinical aspects of global respiratory insufficiency. Med Klin 1997;92(Suppl1):10–13.

858. Kohler D, Schonhofer B. How important is the differentiation between apnea and hypopnea? Respiration 1997;64(suppl):15–21.

859. Arnulf I, Similowski T, Salachas F, et al. Sleep disorders and diaphragmatic function in patients with amyotrophic lateral sclerosis. Am J Respir Crit Care Med 2000;161:849–56.

860. Weinberg J, Klefbeck B, Borg J, Svanborg E. Respiration and accessory muscle activity during sleep in neuromuscular disorders. 8th Journées Internationales de Ventilation á Domicile, abstract 150, March 7, 2001, Hôpital de la Croix-Rousse, Lyon, France.

861. Juan G, Calverley P, Talamo C. Effect of carbon dioxide on diaphragmatic function in human beings. N Engl J Med 1984;310:874–79.

862. Goldstein RS. Hypoventilation: neuromuscular and chest wall disorders. Clin Chest Med 1992;13: 507–21.

863. Redding GJ, Okamoto GA, Guthrie RD, Rollevson D, Milstein JM. Sleep patterns in nonambulatory boys with Duchenne muscular dystrophy. Arch Phys Med Rehabil 1985;66:818–21.

864. Hukins CA, Hillman DR. Daytime predictors of sleep hypoventilation in Duchenne muscular dystrophy. Am J Respir Crit Care Med 2000;161:166–70.

865. Smith PEM, Edwards RHT, Calverley PMA. Ventilation and breathing pattern during sleep in Duchenne muscular dystrophy. Chest 1989;96:1346–51.

866. Soudon P. Ventilation assisté au long cours dans les maladies neuro-musculaire: experience actuelle. Réadaptation Réévalidatie 1987;3:45–65.

867. Ohtake S. Nocturnal blood gas disturbances and treatment of patients with Duchenne muscular dystrophy. Kokyu To Junkan 1990;38:463–69.

868. Smith PEM, Edwards RHT, Calverley PMA. Oxygen treatment of sleep hypoxaemia in Duchenne muscular dystrophy. Thorax 1989;44:997–1001.

869. Guilleminault C, Motta J. Sleep apnea syndrome as a long-term sequelae of poliomyelitis. In: Guilleminault C (ed): Sleep Apnea Syndromes, New York, KROC Foundation, 1978:309–15.

870. Steljes DG, Kryger MH, Kirk BW, Millar TW. Sleep in postpolio syndrome. Chest 1990;98:133–40.

871. Carskadon M, Dement W. Respiration during sleep in the aged human. J Gerontol 1981;36:420–25.

872. George CF, Millar TW, Kryger MH. Identification and quantification of apneas by computer-based analysis of oxygen saturation. Am Rev Respir Dis 1988;137:1238–40.

873. He J, Kryger MH, Zorick FJ, Conway W, Roth T. Mortality and apnea index in obstructive sleep apnea. Chest 1988;94:9–14.

874. Bach JR. Inappropriate weaning and late onset ventilatory failure of individuals with traumatic quadriplegia. Paraplegia 1993;31:430–438.

875. Levy RD, Bradley TD, Newman SL, Macklem PT, Martin JG. Negative pressure ventilation: effects on ventilation during sleep in normal subjects. Chest 1989;65:95–99.

876. Katsantonis GP, Walsh JK, Schweitzer PK, Friedman WH. Further evaluation of uvulopalatopharyngoplasty in the treatment of obstructive sleep apnea syndrome. Otolaryngol Head Neck Surg 1985;93:244–50.

877. Bradley TD, Phillipson EA. Pathogenesis and pathophysiology of the obstructive sleep apnea syndrome. Med Clin N Am 1985;69:1169–85.

878. Bonekat HW, Andersen G, Squires J. Obstructive disordered breathing during sleep in patients with spinal cord injury. Paraplegia 1990;28:392–98.

879. Lombard R Jr, Zwillich CW. Medical therapy of obstructive sleep apnea. Med Clin N Am 1985;69:1317–35.

880. Brown IG, Zamel N, Hoffstein V. Pharyngeal cross-sectional area in normal men and women. J Appl Physiol 1986;61:890–95.

881. Bach JR, Penek J. Obstructive sleep apnea complicating negative pressure ventilatory support in patients with chronic paralytic/restrictive ventilatory dysfunction. Chest 1991;99:1386–93.

882. Bach JR, O'Connor K. Electrophrenic ventilation: a different perspective. J Am Paraplegia Soc 1991;14:9–17.

883. Hodes HL. Treatment of respiratory difficulty in poliomyelitis. In Poliomyelitis: Papers and Discussions Presented at the Third International Poliomyelitis Conference. Philadelphia, Lippincott 1955:91–113.

884. Kimura K, Tachibana N, Kimura J, Shibasaki. Sleep-disordered breathing at an early stage of amyotrophic lateral sclerosis. J Neurol Sci 1999;164:37–43.

885. Flavell H, Marshall R, Thornton AT, Clements PL, Antic R, McEvoy RD. Hypoxia episodes during sleep in high tetraplegia. Arch Phys Med Rehabil 1992;73:623–27.

886. Keenan SP, Ryan CF, Fleetham JA. Sleep disordered breathing following acute spinal cord injury. Am Rev Respir Dis 1993;147:A688.

887. Walker-Engstrom ML, Tegelberg A, Wilhelmsson B, Ringqvist I. 4-year follow-up of treatment with dental appliance or uvulopalatopharyngoplasty in patients with obstructive sleep apnea: a randomized study. Chest 2002;121:739–46.

888. Garrigue S, Bordier P, Jais P, et al. Benefit of atrial pacing in sleep apnea syndrome. N Engl J Med 2002;346:404–12.

889. Marcus CL, Livingston FR, Wood SE, Keens TG. Hypercapnic and hypoxic ventilatory responses in parents and siblings of children with congenital central hypoventilation syndrome. Am Rev Respir Dis 1991;144:136–40.

890. Oren J, Kelly DH, Shannon DC. Long-term follow-up of children with congenital central hypoventilation syndrome. Pediatr 1987:80;375–80.

891. Silverstein D, Michlin B, Sobel HJ, Lavietes MH. Right ventricular failure in a patient with diabetic neuropathy (myopathy) and central alveolar hypoventilation. Respiration 1983;44:460–65.

892. Gold AR, Marcus CL, Dipalo F, Gold MS. Upper airway collapsibility during sleep in upper airway resistance syndrome. Chest 2002;121:1531–40.

893. Guilleminault C, Stoohs R, Kim Y, Chervin R, Black J, Clerk A. Influence of noninvasive positive pressure ventilation on inspiratory muscle activity in obese subjects. Eur Respir J 1997;10:2847–52.

894. Guilleminault C, Stoohs, Clerk A, Cetel M, Maistros P. A cause of excessive daytime sleepiness: the upper airway resistance syndrome. Chest 1993;104:781–87.

895. Yoshida K. Oral appliance therapy for upper airway resistance syndrome. Neurology 2002;87:427–30.

896. Newsom Davis J, Goldman M, Loh L, Casson M. Diaphragm function and alveolar hypoventilation. Q J Med 1976;45:87–100.

897. Dail CW, Affeldt JE. Vital capacity as an index of respiratory muscle function. Arch Phys Med Rehabil 1957;38:383–91.

898. Fromageot C, Lofaso F, Annane D, et al. Supine fall in lung volumes in the assessment of diaphragmatic weakness in neuromuscular disorders. Arch Phys Med Rehabil 2001;82:123–28.

899. Conference on Respiratory Problems in Poliomyelitis, March 12–14, 1952, Ann Arbor, National Foundation for Infantile Paralysis - March of Dimes, White Plains, N.Y.

900. Miller WF. Rehabilitation of patients with chronic obstructive lung disease. Med Clin N Am 1967;51:349–61.

901. De Troyer A, Deisser P. The effects of intermittent positive pressure breathing on patients with respiratory muscle weakness. Am Rev Respir Dis 1981;124:132–37.

902. Estenne M, De Troyer A. The effects of tetraplegia on chest wall statics. Am Rev Respir Dis 1986;134:121–24.

903. De Troyer A, Borenstein S, Cordier R. Analysis of lung volume restriction in patients with respiratory muscle weakness. Thorax 1980;35:603–10.

904. Gibson GJ, Pride NB, Newsom-Davis J, Loh LC. Pulmonary mechanics in patients with respiratory muscle weakness. Am Rev Respir Dis 1977;115:389–95.

905. Enson Y, Giuntini C, Lewis ML, Morris TQ, Ferrer MI, Harvey RM. The influence of hydrogen ion concentration and hypoxia on the pulmonary circulation. J Clin Invest 1964;43:1146–62.

906. Boushy SF, Thompson HK Jr, North LB, Beale AR, Snow TR. Prognosis in chronic obstructive pulmonary disease. Am Rev Respir Dis 1973;108:1373–83.

907. Stoller JK, Ferranti R, Feinstein AR. Further specification and evaluation of a new clinical index for dyspnea. Am Rev Respir Dis 1986;134:1129–34.

908. Woollam CHM. The development of apparatus for intermittent negative pressure respiration (1) 1832-1918. Anaesthesia 1976;31:537–47.

909. Kang SW, Bach JR. Maximum insufflation capacity. Chest 2000;118:61–65.

910. Miller WF. Rehabilitation of patients with chronic obstructive lung disease. Med Clin N Am 1967;51:349–61.

911. (not present)

912. McCool FD, Mayewski RF, Shayne DS, et al. Intermittent positive pressure breathing in patients with respiratory muscle weakness: alterations in total respiratory system compliance. Chest 1986;90: 546–52.

913. Huldtgren AC, Fugl-Meyer AR, Jonasson E, Bake B. Ventilatory dysfunction and respiratory rehabilitation in post-traumatic quadriplegia. Eur J Respir Dis 1980;61:347–56.

914. Marrery M. Chest development as a component of normal motor development: implications for pediatric physical therapists. Pediatr Phys Ther 1991;3:3–8.

915. Perez A, Mulot R, Vardon G, Barois A, Gallego J. Thoracoabdominal pattern of breathing in neuromuscular disorders. Chest 1996;110:454–61.

916. Rideau Y, Delaubier A, Guillou C, Renardel-Irani A. Treatment of respiratory insufficiency in Duchenne's muscular dystrophy: nasal ventilation in the initial stages. Monaldi Arch Chest Dis 1995;50:235–8.

917. Bach JR. New approaches in the rehabilitation of the traumatic high level quadriplegic. Am J Phys Med Rehabil 1991;70:13–20.

918. Bach JR, Alba AS. Noninvasive options for ventilatory support of the traumatic high level quadriplegic. Chest 1990;98:613–19.

919. Frederick C. Noninvasive mechanical ventilation with the iron lung. Crit Care Nurs Clin North Am 1994;6:831–40.

920. Corrado A, Gorini M, De Paola E. Alternative techniques for managing acute neuromuscular respiratory failure. Semin Neurol 1995;15:84–91.

921. Chalmers RM, Howard RS, Wiles CM, Spencer GT. Use of the rocking bed in the treatment of neurogenic respiratory insufficiency. QJM 1994;87:423–9.

922. Goldstein RS, Molotiu N, Skrastins R, Long S, Contreras M. Assisting ventilation in respiratory failure by negative pressure ventilation and by rocking bed. Chest 1987;92:470–74.

923. Bach JR, Bardach JL. Neuromuscular diseases. In: Sipski ML, Alexander CJ (eds). Sexual Function in People with Disability and Chronic Illness: A Health Practitioner's Guide. Gaithersburg, Md, Aspen, 1997:147–60.

924. Lherm T. Ventilation postopératoire non invasive par masque buccal. Ann Fr Anesth Réanim 1998;17:344–47.

925. Leger P, Jennequin J, Gerard M, Robert D. Home positive pressure ventilation via nasal mask for patients with neuromuscular weakness or restrictive lung or chest-wall disease. Respir Care 1989;34:73–79.

926. McDermott I, Bach JR, Parker C, Sortor S. Custom-fabricated interfaces for intermittent positive pressure ventilation. Int J Prosthodont 1989;2:224–33.

927. Leger SS, Leger P. The art of interface: tools for administering noninvasive ventilation. Med Klin 1999;94:35–39.

928. Criner GJ, Travaline JM, Brennan KJ, Kreimer DT. Efficacy of a new full face mask for noninvasive positive pressure ventilation. Chest 1994;106:1109–15.

929. Schonhofer B, Kohler D. Intermittent self-ventilation: therapy of chronic respiratory pump fatigue. Fortschr Med 1995;113:46–48.

930. Netzer N, Sorichter S, Bosch W, Werner P, Lehmann M. The clinical use of an individually fitted nasal mask ("Freiburg Respiratory Mask") within the scope of a case report of controlled BiPAP ventilation. Pneumologie 1997;51Suppl3:798–801.

931. Meduri GU, Abou-Shala N, Fox RC, et al. Noninvasive face mask mechanical ventilation in patients with acute hypercapnic respiratory failure. Chest 1991;100:445–54.

932. Viroslav J, Sortor S, Rosenblatt R. Alternatives to tracheostomy ventilation in high level SCI [abstract]. J Am Paraplegia Soc 1991;14:87.

933. Bach JR, Alba AS. Sleep and nocturnal mouthpiece IPPV efficiency in post-poliomyelitis ventilator users. Chest 1994;106:1705–10.

934. Navalesi P, Fanfulla F, Frigerio P, Gregoretti C, Nava S. Physiologic evaluation of noninvasive mechanical ventilation delivered with three types of masks in patients with chronic hypercapnic respiratory failure. Crit Care Med 2000;28:1785–90.

935. Bach JR, Alba AS. Total ventilatory support by the intermittent abdominal pressure ventilator. Chest 1991;99:630–36.

936. Dougherty G, Davis GM, Gaul M, Diana P. Pneumobelt assisted home ventilation in Duchenne's muscular dystrophy. 4th International Conference on Home Mechanical Ventilation: Book of Abstracts, Enterprise Rhone Alpes International, Lyon, France, March 3–5, 1993.

937. Rochester DF. Respiratory muscle weakness, pattern of breathing, and CO_2 retention in chronic obstructive pulmonary disease. Am Rev Respir Dis 1991;143:901–03.

938. Laier-Groeneveld G, Schucher B, Criee CP. The etiology of chronic hypercapnia. Med Klin 1997;92 Suppl 1:33–38.

939. Diaz O, Iglesia R, Ferrer M, et al. Effects of noninvasive ventilation on pulmonary gas exchange and hemodynamics during acute hypercapnic exacerbations of chronic obstructive pulmonary disease. Am J Respir Crit Care Med 1997;156:1840–45.

940. Pankow W, Hijjeh N, Schuttler F, et al. Influence of noninvasive positive pressure ventilation on inspiratory muscle activity in obese subjects. Eur Respir J 1997;10:2847–52.

941. Schonhofer B, Geibel M, Haidl P, Kohler D. Daytime mechanical ventilation in chronic ventilatory insufficiency (German). Med Klin 1999;94:9–12.

942. Servera E, Perez M, Marin J, Vergara P, Castano R. Noninvasive nasal mask ventilation beyond the ICU for an exacerbation of chronic respiratory insufficiency. Chest 1995;108:1572–76.

943. Feldmeyer F, Randerath W, Ruhle KH. Time course of ventilatory drive in patients with kyphoscoliosis before and during intermittent ventilation (German). Pneumologie 1999;53:S93–S94.

944. Rochester DF, Braun NMT, Laine S. Diaphragmatic energy expenditure in chronic respiratory failure: the effect of assisted ventilation with body respirators. Am J Med 1977;63:223–32.

945. Carrey Z, Gottfried SB, Levy RD. Ventilatory muscle support in respiratory failure with nasal positive pressure ventilation. Chest 1990;93:150–58.

946. Jimenez JFM, Sanchez de Cos Escuin J, Vicente CD, Valle MH, Otero FF. Nasal intermittent positive pressure ventilation: analysis of its withdrawal. Chest 1995;107:382–88.

947. Thorens JB, Ritz M, Reynard C, et al. Haemodynamic and endocrinological effects of noninvasive mechanical ventilation in respiratory failure. Eur Respir J 1997;11:2553–59.

948. Schlenker E, Feldmeyer F, Hoster M, Ruhle KH. Effect of noninvasive ventilation on pulmonary artery pressure in patients with severe kyphoscoliosis. Med Klin 1997;92 Suppl 1:40–44.

949. Sinha R, Bergofsky EG. Prolonged alteration of lung mechanics in kyphoscoliosis by positive hyperinflation. Am Rev Respir Dis 1972;106:47–57.

950. Hoeppner VH, Cockcroft DW, Dosman JA, Cotton DJ. Nighttime ventilation improves respiratory failure in secondary kyphoscoliosis. Am Rev Respir Dis 1984;129:240–43.

951. Banzett RN, Lansing RW, Reid MB, Adams L, Brown R. Air hunger arising from increased PCO_2 in mechanically ventilated quadriplegics. Respir Physiol 1989;l76:53–68.

952. Manning HL, Shea SA, Schwartzstein RM, et al. Reduced tidal volume increases air hunger at fixed pCO_2 in ventilated quadriplegics. Respir Physiol 1992;90:9–30.

953. Patterson JL, Mullinax PF, Bain T, Kreuger JJ, Richardson DW. Carbon dioxide-induced dyspnea in a patient with respiratory muscle paralysis. Am J Med 1962;32:811–16.

954. Wright GW, Branscomb BV. The origin of the sensations of dyspnea. Tr Am Climat & Clin A 1954;66:116–25.

955. Fowler WS. Breaking point of breath holding. J Appl Physiol 1954;6:539–45.

956. Opie LH, Smith AC, Spalding JM. Conscious appreciation of the effects produced by independent changes of ventilation volume and of end-tidal pCO_2 in paralyzed patients. J Physiol 1959;149: 494–99.

957. Rahn H, Bahnson HT, Muxworthy JF, Hagen JM. Adaptation to high altitude: changes in breath-holding time. J Appl Physiol 1953;6:154–57.

958. Ohi M, Chin K, Hirai M, et al. Oxygen desaturation following voluntary hyperventilation in normal subjects. Am J Respir Crit Care Med 1994;149:731–38.

959. Tzeng AC, Bach JR. Prevention of pulmonary morbidity for patients with neuromuscular disease. Chest 2000;118:1390–96.

960. Bach JR. Alternative methods of ventilatory support for the patient with ventilatory failure due to spinal cord injury. J Am Paraplegia Soc 1991;14:158–74.

961. Berggren L, Eriksson I, Mollenholt P, Sunzel M. Changes in respiratory pattern after repeated doses of diazepam and midazolam in healthy subjects. Acta Anaesthesiol Scand 1987;31:667–72.

962. Gleeson K, Zwillich CW, White DP. The influence of increasing ventilatory effort on arousal from sleep. Am Rev Respir Dis 1990;142:295–300.

963. Mortimore IL, Bradley PA, Murray JAM, Douglas NH. Uvulopalatopharyngoplasty may compromise nasal CPAP therapy in sleep apnea syndrome. Am J Respir Crit Care Med 1996;154:1759–62.

964. Meyer TJ, Pressman MR, Benditt J, et al. Air leaking through the mouth during nocturnal nasal ventilation: effect on sleep quality. Sleep 1997;20:561–69.

965. Strohl KP, Redline S. Nasal CPAP therapy, upper airway activation, and obstructive sleep apnea. Am Rev Respir Dis 1986;134:555–58.

966. Wysocki M, Tric L, Wolff MA, et al. Noninvasive pressure support ventilation in patients with acute respiratory failure. Chest 1993;103:907–13.

967. Takasaki Y, Kamio K, Okamoto M, et al. Altered arousability in non-REM sleep during sleep progression in patients with moderate to severe obstructive sleep apnea. Am Rev Resp Dis 1993;147:A513.

968. Nakayama T, Saito Y, Yatabe K, Uchiyama T, Kawai M. The usefulness of tracheostomy in Duchenne muscular dystrophy ventilated by a chest respirator (in Japanese). Rinsho Shinkeigaku 1999;39: 606–09.

969. Jounieaux V, Parreira VF, Delguste P, Aubert G, Rodenstein DO. Nasal mask pressure waveform and inspiratory muscle rest during nasal assisted ventilation. Am J Respir Crit Care Med 1997;155:2096–2101.

970. Parreira VF, Delguste P, Jounieaux V, Aubert G, Dury M, Rodenstein DO. Effectiveness of controlled and spontaneous modes in nasal two-level positive pressure ventilation in awake and sleep normal subjects. Chest 1997;112:1267–77.

971. Parriera VF, Delguste P, Jounieaux V, Aubert G, Dury M, Rodenstein DO. Glottic aperature and effective minute ventilation during nasal two-level positive pressure ventilation in spontaneous mode. Am J Respir Crit Care Med 1996;154:1857–63.

972. Delguste P, Aubert-Tulkens G, Rodenstein DO. Upper airway obstruction during nasal intermittent positive pressure ventilation in sleep. Lancet 1991;338:1295–97.

973. Sanna A, Veriter C, Stanescu D. Expiratory supraglottic obstruction during muscle relaxation. Chest 1995;108:143–49.

974. Malhotra A, Pillar G, Fogel R, Beauregard J, Edwards J, White DP. Upper-airway collapsibility: measurements and sleep effects. Chest 2001;120:156–61.

975. Ahmadian JL, Heller SL, Nishida T, Altman KW. Myotonic dystrophy type 1 presenting with laryngeal stridor and vocal fold paresis. Nuscle Nerve 2002;25:616–8.

976. Pepin JL, Leger P, Veale D, et al. Side effects of nasal continuous positive airway pressure in sleep apnea syndrome: study of 193 patients in two french sleep centers. Chest 1995;107:375–81.

977. Richards GN, Cistulli PA, Gunnar Ungar R, Berthon-Jones M, Sullivan CE. Mouth leak with nasal continuous positive airway pressure increases nasal airway resistance. Am J Respir Crit Care Med 1996;154:182–86.

978. Yamada S, Nishimiya J, Kurokawa K, Yuasa T, Masaka A. Bilevel nasal positive airway pressure and ballooning of the stomach. Chest 2001;119:1965–66.

979. Diaz Lobato S, Tejero Garcia MT, Ruiz Cobos A, Villasante C. Changing ventilator: an option to take into account in the treatment of persistent vomiting during nasal ventilation. Respiration 1998;65: 481–2.

980. Marcy TW. Barotrauma: detection, recognition, and management. Chest 1993;104:578–84.

981. Gammon RB, Shin MS, Buchalter SE. Pulmonary barotrauma in mechanical ventilation. Chest 1992;102:568–72.

982. Choo-Kang LR, Ogunlesi FO, McGrath-Morrow SA, Crawford TO, Marcus CL. Recurrent pneumothoraces associated with nocturnal noninvasive ventilation in a patient with muscular dystrophy. Pediatr Pulmonol 2002;34:73–8.

983. Bitto T, Mannion JD, Stephenson LW, et al. Pneumothorax during positive-pressure mechanical ventilation. J Thorac Cardiovasc Surg 1985;89:585–91.

984. Kolobow T, Moretti MP, Fumagalli R, et al. Severe impairment in lung function induced by high peak airway pressures during mechanical ventilation: an experimental study. Am Rev Respir Dis 1987;135: 312–15.

985. Haake R, Schlichtig R, Ulstad DR, Henschen RR. Barotrauma: pathophysiology, risk factors, and prevention. Chest 1987;91:608–13.

986. Manning HL. Peak airway pressure: why the fuss? Chest 1994;105:242–47.

987. Dreyfuss D, Soler P, Basset G, Saumon G. High inflation pressure pulmonary edema: respective effects of high airway pressure, high tidal volume, and positive end-expiratory pressure. Am Rev Respir Dis 1988;137:1159–64.

988. Dreyfuss D, Basset G, Soler P, Saumon G. Intermittent positive-pressure hyperventilation with high inflation pressures produces pulmonary microvascular injury in rats. Am Rev Respir Dis 1985;132:880–84.

989. Hill NS. Complications of noninvasive ventilation. Respir Care 2000;45:480–81.

990. Laraya-Cuasay L, Mikkilimeni S. Respiratory conditions and care. In: Rosenthal SR, Sheppard JJ, Lotze M (eds): Dysphagia and the Child with Developmental Disabilities. Singular Publishing, San Diego, 1995:227–52.

991. Arvedson J, Rogers B, Buck G, Smart P, Msall M. Silent aspiration prominent in children with dysphagia. Int J Pediatr Otorhinolaryngol 1994;28:173–81.

992. Loughlin GM. Respiratory consequences of dysfunctional swallowing and aspiration. Dysphagia 1989;3:126–30.

993. Lazowick D, Meyer TJ, Pressman M, Peterson D. Orbital herniation associated with noninvasive positive pressure ventilation. Chest 1998;113:841–43.

994. Webber BA, Pryor JA. Physiotherapy skills: techniques and adjuncts. In Webber BA, Pryor JA (eds): Physiotherapy for Respiratory and Cardiac Problems. Churchill Livingstone, London, 1993;113.

995. Hansen LG, Warwick WJ, Hansen KL. Mucus transport mechanisms in relation to the effect of high frequency chest compression (HFCC) on mucus clearance. Ped Pulmonol 1994;17:113–18.

996. Harding J, Kemper M, Weissman C. Pressure support ventilation attenuates the cardiopulmonary response to an acute increase in oxygen demand. Chest 1995;107:1665–72.

997. Hess DR. The evidence for secretion clearance techniques. Respir Care 2001;46:1276–92.

998. Currie DC, Munro C, Gaskell D, Cole PJ. Practice, problems and compliance with postural drainage: a survey of chronic sputum producers. Br J Dis Chest 1986;80:249–53.

999. Birnkrant DJ, Pope JF, Lewarski J, Stegmaier J, Besunder JB. Persistent pulmonary consolidation treated with intrapulmonary percussive ventilation: a preliminary report. Pediatr Pulmonol 1996;21:246–9.

1000. Tomkiewicz RP, Biviji AA, King M. Effects of oscillating air flow on the rheological properties and clearability of mucous gel stimulants. Biorheology 1994;31:511–20.

1001. Dasgupta B, Tomkiewicz RP, Boyd WP, Brown NE, King M. Effects of combined treatment with rhDNAase and airflow oscillations on spinnability of cystic fibrosis sputum in vitro. Pediatr Pulmonol 1995;20:78–82.

1002. Chang HK, Weber ME, King M. Mucus transport by high frequency nonsymetrical airflow. J Appl Physiol 1988;65:1203–09.

1003. Haberman PB, Green JP, Archibald C, et al. Determinants of successful selective tracheobronchial suctioning. N Engl J Med 1973;289:1060–63.

1004. Hanley MV, Rudd T, Butler J. What happens to intratracheal saline instillations. Am Rev Respir Dis 1978;117(suppl):124.

1005. Ishikawa Y, Ishikawa Y, Minami R. The effect of nasal IPPV on patients with respiratory failure during sleep due to Duchenne muscular dystrophy. Clin Neurol 1993;33:856–61.

1006. Kirby NA, Barnerias MJ, Siebens AA. An evaluation of assisted cough in quadriparetic patients. Arch Phys Med Rehabil 1966;47:705–10.

1007. Bach JR, Smith WH, Michaels J, et al. Airway secretion clearance by mechanical exsufflation for postpoliomyelitis ventilator assisted individuals. Arch Phys Med Rehabil 1993;74:170–77.

1008. Sortor S, McKenzie M. Toward Independence: Assisted Cough [video], BioScience Communications of Dallas Inc, 1986.

1009. Newth CJL, Asmler B, Anderson GP, Morley J. The effects of varying inflation and deflation pressures on the maximal expiratory deflation flow-volume relationship in anesthetized Rhesus monkeys. Am Rev Respir Dis 1991;144:807–13.

1010. Operator's and Technical Reference Manual. 840 Ventilator System, Nellcor Puritan Bennett, Carlsbad, Ca, 1998:10–11.

1011. Nomori H, Horio H, Suemasu K. Pressure-controlled ventilation via a minitracheostomy tube: experimental study using a mechanical lung model. Surg Today 2001;31:780–4.

1012. Garstang SV, Kirshblum SC, Wood KE. Patient preference for in-exsufflation for secretion management with spinal cord injury. J Spinal Cord Med 2000;23:80–85.

1013. Freitag L, Long WM, Kim CS, Wanner A. Removal of excessive bronchial secretions by asymmetric high-frequency oscillations. J Appl Physiol 1989;67:614–19.

1014. Singer M, Vermaat J, Hall G, Latter G, Patel M. Hemodynamic effects of manual hyperinflation in critically ill mechanically ventilated patients. Chest 1994;106:1182–87.

1015. Beck GJ, Scarrone LA. Physiological effects of exsufflation with negative pressure. Dis Chest 1956;29:1–16.

1016. Bach JR. Noninvasive respiratory muscle aids and intervention goals. In: Bach JR (ed). Noninvasive Mechanical Ventilation. Philadelphia, Hanley and Belfus 2002:129–164.

1017. Chatwin M, Ross E, Hart N, Nickol AH, Polkey M, Simonds AK. Cough augmentation with mechanical in-exsufflation in adults and children with neuromuscular weakness. Europ Respir J (in press).

1018. Bickerman HA. Exsufflation with negative pressure: elimination of radiopaque material and foreign bodies from bronchi of anesthetized dogs. Arch Int Med 1954;93:698–704.

1019. Siebens AA, Kirby NA, Poulos DA. Cough following transection of spinal cord at C-6. Arch Phys Med Rehabil 1964;45:1–8.

1020. Barach AL, Beck GJ. Exsufflation with negative pressure: physiologic and clinical studies in poliomyelitis, bronchial asthma, pulmonary emphysema and bronchiectasis. Arch Int Med 1954;93:825–41.

1021. Barach AL, Beck GJ, Smith RH. Mechanical production of expiratory flow rates surpassing the capacity of human coughing. Am J Med Sci 1953;226:241–48.

1022. Beck GJ, Barach AL. Value of mechanical aids in the management of a patient with poliomyelitis. Ann Int Med 1954;40:1081–94.

1023. Beck GJ, Graham GC, Barach AL. Effect of physical methods on the mechanics of breathing in poliomyelitis. Ann Intern Med 1955;43:549–66.

1024. Williams EK, Holaday DA. The use of exsufflation with negative pressure in postoperative patients. Am J Surg 1955;90:637–40.

1025. Sammon K, Menon S, Massery M, Cahalin I. A pilot clinical investigation comparing the effects of the mechanical in-exsufflator to suctioning and chest physical therapy in persons with difficulty mobilizing pulmonary secretions. Cardiopulmonary Physical Therapy (abstract) 1998;9:22–23.

1026. Henderson CE, Jackson AB. A comparison of outcomes of using the in-exsufflator with traditional respiratory management in patients with spinal cord injury. JSCM 2002;25:533–34.

1027. Kobavashi I, Perry A, Rhymer J, et al. Relationships between the electrical activity of genioglossus muscle and the upper airway patency: a study in laryngectomised subjects. Respir Crit Care Med 1994;149:A148.

1028. Colebatch HJH. Artificial coughing for patients with respiratory paralysis. Australasian J Med 1961;10:201–12.

1029. Cherniack RM, Hildes JA, Alcock AJW. The clinical use of the exsufflator attachment for tank respirators in poliomyelitis. Ann Intern Med 1954;40:540–48.

1030. Barach AL. The application of pressure, including exsufflation, in pulmonary emphysema. Am J Surg 1955;89:372–82.

1031. Rennie H, Wilson JAC. A coughing-belt. Lancet 1983;1:138–39.

1032. Dail C, Rodgers M, Guess V, Adkins HV. Glossopharyngeal Breathing, Rancho Los Amigos Department of Physical Therapy, Downey, Ca, 1979.

1033. Dail CW, Affeldt JE. Glossopharyngeal breathing [video]. Los Angeles: Department of Visual Education, College of Medical Evangelists, 1954.

1034. Webber B, Higgens J. Glossopharyngeal breathing—what, when and how? (video) Aslan Studios Ltd., Holbrook, Horsham, West Sussex, England, 1999.

1035. Nathanson BN, Yu DG, Chan CK. Respiratory muscle weakness in Charcot-Marie-Tooth disease. Arch Intern Med 1989;149:1389–91.

1036. Lindahl SG, Yates AP, Hatch DJ. Relationship between invasive and noninvasive measurements of gas exchange in anesthetized infants and children. Anesthesiology 1987;66:168–75.
1037. Morley TF, Giaimo J, Maroszan E, et al. Use of capnography for assessment of the adequacy of alveolar ventilation during weaning from mechanical ventilation. Am Rev Respir Dis 1993;148: 339–44.
1038. Wiedemann HP, McCarthy K. Noninvasive monitoring of oxygen and carbon dioxide. Clin Chest Med 1989;10:239–54.
1039. Plewa MC, Sikora S, Engoren M, et al. Evaluation of capnography in nonintubated emergency department patients with respiratory distress. Acad Emerg Med 1995;2:901–08.
1040. Hadjikoutis S, Wiles CM. Venous serum chloride and bicarbonate measurements in the evaluation of respiratory function in motor neuron disease. QJM 2001;94:491–502.
1041. Partridge BL. Use of pulse oximetry as a noninvasive indicator of intravascular volume status. J Clin Monit 1987;3:263–68.
1042. Watson L, Colbert F, Topley L, Kinnear W. Initiation of non-invasive ventilation as an out-patient. 8th Journées Internationales de Ventilation á Domicile, abstract 46, March 7, 2001, Hôpital de la Croix-Rousse, Lyon, France.
1043. Welch JR, DeCesare R, Hess D. Pulse oximetry: instrumentation and clinical applications. Respir Care 1990;35:584–94.
1044. Marini JJ, Hotchkiss JR, Bach JR. Noninvasive ventilation in the acute care setting. In: Bach JR (ed). Noninvasive Mechanical Ventilation. Philadelphia: Hanley & Belfus 2002:223–240.
1045. Laier-Groeneveld G, Criee CP. Epidemiology and diagnosis of intermittent self-ventilation (in German). Med Klin 1997;(92 Suppl)1:2–8.
1046. Rubini F, Zanotti E, Nava S. Monaldi Arch Chest Dis 1994;49:527–29.
1047. Nagato I, Miura T, Ishikawa Y, Ishikawa Y, Minami R. Respiratory physical therapy for extubation in a patient with Duchenne muscular dystrophy and acute respiratory failure. Japanese Pediatric Pulmonology 2001;12:24–30.
1048. Niranjan V, Bach JR. Spinal muscular atrophy type 1: a noninvasive respiratory management approach. Chest 2000;117:1100–05.
1049. Forte V, Cole P, Crysdale WS. Objective assessment of upper airway resistance in the tracheotomized patient. J Otolaryngol 1986;15:359–61.
1050. Viroslav J, Rosenblatt R, Morris-Tomazevic S. Respiratory management, survival, and quality of life for high-level traumatic tetraplegics. 1996;3:313–22.
1051. Gomez-Merino E, Bach JR. Duchenne muscular dystrophy: prolongation of life by noninvasive respiratory muscle aids. Am J Phys Med Rehabil 2002;81:411–15.
1052. Cantas-Yamsnan M, Sanchez I, Kesselman M, Chernick V. Morbidity and mortality patterns of ventilator-dependent children in a home care program. Clin Pediatr 1993;32:706–13.
1053. Khan Y, Heckmatt JZ. Obstructive apnoeas in Duchenne muscular dystrophy. Thorax 1995;50:1123.
1054. Sato K, Ishikawa Y, Ishikawa Y, Izumi T, Okabe M, Minami R. Fukuyama type congenital muscular dystrophy in its advanced stage: effectiveness of mechanical ventilation system. No To Hattatsu 2002;34:330–5.
1055. Begin R, Bureau MA, Lupien L, Lemieux B. Control and modulation of respiration in Steinert's myotonic dystrophy. Am Rev Respir Dis 1980;121:281–80.
1056. Manni R, Zucca MR, Martinetti C, et al. Hypersomnia in dystrophia myotonica: a neurophysiological and immunogenetic study. Acta Neurol Scand 1991;84:498–502.
1057. Lopez-Esteban P, Peraita-Adrados R. Sleep and respiratory disorders in myotonic dystrophy of Steinert. Neurologia 2000;15:102–8.
1058. Tejero G, Langevin B, Petitjean T, et al. Long term home mechanical ventilation in myotonic dystrophy: follow-up and compliance. 8th Journées Internationales de Ventilation á Domicile, abstract 129, March 7, 2001, Hôpital de la Croix-Rousse, Lyon, France.
1059. Nugent AM, Smith IE, Shneerson JM. Domiciliary-assisted ventilation in patients with myotonic dystrophy. Chest 2002;121:459–464.
1060. van der Meche FG, Bogaard JM, van der Sluys JC, Schimsheimer RJ, Ververs CC, Busch HF. Daytime sleep in myotonic dystrophy is not caused by sleep apnoea. J Neurol Neurosurg Psychiatry 1994;57:626–8.
1061. Damian MS, Gerlach A, Schmidt F, Lehmann E, Reichmann H. Modafinil for excessive daytime sleepiness in myotonic dystrophy. Neurology 2001;56:794–6.
1062. Antonini G, Morino S, Fiorelli M, Fiorini M, Giubilei F. Selegiline in the treatment of hypersomnolence in myotonic dystrophy: a pilot study. J Neurol Sci 1997;147:167–9.

1063. Liistro G, Veriter C, Dury M, Aubert G, Stanescu D. Expiratory flow limitation in awake sleep-disordered breathing subjects. Eur Respir J 1999;14:185–90.

1064. Buhr-Schinner H, Laier-Groeneveld G, Criee CP. Amyotrophic lateral sclerosis and intermittent self-ventilation therapy: indications and follow up. Med Klin 1995;90 Suppl 1:49–51.

1065. Giess R, Naumann M, Werner E, et al. Injections of botulinum toxin A into the salivary glands improve sialorrhoea in amyotrophic lateral sclerosis. J Neurol Neurosurg Psychiatry 2000;69:121–23.

1066. Winterholler MG, Heckmann JG, Hecht M, Erbguth FJ. Recurrent trismus and stridor in an ALS patient: successful treatment with botulinum toxin. Neurology 2002;58:502–3.

1067. Bach JR, Intintola P, Alba AS, Holland I. The ventilator-assisted individual: cost analysis of institutionalization versus rehabilitation and in-home management. Chest 1992;101:26–30.

1068. Celikel T, Sungur M, Ceyhan B, Karakurt S. Comparison of intermittent positive pressure ventilation with standard medical therapy in hypercapnic acute respiratory failure. Chest 1998;114: 1636–42.

1069. Benhamou D, Muir JF, Melen B. Mechanical ventilation in elderly patients. Monaldi Arch Chest Dis 1998;53:547–51.

1070. Guerin C, Girard R, Chemorin C, De Varax R, Fournier G. Facial mask noninvasive mechanical ventilation reduces the incidence of nosocomial pneumonia: a prospective epidemiological survey from a single ICU. Intensive Care Med 1997;10:1024–32.

1071. Winslow C, Bode RK, Felton D, Chen D, Meyer PR Jr. Impact of respiratory complications on length of stay and hospital costs in acute cervical spine injury. Chest 2002;121:1548–54.

1072. Bach JR, Hunt D, Horton JA III. Traumatic tetraplegia: noninvasive respiratory management in the acute setting. Am J Phys Med Rehabil 2002;81:792–7.

1073. Devereaux K. Bridging the information gap. RRTC/NMD Program Overview 1998–2003. NIDRR Rehabilitation Research and Training Center in Neuromuscular Diseases at UC Davis: http://www.rehabinfo.net/Clearinghouse/Virtual Library/Index.html

1074. Bach JR, Niranjan V. Noninvasive ventilation in pediatrics. In: Bach JR (ed). Noninvasive Mechanical Ventilation. Philadelphia, Hanley and Belfus 2002:203–222.

1075. Shneerson JM. Home mechanical ventilation in children: techniques, outcomes and ethics. Monaldi Arch Chest Dis 1996;51:426–30.

1076. Payton P, Padgett D, van Stralen D, Newsom H. Incidence of tracheostomy dislodgements in a pediatric subacute facility. 8th Journées Internationales de Ventilation á Domicile, abstract 111, March 7, 2001, Hôpital de la Croix-Rousse, Lyon, France.

1077. de Lemos RA. Management of pediatric acute hypoxemic respiratory insufficiency with bilevel positive pressure nasal mask ventilation. Chest 1995;108:894–95.

1078. Barois A, Bataille J, Estournet B. La ventilation á domicile par voie buccale chez l'enfant dans les maladies neuromusculaires. Agressologie 1985;26:645–49.

1079. Barois A, Estournet B, Duval-Beaupere G, Bataille J, Leclair-Richard D. Amyotrophie spinale infantile. Rev Neurol (Paris) 1989;145:299–304.

1080. Milane J, Bertrand P, Montredon C, Jonquet O, Bertrand A. Intéret de l'assistance ventilatoire abdomino-diaphragmatique dans la réadaptation des grands handicapés respiratoire. In: Simon L (ed.): Actualities en Rééducation Fonctionel et Réadaptation, 15th volume, Masson, 1990.

1081. Milane J, Bertrand A. Indications de la ventilation par prothèse extra-thoracique. Bull Eur Physiopathol Respir 1986;22:37–40.

1082. Klonin H, Bowman B, Peters M, Raffeeq P, et al. Negative pressure ventilation via chest cuirass to decrease ventilator-associated complications in infants with acute respiratory failure: a case series. Respir Care 2000;45:486–90.

1083. Padman R, Lawless S, von Nessen S. Use of bilevel positive airway pressure by nasal mask in the treatment of respiratory insufficiency in pediatric patients: preliminary investigation. Pediatr Pulmonol 1994;17:119–23.

1084. Niranjan V, Bach JR. Noninvasive management of pediatric neuromuscular ventilatory failure. Crit Care Med 1998;26:2061–65.

1085. Hardart MK, Burns JP, Truog RD. Respiratory support in spinal muscular atrophy type 1: a survey of physician practices and attitudes. Pediatrics 2002;110:E24.

1086. Sakakihara Y, Kubota M, Kim S, Oka A. Long-term ventilator support in patients with Werdnig-Hoffmann disease. Pediatr Int 2000;42:359–63.

1087. Iannaccone ST, Guilfoile T. Long-term mechanical ventilation in infants with neuromuscular disease. J Child Neurol 1988;3:30–32.

1088. von Gontard A, Zerres K, Backes M, Laufersweiler-Plass C, Wendland C, Melchers P, Lehmkuhl G, Rudnik-Schoneborn S. Intelligence and cognitive function in children and adolescents with spinal muscular atrophy. Neuromuscul Disord 2002;12:130–6.

1089. Birnkrant DJ, Pope JF, Martin JE, Repucci AH, Eiben RB. Treatment of type 1 spinal muscular atrophy with noninvasive ventilation and gastrostomy feeding. Pediatr Neurol 1998;18:407–10.

1090. Chiswick ML, Milner RD. Crying vital capacity: measurement of neonatal lung function. Arch Dis Child 1976;51:22–27.

1091. Tobias JD, Meyer DJ. Noninvasive monitoring of carbon dioxide during respiratory failure in toddlers and infants: end-tidal versus transcutaneous carbon dioxide. Anesth Anag 1997;85:55–58.

1092. Goldberg AI. The Illinois plan: report of the Surgeon General's workshop, DHHS Publ PHS-83-50194, Washington, D.C., Department of Health and Human Services, 1983:20.

1093. Burr BH, Guyer B, Todres ID, Abraham B, Chiodo I. Home care for children on respirators. N Engl J Med 1983;309:1319–23.

1094. Kettrick RG. The Pennsylvania program: report of the Surgeon General's workshop, DHHS Publ PHS-83-50194, Washington, D.C., Department of Health and Human Services, 1983:13.

1095. Fortenberry JD, DelToro J, Jefferson LS, Evey L, Haase D. Management of pediatric acute hypoxemic respiratory insufficiency with bilevel positive pressure nasal mask ventilation. Chest 1995;108:1059–64.

1096. National Center for Health Statistics: Vital Statistics of the United States, 1985, volume III, Marriage and Divorce, DHHS Publication No. (PHS) 89-1103. Public Health Service, Washington. U.S. Government Printing Office, 1989:4–23,4–24.

1097. Rudnik-Schoneborn S, Zerres K, Ignatius J, Rietschel M. Pregnancy and spinal muscular atrophy. J Neurol 1992;239:26–30.

1098. Fowler WM Jr, Abresch RT, Koch TR, Brewer ML, Bowden RK, Wanlass RL. Employment profiles in neuromuscular diseases. Am J Phys Med Rehabil 1997;76:26–37.

1099. Andries F, Wevers CW, Wintzen AR, Busch HF, Howeler CJ, de Jager AE, Padberg GW, de Visser M, Wokke JH. Vocational perspectives and neuromuscular disorders. Int J Rehabil Res 1997;20:255–73.

1100. Bach JR, Campagnolo D. Psychosocial adjustment of post-poliomyelitis ventilator assisted individuals. Arch Phys Med Rehabil 1992;73:934–39.

1101. Bach JR, Campagnolo DI, Hoeman S. Life satisfaction of individuals with Duchenne muscular dystrophy using long-term mechanical ventilatory support. Am J Phys Med Rehabil 1991;70:129–35.

1102. Campbell A, Converse PE, Rodgers WL. The Quality of American Life: Perceptions, Evaluations and Satisfactions. New York, Russell Sage Foundation, 1976:37–113.

1103. Flanagan JC. Measurement of quality of life: current state of the art. Arch Phys Med Rehabil 1982;63:56–59.

1104. Kammann R, Christie D, Irwin R, Dixon G. Properties of an inventory to measure happiness (and psychological health). New Zealand Psychologist 1979;8:1–9.

1105. Neudert C, Wasner M, Borasio GD. Different approaches to quality of life assessment: a randomised study in patients with amyotrophic lateral sclerosis. ALS and Other Motor Neuron Diseases 2000;1:9.

1106. Armon C, Dhanji TA, Davies VL, et al. Patients' perspectives regarding the relative importance of the direct consequences of ALS: implications for measuring their quality of life using the ALSQOL-11. ALS and Other Motor Neuron Disorders 2000;1:36.

1107. Pearlman RA, Jonsen A. The use of quality-of-life considerations in medical decision making. J Am Geriatr Soc 1985;33:344–52.

1108. Bach JR. Ventilator use by muscular dystrophy association patients: an update. Arch Phys Med Rehabil 1992;73:179–183.

1109. Crane D. Sanctity of Social Life: Physicians' Treatment of Critically Ill Individuals. New York, Russell Sage Foundation, 1975.

1110. Whiteneck GG, Charlifue MA, Frankel HL, et al. Mortality, morbidity, and psychosocial outcomes of persons spinal cord injured more than 20 years ago. Paraplegia 1992;30:617–30.

1111. Whiteneck GG, Carter RE, Charlifue SW, Hall KM, Menter RR, Wilkerson MA, Wilmot CB. A collaborative study of high quadriplegia. Craig, CO, Rocky Mountain Regional Spinal Cord Injury System report to the National Institute of Handicapped Research, 1985:29–33.

1112. Bach JR, Tilton M. Life satisfaction and well-being measures in ventilator assisted individuals with traumatic tetraplegia. Arch Phys Med Rehabil 1994;75:626–32.

1113. Eisenberg MG, Saltz CC. Quality of life among aging spinal cord injured persons: long term rehabilitation outcomes. Paraplegia 1991;29:514–20.

1114. Narayanaswami P, Bertorini TE, Pourmand R, Horner LH. Chronic ventilatory support in neuro-muscular diseases: patient acceptance and quality of life. Abstract. J Neuro Rehab 1998;12:39.

1115. Auriant I, Dazord A, Andronikof-Sanglade A, Benony H, Kovess V, Jaillard P, Charpack Y, Raphael JC. Assessment of satisfaction for Duchenne muscular dystrophy patients submitted to home mechanical ventilation. 8th Journées Internationales de Ventilation à Domicile, abstract 117, March 7, 2001, Hôpital de la Croix-Rousse, Lyon, France.

1116. Cazzoli PA, Oppenheimer EA. Use of nasal and tracheostomy positive pressure ventilation in patients with ALS: changing patterns and outcomes. (abstract) Neurology 1998;50(Suppl4): A417–18.

1117. Ganzini L, Johnston WS, McFarland BH, Tolle SW, Lee MA. Attitudes of patients with amyotrophic lateral sclerosis and their care givers toward assisted sucide. N Engl J Med 1998;339:967–73.

1118. Schonhofer B, von Sydow K, Nietsch M, Suchi S, Kohler D, Jones P. Sexuality in patients with NIV for chronic respiratory failure. 8th Journées Internationales de Ventilation à Domicile, abstract 58, March 7, 2001, Hôpital de la Croix-Rousse, Lyon, France.

1119. Leonard C, Criner GJ. Swallowing function in patients with tracheostomy receiving prolonged mechanical ventilation. 8th Journées Internationales de Ventilation à Domicile, abstract 57, March 7, 2001, Hôpital de la Croix-Rousse, Lyon, France.

1120. Laurie G. Ventilator users, home care, and independent living: an historical perspective. In: Kutscher AH, Gilgoff I (eds): The Ventilator: Psychsocial and Medical Aspects. New York, Foundation of Thanatology 2000:147–51.

1121. Purtilo R. Ethical Issues in the treatment of chronic ventilator-dependent individuals. Arch Phys Med Rehabil 1986;67:718–21.

1122. Kolata G. Ethicists struggle to judge the 'value' of life. New York Times, November 24, 1992:C3.

1123. Jonsen R, Siegler M, Winslade WJ. Clinical Ethics: A Practical Approach to Ethical Decisions in Clinical Medicine. New York, Macmillan, 1982.

1124. Goldstein RS, Gort EH. Home mechanical ventilation: demographics and user perspectives. Chest 1995;108:1581–86.

1125. Dracup K, Raffin T. Withholding and withdrawing mechanical ventilation: assessing quality of life. Am Rev Respir Dis 1989;140:S44–S46.

1126. Moss AH, Oppenheimer EA, Casey P, et al. Patients with amyotrophic lateral sclerosis receiving long-term mechanical ventilation: advance care planning and outcomes. Chest 1996;110:249–55.

1127. McDonald ER, Hillel A, Wiedenfeld SA. Evaluation of the psychological status of ventilatory-supported patients with ALS/MND. Palliat Med 1996;10:35–41.

1128. Gelinas DF, O'Connor P, Miller RG. Quality of life for ventilator-dependent ALS patients and their caregivers. J Neurol Sci 1998;160:S134–S136.

1129. Zola IK. Social and cultural disincentives to independent living. Arch Phys Med Rehabil 1982;63: 394–97.

1130. Trieschmann RB. Spinal cord injuries: psychological, social and vocational rehabilitation. ed. 2. New York, Demos, 1988:107–14.

1131. Gill C. "Right to die" threatens our right to live safe and free. Mainstream 1992:32–36.

1132. Schnur S, Holland I. Concepts-a unique approach to personal care attendants. Rehabilitation Gazette 1987;28:10–11.

1133. Sabatino CP. Final report: lessons for enhancing consumer-directed approaches in home care. Commission on Legal Problems of the Elderly, Washington, American Bar Association, 1990.

1134. Kafka R. ADAPT attendant services free our people. National ADAPT (American Disabled for Attendant Programs Today), Denver CO.

1135. Goldberg AI, Alba AS, Oppenheimer EA, Roberts E. Personal care attendants for people using mechanical ventilation at home. (letter) Chest 1990;98:1543.

1136. Make BJ, Gilmartin ME. Rehabilitation and home care for ventilator-assisted individuals. Clinics Chest Med 1986;7:679–91.

1137. Litvak S, Heumann JE. Attending to America: personal assistance for independent living-the national survey of attendant services programs in the United States. Berkeley, CA, World Institute on Disability, 1987.

1138. Attendant Services Network. Personal Assistance for Independent Living. World Institute on Disability, Oakland, CA, Fall 1988.

1139. World Institute on Disability & Rutgers University Bureau of Economic Research: The need for personal assistance. Oakland, World Institute on Disability.

1140. Gibson B. Long-term ventilation for patients with Duchenne muscular dystrophy: physicians' beliefs and practices. Chest 2001;119:940–46.

1141. Ziter FA, Allsop KG. Comprehensive treatment of childhood muscular dystrophy. Rocky Mountain Med J 1975;329–333.

1142. Smith PEM, Calverley PMA, Edwards RHT, Evans GA, Campbell EJM. Practical problems in the respiratory care of individuals with muscular dystophy. N Engl J Med 1987;316:1197–1204.

1143. Goldblatt D. Decisions about life support in amyotrophic lateral sclerosis. Semin Neurol 1984;4:104–10.

1144. Marik PE, Varon J, Lisbon A, Reich HS. Physicians' own preferences to the limitation and withdrawal of life-sustaining therapy. Resuscitation 1999;42:197–201.

1145. Borasio GD, Voltz R. Discontinuation of mechanical ventilation in patients with amyotrophic lateral sclerosis. J Neurol 1998;245:717–22.

1146. Bach JR, Vega J, Majors J, Friedman A. Spinal muscular atrophy type 1 quality of life. Am J Phys Med Rehabil (in press).

1147. Lanzi G, Balottin U, Borgatti R, Ottolini A. Relational and therapeutic aspects of children with late onset of a terminal disease. Childs Nerv Syst 1993;9:339–42.

1148. Freed MM. Quality of life: the physician's dilemma. Arch Phys Med Rehabil 1984;65:109–11.

J. H. Emerson Co., Cambridge, MA: Cough-Assist™

Fisher-Paykel Inc., Laguna Hills, CA: Oracle™

LouSal Enterprises, Inc., www.roezit.com: RoEzit™

Mallincrodt-Puritan-Bennett Inc., Pleasanton, CA: Adam circuit™; the LP-10™, LP-20™, and Achieva™ portable volume ventilators; Lipseal™

Olympic Medical Inc., Seattle: Olympic™ button for tracheostomy tubes

Passy-Muir Inc., Irvine, CA: Passy-Muir valve™

Pulmonetic Systems Inc., Colton, CA: LTV-900™, LTV-950™

Respironics International Inc., Murrysville, PA: Lipseal™; Exsufflation-Belt™; Whisper-Swivel™; PLV-100™, PLV102™ portable volume ventilators; BiPAP-ST™ Harmony™; Synchrony™ bi-level positive airway pressure machines; 15- and 22-mm angled mouth pieces Reference 4-730-00.

Versa-Med Inc., Rochelle Park, N.J.: I-Vent™

Versitilt Inc., Portland, Or: Tilt-in-Space™

Index

Page numbers in **boldface** indicate complete chapters.